Optimizing Women's Health *through* Nutrition

Optimizing Women's Health *through* Nutrition

Edited by

Lilian U. Thompson
Wendy E. Ward

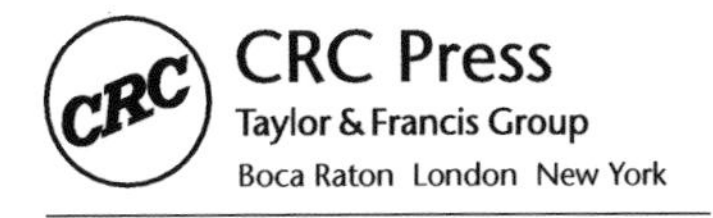

CRC Press is an imprint of the
Taylor & Francis Group, an **informa** business

CRC Press
Taylor & Francis Group
6000 Broken Sound Parkway NW, Suite 300
Boca Raton, FL 33487-2742

First issued in paperback 2019

ISBN-13: 978-1-4200-4300-6 (hbk)
ISBN-13: 978-0-367-38813-3 (pbk)

Library of Congress Cataloging-in-Publication Data

Optimizing women's health through nutrition / edited by Lilian U. Thompson and Wendy E. Ward.
p. ; cm.
Includes bibliographical references.
ISBN-13: 978-1-4200-4300-6 (hardcover : alk. paper)
ISBN-10: 1-4200-4300-5 (hardcover : alk. paper)
1. Women--Nutrition. 2. Women--Diseases--Nutritional aspects. 3. Nutrition--Sex differences. 4. Sex factors in disease. I. Thompson, Lilian U. II. Ward, Wendy E.
[DNLM: 1. Nutrition Physiology. 2. Diet Therapy. 3. Disease--etiology. 4. Sex Factors. 5. Women's Health. QU 145 O62 2008]

RA778.O583 2008
613'.04244--dc22 2007025616

Visit the Taylor & Francis Web site at
http://www.taylorandfrancis.com

and the CRC Press Web site at
http://www.crcpress.com

Dedication

This book is dedicated to our mothers, daughters, and granddaughters, with the hope that women's health will be optimized, at least in part, by applying what is learned through a nutrition approach to overall health.

Contents

SECTION I
INTRODUCTION

SECTION II
NORMAL NUTRITION

SECTION III
NUTRITION IN CHRONIC DISEASE AND VARIOUS CONDITIONS

SECTION IV CONCLUSION

Preface

Sex-based nutrition is a new and exciting area of health research. While it is widely known that women and men have biological and physiological differences throughout the life cycle, most studies have not considered how these differences affect susceptibility to diseases and metabolic responses to dietary treatments. Without question, there is a need to understand these differences so as to optimize health among women.

The overall aim of *Optimizing Women's Health through Nutrition* is to expand our knowledge regarding sex-based nutrition and medicine. This aim is achieved by first describing recent research on biological and physiological differences among men and women, and how these differences translate into varying disease trends between sexes (Chapters 1 and 2). The subsequent chapters describe the nutritional needs of women during the life cycle, particularly during adolescence, pregnancy and lactation, premenopause, and menopause and midlife stages (Chapters 3 through 6). Section III focuses on recent research into each of the common major diseases or conditions that specifically affect the health of women, with emphasis on the role of nutrition in disease risk reduction as well as management and treatment of the disease (Chapters 7 through 18). In selecting the diseases and conditions to be covered in this section, greater focus was given to those in which women are more vulnerable or have a higher incidence than do men. Section IV identifies areas for future research. Strategic areas of investigation are discussed for researchers and health professionals involved with disease prevention and treatment in women, for government regulators involved in setting public health policy, and for the food industry involved in developing novel foods targeted specifically for prevention or treatment of diseases in women to enhance women's health (Chapter 19).

Optimizing Women's Health through Nutrition is a research-based, extensively referenced book, which includes the most recently published, cutting edge work that will guide and stimulate more work, and ultimately lead to more effective nutritional strategies for women's health. The contributors are internationally recognized leaders in the field.

We thank the authors for generously sharing their expertise and time despite their very busy schedules. We thank Randy Brehm and Jill Jurgensen for their support and editorial assistance at Taylor & Francis. We thank our loving families who are always supportive and patient as we pursue our research endeavors.

Editors

Dr. Lilian U. Thompson obtained her PhD from University of Wisconsin in Madison. She is now emeritus professor in the Department of Nutritional Sciences, Faculty of Medicine, University of Toronto, Canada. She is internationally recognized for her research on components of plant foods responsible for their health benefits and/or adverse effects, their interactions with drugs, and the mechanisms of their actions, particularly in relation to breast cancer and other chronic diseases of women. She has published numerous papers in peer-reviewed journals, book chapters, and co-edited the book *Food-Drug Synergy and Safety*, and the first and second editions of *Flaxseed in Human Nutrition*. She has presented numerous invited papers at conferences and symposia and has served on several research granting councils and expert committees.

Dr. Wendy E. Ward obtained a PhD in medical science from McMaster University, Canada, held a National Institute of Nutrition postdoctoral fellowship at the University of Toronto, and is currently a professor in the Department of Nutritional Sciences, Faculty of Medicine, University of Toronto. Her research is focused on the mechanisms by which dietary estrogens and fatty acids regulate bone metabolism, with the long-term goal of developing dietary strategies that protect against fragility fracture. She has published many peer-reviewed articles in the area of nutrition and bone health and book chapters on nutrition and women's health issues, particularly osteoporosis. She recently co-edited a book titled *Food-Drug Synergy and Safety*, and has authored textbook chapters on the topics of micronutrients, herbal preparations, and nutritional supplements. Dr. Ward was a recipient of a Future Leader Award from the International Life Sciences Institute.

Contributors

Marci Goldstein Adams
Evanston Northwestern Healthcare
Department of Obstetrics and Gynecology
Evanston, Illinois

Christina P.C. Borba
Department of Behavioral Sciences
and Health Education
Rollins School of Public Health
Emory University
Atlanta, Georgia

Bette J. Caan
Etiology and Prevention Research
Division of Research
Kaiser Permanente Medical Program
Oakland, California

Aedin Cassidy
School of Medicine, Health Policy
and Practice
University of East Anglia
Norwich, United Kingdom

Leslie G. Cleland
Rheumatology Unit
Royal Adelaide Hospital
Adelaide, South Austraila

Peter Clifton
CSIRO Human Nutrition
and University of Adelaide
Adelaide, South Australia

Jennifer Evans
International Center for Eye Health
London School of Hygiene
and Tropical Medicine
London, England

Peter C. Fritz
Reconstructive Periodontics and
Implant Surgery Clinic
Fonthill, Ontario, Canada

Jayne A. Fulkerson
School of Nursing
University of Minnesota
Minneapolis, Minnesota

Stacie E. Geller
Department of Obstetrics
and Gynecology
College of Medicine Center of
Excellence in Women's Health
University of Illinois at Chicago
Chicago, Illinois

David C. Henderson
Massachusetts General Hospital
Harvard Medical School
Freedom Trail Clinic
Boston, Massachusetts

Lisa A. Houghton
School of Nutrition & Dietetics
Acadia University
Wolfville, Nova Scotia, Canada

Sara Hutchison
Institut für Psychologie
Universität Bern
Bern, Switzerland

Richard E. Kreipe
Division of Adolescent Medicine
Department of Pediatrics
Golisano Children's Hospital at Strong
Rochester, New York

Nicole Larson
Division of Epidemiology and Community Health
School of Public Health
University of Minnesota
Minneapolis, Minnesota

Linda A. Lee
School of Medicine
Johns Hopkins University
Towson, Maryland

Marianne J. Legato
The Foundation for Gender-Specific Medicine, Inc. MJL
Columbia University College of Medicine
New York, New York

Alice H. Lichtenstein
Cardiovascular Nutrition Laboratory
Jean Mayer USDA Human Nutrition Research Center on Aging
Tufts University
Boston, Massachusetts

Nirupa R. Matthan
Cardiovascular Nutrition Laboratory
Jean Mayer USDA Human Nutrition Research Center on Aging
Tufts University
Boston, Massachusetts

Gerard E. Mullin
Division of Gastroenterology and Hepatology
Johns Hopkins Hospital
Baltimore, Maryland

Deborah L. O'Connor
Department of Nutritional Sciences
Faculty of Medicine
University of Toronto, and Hospital for Sick Children
Toronto, Ontario, Canada

Pasqualina Perrig-Chiello
Institut für Psychologie
Universität Bern
Bern, Switzerland

Paula Skidmore
School of Medicine, Health Policy and Practice
University of East Anglia
Norwich, United Kingdom

Hannes B. Staehelin
Memory Clinic
Universitätsspital Basel
Basel, Switzerland

Lisa K. Stamp
Department of Medicine
University of Otogo
Christ Church, New Zealand

Jamie Stang
Division of Epidemiology and Community Health
School of Public Health
University of Minnesota
Minneapolis, Minnesota

Mary Story
Division of Epidemiology and Community Health
School of Public Health
University of Minnesota
Minneapolis, Minnesota

Laura Studee
College of Medicine Center of Excellence in Women's Health
University of Illinois at Chicago
Chicago, Illinois

Lilian U. Thompson
Department of Nutritional Sciences
Faculty of Medicine
University of Toronto
Toronto, Ontario, Canada

Cynthia A. Thomson
Department of Nutritional Sciences
Arizona Cancer Center
University of Arizona
Tucson, Arizona

Sophie Bucher Della Torre
Division of Adolescent Medicine
Department of Pediatrics
Golisano Children's Hospital at Strong
Rochester, New York

Janet A. Vogt
Department of Nutritional Sciences
Faculty of Medicine
University of Toronto
Toronto, Ontario, Canada

Wendy E. Ward
Department of Nutritional Sciences
Faculty of Medicine
University of Toronto
Toronto, Ontario, Canada

Thomas M.S. Wolever
Department of Nutritional Sciences
Faculty of Medicine
University of Toronto
Toronto, Ontario, Canada

Section I

Introduction

1 Need to Optimize the Health of Women

Lilian U. Thompson and Wendy E. Ward

CONTENTS

1.1 INTRODUCTION

Without question, there are specific diseases for which women are more susceptible compared with men. The biological basis for these differences, including the cellular and molecular mechanisms, is often not identified or understood but nonetheless it is widely known that differences in disease incidence and risk exist between men and women. Some of these differences are summarized in Table 1.1 [1,2]. While more heart attacks occur in men, more deaths occur in women within a year after a heart attack. Similarly, while fewer women experience a stroke, more women will die as a result. Depression, irritable bowel syndrome, osteoporosis, osteoarthritis, and auto-immune diseases such as rheumatoid arthritis, lupus, and fibromyalgia are all the more common in women compared with men. There is a need to better understand the sex-based differences in the biology, physiology, and disease risks, and to better understand the unique role of nutrition in the maintenance of good health and the management of chronic diseases.

1.2 SEX-BASED DIFFERENCES IN BIOLOGY AND PHYSIOLOGY

Most previous health-related studies have not focused on sex-based differences. In the past, researchers have often referred to the "70 kg man" as the reference standard from which treatments for women are based. However, there are differences in the biology and physiology between sexes that then determine their susceptibility to disease in response to biological stimuli, including medical treatments and dietary interventions.

TABLE 1.1
Differences in Disease Incidence and Risk between Women and Men

Disease	Men vs. Women
Cardiovascular disease	Heart disease: Men have more, but women are more likely to die within a year after a heart attack; women tend to get heart disease 7–10 years later than men Stroke: Women have fewer strokes but are more likely to die from them than men; women are generally older than men when they have a stroke
Depression	Twice as common in women
Migraine headaches	At least twice as common in women
Irritable bowel syndrome	More common in women
Cancer	Cancer of the lungs, kidneys, bladder, and pancreas are more common in men; thyroid and breast cancer is more common in women
Osteoporosis	More common in women
Rheumatoid arthritis	Two to three times more common in women
Osteoarthritis	Three times more common in women
Lupus	Nine times more common in women
Fibromyalgia	Nine times more common in women

Source: Adapted from Bren, L., *FDA Consum. Mag.*, 39, 10, 2005 and http://www.fda.gov/fdac/features/2005/405_sex.html.

Men and women differ in their life span, with women having longer lives than men. For example, there are ~560 supercentanarians (i.e., 110 years old) worldwide and almost 90% are women [3]. However, although women have lower mortality rates, they have more severe chronic diseases, a greater number of disability days particularly due to arthritis, more frequent doctor visits, and longer hospital stays [3]. This pattern of longevity appears to be common even in some animals, including the chimpanzees, tarantulas, and honey bees but does not occur in all species [3]. For example, male guinea pigs and golden hamsters live longer than their female counterparts. Several hypotheses have been suggested to explain sex-based differences in longevity [3]. These hypotheses, shown in Table 1.2, include a more active immune function and higher levels of estrogen in females, lower hormone activity, attenuated insulin-like growth factor-1 signaling pathways, lower oxidative stress in females, and a compensatory effect of the second X chromosome in females [3]. However, support for these hypotheses is somewhat weak and inconsistent, and thus identify the need for future research to provide a thorough understanding of this sex-based difference on longevity.

At least some of the differences in disease susceptibility relate to dramatic shifts in sex steroid hormones at distinct periods of the life cycle. It is a well-established fact that osteoporosis often develops as a result of the cessation of endogenous estrogen production at menopause [4]. In addition, rheumatoid arthritis often remits during pregnancy with a subsequent relapse postpartum, corresponding to fluctuations in sex steroids [5,6]. It is also known that pregnancy is a common stage of the life cycle when symptoms of periodontal disease appear [7]. Some mental health

TABLE 1.2
Hypotheses Regarding the Mechanisms Whereby Females Live Longer than Males

Hypothesis	Some Evidence For and Against[a]
Female has more active immune system	Lower disease incidence in females is not solely due to difference in immune system
High estrogen in female is protective	Female mammals such as short finned pilot whales, which undergo a true menopause, live longer than the males
Male has XY chromosome; female has XX chromosome; lack of second X chromosome shortens life span	Female longevity is not universal in the animal kingdom: e.g., male guinea pigs and golden hamsters live longer than females
Females have lower activity of growth hormone and insulin-like growth factor-1 signaling cascade	This relationship has been reported in fruit flies, *C. elegans*, and mice, but is yet to be demonstrated in humans
Lower oxidative stress in females	In humans, free radical formation is higher in males than in females. However, in mice, free radical production is higher in males and they live longer than females
Larger animals have shorter life spans	In some species with larger males, e.g., guinea pigs, and in some species with larger females, e.g., golden hamsters, the males live longer

Source: Adapted from Austed, S.N., *Gend. Med.*, 3, 79, 2006.

[a] Some evidence based on observations from animal species.

disorders may also be associated with hormonal fluctuations [8–10]. Figure 1.1 summarizes the relative changes in sex steroid hormones and the ages when some of these chronic diseases or conditions occur, recur, or are attenuated [11,12].

As previously discussed by others [13–15], there are other sex differences at the cellular, tissue, organ, and system level that then determine how men and women respond to environmental stimuli, including drugs and dietary components. It is known that the metabolism of drugs differs among women and men, in part due to differences in activity of liver enzymes responsible for drug processing. In turn, this alters both the drug effectiveness and toxicity between men and women. The metabolism can also differ between men and women because of differences in the rate of absorption of drugs and nutrients as they pass through the gastrointestinal tract, the smaller body weight and organ size of women, endogenous hormones activity, and the drug and body waste elimination by the kidney, which is slower in women compared with men. More sex-based differences in the biology of the gastrointestinal tract are described in Chapter 2.

The 2001 Report of the Committee on Understanding the Biology of Sex and Gender Differences, Institute of Medicine, titled "Exploring the Biological Contributions to Human Health: Does Sex Matter?" [14], resulted in clear recommendations,

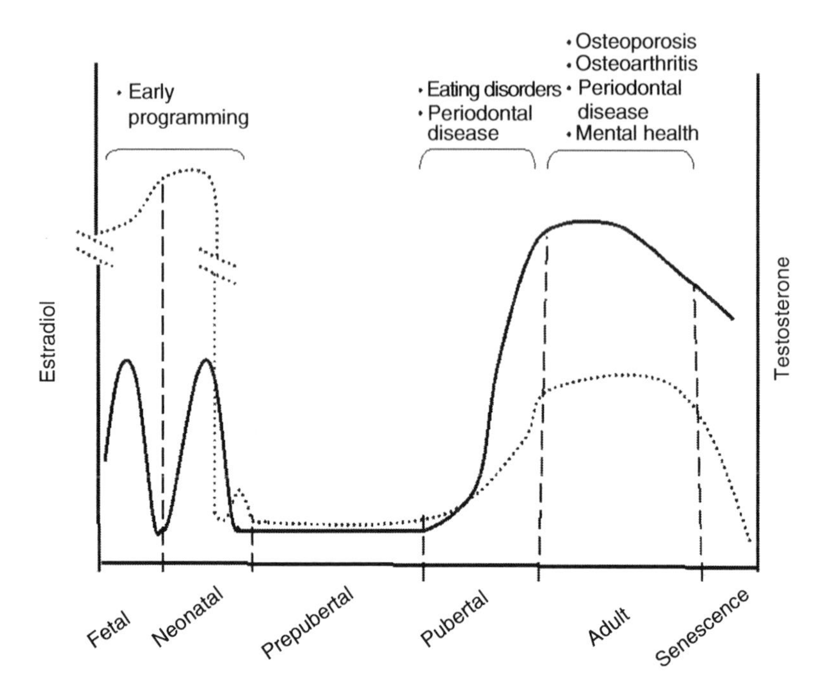

FIGURE 1.1 Both men and women experience significant changes in serum testosterone and estrogen, respectively, throughout the life cycle. A woman's susceptibility to specific diseases may be increased at distinct stages of the life cycle in which marked changes in circulating estrogen occur. The dotted line represents the changes in circulating estrogen in females and the solid line represents changes in circulating testosterone in males throughout the life cycle. In addition, pregnancy is a time in which specific states such as rheumatoid arthritis and periodontal disease may remit or worsen, respectively. (Adapted from Reinwald, S. and Weaver, C.M., *J. Nat. Prod.*, 69, 450, 2006 and http://physiology.lf2.cuni.cz/teaching/lecturenotes/reprod/sld052.htm.)

and in essence a framework, for elucidating how sex modulates susceptibility to specific diseases and overall health (Table 1.3). The impetus for this report arose from recognition of the paucity of studies that specifically examined susceptibility of diseases from a sex-specific approach.

1.3 SEX-BASED DIFFERENCES IN DISEASES AND NUTRITION

It is known that at least some of the diseases that women are particularly vulnerable to, i.e., cardiovascular disease, osteoporosis, depression, rheumatoid arthritis, can be favorably influenced by nutrition, or specific foods or food components. Diets low in saturated fat, and rich in fiber, whole grains, n-3 fatty acids, fruits and vegetables are protective against cardiovascular disease [16–18]. Similarly, bone health is influenced by calcium and Vitamin D intakes throughout the life cycle [19,20].

TABLE 1.3
Summary of the Recommendations of the Committee on Understanding the Biology of Sex and Gender Differences, Institute of Medicine

Promote research on sex at the cellular level
Study sex differences from womb to tomb
Mine cross-species information
Investigate natural variations
Expand research on sex differences in brain organization and function
Monitor sex differences and similarities for all human diseases that affect both sexes
Clarify use of the terms sex and gender
Support and conduct additional research on sex differences
Make sex-specific data more readily available
Determine and disclose the sex or origin of biological research materials
Longitudinal studies should be conducted and should be constructed so that their results can be analyzed by sex
Identify the endocrine status of research subjects
Encourage and support interdisciplinary research on sex differences
Reduce the potential for discrimination based on identified sex differences

Source: Adapted from Exploring the Biological Contributions to Human Health: Does Sex Matter? Report of the Committee on Understanding the Biology of Sex and Gender Differences, Institute of Medicine (IOM), 2001.

In addition, calcium improves the efficacy of hormone replacement therapy at preserving bone mass in postmenopausal women [20,21]. Mental health outcomes such as depression scores are improved with vitamin supplementation, particularly folate, and omega-3 fatty acids [22–25]. Symptoms of rheumatoid arthritis are attenuated with fish oil intervention, such that traditional drug doses can be reduced [26,28–30]. Moreover a vegetarian or vegan diet may also be useful for improving quality of life in individuals with rheumatoid arthritis [27].

Foods or food components may modulate disease onset or progression via direct hormonal mechanisms, modulation of hormone activity, attenuation of inflammatory response, antioxidant activity, or other mechanisms not yet identified. Many diseases are thought to occur as a result of inflammatory responses. Thus, n-3 fatty acids, particularly long chain polyunsaturated fatty acids abundant in fish oil, have been the subject of extensive investigation in a variety of diseases, including cardiovascular disease, osteoporosis, inflammatory bowel disease, and even periodontal disease. Studies also suggest that oxidative stress may have a role in mental health disorders, and have led to the hypothesis that supplementation with antioxidant micronutrients may delay or lessen symptoms of depression, schizophrenia, and development of dementia and Alzheimer's disease [31–35].

Combining knowledge regarding sex-based medicine with the fact that nutrient requirements are sex-specific, and the knowledge that nutrition has a critical role in human health, suggests that a sex-specific response to nutritional interventions likely exists. Indeed, there is an emerging knowledge that women and men may respond differently to nutritional interventions. In general, women and men have different nutrient requirements and respond differently to drugs and other biological stimuli.

1.4 AIMS OF THE BOOK

The overall aim of this book is to provide examples of sex-based nutrition. The specific aims are:

- To provide an overview of differences in the biology and physiology between males and females. It is not the intent to provide all details of the differences but to provide examples that then justifies a need for separate evaluation of the needs of women.
- To describe the nutrient needs of women at the various stages of the life cycle.
- To provide a better understanding of the diseases that affect women more than men and how nutrition may help reduce the risk and help manage those diseases.
- To recommend ways of optimizing the health of women through nutrition, and to provide guidance for future research and action.

Considering these aims, the book was divided into four sections. The first section of this book, the introductory chapters, includes the present chapter and Chapter 2, in which differences in the sex biology of the gastrointestinal tract are discussed to help in the understanding of the differences in nutrient needs in health and disease.

The chapters in the second section discuss the nutritional needs of healthy women at various stages of the life cycle, i.e., adolescence, pregnancy and lactation, premenopause, menopause, and midlife. Throughout these chapters, the nutritional needs of women, where appropriate, are differentiated from the needs of men.

The chapters in the major section, Section 3, discuss nutrition in chronic diseases (cardiovascular disease, metabolic syndrome and Type II diabetes, breast and ovarian cancer, osteoporosis and osteoarthritis, rheumatoid arthritis, irritable bowel syndrome) and other conditions such as obesity, mental health (Alzheimer's disease and dementia, eating disorders, depression, and other psychiatric disorders), eye health, and oral health. These chapters follow a standard format of discussion:

- Etiology of the disease or condition, emphasizing aspects that are unique to women.
- How foods or food components modulate the disease process in women based on the most recent scientific literature. Depending on the specific disease and the scientific information that exists, discussion of nutritional interventions that are appropriate for disease prevention, treatment, and different nutritional interventions at various stages of the disease process

is included. Throughout this section, specific responses that are different or unique to women are identified.
- Identification of areas for future research based on remaining unanswered questions.

Section 4, the concluding chapter, summarizes the main findings for each disease state and suggests further areas of future research for researchers, and identifies pertinent issues for health professionals involved with disease prevention and treatment in women; for government regulators involved in setting public health policy; and for the food industry involved in developing novel foods targeted specifically for prevention or treatment of diseases in women.

1.5 CONCLUSION

It can be argued that the old adage "With knowledge comes power" applies to sex-based nutrition. The more we know about women and their unique biology, the greater is the opportunity for optimizing life expectancy, and importantly, the quality of life. Without ensuring improved quality of life, there is little motivation to increase life span. Although women, in general, live several years longer than men, women suffer from chronic and debilitating conditions for a greater extent of their older years. A key goal of this book is to foster interest in the unique role that sex-based nutrition has in both the prevention and management of chronic diseases. It is hoped that this book is a catalyst that encourages scientists to design and conduct studies that will identify the benefits of approaching health through sex-based nutrition.

REFERENCES

1. Bren, L., Does sex make a difference? *FDA Consum. Mag.*, 39, 10, 2005.
2. http://www.fda.gov/fdac/features/2005/405_sex.html.
3. Austad, S.N., Why women live longer than men: Sex differences in longevity, *Gend. Med.*, 3, 79, 2006.
4. Brown, J.P. and Josse, R.G., Clinical practice guidelines for the diagnosis and management of osteoporosis, *Can. Med. Assoc. J.*, 167, S1, 2003.
5. Brennan, P. et al., Are both genetic and reproductive associations with rheumatoid arthritis linked to prolactin? *Lancet*, 348, 106, 1996.
6. Silman, A., Kay, A., and Brennan, P., Timing of pregnancy in relation to the onset of rheumatoid arthritis, *Arthritis Rheum.*, 35, 152, 1992.
7. Xiong, X. et al., Periodontal disease and adverse pregnancy outcomes: A systematic review, *Brit. J. Obstet. Gynecol.*, 113, 135, 2006.
8. Hafner, H., Gender differences in schizophrenia, *Psychoneuroendocrinology*, 2, 17, 2003.
9. Klump, K.L., Gobrogge, K.L., Perkins, P.S., Thorne, D., Sisk, C.L., and Breedlove, S.M., Preliminary evidence that gonadal hormones organize and activate disordered eating, *Psychol. Med.*, 36, 539, 2006.
10. Klump, K., Gene-environment interactions, *Eat. Disord. Rev.*, 17, 2, 2006.
11. Reinwald, S. and Weaver, C.M., Soy isoflavones and bone health, *J. Nat. Prod.*, 69, 450, 2006.
12. http://physiology.lf2.cuni.cz/teaching/lecturenotes/reprod/sld052.htm.

13. Federman, D.D., The biology of human sex difference, *New Engl. J. Med.*, 354, 1507, 2006.
14. Exploring the Biological Contributions to Human Health: Does Sex Matter? Report of the Committee on Understanding the Biology of Sex and Gender Differences, Institute of Medicine (IOM), 2001.
15. Gochfeld, M., Framework for gender differences in human and animal toxicology, *Environ. Res.*, 104, 4, 2007.
16. Expert Panel on Detection Evaluation and Treatment of High Blood Cholesterol in Adults, Executive Summary of The Third Report of The National Cholesterol Education Program (NCEP), Expert Panel on Detection, Evaluation, and Treatment of High Blood Cholesterol in Adults (Adult Treatment Panel III), *JAMA.*, 285, 2486, 2001.
17. Lichtenstein, A.H. et al., Diet and lifestyle recommendations revision 2006: A scientific statement from the American Heart Association Nutrition Committee, *Circulation*, 114, 82, 2006.
18. Mosca, L. et al., Evidence-based guidelines for cardiovascular disease prevention in women, *J. Am. Coll. Cardiol.*, 43, 900, 2004.
19. Heaney, R.P. and Weaver, C.M., Newer perspectives on calcium nutrition and bone quality, *J. Am. Coll. Nutr.*, 26(Suppl 6), 574S, 2005.
20. Nieves, J.W. et al., Calcium potentiates the effect of estrogen and calcitionin on bone mass: Review and analyses, *Am. J. Clin. Nutr.*, 67, 18, 1998.
21. Shea, B., Meta-analyses of therapies for postmenopausal osteoporosis. VII. Meta-analysis of calcium supplementation for the prevention of postmenopausal osteoporosis, *Endocr. Rev.*, 23, 552, 2002.
22. Kaplan, B.J. et al., Effective mood stabilization with a chelated mineral supplement: An open-label trial in bipolar disorder, *J. Clin. Psychiatry*, 62, 936, 2001.
23. Puri, B.K. et al., Eicosapentaenoic acid in treatment-resistant depression associated with symptom remission, structural brain changes and reduced neuronal phospholipid turnover, *Int. J. Clin. Pract.*, 55, 560, 2001.
24. Stoll, A.L. et al., Omega 3 fatty acids in bipolar disorder: A preliminary double-blind, placebo-controlled trial, *Arch. Gen. Psychiatry*, 56, 407, 1999.
25. Nemets, B., Stahl, Z., and Belmaker, R.H., Addition of omega-3 fatty acid to maintenance medication treatment for recurrent unipolar depressive disorder, *Am. J. Psychiatry*, 159, 477, 2002.
26. Belch, J.J. et al., Effects of altering dietary essential fatty acids on requirements for non-steroidal anti-inflammatory drugs in patients with rheumatoid arthritis: A double blind placebo controlled study, *Ann. Rheum. Dis.*, 47, 96, 1988.
27. Muller, H., de Toledo, W., and Resch, K.-L., Fasting followed by vegetarian diet in patients with rheumatoid arthritis: A systematic review, *Scand. J. Rheumatol.*, 30, 1, 2001.
28. Lau, C.S., Morley, K.D., and Belch, J.J.F., Effects of fish oil supplementation on non-steroidal anti-inflammatory requirement in patients with mild rheumatoid arthritis—a double blind placebo controlled trial, *Br. J. Rheumatol.*, 32, 982, 1993.
29. Skoldstam, L. et al., Effect of six months of fish oil supplementation in stable rheumatoid arthritis. A double-blind, controlled study, *Scand. J. Rheumatol.*, 21, 178, 1992.
30. Kjeldsen-Kragh, J. et al., Dietary omega-3 fatty acid supplementation and naproxen treatment in patients with rheumatoid arthritis, *J. Rheumatol.*, 19, 1531, 1992.
31. Gonzalez-Gross, M., Marcos, A., and Pietrzik, K., Nutrition and cognitive impairment in the elderly, *Brit. J. Nutr.*, 86, 313, 2001.
32. Helmer, C. et al., Association between antioxidant nutritional indicators and the incidence of dementia: Results from the PAQUID prospective cohort study, *Europ. J. Clin. Nutr.*, 57, 1555, 2003.

33. Engelhart, M.J. et al., Dietary intake of antioxidants and risk of Alzheimer disease, *JAMA.*, 287, 3223, 2002.
34. Morris, M.C. et al., Dietary intake of antioxidant nutrients and the risk of incident Alzheimer disease in a biracial community study, *JAMA*, 287, 3230, 2002.
35. Sano, M. et al., A controlled trial of selegiline, α-tocopherol, or both as a treatment for Alzheimer's disease, *New Engl. J. Med.*, 336, 1216, 1997.

2 Sex-Specific Biology of the Gastrointestinal Tract

Marianne J. Legato

CONTENTS

2.1 INTRODUCTION

As is the case with every system of the body, the research of the last 15 years has documented the sexual dimorphism of the normal function of the digestive system. From salivary composition and flow rate to the molecular biology of the P450 system that metabolizes drugs, the digestive system has sex-specific, unique characteristics. However, as is the case with all information about the sexual dimorphism of normal human physiology and the pathophysiology of disease, information about the impact of biological sex on gastrointestinal function and on sex-specific nutritional requirements is often rudimentary. Much of it consists of observational data and, less frequently, original investigations about the impact of biological sex on nutritional requirements. Many isolated observations about sex-specific gastrointestinal function are reported almost incidentally and scattered throughout the literature. Recently, however, systematic overviews of what is known about the sex-specific biology of the gastrointestinal tract and the experience of gastrointestinal illnesses have begun to appear in the literature [1,2]. This chapter summarizes some of that information as they may help in the understanding of sex differences in nutrient requirements and in the prevention and management of some chronic diseases.

2.2 MOUTH

More women are "supertasters" compared with men until older age, and prefer foods with less sugar than do men, especially younger men [3]. Some of this increased ability to taste may be the result of women's relatively greater olfactory sensitivity.

The role of saliva is complex and perhaps underestimated; it begins the process of food digestion, defends against hostile invaders such as bacteria, and lubricates the mouth for fluent speech. The composition and flow rates of saliva are sex-specific and, in the case of women, vary with the phases of the menstrual cycle during menses; for example, glucose concentration increases 3–9 fold [4,5]. Electrolyte composition changes over the course of the cycle as well: at the time of ovulation, potassium concentration rises and calcium and sodium levels decrease [6]. Salivary peroxidases also increase at the time of ovulation, perhaps an evolutionary development to help nourish any embryo generated [7]. The buffering capacity of saliva is less in women than in men, particularly during the menstrual period; this, coupled with women's significantly lower salivary flow rates may contribute to a higher incidence of halitosis due to increased oral bacterial fermentation. Depression, twice as common in women as in men, also lowers salivary flow rates, possibly due at least in part to diminished food intake and the impact of psychotropic medication [8]. Interestingly, women have 1.5–2.0 fold lower levels of salivary cortisol than men after experiencing a stressful situation, although their levels rise during 25th week of gestation and remain high until gestation [9].

2.3 ESOPHAGUS AND STOMACH

The esophagus is shorter in women than in men [10] and women describe more pain on distention of this organ. Its peristaltic activity is higher and more vigorous in women. The higher occurrence of Barrett's esophagus in men may be the consequence of an increased level of the protective "shock" protein Hsp27 in the women esophageal mucosa [11]. The incidence of gastroesophageal reflux increases during pregnancy, due to the impact of higher than usual levels of progesterone on the lower esophageal sphincter [12]. Women have less gastric acid than men, probably the consequence of their smaller parietal cell mass. Testosterone stimulates the parietal cells of the stomach and estrogen suppresses acid secretion. Women have higher levels of the hormone gastrin, on the other hand, their parietal cells are less sensitive to gastrin than those of men. The impact of protein pump inhibitors on gastric acid secretion may be greater in women, as documented in a study investigating the degree of proton pump inhibitor in a small sample of men and women. A higher enterochromaffin-like cell density in older women may be associated with higher rates of gastritis than is the case for older men [13]. Some cancers of the stomach have estrogen or progesterone receptors or both and survival rates are impacted by the levels of circulating hormones in affected patients [14]. Trials of tamoxifen in patients with gastric cancer have been mounted in an effort to treat gastric cancer but have not proven to prolong survival [15].

There is a significant variability of intestinal contractility, including that of the stomach, as a function of the cyclic endocrine levels of women. Menstruating women have a slower emptying time than during the luteal phase of their cycle and even in nonmenstruating females solids take a third longer and liquids twice as long to leave the stomach compared with men [16].

Bloating and belching is more common in women after eating, probably reflecting the impact of progesterone on gut motility [17]. Pregnancy is accompanied by an elevation of progesterone, human chorionic gonadotrophin [2], and a decrease in motilin [18]. All of these variations contribute to abdominal bloating, nausea, and constipation that are so common during pregnancy. These fluctuations disturb the normal gut rhythm that disturbs the amplitude, frequency, and direction of the contractions that propel food forward through the digestive tract.

2.4 PANCREAS AND GALL BLADDER

The composition of bile differs in men and women [19]. Estrogen and progesterone both increase the amount of cholesterol in bile. The high levels of progesterone during pregnancy slow gall bladder emptying, accounting for the increased frequency of gallstones in susceptible gravid individuals. A sex difference in the break-down products of bile has been incriminated in the higher incidence of inflammatory bowel disease in women as well as their higher risk of colon cancer compared with men [19]. Women who have had a cholecystectomy have a higher risk for colon cancer, possibly due to the continuous secretion of bile into the intestinal tract [20]. The higher incidence of pancreatic cancer in men (it is 3 times more frequent in men as in women) has been linked to the impact of testosterone on the pancreas [21]. Twice as high levels of 5-α reductase, which converts testosterone to its more potent form (5-α dihydrotestosterone), have been identified in men with pancreatic cancer [22]. The sex-specific male risk decreases with age, and there is no difference after the age of 70. Because estrogen and progesterone are protective against this malignancy, it is intriguing to consider the use of hormone therapy in patients afflicted with this almost inevitably fatal disease.

2.5 ENTERIC NERVOUS SYSTEM

One of the most exciting developments in gastrointestinal research is the description of the complex and independent system of innervation of the gut, the *enteric nervous system*. It is this nervous system, with its extensive connections to the central nervous system via the vagal nerve and the similarity of its neurotransmitters to those of the brain, that paces and modulates the phasic contractile activity of the intestine. There are several similarities to the central nervous system: there are over 30 neurotransmitters including serotonin that function to integrate its activity and the cells that support the support system encasing the axons of working neurons resemble astrocytes. In fact, lesions that are found in the brain in Alzheimer's and Parkinson's diseases are also present in the enteric nervous system of affected individuals [23]. The parallel between the enteric nervous system and the conducting system of the heart, also modulated by central nervous system activity, is of great interest. The higher incidence of functional bowel disease in women may one day be explained by sex-specific differences and disturbances in the innervation of the intestine. Many of the cyclic variations in intestinal activity that occur with the menstrual cycle may be due to the impact of circulating hormones on enteric nervous system activity. Patients put on oral contraceptives often experience an exacerbation of their symptoms [24], while postmenopausal women put on estrogen replacement therapy alone showed no such intensification of symptoms [25]. Progesterone may well be the culprit in the premenstrual exacerbation of bowel dysfunction in the female patient. Research on the sex-specific activity of the enteric nervous system has not yet been extensive enough to modify patient treatment. It is clear, however, that psychotropic drugs like the serotonin reuptake inhibitors often have a profound effect on gut as well as on mood.

2.6 LIVER

Any discussion of the sex-specific aspects of the gastrointestinal tract must include the observation of the sexual dimorphism in the metabolism of hormones, medications, and other substances by the liver. In general, males have a higher concentration of microsomal oxidative enzymes and females more microsomal reductive enzymes [26]. These metabolic patterns are imprinted in utero [27]. This sex-specific pattern of drug metabolism is related to the pattern of secretion of growth hormone, which is pulsatile in males but steady in females [1]. During pregnancy, functional hepatic blood flow decreases with a resultant decrease in the hepatic clearance of some substances [1]. The sex-specificity of drug metabolism diminishes with age [28], probably because of changes in hormonal levels.

The cytochromes P450 modulate the metabolism of drugs in the liver; they are a family of oxidative enzymes and their activity varies in some cases between men and women. Women have a higher activity, for example, of CYP3A4, and drugs (diazepam and erythromycin) cleared by this enzyme are cleared more quickly in women [29]. Alcohol is metabolized less efficiently in women than in men, in part because of a difference in levels of gastric alcohol dehydrogenase between the sexes [30]. Data on the success of female–male liver transplantation uniformly indicate that failure rates are highest in this group (increased 3.7 fold), while male–male, male–female, and female–female transplants were much more likely to succeed [31]. Data from studies on kidney and heart transplant recipients in a large European study showed the same trend in transplant failure, with female–male donations least likely to succeed [32]. Most investigators attributed this interesting finding to differences in sex hormone levels and receptor biology within the grafted tissue.

2.7 CONCLUSION AND FUTURE RESEARCH

Most of the data that have been accumulated about the sex-specific biology of the gastrointestinal tract concern the profile of illnesses that occur with different frequency in the two sexes. Less available are solid data about the sex-specificity of normal gastrointestinal physiology and how it might influence not only nutritional requirements, but also the prevention and treatment of chronic diseases, particularly of the gastrointestinal tract. There is no question that the sex hormones play an important role in determining the characteristics of the digestive system, and that the hormonal milieu of women, with its monthly fluctuation and the special state of pregnancy further modify those characteristics. With aging, many of the sex-specific differences in gastrointestinal physiology and in nutritional recommendations disappear. Hopefully, as the general interest of the academic community in gender-specific medicine continues to expand, the information about the unique characteristics of this important system in men and women can be refined and enlarged in future research.

REFERENCES

1. Karlstadt, R.G., Hogan, D.L., and Foxx-Orenstein, A., Normal physiology of the gastrointestinal tract and gender differences. In: Legato, M.J., ed. *The Principles of Gender-Specific Medicine*, Elsevier Academic Press, NY 2004. pp 377–396.
2. Karlstadt, R.G., Gender-based biology and the gastrointestinal tract, *J. Gend. Spec. Med.*, 3, 41, 2000.
3. Bartoshuk, L.M. et al., PTC/PROP tasting: anatomy, psychophysics and sex effects, *Physiol. Behav.*, 56, 1165, 1994.
4. Prosser, C.G. and Hartmann, P.F., Saliva and breast milk composition during the menstrual cycle of women, *Aust. J. Exp. Biol. Med. Sci.*, 61, 265, 1983.
5. Percival, R.S. et al., Flow rates of resting whole and stimulated parotid saliva in relation to age and gender, *J. Den. Res.*, 73, 1416, 1994.
6. Puskulian, L., Salivary electrolytes change during the normal menstrual cycle, *J. Den. Res.*, 51, 1212, 1972.
7. Cockle, S.M. and Harkeness, R.A., Changes in salivary peroxidase and polymorphonuclear leukocyte enzyme activities during the menstrual cycle, *BJOG: An. Int. J. Obstet. Gyn.*, 85, 776, 1978.
8. Bergdahl, M. and Bergdahl, J., Low unstimulated salivary flow and subjective oral dryness: association with medication, anxiety and stress, *J. Dental Res.*, 79, 1652, 2000.
9. Scott, E.M. et al., The increase in plasma and saliva cortisol levels in pregnancy is not due to the increase in corticosteroid binding globulin levels, *J. Clin. Endocrinol. Metab.*, 71, 639, 1990.
10. Li, Q. et al., Manometric determination of esophageal length, *Am. J. Gastroenterol.*, 89, 722, 1994.
11. Soldes, O.S. et al., Differential expression of Hsp27 in normal oesophagus. Barrett's metaplasia and oesophageal adenocarcinomas, *Brit. J. Cancer*, 79, 595, 1999.
12. Ulmsten, U. and Sundstrom, G., Esophageal manometry in pregnant and nonpregnant females, *Am. J. Obstet. Gyn.*, 32, 260, 1978.
13. Green, D.M. et al., Enterochromaffin-like cell populations in human fundic mucosa: quantitative studies of their variations with age, sex and plasma gastrin levels, *J. Path.*, 157, 235, 1989.
14. Matsui, M. et al., The prognosis of patients with gastric cancer possessing sex hormone receptors, *Surg. Today*, 22, 421, 1992.
15. Harrison, J.D. et al., The effect of tamoxifen and estrogen receptor status on survival in gastric carcinoma, *Cancer*, 64, 1007, 1989.
16. Caballero-Plasencia, A.M. et al., Are there changes in gastric emptying during the menstrual cycle? *Scand. J. Gastroenterol.*, 34, 772, 1999.
17. Camilleri, M. et al., A US national survey of upper gastrointestinal symptoms in 21,000 community participants, *Gastroenterology*, 118, Abstract 851, 2000.
18. Christofides, N. et al., Decreased plasma motilin concentration in pregnancy, *Br. Med. J.*, 285, 1453, 1982.

19. McMichael, A.J. and Potter, J.D., Host factors in carcinogenesis: certain bile-acid metabolic profiles that selectively increase the risk of proximal colon cancer, *J. Nat. Cancer Inst.*, 75, 185, 1985.
20. Giovannucci, E. et al., A meta-analysis of cholecystectomy and risk of colo-rectal cancer, *Gastroenterology*, 105, 286, 1993.
21. Andren-Sandberg, A. et al., Other risk factors for pancreatic cancer: hormonal aspects, *Ann. Oncol.*, 10(4), 131, 1999.
22. Andren-Sandberg, A., Androgen influence on exocrine pancreatic cancer, *Int. J. Pancreatol.*, 4, 363, 1989.
23. Ashraf, W. et al., Dopaminergic defect of enteric nervous system in Parkinson's disease patients with chronic constipation, *Lancet*, 346, 861, 1995.
24. Heitkemper, M.M. et al., Symptoms across the menstrual cycle in women with irritable bowel syndrome, *Am. J. Gastroenterol.*, 98, 420, 2003.
25. Triadafilopoulos, G. et al., Bowel dysfunction in postmenopausal women, *Women's Health*, 27, 55, 1998.
26. Van Thiel, D.H. and Gavaler, J.S., Pregnancy-associated sex steroids and their effects on the liver, *Sem. Liver Dis.*, 7, 1, 1987.
27. Eagon, P.K. et al., Estrogen and androgen receptors in the liver: their role in liver disease and regeneration, *Sem. Liver Dis.*, 12, 59, 1985.
28. Demyan, W.F. et al., Estrogen sulfotransferase of the rat liver. Complementary DNA > cloning and age and sex-specific regulation of messenger RNA, *Molec. Endocrin.*, 6, 589, 1992.
29. Greenblatt, D.J. et al., Oxazepam kinetics: effects of age and sex, *J. Pharm. Exp. Ther.*, 215, 86, 1980.
30. Frezza, M. et al., High blood alcohol levels in women. The role of decreased gastric alcohol dehydrogenase activity and first pass metabolism, *N. Engl. J. Med.*, 322, 95, 1990.
31. Kahn, D. et al., Gender of donor influences outcome after orthotopic liver transplantation in adults, *Dig. Dis. Sci.*, 38, 1485, 1993.
32. Zeier, M. et al., The effect of donor gender on graft survival, *J. Am. Nephrol.*, 12, 2570, 2002.

Section II

Normal Nutrition

3 Adolescence

Nicole Larson, Jayne A. Fulkerson, Jamie Stang, and Mary Story

CONTENTS

3.1 INTRODUCTION

The nutritional requirements of females are greater during adolescence than at any other time of life [1]. A healthful diet that provides adequate amounts of all essential nutrients is critical to support the rapid physical growth and development that characterizes adolescence. In addition, a nutritious diet reduces risk for problems such as iron deficiency anemia, maturational delay, overweight, poor bone mineralization, and poor school performance. The eating behaviors established during adolescence often influence eating behaviors during adulthood, and thus further impact on long-term health status [2]. For example, a diet composed primarily of fruits and vegetables, whole grains, low-fat dairy products, and lean protein foods, and that is low in saturated and trans fat may reduce risk for the development of heart disease [3]. Similarly, a diet including adequate calcium and vitamin D may reduce risk for the development of osteoporosis [4]. Several conditions and nutrition concerns are particularly relevant for adolescent females. In addition, some eating habits common among adolescent females impact nutritional intake and warrant attention.

This chapter will review the nutritional needs of adolescent females in the contexts of growth and development and the promotion of good health. Special consideration will be given to gaps between the current dietary practices of adolescent females and recommendations for health as well as important differences between adolescent females and males. Finally, common eating behaviors and special health conditions among adolescent females and their impact on nutritional intake will be discussed along with interventions for promoting healthy eating.

3.2 GROWTH AND DEVELOPMENT

Physical, social, and cognitive development during adolescence is complex and dramatic [1]. The simultaneous but asynchronous changes within each developmental stream have many implications for nutritional health. Rapid physical growth increases energy and nutrient requirements [3]. Social developmental tasks such as developing an independent identity and the increasing importance of peer acceptance may lead adolescents to adopt unhealthy eating or weight-control behaviors [1,5]. Limited abstract reasoning and problem-solving skills characteristic of cognitive development in early adolescence may further increase the risk of poor nutrition [1]. Adolescents' limited ability to think about possibilities makes it difficult for them to grasp relationships between present nutrition behavior and long-term health. Likewise, before advanced problem-solving skills are developed, it is difficult for adolescents to identify ways of overcoming barriers to healthy eating. The combination of elevated nutritional needs, increasing autonomy, and immature cognitive abilities places adolescent females at particular nutritional risk. It is therefore essential that persons who provide health supervision for adolescents develop a thorough understanding of adolescent development.

3.2.1 Physical Growth and Development

Puberty marks the beginning of physical growth and development during adolescence. Although the ordering of events in the progression through puberty is highly consistent, the timing and tempo of pubertal changes are characterized by considerable variability with the age of pubertal onset approximating a normal distribution [6]. This variability is driven by many factors, including genetics, environmental factors, general health, and nutrition. For example, some data suggest that females of African American descent may experience puberty earlier than Mexican American or non-Hispanic white females [7–9]. Undernutrition and lower body fat are related to later maturation while moderate overweight is related to early maturation [8,10,11]. Improvements in health and nutrition over the past several generations are thought to be, at least in part, responsible for the secular decline in age at puberty, which has been documented in the population [7].

3.2.1.1 Pubertal Milestones and Sexual Maturation

The appearance of breast buds is the first visible sign of physical development in females. In the United States, breast development begins around the age of 10 years, but some studies have reported ethnic or racial variations. For example, breast buds appear at an average age of 9.5 years in African American females, 9.8 years in Mexican American females, and 10.3 years in non-Hispanic white females [9]. Approximately 6 months later, sparse pubic hair appears. The progression of these secondary sexual characteristics is often described by referring to the sexual maturation rating (SMR) stages [12]. By evaluating breast and pubic hair development and making comparison with the SMR, a practitioner can quickly assess pubertal maturation independent of chronological age. Such an assessment is important because nutritional requirements most closely correspond with stage of pubertal maturation. An SMR of 1 represents prepubertal development, an SMR of 2 represents the beginning of pubertal development, an SMR of 3 or 4 represents ongoing development, and an SMR of 5 represents secondary sexual characteristics, which are fully developed.

The pubertal growth spurt begins shortly after the appearance of pubic hair at SMR Stage 3 of breast development [6]. During this time, as gains in height and weight are made, the female reproductive organs (i.e., uterus, vagina, and ovaries) also continue to mature. Height velocity peaks and then decelerates rapidly prior to menarche, which occurs at an average age of 12–13 years among US females [9]. For up to 2 years after menarche, menstrual cycles may be anovulatory and irregular. Male development proceeds in a similar pattern but starts nearly 2 years later and typically follows a slower tempo [6]. Genital development (i.e., changes in the size and coloring of the testes and scrotum) is used in place of breast development to assess sexual maturation among males. The adolescent growth spurt occurs at a later stage of sexual maturation among males than among females at SMR Stage 4 of genital development [6].

3.2.1.2 Peak Height Velocity

During childhood, growth is consistent, occurring at a rate of ~5–6 cm (2.5 in.) per year until just prior to puberty [13]. A slight "preadolescent dip" in linear growth is typical but the growth rate increases again once puberty begins [13]. The velocity of growth increases until it peaks in females around the age of 11.5 years, at an average rate of 8 cm/year [6]. Peak growth continues for only 6–12 months and then decelerates after menarche. If menarche occurs at the average age of about 12–13 years, females will gain only 7 cm in height after menarche. However, if menarche comes early or late, then more or less growth will be correspondingly observed after menarche. The outcome of linear growth during adolescence is an impressive gain of the final 15%–20% of adult height, but several gender differences in the pattern of linear growth produce an average height advantage of 13 cm for males [13,14]. These differences include two additional years of prepubertal growth before the adolescent growth spurt, a greater velocity of peak growth (9 cm/year), and a longer duration of peak growth [6].

3.2.1.3 Peak Weight Velocity and Changes in Body Composition

In addition to the remarkable gains in height during adolescence, young people also gain 50% of their ideal adult body weight [14]. Among females, peak gains in weight of 8.3 kg (18.3 lb) per year are made 3–6 months later than peak gains in height [13]. Some additional weight gain is normal after menarche, but the rate of weight gain decelerates considerably in a manner similar to changes in height velocity. Unlike females, males experience peak gains in weight and height at about the same time. Males add more weight (9 kg or 19.8 lb) per year at the peak of weight gain but, under the influence of testosterone, tend to gain more lean muscle mass than females [13]. During adolescence, females accrue 1.14 kg fat mass/year while males maintain their fat mass. Consequently, males decrease their percentage of body fat by 1.15 kg/year [13].

3.2.1.4 Bone Mineral Accrual

Despite the dimorphic effects of testosterone and estrogen on body composition, both hormones promote the deposition of bone mineral during puberty [13]. Testosterone acts directly on bone to promote its formation and indirectly by promoting muscle growth, which places stress on bone to further increase growth [15]. Estrogen prevents the breakdown of bone and stimulates its formation [15]. At the end of puberty, estrogen also promotes fusion of the epiphyseal plates, therefore halting further growth in height [13]. The period of peak bone mineral accrual for females is early in adolescence and for males tends to be later during middle adolescence. Males tend to gain more bone mineral than do females at every age; however, by the age of 18, female and male adolescents have accrued more than 90% of their peak bone mass if pubertal development is completed at the normal time [13,16]. Delayed puberty may lead to a reduction in adult bone mineral density and consequently an increased risk of osteoporosis [13]. Additional factors that influence the accrual of bone mass include genetic potential, weight-bearing physical activity, cigarette smoking, alcohol consumption, and nutritional intake [4]. Nutritional factors associated with bone mineral accrual include intakes of vitamin D, calcium, and food components, which may interfere with the retention of calcium (e.g., alcohol, caffeine, oxalates, phytates, sodium) [4].

3.2.2 Social and Emotional Development

Adolescence is the first time when young people have the ability to think through who they are and who they want to become [17]. The myriad of physical changes adolescent females experience can greatly influence their self-perceptions and how they feel about themselves in a positive or negative way. While parents continue to be valued role models, as females progress through adolescence, it is developmentally appropriate for them to establish increasing independence from family and for peer norms to grow in importance [1]. Therefore, comments from parents and peers about physical appearance have the potential to greatly influence views of self during adolescence. Negative appraisals of appearance, especially body weight, can lead to the development of disordered eating behaviors. A high value on acceptance by one's peer group may also impact the food choices of adolescents. Adolescent females may feel pressure to eat high-fat, high-sugar foods and beverages if they are frequently consumed by friends. Alternatively, adolescents may feel pressure to diet or restrict their energy intake if their peer group engages in these unhealthy behaviors.

3.2.3 Cognitive Development

Adolescence is also characterized by development of the cognitive skills needed to think hypothetically and abstractly [1]. Young adolescents (11–14 years) tend to focus only on the concrete and present reality. During this stage, adolescent females typically have difficulty grasping relationships between their current nutrition behavior and future health, understanding intangible concepts, and solving problems that require thinking about multiple aspects of a situation at once [1]. As the transition is made to middle adolescence (15–17 years), cognitive skills become more advanced and adolescents more often display the ability to think about possibilities and multiple aspects of a problem. The initial development of abstract thinking skills leads to heightened self-consciousness and adolescents begin to worry not only about their own thoughts but what others are thinking about them and their behavior [17]. In particular, adolescent females may become more concerned with what others think about their appearance, weight, and food choices. By the time they reach late adolescence (18–21 years), most females have developed advanced cognitive skills. In this stage, adolescent females can more often identify ways to overcome barriers to making changes in their eating behavior [1]. However, even at this stage of development, adolescents may not consistently apply advanced cognitive skills when faced with highly stressful situations.

3.3 NUTRITIONAL NEEDS AND DIETARY INTAKE

Energy and nutrient requirements are high during adolescence to support the rapid growth and development just described. The dietary reference intakes (DRIs) are a set of four reference values useful for planning and evaluating the nutrient intakes of healthy people. While most DRIs are not based on actual experimental studies in adolescents, the reference values provide the best estimates for nutritional requirements of adolescent females. Reference values for adolescents were extrapolated based on data from experimental studies in adults or derived from population intake levels. Recommended dietary allowances (RDAs), adequate intakes (AIs), and tolerable upper intake levels (ULs) are useful for evaluating the diets of individuals and estimated average requirements (EARs) are best used to evaluate the diets of populations [18].

- RDAs represent daily intake levels sufficient to meet the needs of nearly all persons (97%–98%) in a particular life-stage and gender group.
- EARs correspond to daily intake levels sufficient to meet the needs of only 50% of persons in a particular life-stage and gender group. The percentage of a population having intakes of a given nutrient below the EAR can be taken to represent the prevalence of inadequacy for that nutrient.
- AIs are used in place of RDAs and EARs when there is not a sufficient amount of scientific evidence to support their establishment.
- ULs represent the highest level of usual intake that is likely to pose no risk of adverse health effects for nearly all (97%–98%) individuals in a life-stage and gender group. However, as intakes of a nutrient increase above the UL, the potential increases for adverse health effects to occur.

In addition to these four reference values for nutrient intakes, the Institute of Medicine has developed estimated energy requirement (EER) levels for planning and evaluating calorie intakes based on age, sex, and physical activity level [19]. Finally, acceptable macronutrient distribution ranges (AMDRs) were established to provide guidance on the proportion of total calories that should be consumed as protein, carbohydrate, and fat to prevent chronic disease and ensure sufficient nutrient intake [19].

These reference values are categorized according to chronological age rather than stage of maturational development; therefore, practical application of the values in relation to adolescents should be informed by an understanding of how nutritional needs parallel rates of growth. Because of the rapid physiologic growth that occurs during adolescence, total energy and nutrient requirements are greater than during any other period in the life cycle. The greatest nutrient demands occur during the period of peak growth velocity. As reviewed in the first section of this chapter, the period of peak growth and peak nutrient requirements tend to occur a few years earlier among females than among males. Also, as adolescent males experience greater increases in height, weight, and lean body mass than do females, the magnitude increase in nutritional requirements is smaller for females than for males.

While the micronutrient needs of females and males of the same age are very similar prior to the arrival of puberty, notable gender differences emerge in these requirements during adolescence. Sex differences in requirements are driven by sex-specific changes in body composition and the onset of menstruation in females during puberty. For example, menstruation creates an additional demand for iron

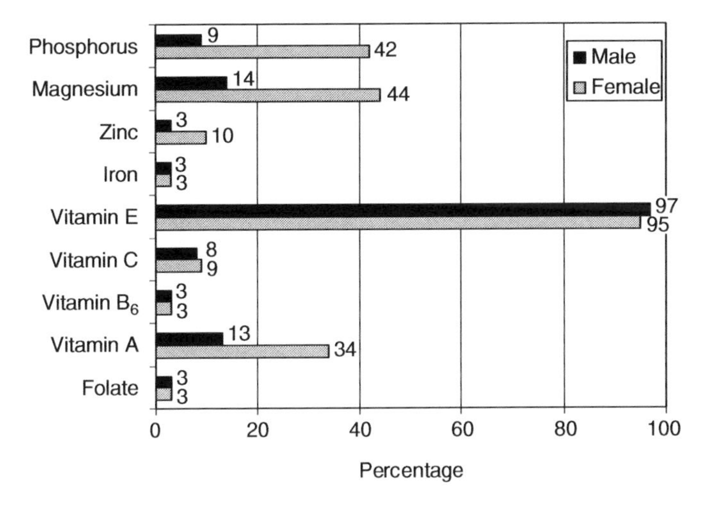

FIGURE 3.1 Percentage of females and males aged 9–13 years whose usual dietary intake is less than the estimated average requirement (EAR). EARs correspond to daily intake levels sufficient to meet the needs of 50% of persons in a particular life-stage and gender group. The percentage of a population having intakes of a given nutrient below the EAR can be taken to represent the prevalence of inadequacy for that nutrient. (Data from Moshfegh, A., Goldman, J., and Cleveland, L., *What We Eat in America, NHANES 2001–2002: Usual Nutrient Intakes from Food Compared to Dietary Reference Intakes*, U.S. Department of Agriculture, Agricultural Research Service, Beltsville, MD, 2005.)

and females have greater requirements than males after menarche. In contrast, females generally have lower requirements than males for the nutrients magnesium, zinc, niacin, riboflavin, thiamin, vitamin A, and vitamin B_6 [20–22]. Relative to these requirements, national nutrition data indicate that many adolescents have marginal or inadequate intakes for several nutrients [23]. These data further suggest that females more often have poor nutritional intake than do males, particularly for phosphorus (9–18 years), magnesium (9–18 years), zinc (9–18 years), iron (14–18 years), vitamin C (14–18 years), vitamin B_6 (14–18 years), vitamin A (9–13 years), and folate (14–18 years) (Figures 3.1 and 3.2).

The 2005 Dietary Guidelines for Americans (Dietary Guidelines) and the US Department of Agriculture (USDA) food guidance system, MyPyramid, provide mainly food-based recommendations complimentary to the reference values and ranges for nutrient intake (i.e., DRIs, AMDRs) developed by the Institute of Medicine [24,25]. The Dietary Guidelines are a set of science-based recommendations established on the principle that nutritional needs should be met primarily from foods and beverages. Recommendations of greatest relevance for adolescent females are outlined in Table 3.1. MyPyramid also provides guidance in the form of meal patterns to help individuals meet their total nutrient needs without consuming calories or other dietary components (e.g., trans fat) in excess. This guidance is based on the energy and nutrients provided by foods from five groups, including

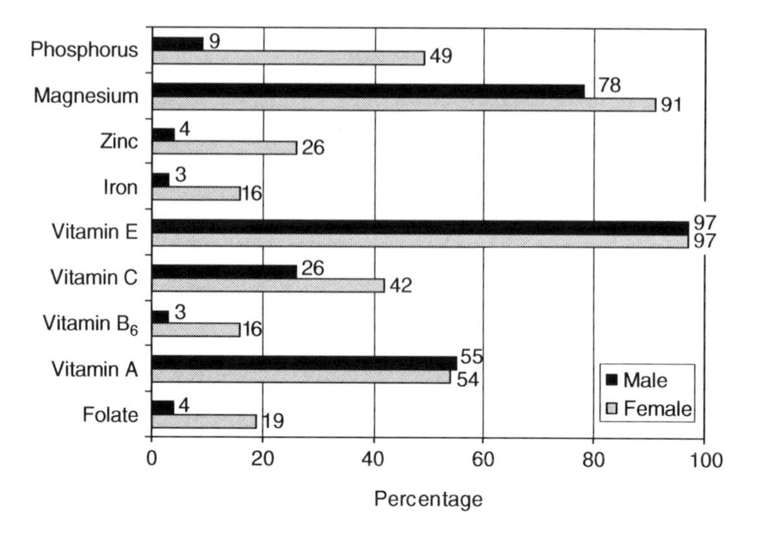

FIGURE 3.2 Percentage of females and males aged 14–18 years whose usual dietary intake is less than the estimated average requirement (EAR). EARs correspond to daily intake levels sufficient to meet the needs of 50% of persons in a particular life-stage and gender group. The percentage of a population having intakes of a given nutrient below the EAR can be taken to represent the prevalence of inadequacy for that nutrient. (Data from Moshfegh, A., Goldman, J., and Cleveland, L., *What We Eat in America, NHANES 2001–2002: Usual Nutrient Intakes from Food Compared to Dietary Reference Intakes*, U.S. Department of Agriculture, Agricultural Research Service, Beltsville, MD, 2005.)

(1) grains, (2) vegetables, (3) fruits, (4) milk, and (5) meats and beans. National nutrition data indicate many adolescents consume less than the recommended number of servings from these food groups (Figure 3.3) [26]. Although oils, solid fats, and added sugars are not considered to be part of any food group, MyPyramid additionally provides guidance for these dietary components.

3.3.1 Energy and Discretionary Calories

EERs for adolescents represent the amount of energy they require to support activity and normal pubertal growth and development. Individuals' energy requirement is influenced by their basal metabolic rate, which is closely associated with lean body mass. Separate EER equations have been developed for males and females because males experience greater increases in lean body mass, height, and weight during adolescence. The equation developed for estimating energy requirements of adolescent females (Equation 3.1) includes an allowance for growth of 25 cal (kcal) per day [19]. Average energy requirements of adolescent females that were calculated using an average height for age and healthy weight for height are provided in Table 3.2.

TABLE 3.1
Selected Recommendations from the 2005 Dietary Guidelines for Americans

Consume adequate nutrients within calorie needs

Consume a variety of nutrient-dense foods and beverages within and among the basic food groups while choosing foods that limit the intake of saturated and trans fats, cholesterol, added sugars, salt, and alcohol

Meet recommended intakes within energy needs by adopting a balanced eating pattern

Females of childbearing age. Eat foods high in heme iron and consume iron-rich plant foods or iron-fortified foods with an enhancer of iron absorption, such as vitamin C-rich foods. Consume adequate synthetic folic acid daily (from fortified foods or supplements) in addition to food forms of folate from a varied diet

Achieve and maintain a healthy weight

Maintain body weight in a healthy range by balancing calories from foods and beverages with calories expended

Those who need to lose weight. Aim for a slow, steady weight loss by decreasing calorie intake while maintaining an adequate nutrient intake and increasing physical activity

Overweight persons with chronic diseases or on medication. Consult a healthcare provider about weight-loss strategies prior to starting a weight-reduction program to ensure appropriate management of other health conditions

Consume adequate amounts from food groups that contribute to health

Consume a sufficient amount of fruits and vegetables while staying within energy needs

Choose a variety of fruits and vegetables each day. In particular, select from all five vegetable subgroups (dark green, orange, legumes, starchy vegetables, and other vegetables) several times a week

Consume 3 cups/day of fat-free or low-fat milk or equivalent milk products

Children and adolescents. Consume whole-grain products often; at least half the grains should be whole grains, with the rest of the recommended grains coming from enriched or whole-grain products

Consume fat in moderation and make wise choices

Consume less than 10% of calories from saturated fatty acids and less than 300 mg/day of cholesterol, and keep trans fatty acid consumption as low as possible

Children and adolescents (4–18 years). Keep total fat intake between 25% and 35% of calories, with most fats coming from sources of polyunsaturated and monounsaturated fatty acids, such as fish, nuts, and vegetable oils

When selecting and preparing meat, poultry, dry beans, and milk or milk products, make choices that are lean, low-fat, or fat-free

Limit intake of fats and oils high in saturated or trans fatty acids, and choose products low in such fats and oils

Choose carbohydrates wisely

Choose fiber-rich fruits, vegetables, and whole grains often

Choose and prepare foods and beverages with little added sugars or caloric sweeteners

Prevent dental caries by practicing good oral hygiene and consuming sugar- and starch-containing foods and beverages less frequently

Consume sodium in moderation and choose potassium-rich foods

Consume less than 2300 mg (~1 tsp of salt) of sodium per day

Choose and prepare foods with little salt. At the same time, consume potassium-rich foods, such as fruits and vegetables

Source: From U.S. Department of Health and Human Services, U.S. Department of Agriculture. *Dietary Guidelines for Americans 2005.* http://www.healthierus.gov/dietaryguidelines (accessed Nov 2006).

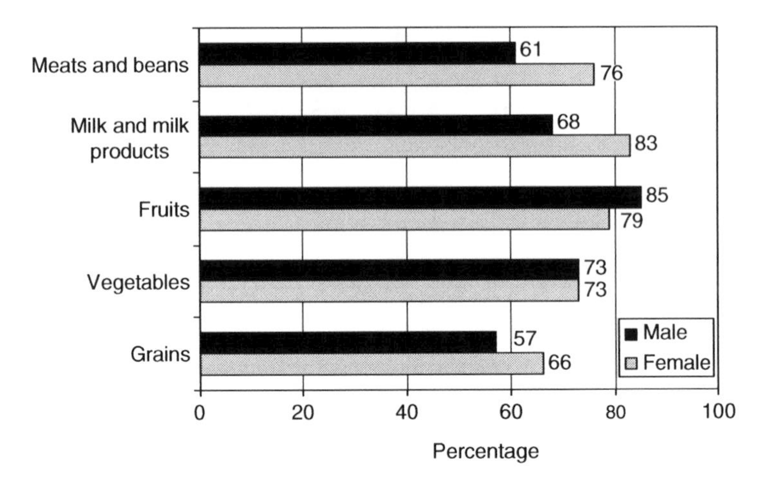

FIGURE 3.3 Percentage of female and male adolescents aged 12–19 years with food group intakes less than recommended based on energy intake and age. (Data from Cook, A. and Friday, J., *Pyramid Servings Intakes in the United States 1999–2002, 1 Day*, Agricultural Research Service, U.S. Department of Agriculture, Beltsville, MD, 2005.)

TABLE 3.2
Estimated Daily Energy (Calorie) Needs of Adolescent Females[a]

	Activity Level		
Age (Years)	**Sedentary[b]**	**Low Active[c]**	**Active[d]**
11	1600	1800	2000
12	1600	2000	2200
13	1600	2000	2200
14	1800	2000	2400
15	1800	2000	2400
16	1800	2000	2400
17	1800	2000	2400
18	1800	2000	2400

Source: From U.S. Department of Agriculture, Center for Nutrition Policy and Promotion. MyPyramid.gov. *Steps to a Healthier You.* http://www.mypyramid.gov (accessed Nov 2006).

[a] Estimated for a person of average height who is at a healthy weight.
[b] Activity level defined by the inclusion of less than 30 min a day of moderate physical activity in addition to daily activities.
[c] Activity level defined by the inclusion of at least 30 min and up to 60 min a day of moderate physical activity in addition to daily activities.
[d] Activity level defined by the inclusion of 60 or more min a day of moderate physical activity in addition to daily activities.

EER for female adolescent 9–18 years is

$$\text{EER} = 135.3 - 30.8 \times \text{Age (years)} + \text{PA} \times [10.0 \times \text{Weight (kg)} + 934 \times \text{Height (m)}] + 25 \text{ (kcal/day for energy deposition)} \quad (3.1)$$

Physical activity coefficient (PA):

1. Sedentary = 1.00, less than 30 min a day of moderate physical activity in addition to daily activities.
2. Low active = 1.16, at least 30 min and up to 60 min of daily moderate physical activity in addition to daily activities.
3. Active = 1.31, at least 60 min of daily moderate physical activity in addition to daily activities.

Accurately assessing the energy needs of adolescents is important as energy intake must be balanced with energy expenditure to support growth and avoid excessive weight gain or weight loss. If adolescents chronically consume an inadequate level of energy intake, linear growth may be compromised and sexual maturation delayed. Alternatively, if energy intake chronically exceeds requirements, then excess weight gain will occur. National data indicate 16% of adolescent females are overweight and are therefore likely consuming excess calories [27]. The top sources of energy in the United States are high-calorie, low-nutrient foods and beverages such as sweets and carbonated soft drinks, indicating efforts to prevent overweight should focus on helping adolescents meet their nutritional needs with more nutrient-dense choices (e.g., lean meats, fat-free milk) [28].

The MyPyramid food guidance system recommends that individuals choose mostly nutrient-dense options when selecting foods and beverages within each food group. Recommended meal patterns are based on the nutrients and energy that would be provided by consuming foods and beverages in this form. Meal patterns appropriate for adolescent females with different energy needs are shown in Table 3.3. A specific number of discretionary calories are also recommended, which are equal to the difference between an individual's EER and the calories provided by the recommended servings of grains, vegetables, fruits, milk, meats and beans, and oils on their meal pattern [25]. Discretionary calories might be consumed in one of several ways, including (1) eating more nutrient-dense foods from within any food group; (2) selecting some foods that are in a form containing additional fat or sugar (e.g., 2% milk, sweetened cereal); (3) adding solid fats (e.g., butter) or sweeteners (e.g., syrup, sugar) to foods and beverages; or (4) eating or drinking items that provide only fat or sugar (e.g., candy, soft drinks).

3.3.2 Macronutrients

3.3.2.1 Protein

Protein requirements are increased during adolescence to support the accrual of lean body mass as well as the maintenance of existing lean body mass. Peak periods of linear growth and weight gain require the greatest protein intake. Therefore, protein

TABLE 3.3
Recommended Food Intake Patterns for Selected Calorie Levels[a]

	Daily Amount of Food from Each Group				
Calorie Level	**1600**	**1800**	**2000**	**2200**	**2400**
Fruits	1.5 cups	1.5 cups	2 cups	2 cups	2 cups
Vegetables	2 cups	2.5 cups	2.5 cups	3 cups	3 cups
Grains	5 oz-eq	6 oz-eq	6 oz-eq	7 oz-eq	8 oz-eq
Meats and beans	5 oz-eq	5 oz-eq	5.5 oz-eq	6 oz-eq	6.5 oz-eq
Milk	3 cups	3 cups	3 cups	3 cups	3 cups
Oils	5 tsp	5 tsp	6 tsp	6 tsp	7 tsp
Discretionary calorie allowance[b]	132	195	267	290	362

Examples and recommended amounts

Fruit Group: $\frac{1}{2}$ cup serving = 1 medium piece of whole fruit, $\frac{1}{2}$ cup of cut-up fruit, ¼ cup of dried fruit, or 4 oz of 100% fruit juice

Vegetable Group: $\frac{1}{2}$ cup serving = $\frac{1}{2}$ cup of raw or cooked vegetables, 1 cup of raw leafy greens, or 4 oz of 100% vegetable juice

Grains: 1 oz-equivalent (oz-eq) = 1 slice of bread, 1 cup of ready-to-eat cereal, or $\frac{1}{2}$ cup of cooked rice, pasta, or cooked cereal

Meats and beans: 1 oz-eq = 1 oz of lean meat, poultry, or fish, 1 egg, 1 tablespoon of peanut butter, ¼ cup of cooked beans, or $\frac{1}{2}$ oz of nuts or seeds

Milk: 1 cup = 1 cup of milk or yogurt, $1\frac{1}{2}$ oz of natural cheese, or 2 oz of processed cheese

Oils: 1 tsp of oils like canola, corn, olive, soybean, and sunflower oil or foods that are mainly oil, including mayonnaise, certain salad dressings, and soft margarine

Source: From U.S. Department of Agriculture, Center for Nutrition Policy and Promotion. MyPyramid.gov. *Steps to a Healthier You.* http://www.mypyramid.gov (accessed Nov 2006).

[a] Nutrient and energy contributions from each group are calculated according to the most nutrient-dense forms of foods in each group (e.g., lean meats, fat-free milk).

[b] The remaining amount of calories in a food intake pattern after accounting for the calories needed for all food groups when using forms of food that are fat-free or low-fat and with no added sugars.

requirements of females per unit of height tend to be greatest between the ages of 11–14 years and for males tend to be greatest between the ages of 15–18 years. The protein RDA for preadolescent and adolescent ages 9–13 years is 0.95 g/kg (EAR = 0.76 g/kg) and for adolescent ages 14–18 years is 0.85 g/kg (EAR = 0.71 g/kg) [19]. The AMDR for protein recommends that calories from protein should represent 10%–30% of total energy intake [19].

As for energy, if intakes of protein are consistently poor, then linear growth may be compromised, sexual maturation delayed, or the accumulation of lean body mass reduced. While most adolescents in the United States consume approximately twice the recommended level of protein, 14% of females aged 14–18 years have intakes less than the EAR [23]. It may be more difficult for adolescents living in food-insecure households, following a vegetarian or vegan diet, or severely restricting their energy intake to achieve AIs of protein. Lean meats, eggs, milk, and milk products are key sources of protein.

3.3.2.2 Carbohydrate and Fiber

The RDA for carbohydrate throughout adolescence is 130 g (EAR = 100 g) and the AMDR recommends that 45%–65% of total calories be consumed as carbohydrate [19]. An additional recommendation for carbohydrate is to limit added sugars to no more than 25% of total energy intake [19]. National nutrition data indicate that adolescent females consume 55% of their energy intake as carbohydrate and the majority of females (>97%) consume more than adequate amounts of carbohydrate [23,29]. However, a large proportion (20%) of carbohydrate intake comes from sweeteners and added sugars with little nutritional value [26]. Conversely, intakes of carbohydrate-rich foods that provide fiber and other important nutrients (e.g., fruit, vegetables, whole grains, and legumes) are less than recommended [26]. Less than 3% of adolescent females have fiber intakes that exceed the adequate intake level of 26 g [23]. In contrast to the MyPyramid meal patterns for adolescent females (Table 3.3), which include three to four servings of fruit and four to six servings of vegetables per day, approximately one-third of adolescent females consume less than one serving of fruit daily and 57% consume less than one serving of vegetables [26].

3.3.2.3 Fat and Cholesterol

Given a lack of evidence to suggest that a defined intake level of fat is needed to prevent obesity or chronic diseases, no RDA or EAR has been set for total fat intake [19]. However, the AMDR for young people aged 4–18 years recommends that 25%–35% of total calories be consumed as fat and AIs have been established for the essential fatty acids, linoleic acid (9–13 years = 10 g/day; 14–18 years = 11 g/day) and α-linolenic acid (9–13 years = 1.0 g/day; 14–18 years = 1.1 g/day) that are consistent with median intakes in populations free of deficiency symptoms. Additional macronutrient recommendations further provide guidance for cholesterol, saturated fat, and trans fat intake. To reduce chronic disease risk it is recommended that these dietary components be kept to a minimum while maintaining a nutritionally adequate diet. The Dietary Guidelines specifically recommend limiting saturated fat to less than 10% of total calories and cholesterol to less than 300 mg/day [24].

National nutrition data indicate that while intakes of saturated fat exceed these guidelines, average fat and cholesterol intakes of adolescent females are in line with current recommendations. As a group, adolescent females consume ~32% of total calories as fat, 11% of total calories as saturated fat, and 200 mg cholesterol/day [29]. To limit intake of saturated and trans fat, liquid plant oils (e.g., olive oil, canola oil, sunflower oil) should be emphasized in the diet over solid and partially-hydrogenated oils. While oils are high in calories (9 kcal/g), they are also key sources of essential fatty acids and vitamin E.

3.3.3 Micronutrients

In addition to the macronutrients, several micronutrients are important for adolescent growth and development. Reference intakes for micronutrients increase steadily through childhood and into adolescence and during periods of rapid growth there is a particular demand for iron, zinc, calcium, and folate. Relative to current recommendations, national nutrition data indicate several problem nutrients, especially among those aged 14–18 years [23]. Data indicate poor intakes of folate, vitamins A, B_6, C, and E, calcium, iron, zinc, magnesium, and phosphorus among many adolescent females (Figures 3.1 and 3.2) [23]. Male adolescents have similarly poor intakes of vitamins A and E, but in regard to most nutrients, females are more likely to have poor intakes [23]. Requirements for nutrients of particular importance during periods of rapid growth and population intakes of these nutrients are discussed in greater detail below.

3.3.3.1 Calcium

The calcium AI level established for adolescents aged 9–18 years is 1300 mg [20]. Adequate calcium intake is especially important during adolescence to support the rapid expansion of bone mass. Starting around 12.5 years, adolescent females accumulate 40%–45% of peak bone mass over a period of 3–4 years [4]. Although the period of peak accrual for adolescent males starts nearly 2 years later (around 14 years), males gain a similar proportion of their peak bone mass during adolescence [4,16]. Observational research suggests that achieving adequate calcium intake during this period of peak accrual may reduce the risk of fractures in adolescents [30]. If adequate calcium intake is further maintained throughout adolescence and bone mass accretion is optimized, then osteoporosis in adulthood will also be reduced [15,20]. The skeleton stores the majority (99%) of total body calcium; therefore, the increased calcium required for expansion of bone mass cannot be supplied by body stores and must be met entirely by dietary intake [4].

In the absence of an established EAR it is more difficult to determine the prevalence of inadequate calcium intake; however, national nutrition data indicate less than 10% of adolescent females have intakes greater than the AI value [23]. A greater proportion of adolescent males than females achieve intakes greater than the AI value, but the proportion of males meeting the recommendation is still less than 50% [23]. Good dietary sources of calcium include milk, other dairy products, dark green vegetables, and fortified foods such as juice, breakfast cereals, and bread. While calcium is best absorbed from dietary sources, especially dairy products, adolescents who are unable to achieve the recommendation may benefit from taking supplements. Calcium supplements (e.g., calcium carbonate, calcium citrate) are readily available and absorption is improved when taken with food in doses no greater than 500 mg.

3.3.3.2 Iron and Zinc

Consuming adequate amounts of iron and zinc is important during adolescence to support the expansion of blood volume as well as gains in lean muscle and bone tissue. Females further require additional iron after menarche to cover menstrual losses. Therefore, the established RDA for iron is higher for adolescent females aged 14–18 years (RDA = 15 mg; EAR = 7.9 mg) than for males aged 14–18 years (RDA = 11 mg; EAR = 7.7 mg) or females aged 9–13 years (RDA = 8 mg; EAR = 5.7 mg) [21]. The recommended amount for a female should be adjusted up (2.5 mg) if she starts menstruating before the age of 14 years and likewise adjusted down if she does not start menstruating by 14 years [21]. The RDA for zinc is 8 mg (EAR = 7 mg) for females aged 9–13 years and 9 mg (EAR = 7.3 mg) for females 14–18 years [21]. Consequences of poor iron intake include anemia, poor exercise tolerance, and impaired cognitive abilities while poor zinc intake may delay growth and sexual maturation [21,31].

Although iron needs may be partially met by mobilizing any body stores, national nutrition data indicate poor iron intake may be a problem for 16% of adolescent females aged 14–18 years [23]. Poor zinc intake may be a problem for an even greater proportion of adolescent females aged 14–18 years (26%) as well as females aged 9–13 years (10%) but is uncommon among adolescent males aged 9–18 years ($\leq$4%) [32]. Meat, fish, poultry, legumes, nuts, seeds, green leafy vegetables, whole grains, and fortified cereals are all good sources of iron. However, the nonheme iron found in plant sources has a much lower bioavailablity than the heme iron found predominantly in meat, fish, and poultry. To enhance the absorption of nonheme iron from plant foods, they should be consumed with sources of heme iron or vitamin C. Good sources of zinc include red meat, shellfish, whole grains, and fortified breakfast cereals.

3.3.3.3 Folate

Another micronutrient of particular significance during periods of rapid growth is folate. Folate is required for reactions that synthesize nucleotides and proteins and plays an important role in promoting the normal formation of red blood cells. The RDA for folate is 300 μg dietary folate equivalents (EAR = 250 μg) for females aged 9–13 years and 400 μg dietary folate equivalents (330 μg) for females aged 14–18 years [22]. However, as considerable evidence has linked maternal folate intake early in pregnancy with neural tube defects among her offspring, it is recommended that after menarche all females should consume 400 μg dietary folate equivalents from supplements or fortified foods (in addition to the folate consumed from food sources) to ensure proper nutrition in the event of a pregnancy. Although recommendations for folate intake are similar for females and males, national nutrition data indicate that females 14–18 years more often have poor intakes than males in the same age group [23]. Nearly 20% of adolescent females aged 14–18 years have intakes less than the EAR. Good sources of folate include dark green leafy vegetables, fruits, legumes, and fortified grains.

3.4 COMMON EATING BEHAVIORS

Micronutrient intake varies by eating habits. Eating behaviors influence the types and amounts of foods eaten and therefore impact micronutrient intakes. As a group, adolescent females engage in certain eating behaviors more often than younger children, including dieting, eating away from home, meal skipping, and snacking. These common eating behaviors and family meal patterns have several implications for dietary intake.

3.4.1 Dieting and Weight-Control Practices

Dieting and other weight-control practices are particularly common behaviors among adolescent females. In a recent national survey of high school students, 46% reported they were trying to lose weight [33]. More females than males reported they were dieting to lose or maintain weight (55% vs. 27%), and females were also more likely to report the use of extreme methods to lose weight, such as taking diet pills (8% vs. 5%), taking laxatives, or vomiting (6% vs. 3%) in the past month [33]. Changes in body shape and size during adolescence may lead to increased body dissatisfaction and thereby prompt efforts to lose weight [1]. In addition, research indicates several other factors may play a role in the decision to attempt weight loss during this period of life. Factors that have been associated with increased dieting and use of weight-control behaviors among adolescents include peer dieting [5,34], parental weight concerns [35,36], weight teasing [37], and media exposure [35,38,39]. Media that discusses dieting or weight loss is particularly problematic as adolescent females may not have developed the skills to critically respond to the persuasive techniques of weight-loss advertisements that are not obviously deceptive [40].

Some weight-control behaviors have been related to improved dietary intake; however, dieting and the use of weight-control practices are also strongly related to several undesirable outcomes. Females who report using moderate or more healthful dieting practices such as exercising, eating more fruits and vegetables, eating fewer sweets, and eating fewer high-fat foods may have a better diet quality than nondieters or females using unhealthful weight-control practices [41,42]. In contrast, unhealthful dieting and weight-control practices (e.g., skipping meals, taking diet pills) are related to poor intakes of fruit, vegetables, grains, and several micronutrients (i.e., calcium, iron, vitamins A, C, and B_6, folate, and zinc) [42]. Further, dieting during adolescence predicts the onset of depression [43]; the initiation of extremely unhealthy weight-control behaviors (e.g., self-induced vomiting, laxative use) [44]; the onset of binge eating and other eating disorders [34,45]; and excess weight gain or the onset of obesity [44,46,47]. Compared with adolescent females who reported no dieting, dieters in one study were found to increase their body mass index (BMI) by an extra 0.6 units over a relatively short period of 5 years [44].

3.4.2 Eating Away from Home

Although US adolescents consume the majority of their total energy intakes at home, national nutrition surveys suggest that on any given day more than 50% of adolescents eat something from a fast-food restaurant [48,49]. Fast-food restaurants are favored by adolescents because they provide (1) relatively inexpensive menu options; (2) an informal social setting for visiting with friends; (3) menu options that can be easily transported on hectic days; and (4) employment for many young people. Fast-food restaurants are often visited by male and female adolescents, but females tend to report less frequent consumption of fast-food than do males [49,50]. Adolescents who report a lower socioeconomic status, playing a team sport, working at least 10 h a week, and a lack of time to eat healthy foods tend to report more frequent consumption of fast-food [50].

As fast-food menu options tend to be less healthful than foods consumed at home, frequent consumption of fast-food may negatively impact on nutritional intake and health. More frequent consumption of fast-food by adolescents has been related to greater intakes of total fat, saturated fat, sodium, and high-fat, high-sugar foods

TABLE 3.4
Menu Options at Fast Food Restaurants

High-Calorie Menu Items	Lower Calorie Alternatives
McDonald's	
Big Mac[a] (560 calories, 30 g fat)	Cheeseburger (310 cal, 12 g fat)
Premium crispy chicken club (680 cal, 29 g fat)	Premium grilled chicken classic (420 cal, 9 g fat)
Large French fries (570 cal, 30 g fat)	Small French fries (250 cal, 13 g fat)
Large soft drink (310 cal, 0 g fat)	8 oz, 1% white milk jug (100 cal, 2.5 g fat)
12 oz Triple Thick Chocolate Shake[a] (440 cal, 10 g fat)	Apple dippers and low-fat caramel dip (100 cal, 1 g fat)
Pizza Hut	
6″ Personal pepperoni pan pizza (640 cal, 29 g fat)	1 slice, 12″ Fit n' Delicious Pizza[b] (160 cal, 4 g fat)
Hot wings and ranch dipping sauce (320 cal, 28 g fat)	Hot wings and lite ranch dressing (180 cal, 13 g fat)
Taco Bell	
Double Decker Taco Supreme[c] (380 cal, 18 g fat)	"Fresco Style" crunchy taco[d] (150 cal, 7 g fat)
Nachos Bell Grande[c] (790 cal, 44 g fat)	Nachos (320 cal, 20 g fat)
Fiesta Taco Salad[c] (860 cal, 46 g fat)	Fiesta Taco Salad, no shell[c] (490 cal, 25 g fat)
Grilled stuft steak burrito (690 cal, 27 g fat)	"Fresco Style" Steak Burrito Supreme[c,d] (350 cal, 9 g fat)

Source: From McDonald's USA Nutrition Information, http://www.mcdonalds.com/usa/eat/nutrition_info.html (accessed Nov 2006); Pizza Hut Nutrition Information, http://www.pizzahut.com/menu/nutritioninfo.asp (accessed Nov 2006); and Taco Bell Printable Nutrition Guide, http://www.yum.com/nutrition/documents/tb_nutrition.pdf (accessed Nov 2006).

[a] Registered trademark of the McDonald's Corporation, Oak Brook, Illinois.
[b] Registered trademark of Pizza Hut, Inc., Dallas, Texas.
[c] Registered trademark of the Taco Bell Corporation, Irvine, California.
[d] Item topped with a mix of diced tomatoes, onions, and cilantro instead of sauce or cheese.

such as French fries and soft drinks [49–51]. In addition, more frequent consumption of fast-food is related to lower intakes of healthful foods (e.g., fruits, vegetables, and milk) and health-promoting food components (e.g., calcium, vitamins A and C, and fiber) [49,50,52]. Because fast-food menu options are often high in fat or sugar and offered in large portion sizes, menu options are often high in calories (Table 3.4). Healthful food choices (e.g., low-fat milk, fruit) and lower calorie options are sometimes available but, fast-food meals may easily provide all or nearly all of the energy an adolescent female requires for the entire day at just one meal. Adolescents may not compensate for the additional calories consumed from fast-food meals at other meals throughout the day [53]; therefore, if they regularly consume fast-food, the development of overweight will be promoted. Research in adolescent females has shown fast-food consumption is positively associated with increases in weight over time [54].

3.4.3 Family Meals

In contrast to the negative implications of frequent fast-food consumption for nutritional intake, having regular meals with family (i.e., family meals) is associated with better diet quality and improved psychosocial health. When parents and adolescents regularly eat together, adolescents are more likely to have diets of higher nutritional quality. Frequency of family meals is related to higher intakes of fruits, vegetables, grains, calcium-rich foods, protein, fiber, and several key micronutrients (i.e., calcium, iron, vitamins A, C, E, and B_6, and folate) [55–57]. In addition, frequent family meals are associated with lower intakes of soft drinks, saturated fat, and trans fat [55–57].

Having regular family meals is associated with the possession of more developmental assets and less frequent engagement in high-risk behaviors, even after taking into account the influence of family relationships and communication. In a nationally representative sample, adolescents who indicated they had regular family dinners (i.e., 5–7 per week) were more likely than adolescents who indicated they had infrequent family dinners (i.e., one or fewer meals per week) to report parents and teachers had high expectations for them, positive self-esteem, a sense of purpose, a strong commitment to learning, and the possession of social resistance skills [58]. Moreover, adolescents who indicated they had regular family dinners were less likely than adolescents who indicated infrequent family dinners to report substance use, school problems, violent or antisocial behavior, sexual intercourse, depressive symptoms, or attempted suicide [58]. Family meals also appear to protect female adolescents from engaging in chronic dieting, unhealthy weight-control behaviors, and binge eating or purging [59].

Despite the many benefits associated with family meals, there is great variability among adolescents in the frequency of having meals with family. On average, adolescents report having four to five meals with their family in a week; however, about one third of adolescents report having less than three meals per week and a similar proportion report having meals with their family at least one time per day [57]. Family meals tend to occur more frequently for adolescents when their family socioeconomic status is higher and when their mother does not work for pay [57]. Younger adolescents attending middle school are more likely to report having frequent family meals than older adolescents attending high school [57]. The majority of adolescents indicate that they enjoy and value eating meals with their family, but conflicting schedules of parents and adolescents present a major barrier to having regular meals together [60,61].

3.4.4 Meal Skipping

Skipping meals can also have an impact on nutritional intake [62]. The frequency of skipping meals increases with age as young people progress through childhood and adolescence [62,63]. Breakfast is the most frequently skipped meal. National nutrition data indicate that breakfast is skipped by 9% of school-aged children (6–8 years), 15% of preadolescents (9–13 years), and approximately one-third of adolescents (14–18 years) [63]. Among adolescents, skipping breakfast is more often reported by females than by males, adolescents with high levels of perceived life stress, and adolescents of lower socioeconomic status [62–65]. Adolescents report lack of time and not being hungry in the morning as barriers to eating breakfast [66]. Several other unhealthy behaviors are also related to meal skipping, including smoking, using unhealthy weight-control methods, a sedentary lifestyle, and high media use [62,67]. Among a large sample of secondary school students, those students who watched four or more hours of television daily were 7 times more likely to skip a meal to watch television, and those who played computer games at least 4 times a week were 9 times more likely to skip a meal to play computer games [67].

The consequences of skipping meals, especially breakfast, include lower daily intakes of micronutrients and compromised academic performance [62]. In general, those who skip breakfast do not consume the micronutrients they fail to consume in the morning at other meals during the day [62]. The nutrients most often reduced when breakfast is skipped include those essential for proper growth and development during adolescence—calcium, iron, and zinc [62].

3.4.5 Snacking

The contribution of snacks, foods, and beverages consumed between meals to the diets of adolescents is considerable and has increased over the past 30 years [68]. Although national nutrition data indicate that slightly more males than females snack, more than 85% of adolescent females consume snacks [68]. Among those who snack, an average of two snacks is consumed per day, representing an increase of 24% in daily snacking occasions since the late 1970s [68]. More frequent snacking is related to meal skipping, more television viewing, lower levels of physical activity, and higher levels of perceived life stress [65,69,70]. Foods and beverages consumed as snacks provide an average of 612 cal/day or approximately one-fourth of daily energy intake [68]. While snacks tend to be more energy dense than meals, snacks tend to be less dense in the key nutrients calcium, iron, zinc, and folate [68]. Given the contribution of snacks to the diets of adolescents, eating healthful foods and beverages (e.g., fruits, vegetables, and low-fat milk) for snacks is of importance. Focus group research in adolescents suggests making healthful options appealing, convenient, inexpensive relative to less nutritious options, and ready availability at home and school promotes their selection [71].

3.5 SPECIAL CONDITIONS AND NUTRITION CONCERNS

Many factors influence the nutritional needs of adolescent females. Overweight, diabetes, eating disorders, iron deficiency anemia, pregnancy, and lactation are common conditions that influence nutrition during adolescence.

3.5.1 Overweight

The growing prevalence of overweight among adolescents in the United States represents a serious threat to the immediate and long-term health of young females. Adolescent overweight, defined here as adolescents who have a BMI equal to or greater than the 95th percentile of the age- and gender-specific Centers for Disease Control (CDC) BMI charts, has more than doubled over the past three decades since the 1970s [72]. In 2003–2004, ~16% of adolescent females (12–19 years) were overweight [27]. In a society that stigmatizes persons who are overweight, overweight female adolescents are at increased risk for low self-esteem, depression, and using unhealthy weight-control behaviors (e.g., smoking cigarettes, vomiting, taking diuretics) [73,74]. Overweight is also associated with increased risk for several adverse chronic health problems, including hypertension, cardiovascular disease, metabolic syndrome, and Type 2 diabetes [75].

While many factors are related to the development of overweight, eating behaviors play a fundamental role in regulating the balance between energy intake and expenditure. Choosing a diet that follows the Dietary Guidelines, reducing the number of meals eaten away from home, and structuring eating times can help to prevent the development of overweight in adolescents along with the inclusion of at least 60 min of daily moderate to vigorous physical activity [76]. See Chapter 7 for a full discussion of nutritional interventions appropriate for the prevention and treatment of overweight.

3.5.2 Diabetes Mellitus

Overweight status increases risk for Type 2 diabetes mellitus and a dramatic increase in the disease has occurred concomitantly with increases in the prevalence of adolescent overweight [76]. In contrast, Type 1 diabetes mellitus is immune-mediated and its etiology is unrelated to weight status. Both forms of diabetes are caused by a disorder of insulin regulation and lead to disturbances in carbohydrate, protein, and fat metabolism. However, Type 1 diabetes is generally characterized by absolute insulin deficiency while persons with Type 2 diabetes often continue to produce some insulin. A 2001 population-based study of physician diagnosed diabetes in young people estimated the crude prevalence of diabetes to be 2.80 cases/1000 adolescents 10–19 years [77]. Type 1 diabetes represented the majority of cases, but Type 2 diabetes, formerly found only in adults, accounted for 0.42 cases/1000 adolescents [77]. The nutritional management of diabetes typically involves carbohydrate counting, and for adolescents with Type 2 diabetes may also encourage weight loss [78]. If diabetes is not closely managed, diabetic ketoacidosis or hypoglycemia may result [78]. Long-term consequences of poor glycemic control include increased risk for heart, eye, and kidney damage [78]. See Chapter 8 for a full discussion of diabetes mellitus.

3.5.3 Eating Disorders

Although full-syndrome eating disorders are less prevalent than overweight, dieting behaviors, and other nutritional concerns of adolescents, they are associated with the highest morbidity and mortality rates among psychiatric disorders. Diagnostic criteria have been established by the American Psychiatric Association for three full-syndrome eating disorders: anorexia nervosa, bulimia nervosa, and binge eating disorder [79].

Anorexia nervosa is characterized by severe weight loss and an intense, irrational fear of becoming fat even though underweight. The disorder occurs in ~1% of adolescents, being more common in females than in males [79]. Related medical complications of the condition include cardiac arrhythmias, compromised linear growth, and impaired bone mineral accretion [80].

Bulimia nervosa is characterized by recurrent, uncontrolled eating episodes involving the consumption of large amounts of food in a short time and followed shortly by compensatory behaviors (e.g., self-induced vomiting, laxative or diuretic abuse, enemas, fasting, and intense exercise). The disorder affects 1%–3% of adolescents [79]. Like anorexia nervosa, bulimia nervosa primarily affects females and may lead to serious cardiovascular complications.

Binge eating disorder is also characterized by recurrent, uncontrolled eating episodes, which involve the consumption of large amounts of food, but the eating episodes are not followed by compensatory behaviors. Despite the significance of this disorder associated with the development of overweight and considerable psychiatric distress, few studies have assessed its prevalence among adolescents [81]. It is likely that most eating disorders have a multifactorial etiology, but dieting appears to be a common precipitating behavior for all three of these disorders [82]. The impact of dieting and restrictive eating habits on nutritional intake is discussed in Section 3.4.1. For a complete discussion of eating disorders see Chapter 17.

3.5.4 Iron Deficiency Anemia

During the rapid growth of adolescence, females are at particular risk for the development of iron deficiency anemia. Iron requirements increase dramatically to support increases in lean body mass, the expansion of total blood volume, and the onset of menses [83]. Iron deficiency, a condition defined by the absence of bone marrow iron stores, progresses to iron deficiency anemia when the deficiency impairs blood production and the concentration of red blood cells in hemoglobin falls (Table 3.5). As a result of increased iron requirements and poor intakes (Figures 3.1 and 3.2), the prevalence of iron deficiency (16%) is higher among females aged 16–19 years than any other group [84]. Among females 12–15 years, the prevalence of iron deficiency (9%) is lower but still greater than the prevalence among adolescent males (5%) [84]. The prevalence of iron deficiency anemia is 2% among females 12–19 years [84]. Risk factors for the development of anemia include following a restrictive vegetarian diet, participating in a strenuous or endurance sport, skipping meals, and following a restrictive weight control diet.

To help prevent iron deficiency, adolescent females should be encouraged to include iron-rich foods such as meat and fortified cereals in their usual diet. Treatment for iron deficiency will typically also include iron supplements of 60–120 mg elemental iron/day [85]. The consequences of iron deficiency for adolescent growth and development are great. Iron deficiency may delay or impair physical growth and compromise cognitive achievements [31,86]. In addition,

TABLE 3.5
Maximum Hemoglobin Concentrations and Hematocrit Values for Female Adolescents[a] Indicating Anemia

Age (Years)	Hemoglobin (<g/dL)	Hematocrit (<%)
12 to <15	11.8	35.7
15 to <18	12	35.9
≥18	12	35.7

Source: From Centers for Disease Control and Prevention, *MMWR*, 47, 1998.

[a] Nonpregnant or lactating females.

iron deficiency and anemia can increase fatigue, impair physical activity and work capacity, and lower resistance to infection [85]. For adolescents who are pregnant, iron deficiency during the first two trimesters further increases risk for a preterm delivery and delivery of a low-birth weight infant [85].

3.5.5 Pregnancy and Lactation

Births to adolescent females have decreased markedly since 1980 [87]. However, adolescent childbearing is not uncommon; the annual rate of births in 2002 was 43 per 1000 adolescent females [87]. To ensure the delivery of a healthy infant and provide for the needs of mothers who may themselves still be growing, a nutritionally adequate diet is critical. Because of poor diet and high nutritional requirements, adolescent females are at increased risk for delivering low-birth weight infants having high rates of mortality during the first year of life. The Institute of Medicine has determined equations for estimating energy intakes that will support the needs of adolescent mothers and healthy fetal development [19]. As changes in total energy expenditure and weight gain are minor during the first trimester, no increase in energy intake is recommended. EERs during the second and third trimesters of pregnancy are determined by summing requirements during the nonpregnant state, a median change in total energy expenditure of 8 cal (kcal) per week, and the energy deposition during pregnancy of 180 cal/day. Energy requirements during lactation take into account the energy required for milk output (500 cal/day) and energy mobilization from tissue stores during the first 6 months postpartum (170 cal/day). EERs for lactating women beyond 6 months postpartum assume weight stability (0 cal mobilized from energy stores) and reduced milk production requiring 400 cal/day.

Higher intakes of protein and micronutrients are also required to support fetal development and milk production. An additional 25 g (EAR = 21 g) of protein per day is recommended for pregnant and lactating adolescents [19]. Vitamin and mineral requirements of pregnant and lactating adolescents are also increased for folate, niacin, riboflavin, thiamin, vitamins A, B_6, B_{12}, and E, iron, magnesium, and zinc [20–22,88]. To meet these requirements, adolescents may require low-dose or prenatal vitamin–mineral supplements. A full discussion of nutritional requirements and concerns during pregnancy and lactation can be found in Chapter 5.

3.6 PROMOTING HEALTHY EATING

This chapter has reviewed considerable gaps between the current dietary practices of female adolescents and nutritional recommendations for health. Efforts are needed to promote healthy eating behaviors and improve the dietary intake of female adolescents. Adolescence is a particularly important time to intervene on dietary intake because adequate nutrition is essential to support rapid growth and eating behaviors established during this period often track into adulthood [2]. Interventions to promote healthy eating in adolescents need to consider the multiple environmental contexts that influence their eating behaviors. Home, school, and community environments each influence on the eating behaviors of adolescent females and offer various opportunities for promoting good nutrition.

3.6.1 Home Environment

It is important that nutrition intervention efforts address the family and home environments of adolescents because this context has a particularly strong influence on eating and weight-related behaviors. Parents can positively influence the behavior of their son or daughter by (1) modeling healthy eating and weight-related behaviors; (2) providing an environment that makes it easy to choose nutritious foods and beverages; and (3) avoiding negative comments about weight. The food choices of adolescents are related to the choices made and modeled by their parents; when parents consume more healthy foods such as fruits, vegetables, and dairy foods, their adolescents also consume greater amounts of the same foods [89,90]. However, it has also been found that adolescents practice unhealthy weight-related behaviors modeled by their parents. When adolescent females observe their parents dieting, they are more likely themselves to use unhealthful weight-control behaviors and to worry about weight gain [91,92].

As adolescents tend to choose snacks that are readily accessible and convenient, parents can also help to improve their adolescent's dietary intake by keeping the kitchen stocked with healthful foods and beverages that are simple to prepare and take "on-the-go" (i.e., prewashed fruit and vegetables, string cheese) [89,93]. Having regular family meals and involving adolescents in meal preparation are opportunities for parents to not only provide a healthful meal but also to model cooking skills and the consumption of nutrient-dense foods and beverages [55,94]. Teasing about weight has been related to increases in binge eating, dieting, and unhealthy weight-control behaviors [37]. Therefore, it is important that parents establish rules to eliminate weight teasing in the home and alternatively focus on encouraging their daughter or son to adopt healthful eating behaviors.

3.6.2 School Environment

Aspects of the school environment with the potential to impact eating behaviors of female adolescents include (1) school food services; (2) school food policies; and

(3) classroom nutrition education. Meals for students are provided through the National School Lunch Program (NSLP) and School Breakfast Program (SBP). These federally sponsored programs, administered by the USDA in conjunction with state and local education agencies, allow students who live in households with incomes between 130% and 185% of the poverty level to receive meals at reduced prices and those from households with incomes 130% of the poverty level or below to receive school meals free of charge. Foods and beverages provided to students through these programs must meet nutritional standards. Meals must provide no more than 30% of energy from fat and less than 10% of energy from saturated fat. In addition, regulations require school lunch meals to provide one-third of the RDAs for protein, vitamin A, vitamin C, iron, calcium, and energy and breakfasts to provide one-fourth of the RDA for these same nutrients. Research evaluating the nutritional impact of these programs has found that participants have higher intakes of most vitamins and minerals than nonparticipants and consume less added sugar [63].

Federal regulations for foods and beverages sold beyond these programs (i.e., competitive foods) are minimal and their availability is high; in a nationally representative survey, 97% of middle schools and 99% of high schools were found to sell foods and beverages through a la carte, vending machines, school stores, or multiple venues [95,96]. Only certain foods and beverages of minimal nutritional value (e.g., carbonated soft drinks, chewing gum, water ices, and hard candy) are prohibited if they are sold in the foodservice area during school meal periods. Unless a school determines more restrictive guidelines as part of its own school wellness policy, the nutritional quality of competitive foods and beverages are largely unregulated. The 2004 Child Nutrition and Special Supplemental Nutrition Program for Women, Infants, and Children (WIC) Reauthorization Act has a provision requiring schools to have a wellness policy that includes nutritional guidelines for items sold outside of the NSLP and SBP; however, schools are not required to make the guidelines for competitive foods and beverages more restrictive than the federal guidelines [97]. Expert groups have developed sample policies for encouraging healthy eating that schools can use as a model in drafting their own wellness policies [98].

The majority of foods and beverages sold through a la carte programs, vending machines, and school stores (i.e., competitive foods) are high-fat or high-sugar items such as salty snacks, sweet baked goods, sugared soft drinks, and candy [95]. Although some nutritious options (e.g., low-fat milk, vegetables, fruit) are available through these venues, they are less likely to be selected when the environment provides ready access to many foods of limited nutritional value. Multiple research studies have found that the availability of competitive food and beverage items may negatively impact the eating habits of young people. These studies have related the availability of competitive foods to higher student intakes of total energy, soft drinks, total fat, and saturated fat and lower intakes of key nutrients (e.g., calcium, vitamin A), fruits, vegetables, and milk [99–101]. School food practices (e.g., foods and beverages are allowed in classrooms; foods and beverages are used as rewards or incentives) allowing greater access to foods and beverages beyond the meal period have been further related to higher BMI values in secondary students [102].

TABLE 3.6
Effective Design Elements of School-Based Nutrition Interventions and Examples from the Teens Eating for Energy and Nutrition at School (TEENS) Intervention

Design Elements	Examples from TEENS
Apply an appropriate theoretical model or framework in planning	Intervention strategies were based on Social Cognitive Theory and addressed individual or personal (e.g., knowledge about nutrition labels), behavioral (e.g., eating breakfast), and environmental factors (e.g., foods and beverages available in school vending machines) identified as correlates of adolescents' dietary intake in prior research
Plan curricula with a behavioral focus. Select developmentally appropriate strategies and messages and tailor these to be culturally appropriate	The classroom educational curricula taught skills for preparing healthy snacks and making nutritious food selections. Goal setting and self-monitoring were included in the curriculum to encourage and reinforce behavior change
Maximize the dose (duration and intensity) of the intervention	Classroom educational lessons were delivered to a cohort of seventh graders across 2 years. Ten 45 min lessons were delivered over 5 weeks in each year of intervention. In addition, peer leaders were trained in delivering classroom lessons
Address the school and home environments in addition to individual behaviors	TEENS staff worked with the school food service to increase the availability of fruits and vegetables in the cafeteria and healthful a la carte snacks Newsletters and coupons encouraging specific behaviors like serving a fruit or vegetable at dinner were sent home with students to share with their families
Partner with families and community groups	School nutrition advisory councils involved school administrators, school staff, students, TEENS staff, and parents of students in collaborative work on school policies related to the availability of healthful foods in schools, food used for fund-raisers, and ways to promote healthier food choices

Source: From Perez-Rodrigo, C., Aranceta, J., *Public Health Nutr.*, 4, 131, 2001; Hoelscher, D., et al., *J. Am. Diet. Assoc.*, 102, S52, 2002; Lytle, L., et al., *Health Educ. Behav.*, 31, 270, 2004; Birnbaum, A., et al., *Health Educ. Behav.*, 29, 427, 2002.

To promote healthy eating, it is recommended that schools develop nutrition guidelines for foods and beverages sold beyond school meals, limit the periods during which students have access to these products, and prohibit their use as incentives for students. In addition, nutrition education is essential to teach the skills necessary for selection of a healthful diet. Students should be educated on using recommendations for healthful eating (e.g., the 2005 Dietary Guidelines for Americans) and preparing both nutritious meals and snacks. To enhance effectiveness, school-based nutrition interventions for adolescents should optimally address all aspects of the school environment and whenever possible also address the home environment. Moreover, involving students in the promotion of healthful foods at school is important to address the influence of peer norms [103–105]. Common elements of effective programs identified through critical reviews of intervention efforts are summarized in Table 3.6 along with illustrative examples from the Teens Eating for Energy and Nutrition at School (TEENS) intervention [103,106–108]. TEENS was a multicomponent intervention developed for students in the seventh and eighth grades with the goal of increasing fruit and vegetable intake and decreasing fat intake to reduce future cancer risk [103,108].

3.6.3 Community Environment

The physical neighborhood environment and community resources also have the potential to greatly impact adolescents' food choices. For example, fast-food restaurants, convenience stores, and vending machines can provide access to high-fat, high-sugar snack foods and beverages. These food outlets are frequently located within a short walking distance of school buildings and community recreation centers making them particularly convenient for adolescents [109]. While few interventions have assessed the impact of modifying the availability of foods and beverages in neighborhood community settings on intakes of adolescents, some work in schools suggests that modifying the availability and price structure of foods can have a considerable influence on food selection [110,111]. In addition, community resources such as after-school programs, community sport teams, and WIC can provide nutrition education and access to healthful foods for adolescents. The physical environment and resources available to adolescents might be addressed by a community coalition or task force. Key members of a community representing restaurants, groceries, retail outlets, recreation facilities, religious organizations, youth groups, libraries, and families can be invited to participate [112]. Once formed, a coalition or task force evaluates needs of the community and works collaboratively for improvements or to develop nutrition programs for adolescents [112].

3.7 CONCLUSION

Adolescent females are at risk for poor nutritional intakes compared with their male counterparts and other age groups in spite of the fact that adolescence is a time when a healthful diet is necessary for optimal growth. Western culture promotes unhealthy eating habits and weight-loss practices, which contribute to nutritional deficiencies and health conditions. Special attention to the promotion of adequate nutrition is needed for adolescent females in all of their surrounding environments, including home, school, and the community.

REFERENCES

1. Story, M., Holt, K., and Sofka, D., eds., *Bright Futures in Practice: Nutrition*, 2nd edn, National Center for Education in Maternal and Child Health, Arlington, VA, 2002.
2. Lien, N., Lytle, L., and Klepp, K., Stability in consumption of fruit, vegetables, and sugary foods in a cohort from age 14 to age 21, *Prev. Med.*, 33, 217, 2001.
3. Gidding, S.S. et al., Dietary recommendations for children and adolescents: A guide for practitioners, *Pediatrics*, 117, 544, 2006.
4. Greer, F., Krebs, N., and the Committee on Nutrition, Optimizing bone health and calcium intakes of infants, children, and adolescents, *Pediatrics*, 117, 578, 2006.
5. Eisenberg, M.E. et al., The role of social norms and friends' influences on unhealthy weight-control behaviors among adolescent girls, *Soc. Sci. Med.*, 60, 1165, 2005.
6. Rosen, D., Physiologic growth and development during adolescence, *Pediatr. Rev.*, 25, 194, 2004.
7. Herman-Giddens, M. et al., Secondary sexual characteristics and menses in young girls seen in office practice: A study from the pediatric research in office settings network, *Pediatrics*, 99, 505, 1997.
8. Freedman, D. et al., Relation of age at menarche to race, time period, and anthropometric dimensions: The Bogalusa Heart Study, *Pediatrics*, 110, e43, 2002.
9. Wu, T., Mendola, P., and Buck, G., Ethnic differences in the presence of secondary sex characteristics and menarche among U.S. girls: The Third National Health and Nutrition Examination Survey, 1988–1994, *Pediatrics*, 110, 752, 2002.
10. Stokic, E., Srdic, B., and Barak, O., Body mass index, body fat mass and the occurrence of amenorrhea in ballet dancers, *Gynecol. Endocrinol.*, 20, 195, 2005.
11. Adair, L. and Gordon-Larsen, P., Maturational timing and overweight prevalence in U.S. adolescent girls, *Am. J. Public Health*, 91, 642, 2001.
12. Tanner, J., *Growth at Adolescence*, Blackwell Scientific Publications, Oxford, 1962.
13. Rogol, A., Roemmich, J., and Clark, P., Growth at puberty, *J. Adolesc. Health*, 31, 192, 2002.
14. Spear, B., Adolescent growth and development, *J. Am. Diet. Assoc.*, 102, S23, 2002.
15. U.S. Department of Health and Human Services, *Bone Health and Osteoporosis: A Report of the Surgeon General*, U.S. Department of Health and Human Services, Office of the Surgeon General, Rockville, MD, 2004.
16. Whiting, S. et al., Factors that affect bone mineral accrual in the adolescent growth spurt, *J. Nutr.*, 134, 696, 2004.
17. Sturdevant, M. and Spear, B., Adolescent psychosocial development, *J. Am. Diet. Assoc.*, 102, S30, 2002.
18. Institute of Medicine, *Dietary Reference Intakes: Applications in Dietary Planning*, National Academy Press, Washington, D.C., 2003.
19. Institute of Medicine, *Dietary Reference Intakes for Energy, Carbohydrate, Fiber, Fat, Fatty Acids, Cholesterol, Protein, and Amino Acids*, National Academy Press, Washington, D.C., 2002.
20. Institute of Medicine, *Dietary Reference Intakes for Calcium, Phosphorus, Magnesium, Vitamin D, and Fluoride*, National Academy Press, Washington, D.C., 1997.
21. Institute of Medicine, *Dietary Reference Intakes for Vitamin A, Vitamin K, Arsenic, Boron, Chromium, Copper, Iodine, Iron, Manganese, Molybdenum, Nickel, Silicon, Vanadium, and Zinc*, National Academy Press, Washington, D.C., 2001.
22. Institute of Medicine, *Dietary Reference Intakes for Thiamin, Riboflavin, Niacin, Vitamin B6, Folate, Vitamin B12, Pantothenic Acid, Biotin, and Choline*, National Academy Press, Washington, D.C., 1998.

23. Moshfegh, A., Goldman, J., and Cleveland, L., *What We Eat in America, NHANES 2001–2002: Usual Nutrient Intakes from Food Compared to Dietary Reference Intakes*, U.S. Department of Agriculture, Agricultural Research Service, Beltsville, MD, 2005.
24. U.S. Department of Health and Human Services and U.S. Department of Agriculture. *Dietary Guidelines for Americans 2005*. http://www.healthierus.gov/dietaryguidelines/ (accessed Nov 2006).
25. U.S. Department of Agriculture and Center for Nutrition Policy and Promotion. MyPyramid.gov. *Steps to a Healthier You*. http://www.mypyramid.gov (accessed Nov 2006).
26. Cook, A. and Friday, J., *Pyramid Servings Intakes in the United States 1999–2002, 1 Day*, Agricultural Research Service, U.S. Department of Agriculture, Beltsville, MD, 2005.
27. Ogden, C.L. et al., Prevalence of overweight and obesity in the United States, 1999–2004, *JAMA*, 295, 1549, 2006.
28. Block, G., Foods contributing to energy intake in the U.S.: Data from NHANES III and NHANES 1999–2000, *J. Food Comp. Anal.*, 17, 439, 2004.
29. Wright, J. et al., *Dietary Intake of Ten Key Nutrients for Public Health, United States: 1999–2000. Advance Data from Vital and Health Statistics; No. 334*, National Center for Health Statistics, Hyattsville, MD, 2003.
30. Wyshak, G. and Frisch, R.E., Carbonated beverages, dietary calcium, the dietary calcium/phosphorus ratio, and bone fractures in girls and boys, *J. Adolesc. Health*, 15, 210, 1994.
31. Halterman, J. et al., Iron deficiency and cognitive achievement among school-aged children and adolescents in the United States, *Pediatrics*, 107, 1381, 2001.
32. Cleveland, L. et al., Dietary intake of whole grains, *J. Am. Coll. Nutr.*, 19, 331S, 2000.
33. Eaton, D.K. et al., Youth risk behavior surveillance—United States, 2005, *MMWR Surveill. Summ.*, 55, 1, 2006.
34. Patton, G. et al., Onset of adolescent eating disorders: Population based cohort study over 3 years, *BMJ*, 318, 765, 1999.
35. Field, A. et al., Peer, parent, and media influences on the development of weight concerns and frequent dieting among preadolescent and adolescent girls and boys, *Pediatrics*, 107, 54, 2001.
36. Field, A. et al., Weight concerns and weight control behaviors of adolescents and their mothers, *Arch. Pediatr. Adolesc. Med.*, 159, 1121, 2005.
37. Haines, J. et al., Weight teasing and disordered eating behaviors in adolescents: Longitudinal findings from Project EAT (Eating Among Teens), *Pediatrics*, 117, e209, 2006.
38. Field, A. et al., Exposure to the mass media and weight concerns among girls, *Pediatrics*, 103, E36, 1999.
39. Utter, J. et al., Reading magazine articles about dieting and associated weight control behaviors among adolescents, *J. Adolesc. Health*, 32, 78, 2003.
40. Hobbs, R. et al., How adolescent girls interpret weight-loss advertising, *Health Educ. Res.*, 21, 719, 2006.
41. Story, M. et al., Dieting status and its relationship to eating and physical activity behaviors in a representative sample of U.S. adolescents, *J. Am. Diet. Assoc.*, 98, 1127, 1998.
42. Neumark-Sztainer, D. et al., Weight-control behaviors among adolescent girls and boys: Implications for dietary intake, *J. Am. Diet. Assoc.*, 104, 913, 2004.
43. Stice, E. et al., Body-image and eating disturbances predict onset of depression among female adolescents: A longitudinal study, *J. Abnorm. Psychol.*, 109, 438, 2000.
44. Neumark-Sztainer, D. et al., Obesity, disordered eating, and eating disorders in a longitudinal study of adolescents: How do dieters fare 5 years later? *J. Am. Diet. Assoc.*, 106, 559, 2006.

45. Stice, E., Presnell, K., and Spangler, D., Risk factors for binge eating onset in adolescent girls: A 2-year prospective investigation, *Health Psychol.*, 21, 131, 2002.
46. Stice, E. et al., Naturalistic weight-reduction efforts prospectively predict growth in relative weight and onset of obesity among female adolescents, *J. Consult. Clin. Psychol.*, 67, 967, 1999.
47. Field, A. et al., Relation between dieting and weight change among preadolescents and adolescents, *Pediatrics*, 112, 900, 2003.
48. Nielsen, S., Siega-Riz, A., and Popkin, B., Trends in food locations and sources among adolescents and young adults, *Prev. Med.*, 35, 107, 2002.
49. Paeratakul, S. et al., Fast-food consumption among U.S. adults and children: Dietary and nutrient intake profile, *J. Am. Diet. Assoc.*, 103, 1332, 2003.
50. French, S.A. et al., Fast food restaurant use among adolescents: Associations with nutrient intake, food choices and behavioral and psychosocial variables, *Int. J. Obes. Relat. Metab. Disord.*, 25, 1823, 2001.
51. Schmidt, M. et al., Fast-food intake and diet quality in black and white girls, *Arch. Pediatr. Adolesc. Med.*, 159, 626, 2005.
52. Bowman, S. et al., Effects of fast-food consumption on energy intake and diet quality among children in a national household survey, *Pediatrics*, 113, 112, 2004.
53. Ebbeling, C. et al., Compensation for energy intake from fast food among overweight and lean adolescents, *JAMA*, 291, 2828, 2004.
54. Thompson, O. et al., Food purchased away from home as a predictor of change in BMI *z*-score among girls, *Int. J. Obes. Relat. Metab. Disord.*, 28, 282, 2004.
55. Gillman, M. et al., Family dinner and diet quality among older children and adolescents, *Arch. Fam. Med.*, 9, 235, 2000.
56. Videon, T. and Manning, C., Influences on adolescent eating patterns: The importance of family meals, *J. Adolesc. Health*, 32, 365, 2003.
57. Neumark-Sztainer, D. et al., Family meal patterns: Associations with sociodemographic characteristics and improved dietary intake among adolescents, *J. Am. Diet. Assoc.*, 103, 317, 2003.
58. Fulkerson, J. et al., Family dinner meal frequency and adolescent development: Relationships with developmental assets and high-risk behaviors, *J. Adolesc. Health*, 39, 337, 2006.
59. Neumark-Sztainer, D. et al., Are family meal patterns associated with disordered eating behaviors among adolescents? *J. Adolesc. Health*, 35, 350, 2004.
60. Fulkerson, J.A., Neumark-Sztainer, D., and Story, M., Adolescent and parent views of family meals, *J. Am. Diet. Assoc.*, 106, 526, 2006.
61. Neumark-Sztainer, D. et al., Family meals among adolescents: Findings from a pilot study, *J. Nutr. Educ. Behav.*, 32, 335, 2000.
62. Rampersaud, G. et al., Breakfast habits, nutritional status, body weight, and academic performance in children and adolescents, *J. Am. Diet. Assoc.*, 105, 743, 2005.
63. Gleason, P. and Suitor, C., Children's diets in the mid-1990s: Dietary intake and its relationship with school meal participation. Special nutrition programs: Report no. CN-01-CD1, U.S. Department of Agriculture, Food and Nutrition Service, Alexandria, VA, 2001.
64. Delva, J., O'Malley, P., and Johnston, L., Racial/ethnic and socioeconomic status differences in overweight and health-related behaviors among American students: National trends 1986–2003, *J. Adolesc. Health*, 39, 536, 2006.
65. Cartwright, M. et al., Stress and dietary practices in adolescents, *Health Psychol.*, 22, 362, 2003.

66. Shaw, M., Adolescent breakfast skipping: An Australian study, *Adolescence*, 33, 851, 1998.
67. Van den Bulck, J. and Eggermont, S., Media use as a reason for meal skipping and fast eating in secondary school children, *J. Hum. Nutr. Dietet.*, 19, 91, 2006.
68. Jahns, L., Siega-Riz, A., and Popkin, B., The increasing prevalence of snacking among U.S. children from 1977 to 1996, *J. Pediatr.*, 138, 493, 2001.
69. Dwyer, J. et al., Adolescents' eating patterns influence their nutrient intakes, *J. Am. Diet. Assoc.*, 101, 798, 2001.
70. Snoek, H. et al., The effect of television viewing on adolescents' snacking: Individual differences explained by external, restrained and emotional eating, *J. Adolesc. Health*, 39, 448, 2006.
71. Neumark-Sztainer, D. et al., Factors influencing food choices of adolescents: Findings from focus-group discussions with adolescents, *J. Am. Diet. Assoc.*, 99, 929, 1999.
72. Ogden, C.L. et al., Prevalence and trends in overweight among U.S. children and adolescents, 1999–2000, *JAMA*, 288, 1728, 2002.
73. Schwartz, M. and Puhl, R., Childhood obesity: A societal problem to solve, *Obes. Rev.*, 4, 57, 2003.
74. Neumark-Sztainer, D. et al., Weight-related concerns and behaviors among overweight and nonoverweight adolescents: Implications for preventing weight-related disorders, *Arch. Pediatr. Adolesc. Med.*, 156, 171, 2002.
75. Styne, D., Childhood and adolescent obesity: Prevalence and significance, *Pediatr. Clin. North Am.*, 48, 823, 2001.
76. Daniels, S. et al., Overweight in children and adolescents: Pathophysiology, consequences, prevention, and treatment, *Circulation*, 111, 1999, 2005.
77. SEARCH for Diabetes in Youth Study Group, The burden of diabetes mellitus among U.S. youth: Prevalence estimates from the SEARCH for diabetes in youth study, *Pediatrics*, 118, 1510, 2006.
78. Kamboj, M. and Draznin, M., Office management of the adolescent with diabetes mellitus, *Prim. Care*, 33, 581, 2006.
79. *Diagnostic and Statistical Manual of Mental Disorders*, 4th edn, American Psychiatric Association, text revision, Washington, D.C., 2000.
80. Katzman, D., Medical complications in adolescents with anorexia nervosa: A review of the literature, *Int. J. Eat. Disord.*, 37, S52, 2005.
81. Wilfley, D., Wilson, G., and Agras, W., The clinical significance of binge eating disorder, *Int. J. Eat. Disord.*, 34, S96, 2003.
82. Fairburn, C. et al., Identifying dieters who will develop an eating disorder: A prospective, population-based study, *Am. J. Psychiatry*, 162, 2249, 2005.
83. Beard, J., Iron requirements in adolescent females, *J. Nutr.*, 130, 440S, 2000.
84. Looker, A. et al., Iron deficiency—United States, 1999–2000, *MMWR*, 51, 897, 2002.
85. Centers for Disease Control and Prevention, Recommendations to prevent and control iron deficiency in the United States, *MMWR*, 47, 1998.
86. Grantham-McGregor, S. and Ani, C., A review of studies on the effect of iron deficiency on cognitive development in childrenn, *J. Nutr.*, 131, 649S, 2001.
87. Hamilton, B. and Ventura, S., Fertility and abortion rates in the United States, 1960–2002, *Int. J. Andrology*, 29, 34, 2006.
88. Institute of Medicine, *Reference Intakes for Vitamin C, Vitamin E, Selenium, and Carotenoids*, National Academy Press, Washington, D.C., 2000.
89. Hanson, N.I. et al., Associations between parental report of the home food environment and adolescent intakes of fruits, vegetables and dairy foods, *Public Health Nutr.*, 8, 77, 2005.

90. Johnson, R., Panely, C., and Wang, M., Associations between the milk mothers drink and the milk consumed by their school-aged children, *Fam. Econ. Nutr. Rev.*, 13, 27, 2001.
91. Keery, H. et al., Relationships between maternal and adolescent weight-related behaviors and concerns: The role of perception, *J. Psychosom. Res.*, 61, 105, 2006.
92. Fulkerson, J. et al., Weight-related attitudes and behaviors of adolescent boys and girls who are encouraged to diet by their mothers, *Int. J. Obes. Relat. Metab. Disord.*, 26, 1579, 2002.
93. Neumark-Sztainer, D. et al., Correlates of fruit and vegetable intake among adolescents. Findings from Project EAT, *Prev. Med.*, 37, 198, 2003.
94. Larson, N.I. et al., Food preparation and purchasing roles among adolescents: Associations with sociodemographic characteristics and diet quality, *J. Am. Diet. Assoc.*, 106, 211, 2006.
95. U.S. Government Accountability Office, *School Meal Programs: Competitive Foods Are Widely Available and Generate Substantial Revenues for Schools*, Report no. GAO-05-563, 2005.
96. Food Research and Action Center. Competitive foods in schools: Child nutrition policy brief. http://www.frac.org (accessed Apr 2006).
97. Food Research and Action Center. Local school wellness policies. http://frac.org/html/federal_food_programs/cnreauthor/wellness_policies.htm (accessed Nov 2006).
98. National Alliance for Nutrition and Activity. Model School Wellness Policies. http://www.schoolwellnesspolicies.org (accessed Nov 2006).
99. Cullen, K. et al., Effect of a la carte and snack bar foods at school on children's lunchtime intake of fruits and vegetables, *J. Am. Diet. Assoc.*, 100, 1482, 2000.
100. Kubik, M. et al., The association of the school food environment with dietary behaviors of young adolescents, *Am. J. Public Health*, 93, 1168, 2003.
101. Templeton, S., Marlette, M., and Panemangalore, M., Competitive foods increase the intake of energy and decrease the intake of certain nutrients by adolescents consuming school lunch, *J. Am. Diet. Assoc.*, 105, 215, 2005.
102. Kubik, M., Lytle, L., and Story, M., Schoolwide food practices are associated with body mass index in middle school students, *Arch. Pediatr. Adolesc. Med.*, 159, 1111, 2005.
103. Birnbaum, A. et al., Are differences in exposure to a multicomponent school-based intervention associated with varying dietary outcomes in adolescents? *Health Educ. Behav.*, 29, 427, 2002.
104. Hamdan, S. et al., Perceptions of adolescents involved in promoting lower-fat foods in schools: Associations with level of involvement, *J. Am. Diet. Assoc.*, 105, 247, 2005.
105. Fulkerson, J. et al., Promotions to increase lower-fat food choices among students in secondary schools: Description and outcomes of TACOS (Trying Alternative Cafeteria Options in Schools), *Public Health Nutr.*, 7, 665, 2004.
106. Hoelscher, D. et al., Designing effective nutrition interventions for adolescents, *J. Am. Diet. Assoc.*, 102, S52, 2002.
107. Perez-Rodrigo, C. and Aranceta, J., School-based nutrition education: Lessons learned and new perspectives, *Public Health Nutr.*, 4, 131, 2001.
108. Lytle, L. et al., School-based approaches to affect adolescents' diets: Results from the TEENS study, *Health Educ. Behav.*, 31, 270, 2004.
109. Austin, S. et al., Clustering of fast-food restaurants around schools: A novel application of spatial statistics to the study of food environments, *Am. J. Public Health*, 95, 1575, 2005.
110. French, S. et al., Pricing strategy to promote fruit and vegetable purchase in high school cafeterias, *J. Am. Diet. Assoc.*, 97, 1008, 1997.

111. French, S. et al., An environmental intervention to promote lower-fat food choices in secondary schools: Outcomes of the TACOS study, *Am. J. Public Health*, 94, 1507, 2004.
112. Stang, J., Story, M., and Kossover, R., Promoting healthy eating and physical activity behavior. In: Stang, J. and Story, M., eds., *Guidelines for Adolescent Nutrition Services*, Center for Leadership, Education, and Training in Maternal and Child Nutrition, Division of Epidemiology and Community Health, School of Public Health, University of Minnesota, Minneapolis, MN, 63, 2005.

4 Premenopause

Paula Skidmore and Aedin Cassidy

CONTENTS

4.1 INTRODUCTION

Optimizing nutritional status during the premenopausal years is critical to maintaining health as women age. In developed countries, women on average live 6–8 years longer than men [1]. Life expectancy for women now exceeds 80 years in at least 35 countries and is approaching this threshold in several other countries [1]. However, the life expectancy of women in countries at different levels of development is markedly different, ranging from just over 50 years in the least developed countries to 60 or 70 years in those undergoing rapid economic development [1]. Since the major preventable causes of morbidity and mortality all take effect over the life cycle, prevention strategies will be most effective when initiated as early in the life course as possible. Improving dietary intake during the premenopausal years can therefore play a key role in reducing risk factors of chronic disease and improving health and quality of life as women age.

We review the current recommended intakes for premenopausal women, and discuss the potential effects dietary intake can have on reducing their risk of a range of diseases associated with this stage of the life cycle and their future health.

4.2 RECOMMENDED INTAKES OF ESSENTIAL NUTRIENTS

Recommended intakes of essential nutrients have been developed in many countries to ensure the health and well-being of their population. These recommended intakes (Tables 4.1 and 4.2) differ slightly from country to country to reflect the relevant characteristics of their population and are formulated by reviewing the evidence from both observational and intervention studies. Intake of each nutrient at its recommended level will ensure that there is an adequate level of the circulating nutrient in the body to maintain health. Hence, each recommended intake will be one that is enough to cure clinical signs of a deficiency disease and to prevent the presence of any signs of these diseases. In the United States, Canada, and UK, these recommended intakes have been in place for decades and are periodically updated, based on the current evidence available [2,3].

These recommended intakes are set at various levels:

- A level that is sufficient to meet the nutritional requirements of nearly all (around 97%) of the healthy population (recommended dietary allowance [RDA] in the United States and Canada, reference nutrient intake [RNI] in UK).
- A level that is sufficient to meet the requirement of half of the healthy individuals in a population (estimated average requirement [EAR]).
- A level that is high enough to meet nutritional requirements but is not too high to pose a risk of adverse health events (tolerable upper intake level in the United States and Canada, Safe Intake in UK).

TABLE 4.1
Recommended Intakes of Macronutrients

	United Kingdom		United States and Canada	
	Women Aged 19–50	Men Aged 19–50	Women Aged 19–50	Men Aged 19–50
Energy (kcal/day)	1940	2550	2000	2400
Saturated fatty acids (% of total energy)	10	10	10	10
Polyunsaturated fatty acids (% of total energy)	6	6	9	9
Monounsaturated fatty acids (% of total energy)	12	12	11	11
Trans fatty acids (% of total energy)	2	2	ND[a]	ND
Total fat (% of total energy)	33	33	35	35
Carbohydrate (% of total energy)	47	47	45–65	45–65
Nonstarch polysaccharides (% of total energy)	18	18	ND	ND
Protein (g/day)	45	55.5	46	56

[a] Not determined.

TABLE 4.2
Recommended Intakes of Micronutrients

	United Kingdom		United States and Canada	
	Women Aged 19–50	Men Aged 19–50	Women Aged 19–50	Men Aged 19–50
Thiamin (mg/day)	0.8	0.9	1.1	1.2
Riboflavin (mg/day)	1.1	1.3	1.1	1.3
Niacin (mg/day)	13	17	14	16
Vitamin B_6 (mg/day)	1.2	1.4	1.3	1.3
Vitamin B_{12} (μg/day)	1.5	1.5	2.4	2.4
Folate (μg/day)	200	200	400	400
Vitamin C (mg/day)	40	40	75	90
Vitamin A (μg/day)	600	700	700	900
Vitamin D (μg/day)	—	—	5	5
Calcium (mg/day)	700	700	1000	1000
Phosphorus (mg/day)	550	550	700	700
Magnesium (mmol/day)	270	300	310/320	400/420
Sodium (mg/day)	1600	1600	1500	1500
Potassium (mg/day)	3500	3500	4700	4700
Chloride (mg/day)	2500	2500	2300	2300
Iron (mg/day)	14.8	8.7	18	8
Zinc (mg/day)	7.0	9.5	8	11
Copper (mg/day)	1.2	1.2	0.9	0.9
Selenium (μg/day)	60	75	55	55
Iodine (μg/day)	140	140	150	150

4.2.1 Energy Intake

Recommended energy intakes are based on age, weight, and energy expenditure and therefore differ between age groups and gender. For example the dietary reference value (DRV) for energy intake for women aged 19–50 is 1940 kcal in the UK and 2000 in the US and Canada, compared with 2550 for UK men and 2500 kcal for men in the US and Canada; the small differences in these values between the UK and the US and Canada are due to slight differences in the calculations used to formulate these EARs. The EARs for men are larger compared with women to take into account differences in both body size and typical amounts of daily physical activity.

4.2.2 Other Micro- and Macronutrients

As DRVs are set based on age, weight, and energy expenditure, some DRVs are larger for men than for women, to take into account the increased energy intake of men, due to their larger size. An example of this is magnesium, where in the UK, the RNI is 270 mg/day for women and 300 mg/day for men. Higher levels are also recommended for men (420 mg/day) compared with women (320 mg/day) in the US and Canada. These higher levels in men are a direct consequence of their higher body weight as the RNI for magnesium is based on the intake per kilogram of body weight per day, as are those for vitamin A. DRVs tend to be larger for pregnant and lactating women to account for the increased needs due to increased body size during pregnancy, the nutritional needs of the fetus, and to incorporate the nutrients given to the child, in breast milk. One exception to this is that the DRV for iron is set at a higher level for premenopausal women, than for men of a similar age, to account for menstrual losses. The RNI for women in the UK is 14.8 mg/day, compared with 8.7 mg/day for men. In the US and Canada, the RNI is 18 mg/day, compared with 8 mg/day for men.

As with the EAR for energy intake, there are slight differences in the RNIs for some micro- and macronutrients between the US and Canada and the UK, e.g., for calcium and potassium. Again, this is because the calculations for each RNI may be based on slightly different body weights. They also take account for population differences, such as ethnic differences, in their respective populations.

4.2.3 Vitamin and Mineral Supplements

Almost 40% of Americans take a vitamin or mineral supplement daily, as they think that their diets do not contain adequate amounts of these micronutrients [4]. However, it is possible to achieve an optimal balance of micronutrients through diet alone. Nutritional deficiency diseases such as scurvy and rickets can occur but these are now rare in the Western world, due to the variety of foods available. Large doses of vitamins may even be harmful—excess vitamin C can cause diarrhea and gastrointestinal disturbances, excess vitamin D can cause hypercalcemia, and excess intakes of vitamin E can cause hemorraghia [2]. For this reason tolerable upper intakes of most vitamins and minerals have been formulated.

Evidence from observational studies found that higher intakes of micronutrients, such as antioxidant vitamins and iron, whether through diet or supplementation were linked to lower levels of cardiovascular disease and all-cause mortality [4–8]. However, when randomized controlled trials were carried out, it was found that supplementation with antioxidant vitamins [7,8], either had little effect on cardiovascular or all-cause mortality and higher doses may even increase mortality. When one consumes a food that is high in a particular nutrient, it is not fully known if the beneficial effects are coming directly from that particular nutrient or from an interaction between this known nutrient and the other constituents of the food. Hence, it is better to obtain all vital nutrients from food, rather than supplements. However, in certain situations, vitamin supplementation may be considered, but it is important that all intakes remain within the recommended levels.

One important exception is recommendations for folic acid for all women of childbearing age who could become pregnant. Recommendations in both the United States and the UK are that these women should consume 400 μg of folic acid/day, and UK recommendations suggest that these levels should be maintained until the 12th week of pregnancy [9]. This increased level of folate intake can be through either improved dietary intake, consumption of fortified foods, or supplements. This increased intake of folic acid is to help prevent neural tube defects (NTD) such as spina bifida and anencephaly, conditions which affect 2500 births in the United States and 4000 in Europe every year [10]. Rates of NTD in the UK and Ireland are the highest in Europe although they have reduced considerably since folic acid supplementation became more widespread [11]. It is thought that by consuming optimal levels of folic acid the incidence of NTD could be halved.

4.3 FOOD INTAKE THROUGH THE MENSTRUAL CYCLE

Several studies indicate that food intake and selection vary during the menstrual cycle [12,13]. The results indicate that during the luteal phase (Days 15–28) of the menstrual cycle the intake of total energy tends to be higher than during the follicular phase (Days 1–14). Patterns of macronutrient selection show less consistency but a number of studies report carbohydrate cravings in the premenstrual phase, particularly in women with premenstrual syndrome [14]. Results from cross-sectional studies support a relationship between both energy and fat ingestion and plasma sex hormone concentrations in premenopausal women [15–18]. In one study, energy intake was associated inversely with plasma androstenedione and dehydroepiandrosterone sulfate (DHEAS), and directly with the probability of a luteal-phase rise in progesterone [19]. For each additional 1 MJ (239 kcal) consumed, androstenedione decreased by 6.0%, DHEAS decreased by 5.1%, and the probability of a progesterone rise increased by 60% [19]. Energy intake (adjusted for ratio of polyunsaturated to saturated fat [P:S] in the diet) was inversely associated with plasma estradiol and estrone during the luteal phase of the menstrual cycle. The potential effects of compounds present in plants on hormonal status have been examined with most studies to date focusing on soy isoflavones. Several carefully controlled metabolic studies showed physiological effects of soy-rich diets on the endocrine regulation of the menstrual cycle and cycle length and led to further investigations which suggested significant effects of soy intervention on hormone metabolism [20,21]. However, more recent long-term free living studies have not shown significant effects of soy intervention on hormonal status and menstrual cycle length [22]. Overall, of the seven intervention studies that controlled for menstrual cycle phase, intakes of isoflavone ranging from 32 to 200 mg/day generally resulted in a decrease in midcycle gonadotrophin levels and a trend towards an increase in menstrual cycle length and reduction in levels of sex steroid hormones [23]. These data suggest that phytochemicals present in plant foods may exert direct effects on menstrual cycle length and hormonal status.

4.4 POTENTIAL EFFECTS OF NUTRITION ON CURRENT HEALTH

4.4.1 IRON

Iron deficiency remains a major health risk worldwide, and significant numbers of premenopausal women are at risk if insufficient dietary iron is available to replace menstrual and other iron losses. In premenopausal women, the most common causes of iron deficiency anemia are menstrual blood loss and pregnancy, and recent data support the concept that identification of individuals with high menstrual losses should be a key component of strategies to prevent iron deficiency [24]. In men and postmenopausal women, iron deficiency anemia occurs predominantly because of gastrointestinal blood loss and malabsorption. Treatment of nutritional iron deficiency anemia includes adequate dietary intake and oral iron supplementation. Dietary iron is found in two forms—heme and nonheme. Heme iron is derived from hemoglobin and is found in poultry, fish, and red meat. Nonheme iron is found in plant foods such as lentils, oats, beans, and spinach. Only around 10%–15% of dietary iron is absorbed, with heme iron being more efficiently absorbed than nonheme iron. Increasing vitamin C intake helps absorption of iron and calcium, while polyphenols, phytates, and tannin can all reduce levels of absorption.

4.4.2 Energy Restriction

The prevalence of amenorrhea is elevated in women who restrict their diets and who undertake intense physical activities [15–18]. The associated hypoestrogenism causes a range of health-related effects including compromised fertility, skeletal demineralization that increases the risk of stress fractures and potential risk of osteoporosis in later life. Restriction in energy intake disrupts menstrual cycle regularity by altering LH pulsatility [25]. Luteal phase length has also been shown to be related to disruption of LH pulsatility following restricted energy availability with greatest disruption in women with shorter luteal phases. Luteal phases shorter than 10 days (determined by basal body temperature and <11 days determined by the LH surge) occur in 35% of biphasic cycles of women in the general population with gynecological ages of 5–15 years [13] but these drop to around 18% of aged 16–20 year olds. Thus, the frequent observation that the prevalence of amenorrhea in athletes declines with age may reflect the age-related decline in the prevalence of short luteal phases.

4.4.3 Premenstrual Syndrome

Premenstrual syndrome (PMS) describes the symptoms that occur during the last part of the luteal phase and gradually subside with menstruation. These symptoms include headache, irritability, insomnia, fatigue, water retention, breast tenderness, fluctuating appetite, anxiety, and depression. Pharmacological treatments for PMS include selective serotonin reuptake inhibitors, gonadotrophin-releasing hormone, anxiolytic agents, and oral contraceptives [26]. Dietary factors may also play an important part in the prevention or reduction of PMS symptoms. There is limited evidence on the role of diets that are high in fat, as there have only been two randomized controlled trials [27,28], both of which had around 30 participants, but both found that high fat diets were associated with increased PMS symptoms. A review of randomized controlled trials investigating complementary and alternative medicine in women of child-bearing age [29] found that of 20 studies that gave vitamin or mineral supplements, 14 focused on B_6 supplementation and 9 of these found that supplementation with B_6 improved PMS symptoms. One study showed no significant effects with vitamin E supplementation and a further three studies showed that calcium supplementation had a positive effect on PMS symptoms.

4.4.4 Overweight

Recent estimates of the burden of disease attributable to obesity by gender provide strong evidence that relative to men, women suffer a disproportionate burden of disease attributable to overweight and obesity [30], predominantly because of differences in health-related quality of life. Overweight men and women lost 270,000 and 1.8 million quality-adjusted life years, respectively, relative to their normal-weight counterparts. Obese men and women lost 1.9 and 3.4 million quality-adjusted life years, respectively, per year [30]. Around 60% of all deaths worldwide are from conditions that are related to overweight and obesity and it is estimated that by 2025, these conditions will account for 75% of all deaths [1]. It is thought that around 300,000 deaths per year in the United States are either directly or indirectly attributed to obesity [4]. Obesity also accounts for a large proportion of all health spending with around $117 billion dollars being spent on treating obesity and its health effects in the United States in 2001 [4].

The higher prevalence of obesity in women than men in most developed countries may be related to the fluctuations in reproductive hormones, which may predispose them to excess weight gain. Studies in experimental animals and women have shown that hormonal changes across the menstrual cycle affect calorie and macronutrient intake and alter 24 h energy expenditure [15–18]. Pregnancy and the menopause are two significant factors in the development of obesity for many women. At the menopause, as well as weight gain, there is a hormonally driven shift in body fat distribution from peripheral to abdominal, which may increase health risks in older women. A recent study investigated the association between changes in weight (both loss and gain in excess of 5% body weight) and risk of breast cancer through the pre- and postmenopausal years [31]. The data suggested that prevention of weight gain between age 18 years and the menopause and of weight loss and maintenance during the premenopausal years resulted in a reduction in risk of breast cancer [31]. Such evidence strongly supports the importance of prevention of weight gain in the premenopausal years.

4.5 POTENTIAL EFFECTS OF NUTRITION ON FUTURE HEALTH OUTCOMES

4.5.1 Prevention of Breast Cancer

Diet is a leading environmental factor in the prevention of breast cancer and research suggests that between 10% and 70% of cancers may be preventable through improving diet [32]. Preventive dietary advice often includes a reduction in alcohol, red meat, and animal fat and increasing the intake of vegetables, fruit and fiber, and their component phytochemicals from various sources. However to date the scientific basis for these recommendations is predominantly derived from epidemiological data, which have increased the knowledge base that provides rationale for various nutritional strategies to contribute to breast cancer prevention. It is also thought that gaining weight in adulthood, rather than during childhood and adolescence, may increase the risk of developing breast cancer [33]. Therefore it may not be absolute weight that is important in the development of breast cancer, but change in size over the life course. It is vital that women eat healthily, in order to achieve and maintain an optimal body size. Alcohol is estimated to be a factor in the development of around 2% of breast cancer cases in the United States and small amounts of alcohol (less than one unit per day) have been found to be associated with higher risk of developing breast cancer in premenopausal women [34]. The effects of fruit and vegetables on breast cancer risk have been inconsistent, but they have been shown to be associated with a reduction of risk for several other types of cancer [35].

4.5.2 Maximization of Bone Mineral Density

Osteoporosis is one of the major chronic conditions affecting health in developed countries. Of the 10 million cases in the United States, over 8 million of these are in women [36]. The WHO definition of this condition is a bone mineral density of more than two standard deviations below the mean of a young adult and 34 million people in the United States are thought to have low bone mass, placing them at increased risk of developing this condition [36]. Osteoporosis is responsible for more than 1.5 million fractures annually in the United States, including over 300,000 hip fractures and 700,000 vertebral fractures [36]. This fracture rate is similar for other countries such as the UK, (60,000 hip fractures and 40,000 vertebral fractures), other Northern European countries, and Australia [36].

Factors that are associated with osteoporosis are genetics, sex hormones, and physical activity. Nutrition plays an important role in the development and progression of osteoporosis. Important micronutrients are vitamins D and K, potassium, and calcium. Peak bone mass, the amount of bone tissue accumulated by the end of skeletal growth, is achieved in the early twenties and is affected by the amount of calcium obtained from the diet and almost all the calcium in the human body is found in bones. Vitamin D enhances calcium absorption in the body. Exposure to sunshine can ensure vitamin requirements are achieved, but such levels of exposure are not often achieved due to the use of protective clothing, sunscreens, and geographical location. If daily sun exposure is not adequate, a diet rich in vitamin D is advised. Vitamin K is involved in the binding of calcium and other minerals to bone. Potassium salts help in the development and attainment of bone mass by counteracting the effects of acids that deplete bone, therefore an adequate intake of potassium from food such as fruits and vegetables is vital for bone health [36].

4.5.3 Prevention of Cardiovascular Disease

Cardiovascular disease (CVD) has traditionally been considered to be a male disease and there is a lack of awareness among the female population about their relative risk of developing CVD [37]. A 2003 survey by the American Heart Association showed that only 13% of women were aware that CVD was the biggest threat to women's health as they age [37]. In America CVD is the leading cause of hospital visits in women and around 40% of all female deaths are due to CVD, almost twice as many as those from cancer [37]. While premenopausal women are thought to be partially protected from CVD, the risk increases with increasing age and 38% of women will die within a year of having their first heart attack, compared with 25% of men of that age [37].

There are numerous risk factors for CVD, and while some of these are not modifiable, such as sex, age, and genetic factors, there are a range of factors that can be changed, and one of these is diet. Decreasing intakes of trans and saturated fatty acids can result in lowering of LDL cholesterol, and oily fish contain the omega-3 fatty acids, eicosapentaenoic acid (EPA), and docosahexaenoic acid (DHA), which have been shown to be beneficial in the prevention of CVD. Increasing intake of fruits and vegetables can increase levels of antioxidants and other phytochemicals, which have been shown to help reduce risk factors for CVD including inflammation and lipoprotein levels. Based on findings from both observational and intervention studies the American Heart association has formulated dietary guidelines for the prevention of CVD that include balancing dietary intake and physical activity, consumption of whole grain and high fiber foods, an increase in fruit and vegetable intake, increased intake of fish for its long chain omega-3 fatty acids, and a reduction in saturated and trans fats, added sugars, and salt [37].

4.6 CONCLUSIONS AND FUTURE RESEARCH

It is of vital importance for women of childbearing age to consume a healthy diet, to help maintain optimal health. Premenopausal women require adequate intakes of iron, to compensate for menstrual cycle losses, and folic acid, to prevent NTD in pregnancy. Further research will be needed to distinguish the independent effects of age and luteal phase length on the susceptibility of the reproductive system to disruption by energy deficiency. Also, chemicals found in fruits and vegetables (phytochemicals), such as resveratrol and genistein, have been found to suppress tumor growth in animal models and this is an area of focus for future research.

The main diet-related challenge in the twenty-first century, for premenopausal women, is to prevent and combat overweight and obesity, as most of the chronic conditions which affect women in this age group are either directly related to dietary intake, or to excess weight, attained by overnutrition. Therefore education is needed to encourage the consumption of low fat diets at a population level, to help reduce the incidence of obesity over the next 10 years. Also, while there is some evidence from shorter term studies of the efficacy of low fat diets for weight loss, in adults, there is a lack of evidence over the longer term. Therefore it is essential that long-term intervention trials, focusing both on diet and exercise interventions are performed with follow-up periods that span years, rather than months.

Optimizing nutritional status during the premenopausal years is critical to maintaining optimal health in the postmenopausal years. Also, while major strides have been made in informing men about their risk of chronic illness and the subsequent prevention strategies for developing these conditions, there is currently a lack of evidence and clear guidance for women, and this needs to be tackled.

REFERENCES

1. http://www.who.int/en/.
2. Committee on Medical Aspects of Food Policy. *Dietary Reference Values for Food Energy and Nutrients for the United Kingdom.* The Stationery Office, London, 1991.

3. *Dietary Guidelines for Americans 2005*. US Government Printing Office, Washington, DC, 2005.
4. http://www.cdc.gov/.
5. van der, A.D.L. et al. Dietary haem iron and coronary heart disease in women. *Eur Heart J*, 26, 257, 2005.
6. Asplund, K. Antioxidant vitamins in the prevention of cardiovascular disease: A systematic review. *J Intern Med*, 251, 372, 2002.
7. Miller, E.R. Meta-analysis: High-dosage vitamin E supplementation may increase all-cause mortality. *Ann Intern Med*, 142, 37, 2005.
8. Vivekananthan, D.P. et al. Use of antioxidant vitamins for the prevention of cardiovascular disease: Meta-analysis of randomised trials. *Lancet*, 361, 2017, 2003.
9. http://www.eatwell.gov.uk/.
10. American Academy of Pediatrics. Committee on Genetics. Folic acid for the prevention of neural tube defects. *Pediatrics*, 104, 325, 1999.
11. Prevention of Neural Tube Defects by Periconceptional Folic Acid Supplementation in Europe. Eurocat Report 2003. http://ec.europa.eu/health/ph-projects/2001/rare-diseases/fp-raredis-2001-a1-01-en.pdf.
12. Cross, G.B. et al. Changes in nutrient intake during the menstrual cycle of overweight women with premenstrual syndrome. *Br J Nutr*, 85, 475, 2001.
13. Vollman, R.F. *The menstrual cycle*. W.B. Saunders Company. Philadelphia: 1977.
14. Dye, L. and Blundell, J.E. Menstrual cycle and appetite control: Implications for weight regulation. *Hum Reprod*, 12, 1142, 1997.
15. Williams, N.I. et al. Strenuous exercise with caloric restriction: Effect on luteinizing hormone secretion. *Med Sci Sports Exerc*, 27, 1390, 1995.
16. Williams, N.I. et al. Evidence for a causal role of low energy availability in the induction of menstrual cycle disturbances during strenuous exercise training. *J Clin Endocrinol Metab*, 86, 5184, 2001.
17. Loucks, A.B. et al. Alterations in the hypothalamic-pituitary-ovarian and the hypothalamic-pituitary-adrenal axes in athletic women. *J Clin Endocrinol Metab*, 68, 402, 1989.
18. Lane, M.A. et al. Energy restriction does not alter bone mineral metabolism or reproductive cycling and hormones in female rhesus monkeys. *J Nutr*, 131, 820, 2001.
19. Dorgan, J.F. et al. Relation of energy, fat, and fiber intakes to plasma concentrations of estrogens and androgens in premenopausal women. *Am J Clin Nutr*, 64, 25, 1996.
20. Cassidy, A., Bingham, S., and Setchell, K.D. Biological effects of a diet of soy protein rich in isoflavones on the menstrual cycle of premenopausal women. *Am J Clin Nutr*, 60, 333, 1994.
21. Duncan, A.M. et al. Soy isoflavones exert modest hormonal effects in premenopausal women. *J Clin Endocrinol Metab*, 84, 192–7, 1999.
22. Maskarinec, G. et al. Effects of a 2-year randomized soy intervention on sex hormone levels in premenopausal women. *Cancer Epidemiol Biomarkers Prev*, 13, 17, 2004.
23. Kurzer, M.S. Hormonal effects of soy in premenopausal women and men. *J Nutr*, 132, 570, 2002.
24. Harvey, L.J. et al. Impact of menstrual blood loss and diet on iron deficiency among women in the UK. *Br J Nutr*, 94, 997, 2005.
25. Loucks, A.B. and Thuma, J.R. Luteinizing hormone pulsatility is disrupted at a threshold of energy availability in regularly menstruating women. *J Clin Endocrinol Metab*, 88, 297, 2003.
26. Rapkin, A.J. New treatment approaches for premenstrual disorders. *Am J Manag Care*, 11, S480, 2005.

27. Barnard, N.D. et al. Diet and sex-hormone binding globulin, dysmenorrhea, and premenstrual symptoms. *Obstet Gynecol*, 95, 245–50, 2000.
28. Jones, D.Y. Influence of dietary fat on self-reported menstrual symptoms. *Physiol Behav*, 40, 483–7, 1987.
29. Fugh-Berman, A. and Kronenberg, F. Complementary and alternative medicine (CAM) in reproductive-age women: A review of randomized controlled trials. *Reprod Toxicol*, 17, 137, 2003.
30. Muennig, P. et al. Gender and the burden of disease attributable to obesity. *Am J Public Health*, 96, 1662, 2006.
31. Harvie, M. et al. Association of gain and loss of weight before and after menopause with risk of postmenopausal breast cancer in the Iowa women's health study. *Cancer Epidemiol Biomarkers Prev*, 14, 656, 2005.
32. http://www.cancer.org/.
33. Kotsopoulos, J. et al. Changes in body weight and the risk of breast cancer in BRCA1 and BRCA2 mutation carriers. *Breast Cancer Res*, 7, R833–43, 2005.
34. Petri, A.L. et al. Alcohol intake, type of beverage, and risk of breast cancer in pre- and postmenopausal women. *Alcohol Clin Exp Res*, 28, 1084, 2004.
35. Vainio, H. and Weiderpass, E. Fruit and vegetables in cancer prevention. *Nutr Cancer*, 54, 111, 2006.
36. http://www.nof.org/.
37. http://www.americanheart.org/.

5 Pregnancy and Lactation

Lisa A. Houghton and Deborah L. O'Connor

CONTENTS

5.1 INTRODUCTION

In pregnancy and lactation, the requirements for energy and most nutrients are elevated, thereby increasing the risk of inadequate intake. Optimal maternal nutrition during all phases of the reproductive cycle—prepregnancy, pregnancy, and lactation—is essential not only for maternal well-being but also for the overall health outcome of the offspring. Suboptimal nutritional status can augment the expression of many reproductive insults, and alter maternal metabolism and reproductive tissue development. The main cause of suboptimal nutritional status and health is a poor quality diet, often due to an inadequate intake or avoidance of animal food sources resulting in micronutrient deficiencies. In contrast, excessive calorie intake may also contribute to poor pregnancy outcome and infant development.

The purpose of this chapter is to highlight the current role that nutrition plays in the well-being of the mother and newborn infant, and the possible influence of nutritional insults on long-term health of the offspring. The current body of evidence regarding key nutrients and the issues surrounding them from preconception through to postpartum will be reviewed. The general guidelines for weight gain during pregnancy and the evidence surrounding postpartum weight retention during lactation will be discussed. The well-known relationship between adequate maternal nutritional status for several micronutrients such as folate, iron and iodine, and abnormal fetal development will be addressed. Less well-established nutrients, Vitamins D, A and zinc may also translate into poor maternal and reproductive outcomes, and the issues surrounding each will be presented individually. Much remains to be done to investigate the impact of inadequate maternal health status during lactation on nutritional health of the mother and infant. Although little data exist evaluating the adverse consequences of micronutrient depletion on maternal health and function during this life cycle period, suboptimal maternal status and nutrient intake can subsequently affect the amount of nutrients secreted in breast milk. Finally, the increasingly popular concept of "early origins of adult disease," whereby nutritional and metabolic exposure during critical periods of early development can result in long-term disease consequences, will be discussed here.

5.2 PRECONCEPTION

5.2.1 FOLATE

Folate is a general term applied to a group of related compounds that are important for DNA synthesis and cell proliferation, and thus are particularly critical during periods of rapid growth [1]. Folate-rich foods include leafy-green vegetables, citrus fruit, and legumes. Fortified foods such as breakfast cereals and vitamin supplements contain folic acid, a synthetic form of folate that is not naturally present in food.

Periconceptional use of folic acid-containing supplements is widely recognized as an effective measure in the prevention of first occurrence and recurrence of neural tube defects (NTDs) [2–5]. In addition, a growing body of evidence suggests that folic acid supplementation during the periconceptional period may also be effective in the reduction of other fetal malformations such as orofacial clefts and congenital heart defects [2,6–9]. In an effort to reduce the risk of NTDs, North American health authorities recommend 400 μg daily folic acid supplement during the periconceptional period for all women of childbearing age [10,11]. For women who previously have had an infant with an NTD, 4 mg/day beginning at least 1 month before conception and continuing through the first trimester is advised [12]. Efforts to educate women on the importance of folic acid supplementation have increased knowledge on the importance of adequate folate intake; however, the translation of this knowledge to actual practice, i.e., daily folic acid supplementation, has been less successful [12–20]. Periconceptional supplementation of folic acid must be implemented before the start of pregnancy, yet ~50% of women have unintended pregnancies [21,22]. Despite educational efforts advising daily folate supplementation of all women capable of becoming pregnant, the prevalence of NTDs remains unchanged in many areas where the food supply has not been fortified with folic acid [23,24]. Mandatory fortification of folic acid in the food supply in countries such as Canada, United States, and Chile has resulted in a reduction of NTDs by 19%–78% [25–29]. Folic acid fortification of cereal grains in Canada and the United States was estimated to provide an additional 100 μg of folic acid to the daily intakes of reproductive age women; therefore, ensuring that this target population receives at least 25% of their recommended folate needs regardless of access to supplements.

5.2.2 Iron

Iron is a component of a number of proteins, including enzymes and hemoglobin. Almost two-thirds of iron in the body is found in hemoglobin, which plays a key role in the transport of oxygen from the environment to tissues throughout the body. Dietary iron is found in one of two forms in foods, heme as found in meat, poultry, and fish, and nonheme, present in various forms in all foods. Heme iron is readily absorbed in the small intestine, while the absorption of nonheme iron is strongly influenced by its solubility and interaction with other food components. The average content of iron in a Western diet is estimated at no more than 5–7 mg iron/1000 kcal [30].

During pregnancy there is a substantial amount of iron required to meet the needs for the fetus and related tissues and for maternal expansion of blood volume. Adequate preconceptional iron reserves may play a role in reducing risk for iron deficiency and anemia during gestation [31]. Reproductive age women often have dietary iron intakes that are too low to offset menstruation losses. Consequently, the overall prevalence of iron deficiency in nonpregnant US women of childbearing age is ~12%, with an increased risk among minority groups (19%–22%) [32]. Iron requirements during pregnancy cannot be met from dietary sources alone, particularly in the latter part of pregnancy. Ideally, to balance the endogenous need for iron, women who normally consume a diet high in heme iron, should have 300 mg or more of iron reserves prior to conception [33]. For those women consuming diets containing only small amounts of heme iron, a higher amount of stored iron is needed. Despite the preservation of iron due to the temporary cessation of menstruation, poor maternal iron stores are difficult to replenish once pregnancy is in progress as a result of a decrease in dietary iron absorption in the first trimester of pregnancy and an increase in iron requirements during the latter part of pregnancy [33,34]. Although the effects of prepregnancy maternal iron status on gestational outcomes are not well defined, clinical trials with nonhuman primate models have demonstrated an association between preconceptional iron supplementation and increased postnatal infant iron stores [35]. Iron status of the infant rhesus monkeys at birth reflected the preconception status of the mother and continued to reflect preconceptional conditions through to 6 months of age.

5.2.3 Maternal Obesity

Maternal obesity is related to a number of adverse outcomes during pregnancy but most complications are generally related to issues of preconceptional obesity rather than excessive weight gain during gestation. Adipose tissue is a highly active endocrine organ secreting a number of hormones that alter the circulation of metabolites, cytokines, and growth factors. There is an increased risk of early miscarriage in obese women compared with normal-weight women [36] as well as increased risk of NTDs (particularly spina bifida), omphalocele, and heart defects [37]. Despite folic acid fortification of North American food supply, increased maternal adiposity continues to be associated with increased risk of NTDs (OR 2.8; 95% CI 1.2–6.6) [38]. Obese women are also at a significantly greater risk of developing preeclampsia and gestational diabetes mellitus compared with nonobese women and this may play a role in the risk of unexplained fetal death [39]. Unfortunately, the prevalence of obesity in North America remains high with recent reports suggesting overall obesity rates of 29% among all racial or ethnic groups of adult women aged 20–39 [40]. Significant differences in obesity prevalence by race or ethnicity is apparent with rates ranging from 24% in non-Hispanic white women to 50% in non-Hispanic black women.

Maternal diet and lifestyle prior to conception can influence the risk of congenital anomalies in her newborn. Clearly, achieving a healthy pregnancy outcome is influenced by a woman's health status prior to conception, yet the challenge lies in that few women seek care prior to conception and many pregnancies are not planned [21]. While there is no doubt that the use of folate during the periconceptional period can result in reductions in NTD, controversy remains over the use of periconceptional multivitamin and mineral supplements for general health. Excessive intakes of essential nutrients during pregnancy can also pose reproductive risks such as the teratogenic effects of high periconceptual Vitamin A intakes and craniofacial malformations and abnormalities of the central nervous system, thymus, and heart [41]. Several key issues still need to be addressed, and at present there is little information concerning what might constitute an optimal micronutrient supplement with respect to which nutrients should be provided and their amount, form, and timing. Women capable of becoming pregnant should consume a varied, well-balanced diet according to Canada's Food Guide to Healthy Eating or the American Food Guide Pyramid. If concerns of nutrient inadequacy arise, the diet should be evaluated. Vitamin and mineral supplementation may be considered together with appropriate dietary modifications as advised by a dietitian or a physician [42]. As a general rule, vitamin and mineral supplementation should never exceed the recommended dietary allowance

(RDA)* for any individual nutrient unless there is a clear benefit of doing so as evaluated by a health professional.

5.3 PREGNANCY

Pregnancy is a dynamic, anabolic process, which can be divided into two distinct developmental stages: embryonic and fetal. During the embryonic period, or the first 14 weeks of gestation, gross development of the fetal anatomical features and placental formation occur. The remaining 26 weeks of gestation are mainly devoted to completing fetal growth and development. Prior to implantation (6–12 days postconception), the embryo is nourished by oviductal and uterine secretions. Maternal–fetal circulatory exchange is not fully established until about 8 weeks of gestation.

5.3.1 Weight Gain

Weight gain in pregnancy is generally considered to be the difference between (1) the woman's weight at the last prenatal visit prior to delivery and her prepregnancy weight or (2) the last prenatal visit and her weight at the first prenatal visit. Weight gain calculated in this fashion represents both fetal (including placenta and amniotic fluid) and maternal tissue (uterus, breasts, blood, extracellular fluid, adipose) accretion [43]. Optimal weight gain ranges published in 1990 by the Institute of Medicine (IOM) were established based on prepregnancy body mass index (BMI) (Table 5.1) [44]. Weight gains within these guidelines are associated with optimal

TABLE 5.1
Institute of Medicine (IOM) Recommendations for Weight Gain during Pregnancy

Preconceptional Body Mass Index (BMI) (kg/m^2)	BMI Classification	IOM Recommended Total Gestational Weight Gain (kg)
<18.5	Underweight	12.5–18
18.5–24.9	Normal weight	11.5–16
25.0–29.9	Overweight	7–11.5
>30.0	Obese	7

Sources: From Committee on Nutritional Status during Pregnancy and Lactation, Institute of Medicine, *Nutrition during Pregnancy*, Washington, DC: National Academy Press, 1990; World Health Organization, *Obesity: Preventing and Managing the Global Epidemic*, Report of a WHO consultation presented at the World Health Organization, June 3–5, 1997, Geneva, Switzerland. Publication WHO/NUT/NCD/98.1.

* Recommended Dietary Allowance, RDA: The average daily dietary nutrient intake level sufficient to meet the nutrient requirements of nearly all (97%–98%) healthy individuals in a particular life stage and gender group.

birth weight and best labor and delivery outcomes. In general, underweight women should aim to gain relatively more weight, and overweight women should aim to gain less weight. Normal-weight women typically gain between 1.0 and 3.5 kg in the first trimester, whereby weight gain increases in the second and third trimester are more steady and incremental [42].

Despite widespread application of these established target weight ranges, a substantial proportion of overweight pregnant women exceed these current goals while women with a low prepregnancy BMI are more likely to gain less than the IOM guidelines [45]. Newborns of mothers with inadequate weight gain are more likely to be premature and of low birth weight or small-for-gestational age [46], and may be predisposed to obesity and metabolic problems later in life [47]. In contrast, rates of large-for-gestational age newborns and caesarean section deliveries tend to be higher when pregnancy weight gain exceeds the recommended guidelines. Research indicates that medically advised weight gain is strongly associated with actual weight gain; however, approximately one-third of women receive no prenatal target weight gain advice [45,48]. Of those who receive weight gain advice, women of higher prepregnancy BMIs are more likely to be advised to overgain while women of lower BMI are more likely advised to undergain, thereby suggesting that some healthcare providers are recommending all pregnant women to gain within the same range [45]. Possible barriers to IOM guideline compliance include lack of awareness, familiarity, and agreement with guidelines [49,50]. Moreover, excessive maternal weight gain in pregnancy has been shown to be predictive of postpartum weight retention, demonstrating a need for greater efforts in promoting appropriate gestation weight gain targets [51,52].

5.3.2 Energy and Macronutrient Needs during Pregnancy

Pregnancy is an anabolic state in which hormonal changes alter and redirect nutrient metabolism to support fetal growth and development, reproductive tissue accretion, and maternal homeostasis. Energy and requirements for most nutrients increase during pregnancy and set requirements are typically estimated by adding an increment to the nonpregnant, nonlactating requirements to adjust for the cost of pregnancy. Over the last decade, the IOM has published a series of reports defining dietary reference intakes (DRIs) for vitamins, minerals, macronutrients, and energy (Table 5.2).

5.3.2.1 Energy

Energy is needed during pregnancy to balance the basal energy expenditure (BEE) attributed to maintenance, the thermic effect of food (TEF) (i.e., food consumption elicits an increase in energy expenditure), and physical activity. In addition, extra energy is needed to allow for the energy cost associated with the deposition of maternal and fetal tissue. BEE increases over the nonpregnant state because of the added metabolism of the uterus and fetus and the increased work of the maternal heart and lungs. In studies of pregnant women, the cumulative changes in BEE throughout pregnancy ranged from 106 to 180 kcal/day [53]. The TEF has shown to

TABLE 5.2
Comparison of Recommended Daily Intakes of Nonpregnant, Nonlactating Adult, Pregnant, and Lactating Women Aged 19–50

	Dietary Reference Intakes[a]					
Nutrient	Adult Women	Pregnancy	% Increase over Adult Women	Lactation	% Increase over Adult Women	Tolerable UL[b,c]
Protein[d] (g)	46	71	54	71	54	N/E
Vitamin C[d] (mg)	75	85	13	120	60	2000
Thiamin[d] (mg)	1.1	1.4	27	1.4	27	N/E
Riboflavin[d] (mg)	1.1	1.4	27	1.6	45	N/E
Niacin[d] (mg NE)	14	18	29	17	21	35
Vitamin B-6[d] (mg)	1.3	1.9	46	2	54	100
Folate[d] (μg DFE)	400	600	50	500	25	1000
Vitamin B-12[d] (μg)	2.4	2.6	8	2.8	17	N/E
Pantothenic acid[e] (mg)	5	6	20	7	40	N/E
Biotin[e] (μg)	30	30	0	35	17	N/E
Choline[e] (mg)	425	450	5	550	29	3500
Vitamin A[d] (μg RE)	700	770	10	1300	86	3000
Vitamin D[e] (IU)	200	200	0	200	0	2000
Vitamin E[b] (mg α-TE)	15	15	0	19	27	N/E
Vitamin K[e] (μg)	90	90	0	90	0	N/E
Calcium[e] (mg)	1000	1000	0	1000	0	2500
Phosphorus[e] (mg)	700	700	0	700	0	3500/4000[f]
Magnesium[d] (mg)	310	350	13	310	0	350
Iron[d] (mg)	18	27	50	9	−50	45
Zinc[d] (mg)	8	11	38	12	50	40
Iodine[d] (μg)	150	220	47	290	93	1100
Selenium[d] (μg)	55	60	9	70	27	400
Fluoride[e] (mg)	3	3	0	3	0	10

[a] Values are from the Institute of Medicine. Abbreviations: NE, niacin equivalents; DFE, dietary folate equivalents; RE, retinol equivalents; TE, tocopherol equivalents; N/E, not established.

[b] Tolerable upper intake level (UL) for pregnancy and lactation, the highest average daily intake level that is likely to pose no risk of adverse health effects to almost all individuals in the general population. As intake increases above the UL, the potential risk of adverse effects may increase.

[c] N/E (not established) indicates that no adverse effects have been associated with excess intake. However, data may be limited, and thus, caution is warranted.

[d] Recommended dietary allowance (RDA), the average daily dietary intake level that is sufficient to meet the nutrient requirements of nearly all (97%–98%) individuals in a life stage and gender group and based on the estimated average requirement (EAR)

[e] Adequate intake (AI), the recommended average daily intake level based on observed or experimentally determined approximations or estimates of nutrient intake by a group of apparently healthy people that are assumed to be adequate. The value used instead of an RDA if sufficient scientific evidence is not available to calculate an EAR.

[f] Tolerable upper intake level for pregnancy and lactation, respectively, reported separately, 14–50 years of age.

be unchanged while the net energy cost of physical activity remains fairly constant [53]. The energy cost of increased tissue mass has been derived from total mean fat (3.7 kg) and assumed protein gain (925 g) in well-nourished, normal-weight pregnant women. Assuming each gram of fat and protein gain costs 9.25 and 5.65 kcal, respectively, the total energy cost of tissue accretion during pregnancy is ~39,862 kcal (180 kcal/day) [53].

Alternatively, energy requirements during pregnancy can be derived from total energy expenditure (TEE) as measured using the doubly labeled water method. This method accounts for the BEE, and energy expended in TEF and physical activity. Longitudinal TEE measurements of free-living pregnant women indicate a median change of 8 kcal/gestational week. Thus, the estimated energy requirement during pregnancy as set by the IOM is derived from the sum of the TEE of a nonpregnant woman plus the median change in TEE of 8 kcal/gestational week plus the energy deposition during pregnancy of 180 kcal/day. Since the TEE increases are minor and very little weight gain is expected to occur during the first trimester, increases in energy intake are recommended only in the second and third trimester of pregnancy. An additional energy requirement of 340 and 452 kcal/day greater than the nonpregnant state are recommended during the second and third trimesters, respectively.

5.3.2.2 Protein

The amount of protein deposited throughout a normal pregnancy is generally agreed to be the sum of the protein components of the fetus, uterus, maternal blood volume and extracellular fluid, placenta, and amniotic fluid. In an average pregnancy involving 12.5 kg of maternal weight, this is equivalent to 925 g protein [54]. Thus, additional protein is needed during pregnancy to allow for both adequate protein deposition and maintenance of the new pregnant tissue. Since only a small amount of protein accretion occurs during the first trimester (as demonstrated by protein turnover studies) [55], the RDA is set at 25 g/day above the protein needs of the nonpregnant women during the second and third trimesters. In total, the RDA for pregnant women is equal to 1.1 g/kg/day, which is the sum of 0.8 g/kg/day for nonpregnant women plus 0.27 g/kg/day for the anticipated amount necessary for protein deposition in pregnancy [53].

5.3.2.3 Fat

Fat is a major source of energy in the diet and facilitates the absorption of fat-soluble vitamins and carotenoids. There are two polyunsaturated fatty acids that are essential in the diet because they cannot be synthesized de novo by humans: linoleic acid (18:2 n-6) and α-linolenic acid (18:3 n-3). In the body, dietary linoleic acid can be desaturated and elongated to long-chain polyunsaturated fatty acid (LCPUFA), arachidonic acid (AA; 20:4 n-6), and α-linolenic acid are converted into docosahexaenoic acid (DHA; 22:6 n-3) and eicosapentaenoic acid (EPA; 20:5 n-3). LCPUFAs are essential for normal fetal development, particularly neural and visual function. n-3 fatty acid deposition in the developing fetal brain and retina initially occurs fairly slowly and then rapidly accumulates during the last trimester of pregnancy [56]. Some, but not all studies suggest a reduction in maternal n-3 fatty acid concentration in the blood during pregnancy with decreased DHA concentrations [57]. It is not clear if this reflects declining DHA concentration due to inadequate n-3 fatty acid intake or reflects normal physiological changes in maternal DHA concentrations. Fetal tissue has active desaturases to allow DHA formation from α-linolenic acid although controversy exists, especially postnatally, whether the amount converted is sufficient [53]. Studies assessing the influence of n-3 fatty acids during pregnancy on length of gestation, infant birth size, preeclampsia, maternal depression, and infant visual function and neurodevelopment vary widely; and, no clear consensus exists to indicate that increasing intakes in pregnant women consuming diets that meet n-3 and n-6 requirements have any physiologically significant benefits to the infant [57].

To date, no official recommendations have been made for the LCPUFA intake of pregnant women. Adequate intakes (AIs)* for essential fatty acids, linoleic acid (13 g/day) and α-linolenic acid (1.4 g/day), in pregnancy are based on the median intakes among pregnant women in the United States [53]. The habitual North American diet usually contains greater amounts of linoleic acid than α-linolenic acid. Foods containing large amounts of α-linolenic acid include canola, flaxseed, and soybean oils, as well as nuts and seeds. Good sources of linoleic acid include corn, sunflower, and peanut oils. In addition to endogenous conversion, DHA and AA can be directly obtained from the diet. DHA is found in marine fatty fish such as salmon, mackerel, and sardines, while meat and eggs are rich sources of AA.

5.3.3 Vitamin and Mineral Needs during Pregnancy

Available data on vitamin and mineral requirements during pregnancy are scarce, and biochemical assessment of status is complex because of lack of pregnancy-specific normal laboratory indexes and hormone-induced changes. Nutrients are redirected to support placenta, fetal, and mammary gland growth. Urinary excretion is increased to accommodate the clearance of both fetal and maternal metabolic waste excretion, and thus is associated with increased excretion of water-soluble vitamins (e.g., folate). Maternal blood volume increases by 35%–40% due primarily to a 40%–50% expansion of plasma volume and a 15%–20% expansion of red blood cell mass. Several micronutrient deficiencies during pregnancy are well established and their contribution to abnormal prenatal development or pregnancy outcome is discussed below. Little attention has been paid to the adverse consequences of micronutrient depletion on maternal health and function during this period. Nutrients most likely to be limiting in the diet are discussed.

5.3.3.1 Vitamin A

Although Vitamin A is essential throughout the entire life cycle, it plays a critical role during rapid cell proliferation and differentiation as occurs during embryonic and fetal development. It is recognized as being essential for normal vision, gene expression, and immune function [41]. The term Vitamin A includes retinol (preformed

---

* Adequate intake, AI: The recommended average daily intake level based on observed or experimentally determined approximations or estimates of nutrient intake by a group (or groups) of apparently healthy people that are assumed to be adequate—used when an RDA cannot be determined.

Vitamin A) and provitamin carotenoids such as β-carotene that are dietary precursors of retinol. Both preformed Vitamin A and carotenoids are found naturally in foods. Vitamin A is found primarily in animal-derived food, especially liver and dairy products, whereas carotenoids are synthesized by a wide variety of plants, and are abundant in darkly colored fruits and vegetables.

There are no direct studies on Vitamin A requirements during pregnancy but placental transfer of Vitamin A between mother and fetus is considerable [41]. An additional 50 μg/day of Vitamin A is needed during pregnancy to provide the amount of Vitamin A assumed to be accumulated by the fetal liver [41]. Vitamin A deficiency is widespread in developing countries, and an insufficient supply during pregnancy is known to increase maternal mortality [58,59] and night blindness [60,61]. Poor maternal Vitamin A status has also been associated with an increased susceptibility to infection with HIV during pregnancy. In contrast, the frequency of hypovitaminosis A is quite low in countries such as North America, and concern for the possible teratogenic effects of high doses of Vitamin A is more evident [62]. The risk of toxicity is greatest in the first trimester of pregnancy. Primary birth defects associated with excess Vitamin A intakes are those involving the cranial neural crest cells leading to craniofacial malformations and abnormalities of the central nervous system (except NTDs), thymus, and heart. Studies evaluating the teratogenecity of Vitamin A before and during pregnancy were used to derive a tolerable upper intake level (UL)* of 3000 μg/day [41]. Interestingly, supplementations with high doses of β-carotene have not been reported to increase the risk of birth defects likely due to its limited absorption in the intestine [63].

5.3.3.2 Vitamin D

Vitamin D refers to a group of fat-soluble seco-sterols that are found in very few foods naturally, and is photosynthesized in the skin of vertebrates by the exposure to ultraviolet B (UVB) radiation [64]. The main biologic function of Vitamin D in humans is to maintain serum calcium and phosphorus concentrations within the normal range to optimize bone health. Significant changes in maternal Vitamin D and calcium metabolism occur during pregnancy to provide the calcium required for fetal bone mineralization. The biologically active metabolite, 1,25-dihydroxy-cholecalciferol, increases in pregnancy whereas the main circulating form of Vitamin D in plasma, 25-hydroxycholecalciferol, generally decreases but is responsive to increased maternal intake [65].

While the AI of 5 μg/day or 200 IU/day of Vitamin D was not increased above nonpregnant requirements, studies in both northern and southern latitudes indicate that many women are deficient in Vitamin D both before and during pregnancy despite supplementation ($\geq$200 IU/day) in some, but not all studies [66]. Vitamin D deficiency during pregnancy may impair the neonatal handling of calcium, resulting in a lower bone mass at birth [67]. Maternal vitamin D insufficiency was recently

* Tolerable upper intake level (UL): The highest average daily nutrient intake level that is likely to pose no risk of adverse health effects to almost all individuals in the general population. As intake increases above the UL, the potential risk of adverse effects may increase.

associated with reduced bone mineral accrual at 9 years, suggesting an effect on skeletal development that continues long after infancy [68]. In addition to the well-established role of Vitamin D in maintaining proper bone mineralization, Vitamin D insufficiency in utero may represent a predisposing factor for the developing fetus to a number of future disease outcomes, such as Type 1 diabetes and autoimmune diseases [69–71].

Most experts agree that the current DRI is too low, and based on current evidence, the AI may be closer to 1000 IU or higher [65,72]. Furthermore, the UL of 2000 IU established by the IOM for Vitamin D in 1997 is also viewed by experts as being too restrictive, and current reports propose a UL of 10,000 IU [73]. As food sources of Vitamin D are scarce, North American population are primarily dependent on fortified foods and dietary supplements to meet their Vitamin D needs, particularly during times of insufficient UVB exposure (i.e., above and below 40° N and 40° S during winter months). In Canada, fluid milk and margarine are the predominant vehicles for Vitamin D fortification, whereas fluid milk and breakfast cereals are the predominant food sources in the United States [74].

5.3.3.3 Folate

Apart from the influence of periconceptional folic acid intake and NTDs, compromised folate status is associated with several negative pregnancy outcomes, including low birth weight, abruption placentae, and risk for spontaneous abortions [75,76]. The recommended intake for folate during pregnancy amounts to 600 μg/day dietary folate equivalents (DFE), exceeding that of the nonpregnant state [1]. Although data suggest a significant improvement in blood folate indexes following folic acid fortification, a recent study indicates that many pregnant women (following closure of the neural tube) are still not meeting their dietary folate requirements from diet alone [77]. In this study when prenatal supplementation or folic acid supplements (~925 μg/day of folic acid) were added to the dietary intake, mean folate intake increased to over 2000 μg/day DFE. For this reason, supplementation of folic acid throughout pregnancy is likely needed, although investigation of a lower prenatal dose (i.e., 1000 μg decreased to 400 μg folic acid) may be worthwhile. In countries without fortification measures or prenatal folic acid supplementation recommendations, gestational folate deficiency likely remains at an increased risk.

5.3.3.4 Iron

The requirements for absorbed iron increase slowly during pregnancy from 1.2 mg/day in the first trimester to 5.6 mg/day in the third trimester [41]. Based on a bioavailability of at least 25%, the recommended dietary intake of iron is increased 50% over the nonpregnant state to 27 mg/day [41]. Although enhanced intestinal iron absorption ($\approx$3 mg/day) occurs, dietary iron intake in most pregnant women is inadequate [78] and supplementation is required to prevent the development of iron deficiency. The overall prevalence of iron deficiency in North America is not well characterized but available data suggest a substantial increased risk in the last trimester, particularly among low-income minority women [79]. Beyond the reduction of iron deficiency anemia during pregnancy [33], early pregnancy iron supplementation may have increased birth weight and lowers the incidence of preterm delivery as demonstrated in a recent clinical trial of iron-replete women randomly assigned to prenatal iron-containing supplements (30 mg/day) from about 12 weeks of gestation compared with women who were assigned to placebo [80]. In contrast, iron supplements and enhanced iron stores have recently been associated with increased risk of gestational diabetes and increased oxidative stress [79]. Further investigation regarding the risks and benefits of prophylactic iron supplementation during gestation (dose, duration, and frequency) is required. Despite the lack of universal endorsement of prophylactic prenatal iron supplementation, data from the National Health and Nutrition Examination Survey, 1988–1994, found that 72% of US women were consuming iron-containing supplements during pregnancy with an average dose (78 mg/day) well above the UL (45 mg/day) [81].

5.3.3.5 Zinc

Zinc functions as a component of numerous enzymes in the maintenance of the structural integrity of proteins and the regulation of gene expression. Zinc is particularly essential during periods of rapid growth and for tissues with rapid cellular differentiation and turnover as occurs during pregnancy. Zinc is widely distributed in the food supply, and thus severe zinc deficiency in developed countries is not common [41]. On the contrary, mild-to-moderate zinc deficiency during pregnancy may be relatively common throughout the world [82]. Few data are available, in part, because the appropriate indicators of zinc status for pregnant women are not well defined. The RDA during pregnancy is based on an additional requirement of 3 mg/day above nonpregnant, nonlactating women [41]. Based on compilation of dietary zinc intake data of pregnant and lactating women, Caulfield and colleagues estimated that ~82% of pregnant women worldwide consume an inadequate intake of zinc compared with the RDA [82]. Mild forms of zinc deficiency during pregnancy have been associated with low birth weight, intrauterine growth retardation, and preterm delivery, although results are far from conclusive [82].

Iron supplementation at levels such as those found in some supplements could interfere with zinc absorption [83]. In 1990, IOM recommended 15 mg of zinc supplementation for women taking more than 30 mg of iron per day [44], although more recent work has found no adverse effect in zinc metabolism when high-dose iron supplementation (100 mg/day iron) was administered in iron-replete pregnant women [84].

5.3.3.6 Iodine

Iodine is an essential component for the production of thyroid hormones, triiodothyronine (T3), and thyroxine (T4), which are involved in many key biochemical reactions, including protein synthesis and energy production. Inadequate supply of thyroid hormone affects growth and development and reproductive function [41]. The major target organs are the developing brain, muscle, heart, pituitary, and kidney. Iodine is secreted in milk and is present in dairy products, marine fish, seaweed and kelp, and a variety of foods grown in iodide-rich soil. Iodized salt is also readily available in North America.

Requirements for iodine are increased in pregnancy to maintain normal metabolism of the women as well as meet the thyroid iodine uptake of the fetus [41]. Suboptimal maternal iodine intake adversely affects both maternal and fetal thyroid function and can affect brain development and intellectual potential. If the iodine deficiency is severe enough, particularly during critical periods of fetal growth and development such as the perinatal period, damage to the developing brain will occur, leading to varying degrees of irreversible mental retardation [85]. This damage appears to increase with the degree of deficiency, resulting in overt endemic cretinism as the severest consequence [85]. The RDA for iodine of 220 μg/day, set by the IOM, is based on the uptake of iodine of the newborn thyroid gland (50–100 μg) [41]. Although dietary iodine intake in North America is generally adequate, the World Health Organization estimates that 20 million people worldwide have neurological impairment resulting from maternal iodine deficiency [86]. Pregnant women at risk for suboptimal intakes should be supplemented with iodine in the form of potassium iodide tablets or iodine-containing prenatal multivitamin preparations. Given that adequate iodine before conception is best, continued efforts for the iodization of salt remain a priority in those countries lacking a universal program.

5.3.4 Impact of Maternal Diet on Early Epigenetic Programming

The influence of maternal nutrition during pregnancy extends well beyond that of the immediate viability and health of the newborn. In fact, chronic adult diseases may have their origin in early fetal life and can be modulated by the in utero metabolic environment. Barker and colleagues initially suggested this latter connection, also known as the 'Barker hypothesis, fetal programming or early origins of adult disease hypothesis' from their observations relating different mortality rates from stroke and cardiovascular diseases in England and Wales in 1968–1978 to earlier rates of neonatal mortality (1921–1925) in the same geographical region. Since low birth weight was the most common cause of infant death, they speculated that environmental influences that impair growth in early fetal life also result in an increased risk for ischemic heart disease [87]. Since this time, extensive human epidemiological studies have extended these initial observations of low birth weight and cardiovascular disease to include associations between early growth patterns and later inappropriate diets to adult disorders such as obesity, hyperlipidemia, Type II diabetes, and hypertension [88]. As a result, the early origins of adult disease hypothesis specifically states that adverse influences early in development, and particularly during in utero, can result in permanent changes in physiology and metabolism. These changes are expected to confer a competitive advantage in order to enhance the offspring's chances of survival in what it expects to be a poor nutritional environment [89]. For example, low birth weight infant may be better suited to survive in an environment of food scarcity; yet, when the postnatal environment is not characterized by nutrient restriction, this programmed advantage becomes a detriment leading to harmful long-term health consequences. Numerous animal model studies employing subtle nutritional imbalances and metabolic disturbances during specific, sensitive, or critical periods of early development also lend support to the underlying basis of programming. Maternal undernutriton and protein restriction in rats, sheep, and guinea pigs have led to a reduction in birth weight, increased blood pressure, and impaired glucose tolerance in the offspring [90,91].

In light of the tremendous interest in fetal programming, research efforts over the past few years have been directed toward understanding the specific biologic mechanisms and stimulus underlying this phenomenon. Of the many proposed mechanisms, the belief that epigenetic modification of gene expression and phenotype by nutritional stimuli in utero is very popular. The term epigenetics, literally meaning "above genetics," is defined as a stable alteration in gene expression that occurs without changes in the DNA sequence [92]. As first illustrated by Conrad Waddington [93] over 40 years ago in his metaphorical epigenetic landscape, each cell of an early embryo can be envisioned as a marble rolling down a hill. Although the topography of the terrain is determined by genes, it is not possible to predict whether the marble will roll to the left or to the right. However, nutrition or other environmental influences during development may be viewed as the "wind" blowing over the epigenetic landscape, thereby potentially diverting the marble into an alternative pathway and affecting the nature of developmental outcome (Figure 5.1) [92].

Methylation of cytosine residues of DNA and posttranslational modifications of the histone proteins associated with the DNA strand is one of the several epigenetic gene regulatory mechanisms that are responsible for establishing and maintaining tissue-specific patterns of gene expression. More specifically, methylation of DNA is associated with a repressive state of chromatin leading to transcriptional repression, and irreversible silencing of genes [94]. Because DNA methylation patterns are largely established in utero, environmental influences during the embryonic and

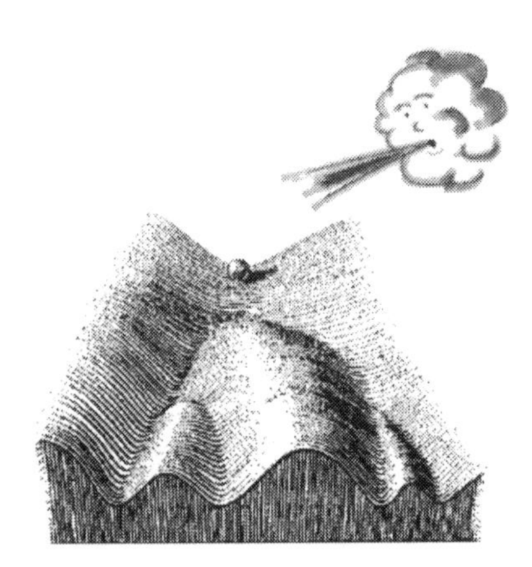

FIGURE 5.1 Subtle environmental influences may affect development outcome via epigenetics. The epigenetic landscape as originally illustrated by Conrad Waddington [93] depicts the stochastic (nondeterministic) nature of development as a marble rolling down a hill. Although the landscape is completely determined by genetic interactions, one cannot determine which developmental pathway will be followed. Nutrition and other environmental influences delivered during a critical developmental period may have a profound impact on final developmental outcome. (From Waterland, R.A., *J. Pediatr.*, 149, S137–S142, copyright Elsevier (2006). With permission.)

fetal environment may induce stable changes in gene expression that may be sustained throughout the life span of the individual. Folate, Vitamin B12, choline, zinc, and methionine all contribute to the methyl pool in the body and specifically to the formation of *S*-adenosylmethionine (SAM) [94] (Figure 5.2). SAM is the universal methyl donor in the body and is specifically responsible for global methylation of DNA. Of the limited studies available, folate and Vitamins B12 and B6 are able to influence the phenotype of a newborn via modulation of DNA methylation. In the mouse model, for example, methylation of DNA in the offspring was shown to be altered by the level of methyl donating nutrients in the maternal diet [95]. Further, supplementation of female yellow agouti (A^{vy}/a) mice with high doses of folic acid,

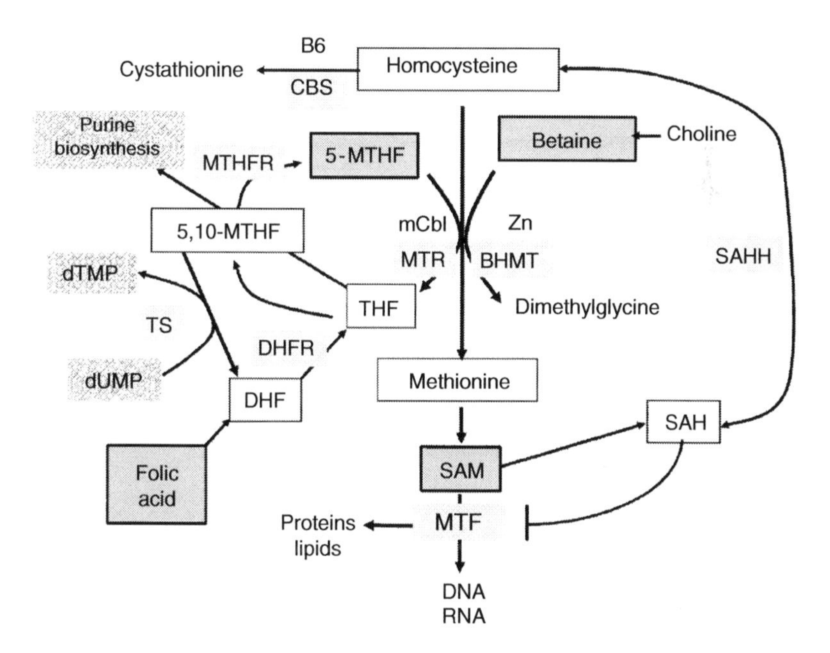

FIGURE 5.2 Methylation pathway. Homocysteine is converted into methionine by two pathways: methionine synthase (MTR), which uses methylcobalamin (mCbl) as a cofactor and acquires a methyl group from the conversion of 5-methyltetrahydrofolate (5-MTHF) into tetrahydrofolate (THF). 5-MTHF is acquired via food folates or folic acid supplementation, which is converted from dihydrofolate (DHF) by dihydrofolate reductase (DHFR) and 5,10-methylenetetrahydrofolate (5,10-MTHF) by methylene tetrahydrofolate reductase (MTHFR). These also participate in DNA synthesis through conversion of dUMP in dTMP by thymidilate synthase (TS) and purine biosynthesis. In selected tissues, methionine can also acquire a methyl group via conversion of betaine to dimethylglycine by betaine homocysteine methyltransferases (BHMT), which use zinc (Zn) as a cofactor. Methionine is further converted to *S*-adenosylmethionine (SAM), the major methyl donor for all methyl transferases (MTF), which add methyl groups to DNA, RNA, lipids, and proteins. SAM is recycled via the intermediate *S*-adenosylhomocysteine (SAH), which is converted to homocysteine in a reversible reaction by *S*-adenosylhomocysteine hydrolase (SAHH). (From the *Ann. Rev. Nutr.*, 22, 2002, by Annual Reviews www.annualreviews.org. With permission.)

Vitamin B12, choline, and betaine beginning 2 weeks prior to conception until parturition resulted in partially silencing the "agouti-gene" and altered the coat color of the offspring [96]. Likewise, dietary supplementation of female mice with methyl donating nutrients before and during pregnancy reduced by half the incidence of tail kinking in *axin fused* mouse [97].

Methylation of DNA in the fetal liver is also altered by low-protein diet during pregnancy in rats [98]. Recent studies suggest that feeding low-protein diets during gestation also produced changes to the methylation status and expression of the glucocorticoid receptor and perioxisomal proliferator-activated receptor-α expression in the offspring of mice [99]. This observation is consistent with epidemiological reports of induction of later hypertension, and impaired fat and carbohydrate metabolism by maternal protein restriction. Furthermore, there is increasing evidence that phenotypic adjustments brought about by fetal programming can be passed on from one generation to the next [100]. This is supported by intergenerational studies showing that the effects of undernutrition during pregnancy influence both the birth weight and glucose tolerance of offspring and subsequent generations [91].

Experimental evidence of nutritional programming from a range of animal studies have led some investigators to speculate that the significant increase in folate intake in North Americans via folic acid fortification program may have unintended deleterious gene-specific epigenetic changes during human embryonic development [101]. For example, it has been hypothesized that elevated amounts of folic acid during the periconceptional period could lead to genetic selection of embryos carrying a mutation (677C→T) in methylenetetrahydrofolate reductase (MTHFR) enzyme [102]. MTHFR irreversibly converts 5,10-methylenetetrahydrofolate (5,10-MTHF) to 5-methyltetrahydrofolate (5-MTHF), which then donates a methyl group to homocysteine to produce methionine (Figure 5.2). When folate intake is insufficient, this TT genotype is associated with elevated homocysteine and aberrant epigenetic processes, both of which are considered to be key factors in vascular disease and cancer [102,103]. Demographical information on the geographical distribution of the allele suggests a possible relationship between the abundance of foods rich in folate and the frequency of the 677C→T allele [102].

Nutritional influences early in the postnatal period may also effect gene-specific epigenetic changes [96]. For example, the link between reduced risk of obesity among children previously breastfed [104,105] suggests that breast milk may have long-term programming effects on appetite regulation. While there are sufficient observational data to support the role of breastfeeding in decreasing later obesity risk, the effect size is relatively modest. There is an urgent need for more research in this area as the field of nutritional epigenomics will play an important role in identifying early life nutritional interventions, or even corrective therapies, aimed at preventing chronic disease in humans.

5.4 LACTATION

Breast milk production, or lactogenesis, is initiated during the last trimester of pregnancy. Milk begins to form, and the lactose and protein content of milk increases. Following parturition, the onset of milk secretion is initiated through the decline in circulating estrogen and progesterone in combination with elevated levels of prolactin. Prolactin is a hormone secreted from the anterior pituitary whose principal action is the promotion of milk production. The initiation of milk secretion does not require infant suckling but by 3–4 days postpartum, the infant must be put to the breast to maintain milk production. Significant changes in both milk composition and volume occur during the first 10 days postpartum. Typical milk production begins with ~50 mL on Day 1 and increases to 500 mL by Day 5, 600 mL by 1 month, and 750–800 mL/day by 4–5 months postpartum [106]. The quantity of milk and its nutritional composition are often used to assess maternal nutritional adequacy in determining the recommended dietary intakes of lactating women (Table 5.2).

The physical and psychosocial benefits of breastfeeding for mothers and infants are well established [107]. Health professionals in North America recommend that infants be exclusively breastfed for the first 6 months of life and then breastfed in combination with complementary foods thereafter until at least the end of the first year of life [108,109]. In the context of developed countries, the most impressive advantage of breastfeeding to the infant is the anti-infective properties of human milk. Bottom line evidence suggests that breastfeeding is associated with decreased incidence of gastrointestinal illness (specifically diarrheal disease) in the infant and likely a trend toward decreased respiratory infection and otitis media in developed countries [110,111].

Although the prevalence of breastfeeding across the continent has risen, the duration of this practice remains short of the recommended targets [107,112]. Health programs can play a significant role in improving both initiation and continuation of breastfeeding. The promotion of breastfeeding by health care professionals should encompass an appreciation for the high nutritive demands of breastfeeding as they are considerably greater than those of pregnancy. The energy cost of lactation in the first 4 months postpartum is equivalent to the total energy cost of pregnancy [113]. Moreover, the mammary gland exhibits metabolic priority for nutrients often at the expense of maternal nutrient stores [113]. The specific energy and nutrient demands of lactation are directly proportional to intensity and duration, and thus evaluation of maternal nutritional status in early lactation may not appropriately reflect status in late lactation (>6 months postpartum).

5.4.1 Energy Needs during Lactation

The majority of studies have shown that the basal metabolic rates of lactating and nonlactating women are similar [53]. The recommended energy intake during the first 6 months of lactation is an additional 500 kcal/day. This is estimated using the factorial approach whereby the cost of milk production is added to the energy requirement of nonpregnant, nonlactating women. Milk production cost is based on a mean milk production of 780 mL/day, energy density of milk of 0.67 kcal/g, and energetic efficiency of milk synthesis (conversion of maternal dietary energy to milk energy) of 80% [53]. In well-nourished women, 170 kcal/day is deducted to account for energy mobilization (0.8 kg/month) from adipose stores laid down during pregnancy. Beyond 6 months postpartum, weight loss is considered minor and total energy cost of milk production is derived solely from diet. Using a reduced milk production volume of 600 mL, recommended energy intake for partially breastfeeding women in the second 6 months of lactation is 400 kcal/day above the nonpregnant, nonlactating energy requirement.

Many nutritional surveys among lactating women generally indicate that the amount of energy consumed is not sufficient to accommodate the increased estimated energy cost of lactation [77]. There may be several reasons for the low published energy intakes, including underreporting of dietary intake and restriction of energy intake in an effort to attain prepregnancy weight [106]. The recommended energy intake for lactation is based on a slow weight loss of ~5 kg during the first 6 months postpartum. Few studies, however, have reported a protective effect of breastfeeding on postpartum weight retention. Weight retention over time has been found to be greater in women who are older, unmarried, or had greater weight gain during pregnancy [114]. Of those studies reporting positive influences of the pattern of postpartum weight retention [114–116], the modest effect warrants minimal emphasis on lactation as a means of minimizing postpartum weight retention.

5.4.2 Vitamin and Mineral Requirements

Similar to energy requirements, recommended intakes for many vitamins and minerals are notably higher in lactation as compared with pregnancy (Table 5.2). Vitamin and mineral recommendations during lactation are mostly determined by estimating the total amount of any given nutrient secreted into milk (milk volume × nutrient concentration in milk) multiplied by a correction factor to account for the maternal bioavailability of the nutrient. This incremental amount is then added to the estimated value of nonpregnant, nonlactating women. This approach, however, may not necessarily be correct as it is difficult to account for variation in the following: (1) maternal nutritional status at the end of pregnancy; (2) intervariability of nutrient content of milk; (3) anabolic requirements of milk production; and (4) temporal changes in milk nutrient content based on the stage of lactation. Vitamin and mineral intakes that do not meet recommended levels have been reported for lactating women [117,118], and nutrient intakes of concern or at risk of inadequacy include folate and B12, Vitamin A, calcium, Vitamin D, iron, and zinc [1,65,77,118–122].

5.4.2.1 Folate and B12

Folate and Vitamin B12 are secreted into human milk, and hence there is an increasing demand for these two vitamins during lactation. Prior to the folic acid fortification of the food supply in North America, a reduction in maternal folate stores during the lactation period was observed secondary to inadequate dietary intakes [123–126]. Despite declining maternal blood folate concentrations, the folate content of breast milk is tightly regulated and has reported to remain stable or even increase as lactation progresses [127]. Therefore, the folate needs of the infant are met regardless of maternal folate nutriture except in cases of severe deficiency, e.g., megaloblastic anemia, which is rare in developed countries. Although recent data reveal improvements in blood folate status of reproductive women following fortification [128], dietary folate intakes during lactation still remain suboptimal for approximately one-third of women as demonstrated in a sample of well-nourished lactating Canadian women [77]. The recommended dietary requirement of folate during lactation is 500 μg/day DFE.

Vitamin B12 is essential for normal blood formation and neurological function. The main dietary sources of Vitamin B12 are animal-based products such as beef, milk, fish, and eggs. Unlike folate, breast milk concentrations of Vitamin B12 are reflective of maternal B12 status, and an insufficient supply of Vitamin B12 during lactation may lead to anemia and neurological damage in both the mother and breastfed infant as has been reported in vegetarians [129,130]. The prevalence of Vitamin B12 deficiency indicates that Vitamin B12 deficiency may be far more prevalent in both developing and developed countries than previously documented [119,131–134]. Maternal dietary intake of Vitamin B12, however, may be more important than maternal stores as demonstrated by several studies of Vitamin B12 deficient infants, whereby maternal plasma concentrations of the vitamin were determined to be normal or low normal [1]. Thus, lactating vegetarian women should be advised that milk is a source of Vitamin B12, while vegan women should be instructed to take a Vitamin B12 supplement or consume foods fortified with Vitamin B12, e.g., breakfast cereals.

5.4.2.2 Vitamin A

Since human milk fed infants consume an average of 400 μg/day of Vitamin A in the first 6 months of life, 400 μg retinoic acid equivalents were added to the EAR for nonpregnant women to ensure adequate dietary supply of Vitamin A. Vitamin A content of breast milk is affected by maternal Vitamin A status and intake. In developed countries, an additional dietary Vitamin A intake to support the needs of lactation is easily achieved by regular consumption of fruits and vegetables. In contrast, the average Vitamin A intake in developing countries is significantly less, and many breastfed infants show signs of depletion [119]. Marginal Vitamin A intake during lactation has also shown to reduce milk iron concentrations due to potential alterations on mammary gland iron transporters [135,136].

5.4.2.3 Calcium

Calcium is required for normal development and maintenance of the skeleton. The principal dietary source of calcium is from milk products (i.e., ~300 mg/250 mL serving of fluid milk) [137]. The calcium for skeletal mineralization of the offspring is supplied by the mother in utero and through breast milk during infancy. At peak lactation, breast milk calcium secretion averages ~200 mg/day. Lactation is known to be accompanied by an upregulation in maternal bone resorption—a strategy for meeting the calcium needs of the nursing infant [138]. This loss of maternal bone appears to be unresponsive to dietary calcium intakes, and epidemiological studies have shown that lost calcium is replaced after cessation of breastfeeding and re-establishment of menses [137]. Many studies have found no associations between lactation history and long-term bone mineral density or fracture risk [139–142]. As a result, there is no evidence that calcium intake in lactating women should be increased above nonlactating women, and thus the AI for calcium during lactation for women aged 19–50 remains set at 1000 mg/day (approximately three to four 250 mL servings of milk). Calcium intakes of lactating women in both developed and developing countries often fail to meet recommended requirements [117,118,141,143].

Calcium requirements for lactating adolescents may be higher than the nonpregnant state to support both lactation and the ongoing growth of the mother. The impact of lactation at a time when the maternal skeleton is still accruing mineral has been the focus of few studies. The evidence to date is insufficient to recommend additional calcium intakes above those of their nonlactating adolescent counterparts.

5.4.2.4 Vitamin D

Literature pertaining to Vitamin D intakes and status of lactating women are scarce. In light of the available evidence in 1997, the US daily recommended AI level for Vitamin D during lactation was set at 200 IU/day [137]. It was concluded that insignificant quantities of maternal circulating Vitamin D and its metabolites were secreted in human milk and hence, there was no reason to expect an increase in maternal Vitamin D requirements during this time period. Over the past decade, important advances have been made in Vitamin D research, and the high prevalence of Vitamin D deficiency in the general population has been well documented [144]. Vitamin D dependent rickets in children and osteomalacia in adults are the most commonly reported adverse effects of deficiency. Sun exposure is the major factor affecting the Vitamin D status of lactating mothers and their infants, and those who live at more northern latitudes are at greater risk of Vitamin D deficiency. Although the appropriate dose of Vitamin D during lactation is unknown, doses <1000 IU/day appear to inadequately maintain normal serum 25-hydroxyvitamin D concentrations, the indicator of nutritional Vitamin D status [65]. Hollis and Wagner [145] showed increased mean circulating 25-hydroxyvitamin D levels in lactating women supplemented with 2000 IU or 4000 IU/day over a 3 month study period. Serum 25-hydroxyvitamin D concentrations of supplemented mothers were all within the mid-normal reference range. Furthermore, the increase in maternal Vitamin D blood status resulted in increased Vitamin D content of breast milk, which produced significant effects on the infants' circulating 25-hydroxyvitamin D concentrations. The potential skeletal and other health benefits of higher recommended intake of Vitamin D supplementation during lactation is worthy of further investigation.

5.4.2.5 Iron

The concentration of iron in human is low, and does not appear to be altered by maternal nutritional status. The recommended iron intake of 9 mg/day during lactation is based on the amount of iron secreted in milk (0.27 mg/day) in addition to basal iron losses (0.85 mg/day). Menstrual losses are not considered as it is assumed that menstruation will not resume until after the 6 month period of exclusively breastfeeding. Re-establishment of menses prior to 6 months postpartum in many lactating women challenges this theoretical derivation of iron requirements. Furthermore, given that a high incidence of iron deficiency anemia during pregnancy, particularly in the third trimester, is well characterized [41], it may be necessary to consider the recovery of iron stores and alleviation of iron deficiency after pregnancy. The consequence of poor maternal iron status postpartum has shown to be related to maternal fatigue, depression, and decreased maternal ability to care and nurture the offspring [120–122]. Despite the well-accepted notion that iron deficiency leads to malaise and fatigue, the mechanism by which iron deficiency alters maternal emotional status and cognition is largely unexplored. Emerging evidence suggests that iron deficiency impacts cognition through a decrease in activity of iron-containing enzymes in the brain [146].

5.4.2.6 Zinc

The average concentration of zinc in human milk exhibits a rapid physiologic decline ranging from 4 mg/L at 2 weeks postpartum to 1.5 mg/L at 12 weeks postpartum [41]. Postpartum involution of the uterus and decreased maternal blood volume release ~30 mg of zinc that has been accumulated during gestation. It is assumed that this provision of endogenous zinc supplies ~1 mg/day to meet maternal zinc needs during lactation. In addition, the fractional absorption of dietary zinc increases nearly two-fold during lactation [147]. In consideration of these physiological adjustments, the average dietary requirement for zinc during lactation increases by 4 mg/day above the nonpregnant, nonlactating adult women. Although severe zinc deficiency is considered to be rare, mild or moderate zinc deficiency is thought to be common worldwide, particularly among women in developing countries or those who consume vegetarian diets [117]. Milk zinc concentrations appear to be tightly regulated and unaltered by maternal zinc supplementation in well-nourished women [148,149]; however, animal studies suggest that marginal zinc nutrition may both decrease milk zinc concentration and compromise milk production [150].

5.5 CONCLUSION

Maternal nutritional requirements during pregnancy and lactation are increased to support fetal and infant growth and development, and deposition and maintenance of maternal tissues. As the estimated increase in energy needs is less than the increased need for most nutrients, dietary choices of pregnant and lactating women must be nutrient dense. Current evidence strongly indicates that some micronutrient needs, such as folate, iron, and Vitamin D during these periods may be difficult to meet from diet alone.

5.6 FUTURE RESEARCH

While multiple micronutrient supplementation in developing countries is likely to be beneficial because of widespread maternal malnutrition, there is lack of consensus on the optimal formulation of micronutrient supplement for pregnant women or recognition of the need to continue these supplements during lactation. Preferably micronutrient deficiencies should be prevented or treated before pregnancy begins. Although it is appreciated that maternal diet plays a key role in reproductive success and potential long-term health outcomes of the mother and infant, including a role as an antecedent to adult diseases, lack of sensitive and specific nutritional biomarkers, and limited data from well-controlled intervention trials underscore the reality that the extent of our knowledge is far from complete. Furthermore, because the nutrient content of breast milk can be affected by the micronutrient status and dietary intake of the mother, a greater emphasis should be directed to the nutritional health of lactating women.

REFERENCES

1. Institute of Medicine, *Dietary Reference Intakes for Thiamin, Riboflavin, Niacin, Vitamin B6, Folate, Vitamin B12, Pantothenic Acid, Biotin and Choline*, National Academy Press, Washington, DC, 1998.
2. Czeizel, A.E. and Dudas, I., Prevention of the first occurrence of neural-tube defects by periconceptional vitamin supplementation, *N. Engl. J. Med.*, 327, 1832, 1992.
3. Kirke, P.N., Daly, L.E., and Elwood, J.H., A randomised trial of low dose folic acid to prevent neural tube defects, *Arch. Dis. Child.*, 67, 1442, 1992.
4. MRC Vitamin Research Group, Prevention of neural tube defects: Results of the Medical Research Council Vitamin Study, *Lancet*, 338, 131, 1991.
5. Berry, R.J. et al., Prevention of neural tube defects with folic acid in China. China–US Collaborative Project for neural tube defect prevention., *N. Engl. J. Med.*, 341, 1485, 1999.
6. Czeizel, A.E. Reduction of urinary tract and cardiovascular defects by periconceptional multivitamin supplementation, *Am. J. Med. Genet.*, 62, 179, 1996.
7. Shaw, G.M. et al., Risks of orofacial clefts in children born to women using multivitamins containing folic acid periconceptionally, *Lancet*, 345, 393, 2007.
8. Loffredo, L.C.M. et al., Oral clefts and vitamin supplementation, *Cleft Palate-Craniofac. J.*, 38, 76, 2001.
9. Itikala, P.R. et al., Maternal multivitamin use and orofacial clefts in offspring, *Teratology*, 63, 79, 2001.
10. McCourt, C., Primary prevention of neural tube defects: Notice from HPB, *Can. Medl. Assoc. J.*, 148, 1451, 1993.
11. U.S. Department of Health and Human Services, Recommendations for the use of folic acid to reduce the number of cases of spina bifida and other neural tube defects, *MMWR Morb. Mortal. Wkly. Rev.*, 4, 1, 1992.
12. Morin, P. et al., Pregnancy planning: A determinant of folic acid supplements use for the primary prevention of neural tube defects, *Can. J. Public Health*, 93, 259, 2002.
13. French, M.R., Barr, S.I., and Levy-Milne, R., Folate intakes and awareness of folate to prevent neural tube defects: A survey of women living in Vancouver, Canada, *J. Am. Diet. Assoc.*, 103, 181, 2003.
14. Carmichael, S.L. et al., The National Birth Defects Prevention Study. Correlates of intake of folic acid-containing supplements among pregnant women, *Am. J. Obstet. Gynecol.*, 194, 203, 2006.
15. Ren, A. et al., Awareness and use of folic acid, and other blood folate concentrations among pregnant women in northern China—An area with a high prevalence of neural tube defects, *Reprod. Toxicol.*, 22, 431, 2006.
16. Knudsen, V.K. et al., Low compliance with recommendations on folic acid use in relation to pregnancy: Is there a need for fortification? *Public Health Nutr.*, 7, 843, 2004.
17. Tam, L.E. et al., A survey of preconceptional folic acid use in a group of Canadian women, *J. Obstet. Gynecol. Can.*, 27, 232, 2005.

18. Center for Disease Control, Use of dietary supplements containing folic acid among women of childbearing age—United States, 2005, *MMWR Morb. Mortal. Wkly. Rep.*, 54, 955, 2005.
19. Goldberg, B.B. et al., Prevalence of periconceptional folic acid use and perceived barriers to the postgestation continuance of supplemental folic acid: Survey results from a Teratogen Information Service, *Birth Defects Res.*, 76, 193, 2006.
20. de Jong-van den Berg et al., Trends and predictors of folic acid awareness and periconceptional use in pregnant women, *Am. J. Obstet. Gynecol.*, 192, 121, 2005.
21. Institute of Medicine, *Best Intentions: Unintended Pregnancy and the Well-Being of Children and Families*, National Academy Press, Washington, DC, 1995.
22. Finer, L.B. and Henshaw, S.K., Disparities in rates of unintended pregnancy in the United States, 1994 and 2001, *Perspect. Sex. Reprod. Health*, 38, 90, 2006.
23. Botto, L.D. et al., International retrospective cohort study of neural tube defects in relation to folic acid recommendations: Are the recommendations working? *Br. Med. J.*, 330, 571, 2005.
24. Botto, L.D. et al., Trends of selected malformations in relation to folic acid recommendations and fortification: An international assessment, *Birth Defects Res.*, 76, 693, 2006.
25. Honein, M.A. et al., Impact of folic acid fortification of the US food supply on the occurrence of neural tube defects, *JAMA*, 285, 2981, 2001.
26. Ray, J.G. et al., Association of neural tube defects and folic acid fortification in Canada, *Lancet*, 360, 2047, 2002.
27. Persad, V.L. et al., Incidence of open neural tube defects in Nova Scotia after folic acid fortification, *Can. Med. Assoc. J.*, 167, 241, 2002.
28. Liu, S. et al., A comprehensive evaluation of food fortification with folic acid for the primary prevention of neural tube defects, *BMC Pregnancy Childbirth*, 4, 20, 2004.
29. Lopez-Camelo, J.S. et al., Reduction of birth prevalence rates of neural tube defects after folic acid fortification in Chile, *Am. J. Med. Genet.*, 135A, 120, 2005.
30. Gropper, S.S., Smith, J.L., and Groff, J.L., *Advanced Nutrition and Human Metabolism*, 4th Thomson Wadsworth, Belmont, CA, 2005.
31. Casanueva, E. et al., Iron and folate status before pregnancy and anemia during pregnancy, *Ann. Nutr. Metab.*, 47, 60, 2003.
32. Centers for Disease Control and Prevention, Iron Deficiency—United States, 1999–2000, *MMWR Morb. Mortal. Wkly. Rep.*, 51, 897, 2002.
33. Bothwell, T.H., Iron requirements in pregnancy and strategies to meet them, *Am. J. Clin. Nutr.*, 72 (suppl), 257S, 2000.
34. Svanberg, B., Iron absorption in early pregnancy—a study of the absorption of non-haeme iron and ferrous iron in early pregnancy, *Acta. Obstet. Gynecol. Scand. Suppl.*, 48, 69, 1975.
35. Lubach, G.R. and Coe, C.L., Preconception maternal iron status is a risk factor for iron deficiency in infant rhesus monkeys (*Macaca mulatta*), *J. Nutr.*, 136, 2345, 2006.
36. Lashen, H., Fear, K., and Sturdee, D.W., Obesity is associated with increased first trimester and recurrent miscarriage: Matched case–control study, *Hum. Reprod.*, 19, 1644, 2004.
37. Watkins, M.L. et al., Maternal obesity and risk factors for birth defects, *Pediatrics*, 111, 1152, 2003.
38. Ray, J.G. et al., Greater maternal weight and the ongoing risk of neural tube defects after folic acid flour fortification, *Obstet. Gynecol.*, 105, 261, 2005.
39. Catalano, P.M., Management of obesity in pregnancy, *Obstet. Gynecol.*, 109, 419, 2007.
40. Ogden, C.L. et al., Prevalence of overweight and obesity in the United States, 1999–2004, *JAMA*, 295, 1549, 2006.

41. Institute of Medicine, *Dietary Reference Intakes for Vitamin A, Vitamin K, Arsenic, Boron, Chromium, Copper, Iodine, Iron, Manganese, Molybdenum, Nickel, Silicon, Vanadium, and Zinc*, National Academy Press, Washington, DC, 2001.
42. Health Canada, Nutrition for a healthy pregnancy. National guidelines for the childbearing years, Minister of Public Works and Government Services Canada, Ottawa, 1999.
43. Butte, N.F. and King, J.C., Energy requirements during pregnancy and lactation, *Public Health Nutr.*, 8, 1010, 5 A.D.
44. Institute of Medicine, *Nutrition during Pregnancy*, National Academy Press, Washington, DC, 1990.
45. Stotland, N.E. et al., Body mass index, provider advice, and target gestational weight gain, *Obstet. Gynecol.*, 105, 633, 2005.
46. Parker, J.D. and Abrams, B., Prenatal weight gain advice: An examination of the recent prenatal weight gain recommendations of the Institute of Medicine, *Obstet. Gynecol.*, 79, 664, 1992.
47. Taylor, P.D. and Poston, L., Developmental programming of obesity, *Exp. Physiol.*, Dec 14 [Epub ahead of print], 2006.
48. Cogswell, M.E. et al., Medically advised, mother's personal target, and actual weight gain during pregnancy, *Obstet. Gynecol.*, 94, 616, 1999.
49. Cabana, M.D. et al., Why don't physicians follow clinical practice guidelines? A framework for improvement, *JAMA*, 282, 1458, 1999.
50. Feig, D.S. and Naylor, C.D., Eating for two: Are guidelines for weight gain during pregnancy too liberal? *Lancet*, 351, 1054, 1998.
51. Muscati, S.K., Gray-Donald, K., and Koski, K.G., Timing of weight gain during pregnancy: Promoting fetal growth and minimizing maternal weight retention, *Int. J. Obes. Relat. Metab. Disord.*, 20, 526, 1996.
52. Polley, B.A., Wing, R.R., and Sims, C.J., Randomized controlled trial to prevent excessive weight gain in pregnant women, *Int. J. Obes.*, 26, 1494, 2002.
53. Institute of Medicine, *Dietary Reference Intakes for Energy, Carbohydrate, Fiber, Fat, Fatty Acids, Cholesterol, Protein, and Amino Acid*, National Academy Press, Washington, DC, 2002.
54. Hytten, F.E. and Leitch, I. *The Physiology of Human Pregnancy*, Blackwell, Oxford, 1971.
55. Thompson, G.N. and Halliday, D., Protein turnover in pregnancy, *Eur. J. Clin. Nutr.*, 46, 411, 1992.
56. Percy, A. et al., Polyunsaturated fatty acid accretion in first- and second-trimester human fetal brain: Lack of correlation with levels in paired placental samples, *Biochem. Mol. Med.*, 59, 38, 1996.
57. Jensen, C.L., Effects of n-3 fatty acids during pregnancy and lactation, *Am. J. Clin. Nutr.*, 83, 1452S, 2006.
58. West, K.P. et al., Double blind, cluster randomised trial of low dose supplementation with vitamin A or β-carotene on mortality related to pregnancy in Nepal. The NNIPS-2 Study Group, *Br. Med. J.*, 318, 570, 1999.
59. Christian, P. et al., Night blindness during pregnancy and subsequent mortality among women in Nepal: Effects of vitamin A and β-carotene supplementation, *Am. J. Epidemiol.*, 152, 542, 2000.
60. Christian, P. et al., Night blindness of pregnancy in rural Nepal—nutritional and health risks., *Int. J. Epidemiol.*, 27, 231, 1998.
61. Katz, J. et al., Night blindness is prevalent during pregnancy and lactation in rural Nepal, *J. Nutr.*, 125, 2122, 1995.
62. Rothman, K.J. et al., Teratogenicity of high vitamin A intake, *N. Engl. J. Med.*, 23, 1369, 1995.

63. Miller, R.K. et al., Periconceptional vitamin A use: How much is teratogenic? *Reprod. Toxicol.*, 12, 75, 1998.
64. Holick, M.F., Vitamin D: New horizons for the 21st century, *Am. J. Clin. Nutr.*, 60, 619, 1994.
65. Hollis, B.W. and Wagner, C.L., Assessment of dietary vitamin D requirements during pregnancy and lactation, *Am. J. Clin. Nutr.*, 79, 717, 2004.
66. Bodnar, L.M. et al., High prevalence of vitamin D insufficiency in black and white pregnant women residing in the northern United States and their neonates, *J. Nutr.*, 137, 447, 2007.
67. Weiler, H. et al., Vitamin D deficiency and whole-body and femur bone mass relative to weight in healthy newborns, *Can. Med. Assoc. J.*, 172, 757, 2005.
68. Javaid, M.K. et al. Maternal vitamin D status during pregnancy and childhood bone mass at age 9 years: A longitudinal study, *Lancet*, 367, 36, 2006.
69. Willer, C.J. et al., Timing of birth and risk of multiple sclerosis: Population based study, *Br. Med. J.*, 330, 120, 2005.
70. Chaudhuri, A., Why we should offer routine vitamin D supplementation in pregnancy and childhood to prevent multiple sclerosis, *Med. Hypotheses*, 64, 608, 2005.
71. Mathieu, C. and Badenhoop, K., Vitamin D and type 1 diabetes mellitus: State of the art, *Trends Endocrinol. Metab.*, 16, 261, 2005.
72. Bischoff-Ferrari, H.A. et al., Estimation of optimal serum concentrations of 25-hydroxyvitamin D for multiple health outcomes, *Am. J. Clin. Nutr.*, 84, 18, 2006.
73. Hathcock, J.N. et al., Risk assessment for vitamin D, *Am. J. Clin. Nutr.*, 85, 6, 2007.
74. Calvo, M.S., Whiting, S.J., and Barton, C.N., Vitamin D fortification in the United States and Canada: Current status and data needs, *Am. J. Clin. Nutr.*, 80 (suppl), 1710S, 2004.
75. Scholl, T.O. and Johnson, W.G., Folic acid: Influence on the outcome of pregnancy, *Am. J. Clin. Nutr.*, 71 (suppl), 1295S, 2000.
76. Tamura, T. and Piccianno, M.F., Folate and human reproduction, *Am. J. Clin. Nutr.*, 83, 993, 2006.
77. Sherwood, K.L. et al., One-third of pregnant and lactating women may not be meeting their folate requirements from diet alone based on mandated levels of folic acid fortification, *J. Nutr.*, 136, 2820, 2006.
78. Turner, R.E. et al., Comparing nutrient intake from food to the estimated average requirements shows middle- to upper-income pregnant women lack iron and possibly magnesium, *J. Am. Diet. Assoc.*, 103, 461, 2003.
79. Scholl, T.O., Iron deficiency during pregnancy: Setting the stage for mother and infant, *Am. J. Clin. Nutr.*, 81, 1218S, 2005.
80. Siega-Riz, A.M. et al., The effects of prophylactic iron given in prenatal supplements on iron status and birth outcomes: A randomized controlled trial, *Am. J. Obstet. Gynecol.*, 194, 512, 2006.
81. Cogswell, M.E., Kettel-Khan, L., and Ramakrishnan, U., Iron supplement use among-women in the United States: Science, policy and practice, *J. Nutr.*, 133, 1974S, 2003.
82. Caulfield, L.E. et al., Potential contribution of maternal zinc supplementation during pregnancy to maternal and child survival, *Am. J. Clin. Nutr.*, 68 (suppl), 499S, 1998.
83. O'Brien, K.O. et al., Influence of prenatal iron and zinc supplements on supplemental iron absorption, red blood cell iron incorporation, and iron status in pregnant Peruvian women, *Am. J. Clin. Nutr.*, 69, 509, 1999.
84. Harvey, L.J. et al., Effect of high-dose iron supplements on fractional zinc absorption and status in pregnant women, *Am. J. Clin. Nutr.*, 85, 131, 2007.

85. Delange, F., Iodine deficiency as a cause of brain damage, *Postgrad. Med. J.*, 77, 217, 2001.
86. Hetzel, B.S., Iodine deficiency and fetal brain damage, *N. Engl. J. Med.*, 331, 1739, 1994.
87. Barker, D.J. et al., Growth in utero, blood pressure in childhood and adult life, and mortality from cardiovascular disease, *Bone Miner. J.*, 298, 564, 1989.
88. Waterland, R.A. and Garza, C., Potential mechanisms of metabolic imprinting that lead to chronic disease, *Am. J. Clin. Nutr.*, 69, 179, 1999.
89. Godfrey, K.M. and Barker, D.J., Fetal nutrition and adult disease, *Am. J. Clin. Nutr.*, 71 (suppl), 1344S, 2000.
90. De Boo, H.A. and Harding, J.A., The developmental origins of adult disease (Barker) hypothesis, *Aust. N. Z. J. Med.*, 46, 4, 2007.
91. McMillen, I.C. and Robinson, J.S., Developmental origins of the metabolic syndrome: Prediction, plasticity, and programming, *Physiol. Rev.*, 85, 571, 2005.
92. Waterland, R.A., Epigenetic mechanisms and gastrointestinal development, *J. Pediatr.*, 149, S137, 2006.
93. Waddington, C.H., *The Strategy of Genes*, Allen & Unwin, London, 1957.
94. Van den Veyver, I.B., Genetic effects of methylation diets, *Ann. Rev. Nutr.*, 22, 255, 2002.
95. Wolf, G.L. et al., Maternal epigenetics and methyl supplements affect agouti gene expression Avy/a mice, *FASEB J.*, 12, 949, 1998.
96. Waterland, R.A. and Jirtle, R.L., Transposable elements: Targets for early nutritional effects on epigenetic gene regulation, *Mol. Cell. Biol.*, 23, 5293, 2003.
97. Waterland, R.A. et al., Maternal methyl supplementation increases offspring DNA methylation at Axin Fused, *Genesis*, 44, 401, 2006.
98. Rees, W.D. et al., Maternal protein deficiency causes hypermethylation of DNA in the livers of rat foetuses, *J. Nutr.*, 130, 1821, 2000.
99. Lillycrop, K.A. et al., Dietary protein restriction of pregnant rats induces and folic acid supplementation prevents epigenetic modification of hepatic gene expression in the offspring, *J. Nutr.*, 135, 1382, 2005.
100. Kelly, T.L. and Trasler, J.M., Reproductive epigenetics, *Clin. Genet.*, 65, 247, 2004.
101. Kim, Y.I., Will mandatory folic acid fortification prevent or promote cancer, *Am. J. Clin. Nutr.*, 80, 1123, 2004.
102. Lucock, M. and Yates, Z., Folic acid—vitamin and pancea or genetic time bomb? *Nat. Rev. Genet.*, 6, 235, 2005.
103. Das, P.M. and Singal, R., DNA methylation and cancer, *J. Clin. Oncol.*, 22, 4632, 2004.
104. Arenz, S. et al., Breast-feeding and childhood obesity—a systematic review, *Int. J. Obes. Relat. Metab. Disord.*, 28, 1247, 2004.
105. Ong, K.K. et al., Size at birth and early childhood growth in relation to maternal smoking, parity and infant breast-feeding: Longitudinal birth cohort study and analysis, *Pediatr. Res.*, 52, 863, 2002.
106. Institute of Medicine, *Nutrition during Lactation*, National Academy Press, Washington, DC, 1991.
107. Position of the American Dietetic Association, Promoting and supporting breastfeeding, *J. Am. Diet. Assoc.*, 105, 810, 2005.
108. American Academy of Pediatrics Working Group on Breastfeeding, Breastfeeding and the use of human milk, *Pediatrics*, 115, 496, 2005.
109. Health Canada, Exclusive Breastfeeding Duration—2004 Health Canada Recommendation, Food & Nutrition, http://www.hc-sc.gc.ca/fn-an/nutrition/child-enfant/infant-nourisson/excl_bf_dur-dur_am_excl_e.html, 2004.

110. Dewey, K.G., Heinig, M.J., and Nommsen-Rivers, L.A., Differences in morbidity between breast-fed and formula-fed infants, *J. Pediatr.*, 126, 696, 1995.
111. Kramer, M.S. et al., Infant growth and health outcomes associated with 3 compared with 6 mo of exclusive breastfeeding, *Am. J. Clin. Nutr.*, 78, 291, 2003.
112. Palda, V.A. et al., Canadian Task Force on Preventive Health Care Interventions to promote breast-feeding: Applying the evidence in clinical practice, *Can. Med. Assoc. J.*, 170, 976, 2004.
113. Picciano, M.F., Pregnancy and lactation: Physiological adjustments, nutritional requirements and the role of dietary supplements, *J. Nutr.*, 133, 1997S, 2003.
114. Janney, C.A., Zhang, D., and Sowers, M., Lactation and weight retention, *Am. J. Clin. Nutr.*, 66, 1116, 1997.
115. Kramer, F.M. et al., Breast-feeding reduces maternal lower-body fat, *J. Am. Diet. Assoc.*, 93, 429, 1993.
116. Dewey, K.G., Heinig, M.J., and Nommsen, L.A., Maternal weight-loss patterns during prolonged lactation, *Am. J. Clin. Nutr.*, 58, 162, 1993.
117. Todd, J.M. and Parnell, W.R., Nutrient intakes of women who are breastfeeding, *Eur. J. Clin. Nutr.*, 48, 567, 1994.
118. Mackey, A.D. et al., Self-selected diets of lactating women often fail to meet dietary recommendations, *J. Am. Diet. Assoc.*, 98, 297, 1998.
119. Allen, L.H., Multiple micronutrients in pregnancy and lactation: An overview, *Am. J. Clin. Nutr.*, 81(suppl), 1206S, 2005.
120. Perez, E.M. et al., Mother-infant interactions and infant development are altered by maternal iron deficiency anemia, *J. Nutr.*, 135, 850, 2005.
121. Beard, J.I. et al., Maternal iron deficiency anemia affects postpartum emotions and cognition, *J. Nutr.*, 135, 267, 2005.
122. Corwin, E.J., Murray-Kolb, L., and Beard, J.L., Low hemoglobin level is a risk factor for postparum depression, *J. Nutr.*, 133, 4139, 2003.
123. Tamura, T., Yoshimura, Y., and Arakawa, T., Human milk folate and folate status in lactating mother's and their infants, *Am. J. Clin. Nutr.*, 33, 193, 1980.
124. Butte, N.F., Calloway, D.H., and Van Duzen, J.L., Nutritional assessment of pregnant and lactating Navajo women, *Am. J. Clin. Nutr.*, 34, 2216, 1981.
125. Sneed, S.M., Zane, C., and Thomas, M.R., The effects of ascorbic acid, vitamin B6, vitamin B12 and folic acid supplementation on the breast milk and maternal nutritional status of low socioeconomic lactating women, *Am. J. Clin. Nutr.*, 34, 1338, 1981.
126. Keizer, S.E., Gibson, R.S., and O'Connor, D.L., Postpartum folic acid supplementation of adolescents: Impact on maternal folate and zinc status and milk composition, *Am. J. Clin. Nutr.*, 62, 377, 1995.
127. O'Connor, D.L., Green, T.J., and Piccianno, M.F., Maternal folate status and lactation, *J. Mammary Gland Biol. Neoplasia*, 2, 279, 1997.
128. Ray, J.G. et al., Increased red cell folate concentrations in women of reproductive age after Canadian folic acid fortification, *Epidemiology*, 13, 238, 2002.
129. Weiss, R., Fogelman, Y., and Bennett, M., Severe vitamin B12 deficiency in an infant associated with a maternal deficiency and a strict vegetarian diet, *J. Pediatr. Hematol. Oncol.*, 26, 270, 2004.
130. Michaud, J.L. et al., Nutritional vitamin B12 deficiency: Two cases detected by routine newborn screening, *Eur. J. Pediatr.*, 151, 218, 1992.
131. House, J.D. et al., Folate and vitamin B12 status of women in Newfoundland at their first prenatal visit, *Can. Med. Assoc. J.*, 162, 1557, 2000.

132. Koebnick, C. et al., Long-term ovo-lacto vegetarian diet impairs vitamin B12 status in pregnant women, *J. Nutr.*, 134, 3319, 2004.
133. Allen, L.H., Vitamin B12 metabolism and status during pregnancy, lactation and infancy., *Adv. Exp. Med. Biol.*, 352, 173, 1994.
134. Stabler, S.P. and Allen, L.H., Vitamin B12 deficiency as a worldwide problem, *Annu. Rev. Nutr.*, 24, 299, 2004.
135. Muslimatun, S. et al., Weekly vitamin A and iron supplementation during pregnancy increases vitamin A concentration of breast milk but not iron status in Indonesian lactating women, *J. Nutr.*, 131, 2664, 2001.
136. Kelleher, S.L. and Lönnerdal, B., Low vitamin A intake affects milk iron level and iron transporters in rat mammary gland and liver, *J. Nutr.*, 135, 27, 2005.
137. Institute of Medicine, *Dietary Reference Intakes for Calcium, Phosphorus, Magnesium, Vitamin D and Fluoride*, National Academy Press, Washington, DC, 1997.
138. Prentice, A., Micronutrients and the bone mineral content of the mother, fetus and newborn, *J. Nutr.*, 133, 1693S, 2003.
139. Koetting, C.A. and Wardlaw, G.M., Wrist, spine and hip bone density in women with variable histories of lactation, *Am. J. Clin. Nutr.*, 48, 1479, 1988.
140. Cummings, S.R. et al., Risk factors for hip fracture in white women: Study of Osteoporotic Fractures Research Group, *N. Engl. J. Med.*, 332, 767, 1995.
141. Jarjou, L.M.A. et al., Randomized, placebo-controlled, calcium supplementation study in pregnant Gambian women: Effects on breast-milk calcium concentrations and infant birth weight, growth and bone mineral accretion in the first year of life, *Am. J. Clin. Nutr.*, 83, 657, 2006.
142. Prentice, A., Calcium in pregnancy and lactation, *Annu. Rev. Nutr.*, 20, 249, 2000.
143. Lovelady, C.A. et al., Effects of dieting on food and nutrient intakes of lactating women, *J. Am. Diet. Assoc.*, 106, 908, 2006.
144. Holick, M.F., High prevalence of vitamin D inadequacy and implications for health, *Mayo Clin. Proc.*, 81, 353, 2006.
145. Hollis, B.W. and Wagner, C.L., Vitamin D requirements during lactation: High-dose maternal supplementation as therapy to prevent hypovitaminosis D for both the mother and nursing infant, *Am. J. Clin. Nutr.*, 80 (suppl), 1752S, 2004.
146. Bodnar, L.M., Cogswell, M.E., and McDonald, T., Have we forgotten the significance of postpartum iron deficiency? *Am. J. Obstet. Gynecol.*, 193, 36, 2005.
147. Fung, E.B. et al., Zinc absorption in women during pregnancy and lactation: A longitudinal study, *Am. J. Clin. Nutr.*, 66, 80, 1997.
148. Krebs, N.F. et al., Zinc supplementation during lactation: Effects on maternal status and milk zinc concentrations, *Am. J. Clin. Nutr.*, 61, 1030, 1995.
149. Chierici, R., Saccomandi, D., and Vigi, V., Dietary supplements for the lactating mother: Influence on trace element content of milk, *Acta Paediatr.*, 88, 7, 1999.
150. Chowanadisai, W., Kellehr, S.L., and Lönnerdal, B., Maternal zinc deficiency raises plasma prolactin levels in lactating rats, *J. Nutr.*, 134, 1314, 2004.

6 Menopause and Midlife

Stacie E. Geller, Marci Goldstein Adams, and Laura Studee

CONTENTS

6.1 INTRODUCTION

The midlife transition is associated with many changes in hormonal and physiological function, some of which are sex related. In women, one of the most dramatic hormonal changes is the striking reduction in estrogen production that accompanies menopause. The word menopause is derived from two Greek roots: mens, meaning monthly, and pause, meaning to stop. It refers specifically to the cessation of menstruation and the termination of fertility, two events which may not happen at the same time.

Technically, menopause is the point at which a woman has her last menstrual period and is therefore no longer fertile. For some time before this, menstrual periods may have occurred without ovulation and may have been getting gradually further apart, or, in some cases, closer together. The perimenopausal period, the time leading up to that final menses, may be as long as 10–15 years, but can vary widely between women. The years following the last menstrual cycle are known as postmenopause and may comprise as much as one-third of a woman's life.

At the menopause, the ovaries stop producing the hormones estrogen and progesterone, which leads to many bodily changes. For example, although estrogen is mainly thought of as a sex hormone, cells in the vagina, bladder, breasts, skin, bones, arteries, heart, liver, and brain all contain estrogen receptors. Prior to menopause, estrogen helps protect a woman's arterial walls from fat and cholesterol buildup by raising the levels of high density lipoproteins (HDL), the "good" cholesterol and lowering the levels of low density lipoproteins (LDL), the "bad" cholesterol. As menopause drives down estrogen levels and as women age, this protection disappears and leaves women as vulnerable to heart disease as men. Aging and declining estrogen levels also affect bone density, putting women at risk for osteoporosis, and contributing to a greater risk of metabolic syndrome [1]. During the perimenopause, women may also experience symptoms such as hot flashes, depression, anxiety, and other changes that can greatly impact their quality of life. These symptoms can vary greatly, with some women having no complaints and others having symptoms for several years.

Despite these changes, it is important to remember that menopause is not a medical condition or a disease but is a natural physiological change and an important stage of life that has special nutritional requirements. As women age, their bodies require less energy overall because of a general decline in physical activity and a loss of lean body mass which in turn slows down metabolism—all of which can lead to weight gain [2,3]. With a proper diet as well as nutritional supplements and exercise, most of the unpleasant side effects of menopause can be minimized if not eliminated, and many chronic health conditions related to aging can be averted or lessened. Following is an overview of food sources, vitamins and minerals, and botanical and dietary supplement (BDS) products thought to be optimal for midlife women.

6.2 HEALTHY EATING

A healthy and well-balanced diet is one of the most important aspects for promoting overall health. However, having a healthy diet is sometimes easier said than done. It is tempting to eat less healthy foods because they might be easier to obtain or prepare, and they may also satisfy a craving. Between family, work, and other obligations, taking time to buy the ingredients for and to cook a healthy meal is often difficult to accomplish on a regular basis.

However, a healthy diet not only helps women feel better and improve over all well-being, it is also linked with a decrease in diseases such as cancer, diabetes, osteoporosis, and heart disease. Therefore, a well-balanced diet is one of the keys to ensuring that the midlife years are as healthy as possible. A healthy eating plan focuses on increasing lean protein and dietary fiber through fruits, vegetables, whole grains, while minimizing sugar, salt, and saturated fats. Following are some of the foods that should be a daily part of any good diet as well as those foods that are best minimized or avoided.

6.2.1 Dietary Fiber

Dietary fiber, also known as roughage or bulk, is probably best known for its ability to prevent or relieve constipation. A high-fiber diet may lower the risk of specific disorders, such as hemorrhoids, irritable bowel syndrome, and the development of small pouches in the colon (diverticular disease).

But fiber can provide other health benefits as well, such as lowering the risk of diabetes and heart disease. Studies have shown that a high-fiber diet, particularly from whole grain sources, can reduce blood pressure, total and LDL cholesterol, and coronary artery disease [4–6]. Research suggests that women who consume a larger proportion of whole grains, as opposed to refined grains, have a reduced risk of death from coronary heart disease, cancer, diabetes, and ischemic stroke [7–12]. Dietary fiber comes from whole grain, fruit, and vegetable sources. The dietary reference intake (DRI) for fiber for women 51–70 years old is 21 g/day.

Eating a high-fiber diet may also help with weight loss. High-fiber diets tend to be less energy dense, which means they have fewer calories for the same volume of food. These foods generally require more chewing time, giving the body time to register satiety, making one less likely to overeat.

Fruits and vegetables are also a good source of dietary fiber and have been shown to decrease heart disease and the risk of stroke [13,14]. It is recommended that women consume more than five servings of fruits and vegetables a day to promote protection from heart disease and stroke.

An interesting side benefit of a high-fiber diet may also be a reduction in the vasomotor symptoms related to menopause. A recent study of breast cancer survivors found that high-fiber intake was associated with a decrease in vasomotor symptoms over a 12 month period [15].

6.2.2 Soy Isoflavones from Food Sources

Although many women use soy isoflavones as a supplement in the form of capsules or tablets, it is always preferable to increase their intake through food sources. Similar to supplements, soy-rich foods may help to alleviate menopause symptoms, although the data related to effectiveness is modest [16]. However, soy-based foods have been associated with decreasing the risk of cardiovascular disease and osteoporosis [17]. Notwithstanding a soy allergy, soy foods are very healthy as they are comprised of protein, antioxidants, phytonutrients, calcium, and folate. The best forms of soy foods are those with the highest amount of isoflavones and protein including whole soybeans, tempeh, textured soy protein, soynuts, soy protein powders, tofu, soymilk, miso, and soy beverages. Isoflavones are also found in brussel sprouts, yams, legumes, and many vegetables and fruits.

However, the actual isoflavone content has to be high enough to produce positive effects. Some foods made from soy protein concentrate, like soy hotdogs, have very little isoflavones due to their processing method. Other products, such as soybean oil and soy sauce, contain no isoflavones at all. To obtain benefits, it is recommended that women consume at least 25 g of soy protein and 30–50 mg of isoflavones daily (equal to 1–2 servings) [18]. Additional information on soy supplements can be found in the BDS section of this chapter.

6.2.3 Dietary Fats

The midlife is a time when many women begin to add unwanted weight and increase their risk for heart disease, stroke diabetes, and many cancers [19]. Eating a diet low in fat is thought to reduce the amount of weight gained during menopause and reduce chronic disease. Fat intake, and particularly saturated fat, is associated with breast cancer risk in postmenopausal women [20–22]. One large-scale trial of women with early stage breast cancer found that those assigned to a low-fat diet (15% of calories or less from fat) were less likely to have a relapse than those not on a low-fat diet [23]. This finding suggests that reducing the amount of dietary fat may not only decrease the risk of breast cancer, but help increase survival after a diagnosis.

Recent research suggests that the total amount of fat in the diet is less important than the type of fat [24]. The Women's Health Initiative (WHI) Dietary Modification Trial found no decrease in risk of cardiovascular disease or risk factors such as improved lipid profiles in women following a low-fat diet [25]. However, women in this study were instructed to reduce their total fat intake and not to reduce the bad fats, i.e., saturated and trans fats. It is these fats that are associated with increased risk of cardiovascular disease and breast cancer. The good fats, i.e., monounsaturated and polyunsaturated fats, lower the risk of cardiovascular disease and cancer.

The key is to substitute good fats for bad fats. In general, women should choose foods low in saturated fat and cholesterol; fat intake should be less than 30% of daily calories. The American Heart Association recommends less than 7% of calories come from saturated fat [26]. Consumption of good fats such as olive oil (a monounsaturated fat) is significantly related to a reduced risk of breast cancer [27]. In the WHI Dietary Modification Trial, although there was no overall reduction in the risk of breast cancer, among women that consumed the highest levels of fat at baseline, those that followed a low-fat diet high in fruits and vegetables did reduce their risk for breast cancer [28]. Table 6.1 provides a summary of dietary fat types, sources, and their effect on blood lipids.

TABLE 6.1
Fat Types and Sources

Type	Sources	Effect on Serum Lipids
Monounsaturated fat	Olives; olive oil, canola oil, peanut oil; cashews, almonds, peanuts, and most other nuts; avocados	Lowers LDL; raises HDL
Polyunsaturated fat (ratio should be 2:1 n-6 to n-3)	—	Lowers LDL; raises HDL
n-3	Oily fish (e.g., sardines, mackerel, tuna), flaxseed oil, some eggs	Lowers triglyceride levels
n-6	Cereals, whole grain breads, vegetable oils (e.g., canola, olive oil)	High n-6 has a negative effect on lipids
Saturated	Whole milk, butter, cheese, and ice cream; red meat; chocolate; coconuts, coconut milk, and coconut oil	Raises both LDL and HDL
Trans	Most margarines; vegetable shortening; partially hydrogenated vegetable oil; deep-fried chips; many fast foods; most commercial baked goods	Raises LDL

6.2.3.1 Trans Fatty Acids

In 2006, the New York City ban on the use of trans fatty acids in restaurants is evidence of the concern associated with their consumption [29]. While avoiding trans fatty acids entirely is most desirable, the American Heart Association recommends that less than 1% of calories consumed should come from trans fatty acids [26]. For a woman consuming 1800 cal/day, this translates to approximately 2 g of trans fats [30]. Trans fatty acids are often found in fast food, margarine, and commercially prepared baked goods. Avoiding products with ingredients that include "shortening," "hydrogenated vegetable oil," or "partially hydrogenated vegetable oil" will also help to eliminate trans fatty acids [30]. US food-labeling requirements indicate that products with less than 0.5 g/serving may call themselves trans-fat free; although this means that small amounts will still be consumed.

Consumption of trans fatty acids has been associated with increased risk of death from coronary heart disease [31], acute myocardial infarction [32], and coronary heart disease [33]. Trans fatty acids elevate bad cholesterol (LDL) and reduce good cholesterol (HDL), thereby negatively affecting the LDL:HDL ratio [34,35]. Trans fats may also contribute to systemic inflammation, insulin resistance, and type 2 diabetes [36,37].

6.2.3.2 n-3 Fatty Acids

Fish and shellfish are rich in n-3 fatty acids and are known to have beneficial effects on blood pressure and cardiovascular disease [38,39]. n-3s may be especially important for women because they effectively reduce triglyceride levels, which are associated with cardiovascular disease [40]. Several studies have found that women who ate more fish and more n-3 fatty acids had a lower risk of coronary heart disease, myocardial infarction (MI), stroke, and death due to coronary heart disease (CHD) [41–43]. Even among postmenopausal women with CHD, fish consumption has been found to be associated with several markers for improvement in coronary artery health [44].

Fish consumption, higher levels of n-3 fatty acid consumption, and high ratios of n-3 to n-6 fatty acids have also been associated with lower risk of breast cancer and female colorectal cancer [45–47]. Other benefits of n-3 fatty acids include decreased risk of cataracts and joint tenderness in individuals with rheumatoid arthritis [48,49]. One study that tested a polyunsaturated fatty acid supplement found that n-3 fatty acids even reduced hot flashes [50].

While there is no DRI for n-3 fatty acids, consuming between 1 and 3 g/day is optimal. That translates to about 3–4 oz of mackerel or herring, or about 8 oz of salmon, albacore, tuna, or lake trout. The American Heart Association 2006 Diet and Lifestyle Recommendations suggest eating at least 2 servings/week of oily fish such as orange roughy, salmon, sardines, or trout [26].

6.2.3.3 n-6 Fatty Acids

n-6 fatty acids are necessary for maintaining skin and hair health. They come from corn and other vegetable oils, beef, milk, and products from other animals that eat corn and grain [51]. However, eating too much n-6 and too little n-3 fatty acids can cause clots and constrict arteries which can increase the risk for heart attacks, increase swelling to worsen arthritis, and aggravates a skin disease called psoriasis [52].

The correct ratio of n-6s and n-3s is about 2:1. However, over the last 50 years in North America, the ratio has changed from 2:1 to 10–20:1. The Western diet includes large amounts of oils that are extracted from plants and used for cooking or in prepared foods. These oils (such as corn oil, safflower oil, cottonseed oil, peanut oil, soybean oil) are primarily n-6s. A "Mediterranean" diet consisting of fish, whole grains, olive oil, and less red meat typically has a better ratio of n-6s to n-3s.

6.3 VITAMINS AND MINERALS

Vitamins and minerals are raw materials that the body must have to meet its daily work and activity demands. They rejuvenate and energize cells and help the functioning of all bodily processes. Deficiencies in vitamins and minerals can lead to brittle bones, unhealthy skin and hair, loose teeth, bleeding gums, and even diseases like scurvy, pellagra, and rickets. Low vitamin and mineral levels can also lead to increased susceptibility to infection, slow healing, decreased mental capacity, fatigue, and chronic diseases such as cardiovascular disease, cancer, and osteoporosis [53].

Most American women have a diet that is adequate to avoid or minimize major health problems. However, it is still possible that many women may not be getting all the nutrients they need. This is especially true if women are continuously trying to minimize caloric intake. In fact, as women age their requirements for certain vitamins and minerals increase and there is a greater chance of deficiencies for certain nutrients. Following is an overview of those vitamins and minerals deemed most important for women's healthy aging.

6.3.1 Antioxidants

Antioxidants are compounds which prevent an excess of free radicals from accumulating in the body. An over abundance of free radicals can lead to health problems associated with aging including cancer and heart disease. For this reason, it is recommended that midlife women eat a diet rich in fruits, vegetables, and whole-grain cereal products which contain high levels of the major antioxidant vitamins: A, C, and E. The role of specific antioxidants in promoting health and preventing cancer and heart disease is discussed in the following sections.

6.3.1.1 Vitamin A

There are two categories of vitamin A: preformed vitamin A and provitamin A carotenoid. Preformed vitamin A is found in animal products such as dairy or meat, and it is absorbed mainly in the form of retinol, one of the most bioavailable forms of vitamin A. Provitamin A carotenoids are found mainly in fruits and vegetables. The carotenoid most readily converted to retinol is β-carotene. The Institute of Medicine (IOM) has set the DRI of vitamin A to 700 mcg/day of retinol activity equivalents (RAE) for adult women, most of which should come from β-carotene. Common food sources of vitamin A, both retinol and β-carotene, are found in Table 6.2.

TABLE 6.2
Food Sources of Vitamin A

Food, Serving Size	mcg RAE/Serving	% of US DRI/Serving
Organ meats (liver, giblets), cooked (3 oz)	1490–9126	212–1390
Sweet potato with peel, baked (1 medium)	1096	156
Pumpkin, canned ($\frac{1}{2}$ cup)	953	136
Spinach, cooked from frozen ($\frac{1}{2}$ cup)	573	82
Collards, cooked from frozen ($\frac{1}{2}$ cup)	489	70
Kale, cooked from frozen ($\frac{1}{2}$ cup)	478	68
Carrot, raw (1 small)	301	43
Winter squash, cooked ($\frac{1}{2}$ cup)	268	38
Cantaloupe, raw (¼ of medium melon)	233	33

DRI = 700 mcg/day RAE[a] for women aged 51–70.

[a] RAE = retinol activity equivalents.

Vitamin A, especially in the form of β-carotene, has been suggested to reduce the risk of some reproductive cancers. Studies of the relationship between vitamin A and the two major postmenopausal cancers, ovarian and breast, have yielded different results. Two of three population-based studies found a reduction in ovarian cancer with increased vitamin A [54–56]. Conversely, two of these studies did not show a reduction in breast cancer risk with vitamin A intake [57–59]. In all of these studies, vitamin A came from dietary sources, not supplements.

Overall, epidemiologic studies show strong evidence that vitamin A protects against heart disease. Several of the studies did not examine diet, but rather used levels of vitamin A in plasma as a proxy for vitamin A intake. Three studies found that higher plasma β-carotene was correlated with a decreased incidence of cardiac events such as infarction [60–62]. However, clinical studies which try to estimate the relationship between dietary vitamin A intake and heart disease are less consistent. One study found no association between vitamin A and deaths due to coronary heart disease [63], however, another study of over 87,000 nurses found increased vitamin A and β-carotene intake associated with a decreased risk of CHD [64].

6.3.1.2 Vitamin C

Vitamin C is required for the growth and repair of body tissues. Since the body does not manufacture vitamin C on its own, it is a required nutrient in the diet. All fruits and vegetables contain some vitamin C, although the quantity can vary greatly. A list of foods high in vitamin C can be found in Table 6.3. The US DRI is 75 mg/day for adult women with a tolerable upper limit of 2000 mg/day. It is important to note that high doses may cause nausea and diarrhea [65].

TABLE 6.3
Food Sources of Vitamin C

Food, Serving Size	mg/Serving	% of US DRI/Serving
Red bell pepper, raw ($\frac{1}{2}$ cup)	142	189
Red bell pepper, cooked ($\frac{1}{2}$ cup)	116	155
Kiwi fruit (1 medium)	70	93
Orange, raw (1 medium)	70	93
Orange juice ($\frac{3}{4}$ cup)	61–93	81–124
Green bell pepper, raw ($\frac{1}{2}$ cup)	60	80
Vegetable juice cocktail ($\frac{3}{4}$ cup)	50	67
Strawberries, raw ($\frac{1}{2}$ cup)	49	65
Cantaloupe, raw (¼ of medium melon)	47	63
Broccoli, raw ($\frac{1}{2}$ cup)	39	52
Broccoli, cooked ($\frac{1}{2}$ cup)	37	49
Kale, cooked from frozen ($\frac{1}{2}$ cup)	27	36

DRI = 75 mg/day for women aged 51–70.

High vitamin C intake has been associated with reduced rates of several types of cancer including oral, esophageal, and stomach cancers in observational studies [66–68]. However, the evidence related to vitamin C intake and breast cancer is mixed and somewhat contradictory. Two meta-analyses have found a decreased risk of breast cancer with higher intakes of vitamin C (over 200 mg/day) versus lower intakes (50 mg/day or less) [69,70]. However, a recent case-control study found an increased risk of breast cancer with higher intakes of vitamin C from both dietary and supplement sources [59]. Other studies have shown no relationship between vitamin C intake and breast cancer risk [57,71,72].

To summarize, although vitamin C is a strong antioxidant, it does not appear to prevent or reduce heart disease. Most studies of dietary intake of vitamin C and heart disease show no benefit with higher consumption and those that do show only a modest benefit [63,73–76]. As a form of secondary prevention, vitamin C has not been shown to reduce progression of heart disease in patients [53]. Notwithstanding, it is an important nutrient for overall good health and should be a consistent part of the daily diet.

6.3.1.3 Vitamin E

Vitamin E, like vitamin A, is a group of compounds with antioxidant activity. The two major compounds are the tocopherols and tocotrienols. The form of vitamin E most commonly found in food and supplements is α-tocopherol. Major dietary sources of vitamin E can be found in Table 6.4. For women 51–70 years old, the DRI is 15 mg. Doses up to 800 mg are tolerated without adverse effects, but can be associated with headache, fatigue, nausea, diarrhea, cramping, weakness, and blurred vision [65]. A meta-analysis has shown that doses greater than 400 IU/day (or 266 mg/day) may increase the risk of all-cause mortality [77].

TABLE 6.4
Food Sources of Vitamin E

Food, Serving Size	mg AT/Serving	% of US DRI/Serving
Fortified ready-to-eat cereals (~1 oz)	1.6–12.8	11–85
Almonds (1 oz)	7.3	49
Mixed nuts (1 oz)	3.1	21
Tomato paste (¼ cup)	2.8	18
Peanut butter (2 tbsp)	2.5	17
Tomato sauce ($\frac{1}{2}$ cup)	2.5	17
Canola oil (1 tbsp)	2.4	16
Peanuts (1 oz)	2.2	15
Avocado, raw ($\frac{1}{2}$ medium)	2.1	14
Olive oil (1 tbsp)	1.9	13
Spinach, cooked from frozen ($\frac{1}{2}$ cup)	1.9	13

DRI = 15 mg/day of α-tocopherol (AT) for women aged 51–70.

Although touted for years for cancer prevention, vitamin E has not been associated with a reduced risk of cancers in women. However, there is evidence from the Nurses Health Study that long-term vitamin E supplementation may reduce the risk of heart disease. Women in this study who took vitamin E supplements containing a median of 208 IU/day for over 2 years had a 44% reduced risk of coronary disease compared to the lowest intake group [73]. Also, a study of over 34,000 postmenopausal women found that vitamin E consumption from food was associated with a lower risk of death from cardiovascular disease [63].

Because of the reported positive association between vitamin E supplementation and heart disease, many clinical trials have investigated this link. In contrast to the observational study results, these trials have not found a positive association between supplementation with vitamin E and heart disease. Two large, randomized trials of high-risk patients found no decrease in cardiovascular events for those taking vitamin E [78,79]. The WHI, a 10 year randomized controlled trial, found no association between vitamin E and the incidence of cardiovascular events in healthy postmenopausal women [80].

Overall, antioxidants are beneficial to health, but seem to be able to do only so much for prevention of disease. High doses of supplementation should be avoided and most women should be able to get a beneficial level of antioxidants with a diet high in fruits and vegetables.

6.3.2 B-Vitamins

The B-vitamins are a group of eight vitamins: vitamin B_1 (Thiamine), vitamin B_2 (Riboflavin), vitamin B_3 (Niacin), vitamin B_5 (Pantothenic acid), vitamin B_6 (Pyridoxine), vitamin B_7 (Biotin), vitamin B_9 (Folate or Folic acid), and vitamin B_{12}. vitamins B_6, B_{12}, and folate are critical for a healthy cardiovascular system because of their action on homocysteines [81]. Increased levels of homocysteine in the blood cause damage to blood vessels and have been linked to cardiovascular disease [82]. Several clinical trials demonstrate that adequate levels of these B-vitamins help to maintain normal homocysteine metabolism [81,83–85].

Most research suggests that B-vitamins can reduce heart disease in a healthy population [86–88]. However, clinical trials have found that supplementation with B-complex does not prevent cardiovascular disease in high-risk populations (e.g., previous MI, vascular disease, chronic renal failure, or diabetes) [89–91].

6.3.2.1 Vitamin B_6

Vitamin B_6 (or pyridoxine) is a component of a large number of enzymes and necessary for body system optimal function. Some important enzymes that require vitamin B_6 are responsible for amino acid (protein) metabolism, formation of essential fatty acids, and formation of some neurotransmitters. Research has shown that vitamin B_6 is beneficial for maintaining nerve health, hormonal balance in premenstrual women, healthy lung function, and improving magnesium absorption into cells [92–94]. The US DRI for B_6 is 1.5 mcg. Over doing of vitamin B_6 supplements can cause temporary nerve problems and can interfere with normal milk production of breast-feeding women [95]. Food sources for B_6 can be found in Table 6.5.

TABLE 6.5
Food Sources of Vitamin B_6

Food, Serving Size	mg/Serving	% of US DRI/Serving
Banana, raw (1 medium)	0.68	45
Garbanzo beans, canned ($\frac{1}{2}$ cup)	0.57	38
Chicken breast, cooked ($\frac{1}{2}$ breast)	0.52	35
Spinach, frozen, cooked ($\frac{1}{2}$ cup)	0.14	9
Tomato juice, canned (6 oz)	0.20	13
Avocado, raw ($\frac{1}{2}$ cup)	0.20	13
Tuna, canned in water, drained solids (3 oz)	0.18	12
Peanut butter (2 tbsp)	0.15	10

DRI = 1.5 mg/day for women aged 51–70.

6.3.2.2 Vitamin B_{12}

B_{12} is an essential nutrient which supports energy and memory, appetite, and digestion. It is important for the maintenance of a healthy nervous system and is considered by many to play an important role as an antiaging nutrient. Many of the functions of vitamin B_{12}, such as building blood cells, promoting DNA synthesis, naturally interfering with inflammation, and strengthening the immune system are fundamental to a healthy body [96]. Marginal vitamin B_{12} deficiency is fairly common, particularly among the elderly and such deficiencies are associated with difficulties in thinking, poor memory, low energy, high homocysteine levels, and a weakened immune system [97–100]. The US DRI for B_{12} is 2.4 mcg. As women age, they do not process B_{12} from food as well as they once did. Therefore it is recommended that older women acquire their DRI of B-vitamins, especially B_{12}, from fortified food and supplements [101]. Food sources for B_{12} can be found in Table 6.6.

TABLE 6.6
Food Sources of Vitamin B_{12}

Food, Serving Size	mcg/Serving	% of US DRI/Serving
Beef, lean, broiled (3 oz)	2.4	100
Yogurt, plain, skim (1 cup)	1.4	58
Tuna, canned in water, drained solids (3 oz)	1.0	42
Milk (1 cup)	0.9	38
Egg, hard boiled (1 whole)	0.6	25
American pasteurized cheese food (1 oz)	0.3	13
Chicken breast, cooked ($\frac{1}{2}$ breast)	0.3	13

DRI = 2.4 mcg/day for women aged 51–70.

6.3.2.3 Folate/Folic Acid

Folate and folic acid are forms of a water-soluble B vitamin. Folate occurs naturally in food and folic acid is the synthetic form of this vitamin that is found in supplements and fortified foods. Folate is necessary for the production and maintenance of new cells and is needed to build normal red blood cells and prevent anemia. Folate is needed to make DNA and RNA, the building blocks of cells; it also helps prevent changes to DNA that may lead to cancer. A recent study found that older adults with higher folate intake from both diet and supplements were 50% less likely to develop Alzheimer's disease. Since folate lowers blood levels of homocysteine, folate may help to decrease the risk of brain atrophy [102].

Leafy greens such as spinach and turnip greens, dry beans and peas, fortified cereals and grain products, and some fruits and vegetables are rich food sources of folate. Some breakfast cereals (ready-to-eat and others) are fortified with 25% or 100% of the daily value (DV) for folic acid. The US DRI for folate is 400 mcg/day. Folic acid consumption should be limited to 1000 mcg/day from all sources, according to the FDA. Food sources for folate can be found in Table 6.7.

6.3.3 Calcium

In women, the amount of bone tissue in the skeleton, known as bone mass, continues to accumulate until around age 30. At that point, bones have reached their maximum strength, known as peak bone mass or peak bone mineral density (BMD). In women, there tends to be minimal change in total bone mass between age 30 and menopause. But in the first few years after menopause, most women experience rapid bone loss, which then slows, but can continue throughout the postmenopausal years [103–105].

Calcium is an essential nutrient for bone health. Several studies have suggested that supplementation with 500–1000 mg/day calcium and 200–400 IU vitamin D can maintain BMD or decrease bone loss. These studies even suggest that for women who were very compliant with treatment, there was also a significant reduction in hip fractures [106,107]. The combination of calcium with vitamin D is critical [108]. A 1994 Consensus Conference at the National Institutes of Health recommended that

TABLE 6.7
Food Sources of Folate/Folic Acid

Food, Serving Size	mcg/Serving	% of US DRI/Serving
Lentils, cooked ($\frac{1}{2}$ cup)	180	45
Asparagus, cooked ($\frac{1}{2}$ cup)	132	33
Spinach, cooked ($\frac{1}{2}$ cup)	131	33
Kidney beans ($\frac{1}{2}$ cup)	115	29
Tomato juice (1 cup)	48	12
Orange (1 medium)	47	12

DRI = 400 mcg/day for women aged 51–70.

TABLE 6.8
Food Sources of Calcium

Food, Serving Size	mg/Serving	% of US DRI/Serving
Dairy sources		
Plain, nonfat yogurt (1 cup)	452	38
Swiss cheese (1.5 oz)	336	28
Ricotta cheese, part skim ($\frac{1}{2}$ cup)	335	28
American cheese, pasteurized, processed (2 oz)	323	27
Mozzarella cheese, part skim (1.5 oz)	311	26
Cheddar cheese (1.5 oz)	307	25
Fat-free (skim) milk (1 cup)	306	25
Nondairy sources		
Soy beverage, calcium fortified (1 cup)	368	31
Collards, cooked from frozen ($\frac{1}{2}$ cup)	178	15
Molasses, blackstrap (1 tbsp)	172	14
Spinach, cooked from frozen ($\frac{1}{2}$ cup)	146	12
Soybeans, green, cooked ($\frac{1}{2}$ cup)	130	11
White beans, canned ($\frac{1}{2}$ cup)	96	8

DRI = 1200 mg/day for women aged 51–70.

peri- and postmenopausal women consume 1500 mg/day through food sources and supplementation [109]. Foods high in calcium include milk, yogurt, cheese, and other dairy products; oysters, sardines, and canned salmon with bones; and dark-green leafy vegetables like spinach and broccoli. Table 6.8 lists good sources of dietary calcium with their respective calcium content.

Many women of peri- and postmenopausal age do not meet the recommended daily dietary calcium intake [110]. Studies have found that among women 50–59 years old, the average calcium intake was 651 mg/day, a little over half the recommended dose. Compliance varies by race with Mexican-American women consuming the highest (701 mg/day) and African-American women the lowest amount (564 mg/day) [111].

For women who wish to supplement their diet with calcium tablets, calcium carbonate or calcium citrate is the most concentrated, and most easily absorbed by the body when taken with food [112]. Synthetic calcium carbonate should be used, rather than natural derivations from bone or shells which may contain lead [112]. Calcium citrate is the preferred source of calcium as it may provide greater protection against bone loss [113]. Absorbability of different calcium compounds is similar when taken with food [114,115]. No more than 500 mg of calcium can be absorbed at a time, so intake should be distributed throughout the day [116]. Eating foods high in vitamin C or taking a supplement can improve absorption of calcium [112].

Calcium intake in excess of the recommended allowances has no recognized health benefits, and more than 2500 mg/day can increase the risk of hypercalcemia (elevated calcium levels in the blood) and chronic overdosing can result in renal or bladder stones [103,116]. It is difficult to know how much calcium to take as supplemental in addition to normal dietary intake. It is generally thought that most women consume about 500–600 mg/day as typical intake from diet, suggesting that supplementation should be about 900–1000 mg/day [117]. For women who consume more of their calcium through food sources, less supplementation is needed.

A large segment of the population is lactose intolerant (cannot digest milk products), especially African-American, American-Indian, and Asian women [118]. In such cases alternatives to the usual source of calcium, such as acidophilus or soy milk, are recommended since they are more digestible [103].

Calcium may have other benefits including protection against certain cancers, although the data are limited. Animal studies have suggested that calcium can protect against colon cancer [119]. Human research has shown similar trends in epidemiological research; however, clinical trials have demonstrated inconsistent results [120–124].

Similarly, there appears to be a promising relationship between calcium and breast cancer risk. Among postmenopausal women, intake of vitamin D and calcium was not found to be associated with increased breast density, a risk factor for breast cancer [125]. There has even been some positive evidence of a protective effect of calcium on breast cancer. Women with higher intake of dietary calcium (>1250 mg/day) were at lower risk of breast cancer than were women who consumed <500 mg/day [126], although the level of protection seemed to diminish with age [46].

Several observational studies have even suggested a relationship between calcium intake and body mass or weight change. Women who reported taking calcium supplements gained significantly less weight over a 10 year period as compared to women who did not take supplements [127]. A weight-loss intervention trial of pre- and postmenopausal women demonstrated that those who consumed 1000 mg/day calcium lost more weight and fat than those not using calcium [128].

6.3.4 Vitamin D

Vitamin D is important for calcium absorption and bone formation. The National Academy of Sciences suggests 400 IU of vitamin D for women 51–70, and 600 IU for women 71 and older. The Osteoporosis Society of Canada recommends that all women over 50 years old consume 800 IU/day. The North American Menopause Society and the National Osteoporosis Foundation suggest that women at risk of vitamin D deficiency because of inadequate sunlight exposure consume up to 800 IU/day [116]. Exposure to sunlight triggers vitamin D synthesis in the skin, but older women do not convert sunlight into essential vitamin D as efficiently as when they were younger [129].

Dietary consumption of vitamin D by adults over 50 is generally low, with only 4% meeting the requirement through food alone. However, even when total intake through food and supplements is considered, only 32% of women 50 years and older meet adequate intake levels [130]. Studies have shown that the benefit of vitamin D supplementation increases with age [131]. Higher than recommended doses of vitamin D can cause kidney stones, constipation, or abdominal pain, particularly in women with existing kidney problems. The IOM indicates that 2000 IU/day is the tolerable upper limit. Table 6.9 provides good food sources for vitamin D.

TABLE 6.9
Food Sources of Vitamin D

Food, Serving Size	mcg/Serving (IU)	% of US DRI/Serving
Salmon, cooked (3 $\frac{1}{2}$ oz)	9 mcg (360 IU)	90
Milk, skim, vitamin D fortified (1 cup)	2.5 mcg (98 IU)	25
Liver, beef, cooked (3 $\frac{1}{2}$ oz)	0.75 mcg (30 IU)	8
Egg (1 whole)	0.63 mcg (25 IU)	6

DRI = 10 mcg/day (or 400 IU) for women aged 51–70.

Supplementing calcium with vitamin D has been shown to have positive effects on bone mineral density, falls, and fracture rate [107,132–135]. Studies comparing calcium and vitamin D supplementation to calcium alone have also found a decrease in the risk of falling for those using both supplements. The additional benefit of vitamin D may be due to an improvement in neuromuscular or musculoskeletal function [136,137].

6.3.5 Iron

Adequate dietary iron is needed for the blood to transport sufficient oxygen throughout the body. Severe iron deficiency can result in anemia, and can impair the body's ability to fight infection [51]. However, over consumption can be toxic, and thus iron supplements should be used with caution. The US DRI for iron is 8 mg/day for women 50 years old and older, and the tolerable upper limit is 45 mg/day. According to National Institutes of Health (NIH), postmenopausal women are at low risk of iron deficiency, and in fact iron stores increase after menopause, in part due to cessation of menstrual periods [138].

Research suggests that perimenopausal women, especially those with frequent or heavy menses, may not meet the recommended intake levels for iron, and African American women appear to have the lowest intake of iron [110]. Vegetarian women may also be at increased risk of iron deficiency, due to the fact that iron from nonheme (non red meat) sources such as beans or lentils is not absorbed as readily [139]. However, most midlife women can get adequate iron through food sources including meats, beans, lentils, soybeans, and spinach.

6.3.6 Magnesium

Magnesium enables the body to metabolize calcium, helping to maintain bone mass [140,141]. Human and animal studies have demonstrated that magnesium deficiency can result in bone loss and that supplementation with magnesium may prevent osteoporosis but this has not been adequately tested in clinical trials [103,141,142]. Magnesium deficiency may also lead to insulin resistance, cardiovascular disease, and may also affect the metabolism of potassium and cholesterol [143,144].

In women with premenstrual syndrome (PMS), magnesium supplementation has been shown to reduce water retention, improve mood, and reduce headaches [145–148]. The US DRI for magnesium for women 51 years and older is 320 mg/day. Good sources of magnesium in food are whole grains, vegetables (broccoli, squash), nuts, and seeds [103]. Dairy products and meats also contribute magnesium to a diet, as well as chocolate and coffee, depending on the amount consumed [103]. "Hard" water contains high concentrations of magnesium, and can be considered a dietary source [103].

6.3.7 Potassium

Potassium is an essential dietary mineral that helps the kidneys function normally. The regulation of potassium concentrations plays a key role in cardiac, skeletal, and smooth muscle contraction, making it an important nutrient for normal heart, digestive, and muscular function [51,149]. Having too much potassium in the blood is called hyperkalemia and having too little in the blood is known as hypokalemia. Proper balance of potassium in the body depends on sodium. Therefore, excessive use of sodium may deplete the body's stores of potassium. Other conditions that can cause potassium deficiency include diarrhea, vomiting, excessive sweating, malnutrition, and use of diuretics. In addition, coffee and alcohol can increase the amount of potassium excreted in the urine. Adequate amounts of magnesium are also needed to maintain normal levels of potassium.

Potassium has also been shown to be associated with bone mineral density, and thus adequate consumption may help to prevent osteoporosis [150,151]. The US DRI for potassium is 4.7 g/day. Fruits (including citrus fruits and raisins), vegetables (especially spinach and potatoes), and nuts (such as almond, cashew, peanut) are good sources of potassium [51].

For most people, a healthy diet rich in vegetables and fruits provides all of the potassium needed. As women age, they become at higher risk for developing hyperkalemia due to decreased kidney function that can occur as one ages [152]. Older women should be cautious when taking medication that may further affect potassium levels in the body, such as medications for water retention, nonsteroidal anti-inflammatory drugs (NSAID), and angiotensin-converting enzyme inhibitors.

6.3.8 Trace Minerals: Zinc and Copper

Trace minerals such as zinc and copper are important in small quantities to ensure good health. It is important to maintain adequate levels of zinc and copper in the diet to prevent and treat osteoporosis. A zinc deficiency is associated with decreases in bone density. Likewise, copper is an important mineral in the normal growth and development of the skeletal system. Zinc and copper are also both important in maintaining proper magnesium balance [144,153]. The DRIs for zinc and copper are 8 mg/day and 900 mcg/day, respectively. Good food sources that contain zinc include nuts, primarily peanuts, brazil nuts and pecans, oats, oysters, pumpkin seeds, rye, and split peas. Food sources that contain copper include buckwheat, crab, liver, mushrooms, peanut butter, seeds and nuts, split peas, and vegetable oils (sunflower, olive).

6.4 BOTANICALS AND DIETARY SUPPLEMENTS

Ever since the results of the WHI, which reported an increased risk of breast cancer and other adverse outcomes associated with the use of hormone therapies, many women are turning to botanical and dietary supplement (BDS) products for relief of menopausal symptoms and prevention and treatment of chronic health conditions associated with aging. Botanical products are derived from plant extracts and women throughout the world have been using these extracts for hundreds of years to treat uterine disorders, menstrual complaints, pregnancy, and childbirth. Most BDS appear to have no toxic effects; however, rigorous long-term safety trials are rare [154,155].

The use of BDS among menopausal women has increased exponentially in recent years [156–158]. In the United States and Britain, surveys show that 80% of peri- and postmenopausal women are current or former users of dietary supplements. In these surveys, a majority of women cited two primary beliefs: (1) BDS supplements were good for one's health and (2) use of these herbal products is natural and safe and therefore cannot hurt them. Consequently, women rarely discuss use of BDS with their health care providers, nor do clinicians ask their patients about use of these therapies [156,159,160].

In most countries of the world, botanicals are not well regulated by federal agencies. In the United States, botanicals are classified by the Dietary Supplement Health Education Act (DSHEA) as dietary supplements, not drugs, and are not intended for diagnosis, prevention, or treatment. Therefore they are not regulated by the Food and Drug Administration (FDA). This classification results in considerable variability of content, standardization, dosage, purity, and possible contamination of available products. The European Food Safety Authority has only recently begun to address the issue of botanical safety and purity regulation for its member states [161]. By contrast, dietary supplements have been scrutinized for safety and efficacy by the German Commission E, a health regulatory body that regulates dietary supplements, for over two decades [162].

Following is an overview of BDS products that are commonly used by peri- and postmenopausal women. These substances are used for complaints of menopause including vasomotor symptoms, depression, anxiety, and poor sleep, as well as for prevention and treatment of health conditions related to aging such as heart disease, osteoporosis, and cognitive problems. Additional information on use of BDS for menopause and related conditions can be found in papers by Geller et al. [16,17,163,164].

6.4.1 Black Cohosh (*Cimicifuga racemosa*)

Black cohosh is a perennial plant native to North America and a member of the buttercup family. It is one of the most commonly used botanicals to treat vasomotor symptoms during perimenopause [165]. Black cohosh contains triterpene glycosides, flavonoids, aromatic acids, and other constituents. Because of its effect on hot flashes, black cohosh was presumed to have estrogenic activity, however, studies show no effect on serum hormone levels (e.g., luteinizing hormone [LH], follicle stimulating hormone [FSH], prolactin, sex hormone binding globulin [SHBG], and estradiol) [166]. Additionally, animal studies using black cohosh extracts have found no estrogenic increases in uterine weight or stimulation of vaginal and breast tissue [167–169]. Recent data, in fact, has demonstrated that black cohosh acts on serotonin receptors which may be the mechanism for relief of hot flashes and improvement in mood [170,171].

Much of the research on black cohosh has been conducted in Germany since the 1940s. The German Commission E has approved the use of 40 mg/day of black cohosh for 6 months for relief of menopausal symptoms, primarily vasomotor symptoms, and mood disorders [172]. Over 15 clinical trials related to vasomotor symptoms have shown very promising results for relief of menopausal symptoms, primarily hot flashes and mood swings [173–188].

However, a recent clinical trial, Herbal Alternatives (HALT) for Menopause Study, tested the efficacy of black cohosh alone or as a multibotanical supplement (black cohosh and a number of other herbs) and did not find a statistically significant effect for either formulation. This study contradicts several randomized clinical trials conducted in over 3000 women using black cohosh for climacteric/vasomotor symptoms [189]. The vast majority of studies found overwhelmingly positive evidence of the efficacy and safety of black cohosh primarily for relief of vasomotor symptoms.

Black cohosh has been reported to have a positive safety profile when used for up to 6 months; however, in Germany, many women use this herbal remedy for longer periods of time with physician oversight [190]. The most commonly reported side effects are mild gastric complaints, which tend to dissipate over time although high doses may cause headaches, vomiting, and dizziness [181].

There have been no documented cases of drug interactions [191]. Of recent concern are a few case reports of liver failure in women using black cohosh [192–195]. It is not clear what the contribution of black cohosh was, if any, in these cases. Many questions remain about the composition and purity of the products that were used as well as the multiple comorbidities and the concomitant medications of the women using black cohosh. The US National Institutes of Health (NIH) has released findings from a workshop on the safety of black cohosh in clinical trials which concluded "at this time there is no known mechanism with biological plausibility that explains any hepatotoxic activity of black cohosh." [196]. They also note that millions of women have taken black cohosh with very few adverse events reported. In contrast to the US, the UK Medicines and Healthcare Products Regulatory Agency (MHRA) announced that it was introducing labeling of products containing black cohosh warning of the possibility of rare liver problems. This coincided with a public safety statement from the European Medicines Agency (EMEA) on black cohosh [197].

Previous studies on both in vitro investigations with breast cancer cells and in vivo data show no stimulation of estrogen-dependent mammary gland tumors with black cohosh [166,168,174–176]. In fact, black cohosh has been suggested for relief of vasomotor symptoms for women with breast cancer who are on tamoxifen, largely because of its presumed serotonergic rather than estrogenic effect. Two of three studies of black cohosh for women on tamoxifen have shown a significant reduction in number and severity of hot flashes as compared to placebo as well as improvement in sleep, fatigue levels, and abnormal sweating [186–188].

There has been almost no research on black cohosh to study health conditions associated with aging such as heart disease, osteoporosis, and fracture, although one study compared the effects of black cohosh, conjugated estrogens, and placebo on menopausal symptoms as well as bone markers. The investigators found that black cohosh had an equivalent effect to conjugated estrogens on significantly improving both menopausal symptoms and bone markers compared to placebo [179].

In summary, black cohosh shows great promise for relief of menopausal symptoms, primarily for the treatment of vasomotor symptoms and perhaps depression with an overall positive safety profile for at least six months and likely longer. However, any women with a history of liver problems should not use black cohosh.

6.4.2 Phytoestrogens (Soy and Red Clover)

Botanicals and dietary supplements can be divided into two broad categories—plants that exhibit "estrogen-like" properties (phytoestrogens which are weak estrogens) and plants that do not exhibit these characteristics. Isoflavones belong to the class of compounds known as phytoestrogens, which have structural and functional similarities to human estrogen, 17-β estradiol [198]. These compounds mimic estrogen but are thousands of times weaker than the hormone. The major phytoestrogens used by women are soy and red clover for treatment of menopausal symptoms and conditions related to aging.

Soy isoflavones have been consumed in large quantities across the world for centuries and are commonly used by midlife women, either in food, protein supplement, or isoflavone tablet form. Soy contains very high amounts of isoflavones, particularly genistein, daidzein, and glycitein. These are readily absorbed and metabolized in the gut and are well tolerated without reported adverse effects [199].

Similar to soy, red clover is a rich source of isoflavones; however, it has a distinct chemical profile from soy with higher levels of *O*-methylated isoflavones, formononetin, and biochanin A, and less daidzein and genistein than soy [200,201]. The commercially available red clover extracts are the hydrolyzed form of the isoflavones to enhance bioavailability by gut bacteria and are easily absorbed in the intestine [202].

6.4.2.1 Menopausal Symptoms

Although isoflavones from soy and red clover are the most heavily studied plant for alleviation of menopausal symptoms, evidence from the more rigorous trials shows, at best, only a modest to minimal effect on vasomotor symptoms [16,203,204]. However, many women continue to use isoflavones as a daily part of their diet because they may have other health benefits beyond that of menopausal symptoms such as prevention and treatment for heart disease, osteoporosis, and cognitive impairments.

6.4.2.2 Prevention and Treatment of Common Complaints of Midlife and Aging

6.4.2.2.1 Heart Disease

Heart disease is a leading cause of death for women throughout the world and many women are trying to control their cholesterol as one means of prevention [205,206]. Several studies have suggested that soy and red clover can reduce overall cholesterol, lower LDL and triglycerides, and raise HDL [17]. The FDA has approved a health claim for isoflavone-rich soy protein stating that consumption of 25 g of soy protein daily can reduce cholesterol levels [18]. The German Commission E has also approved soy (as soy lecithin or soy phospholipid) for hypercholesterolemia [172].

A meta-analysis of 38 controlled human studies (including both men and women) of soy consumption found that individuals who replaced animal protein with soy protein had a significant decrease in overall cholesterol and LDL cholesterol concentrations compared to those who consumed protein from animal sources [207]. Individuals with higher initial serum cholesterol concentrations had a greater absolute and percent change in cholesterol levels compared to people with lower initial cholesterol.

There have been 21 randomized, controlled trials of soy foods, soy supplements, or soy isoflavone supplements for lipid changes specifically in peri- and postmenopausal women and about one-half of the studies found a significant lipid-lowering effect of soy compared to placebo [208–216].

Since red clover contains isoflavones similar to soy, researchers have hypothesized that it would also positively affect lipid profiles. There have been six randomized controlled trials (RCTs) of red clover isoflavones in peri- and postmenopausal women, and five of the six studies found some positive effect of red clover isoflavones on lipids, either increased HDL or decreased triglycerides [217–222].

Thus far, the literature has demonstrated that isoflavones from soy or red clover may be useful for reducing serum cholesterol levels in postmenopausal women. Soy appears to reduce total cholesterol levels and LDL cholesterol, while red clover reduced triglycerides and increased HDL cholesterol. It is important to note that the cholesterol-lowering benefits of soy protein are lost when isoflavones are separated from the protein portion [17].

6.4.2.2.2 Osteoporosis

The incidence of osteoporosis is increasing worldwide as populations age and women are four times more likely than men to develop osteoporosis [223]. By year 2010, 35 million women in the United States alone will either have osteoporosis or be at risk of developing this condition [224]. Soy and red clover have been hypothesized to have a positive effect on bone mineral density as women age [17]. Data from several observational studies has suggested that populations with a high mean intake of dietary soy, such as Japan, have a lower incidence of osteoporotic fractures compared to Western populations [225,226]. However, when comparisons are made between populations, issues such as amount and type of soy consumption, physical activity, and other lifestyle factors limit the results [227,228].

Fourteen randomized, controlled trials have been conducted to examine the effects of soy on bone mineral density (BMD) in peri- and postmenopausal women [208,210,227,229–240]. Seven studies found that BMD was significantly higher after supplementation with isoflavone tablet, isolated soy protein, or soy foods, compared to placebo [210,229–234]. A large cohort study that followed 75,000 Chinese women between the ages of 40 and 70 reported that high soy protein consumption (11–18 g) was linked with a 48% decrease in fractures for women within 10 years of menopause [241]. Similarly, an RCT conducted in China with nonobese, early postmenopausal women found a positive effect of soy isoflavones on attenuating bone loss at the spine and femoral neck [242].

The bone preserving effects of red clover have also been examined, but not as extensively as that of soy. Of the three randomized controlled trials of red clover isoflavones for bone loss, two of the trials demonstrated a positive effect of red clover on bone mineral density [218,219,221]. Although the evidence is still limited, it appears that red clover isoflavones may have a helpful effect on bone mineral density in peri- and postmenopausal women.

6.4.2.2.3 Cognition and Memory

Cognitive problems and forgetfulness are common complaints for peri- and postmenopausal women [243]. Few studies have been published examining the relationship between isoflavones found in soy or red clover on cognitive function in postmenopausal women. Three of the four studies of soy for cognition found a positive effect, with improvements in short-term memory, frontal lobe function, mental flexibility, planning ability, category fluency, and sustained attention [237,244–246]. The only study of red clover isoflavones for cognitive function found no difference between treatment and control groups [222]. It appears that soy isoflavones could have positive effects on cognitive function in postmenopausal women; however, more research is needed for both soy and red clover isoflavones.

6.4.2.3 Side Effects and Safety

The most commonly reported side effects of soy are gastrointestinal complaints such as stomach pain, loose stool, and diarrhea [172]. Soy should be avoided if an allergy exists. Other side effects reported for red clover are mild and include headache, myalgia, and nausea [247].

Overall, isoflavones from both soy and red clover have positive safety profiles. Soy has not been found to increase the risk of endometrial cancer or endometrial hyperplasia [248,249], with one study showing higher intake of soy isoflavones linked to a decreased risk of endometrial cancer. However, one long-term 5 year trial of the effects of soy isoflavone on endometrial tissue found a significantly increased incidence of endometrial hyperplasia in the group taking soy isoflavone. The increased incidence was small (3.7% versus 0%), and no cases of endometrial cancer were reported [250]. Red clover also has a positive safety profile and appears not to negatively affect the endometrium [251], although there have been very few studies that specifically investigated this relationship.

Soy and red clover isoflavones have been studied both in vitro and in animal models to examine the risk of breast cancer. In vitro studies of both soy and red clover isoflavones show that they do not promote breast cell proliferation. Furthermore, animal models show a 25%–50% reduction in tumors for animals consuming soy protein compared to animals consuming other protein sources [252–255].

Human studies show no negative effect on the breast and some have suggested a protective effect of soy on breast tissue. Several case-control studies in Asian countries have demonstrated decreased rates of breast cancer [228,243,256]. It is interesting to note, however, that when Asian women move to the United States, their cancer risk increases. The presumed protective effect of soy isoflavones may have been a combination of several factors including the consumption of soy early in life, a low-fat and high-fiber diet, lower body mass index (BMI), as well as a less sedentary lifestyle. It is important to note that the effect of soy on breast cancer is somewhat controversial. Further research is recommended to determine the safety of soy food and soy isoflavones for women at high risk of breast cancer and breast cancer patients [257].

6.4.3 Other Botanicals Commonly Used for Menopause and Aging

Many other botanicals are commonly used for menopausal complaints as well as prevention for chronic conditions related to aging. These include licorice root (*Glycyrrhiza glabra*), dong quai (*Angelica sinensis*), rhubarb (*Rheum rhaponticum*), chastetree (*Vitex agnus-castus*), wild yam (*Dioscorea villosa*), evening primrose (*Oenothera biennis*), ginkgo (*Ginkgo biloba*), ginseng (*Panax ginseng*), kava (*Piper methysticum*), valerian (*Valeriana officinalis*), motherwort (*Leonurus cardiaca*), and St. John's Wort (*Hypericum perforatum*). Chastetree, wild yam, and evening primrose are more commonly used for premenstrual syndrome (PMS) and early menopausal symptoms. Other botanicals are used primarily for sleep disturbances, nervousness, depression, mood swings, and memory loss (e.g., ginkgo, motherwort, ginseng, valerian, kava, and St. John's wort) [163].

Most of these products have not been studied for safety and efficacy in peri- and postmenopausal women. As such, the findings related to sleep, anxiety, and mood cannot necessarily be extrapolated to the menopausal experience. Additionally, many of the botanicals are used in combination with other extracts, in the form of a multibotanical, of which there is even less data for efficacy and safety. For example, licorice is not often used on its own, but as part of a multibotanical remedy for menopause. Since it is thought that doses as little as 500 mg/day for 7 days are associated with congestive heart failure and most menopausal remedies contain about 150–225 mg of licorice a day, it is important to be aware of the amount of licorice root peri- and postmenopausal women are consuming [258].

6.4.3.1 Menopausal Symptoms

6.4.3.1.1 Dong Quai (Angelica sinensis)

Dong quai is one of the most commonly prescribed Chinese herbs for problems unique to women [259]. It is known as a "female tonic" and is used by herbalists across the world for a variety of menstrual problems (both abnormal menstruation and menopausal symptoms), however, little research has been done to demonstrate the safety and efficacy of dong quai for menopausal symptoms. One study that compared dong quai to placebo for relief of hot flashes found no effect but also showed no stimulation of the endometrium for either group, suggesting a nonestrogenic effect [260]. Another more recent study of a product containing dong quai and chamomile found a significant reductions in hot flashes [261]. Taken alone, dong quai does not appear to be beneficial for menopausal symptoms; however, it is most commonly used in multibotanical formulations and is still considered to be a valuable female tonic by herbalists around the world.

6.4.3.1.2 Rhubarb (*Rheum rhaponticum*)

A rhubarb extract from the roots of Sibiric rhubarb, referred to as rhapontic rhubarb, has been used in Germany for decades for women with menstrual irregularities as well as women with climacteric complaints in peri- and postmenopause. It was approved by the German Commission E in 2005 as a treatment for symptoms associated with menopause. This rhubarb plant originates from Central Asia, was introduced into Europe in the seventeenth century, and has been used in Western Europe, East Asia, and the United States. The mechanism of action of rhubarb is only partially understood. Preliminary results from endometrial cells show no estrogenic activity [262,263].

A recent 12 week clinical trial conducted in Germany evaluated the efficacy and safety of Sibiric rhubarb compared with placebo in perimenopausal women with climacteric complaints. The rhubarb group had significantly decreased number and severity of hot flushes as well as overall improved quality of life, including improved sleep disturbances, depressive mood, irritability, and anxiety. There were no differences in gynecological findings and other clinical parameters including endometrial biopsies, bleeding, weight, blood pressure, pulse, and laboratory safety parameters between the treatment groups. No adverse events were classified as being related to the investigational medication [264]. This study is promising but there is limited clinical data and no long-term safety data on this extract.

It is important to distinguish this particular rhubarb species (*Rheum rhaponticum*) from all the other rhubarb plants (*Rheum palmatum*, *Rheum officinale*). The extract of this rhubarb has a different spectrum of constituents and does not contain any anthraquinones, a concern for liver toxicity, as compared to the other rhubarb extracts which are used as laxatives [264].

6.4.3.1.3 Chastetree (*Vitex agnus-castus*)

Chastetree/Vitex has been approved by German health authorities for PMS, breast tenderness, and irregularities in the menstrual cycle and is often recommended for women in early menopause experiencing irregular menstrual cycles [172]. The progesterone-like effect of Vitex has been verified by endometrial biopsy, analysis of blood hormone levels, and examination of vaginal secretions [265]. The majority of research has been limited to PMS and breast tenderness and very little is known about the efficacy related to menopausal symptoms. The only study of Chastetree alone in peri- and postmenopausal women reported improvement in mood and hot flashes, although the study had no placebo or comparison group [266]. Most often, when Chastetree is used for menopause it is in combination with black cohosh and other herbs.

6.4.3.1.4 Wild Yam (*Dioscorea villosa*)

Wild yam has historically been used for menstrual cramps and postpartum pain. The only RCT of topical wild yam cream showed no difference in alleviation of menopausal symptoms or serum/salivary hormone levels compared to placebo [267]. Despite promotional claims, wild yam does not appear to convert to progesterone when taken internally or applied topically and although popular for menopause, there is no evidence of benefit.

6.4.3.1.5 *Evening Primrose (Oenothera biennis)*

Evening primrose contains gamma-linolenic acid which is believed to reduce vasomotor symptoms [268]. The only RCT of evening primrose for menopausal symptoms found no differences in the reduction of hot flashes between the placebo and evening primrose groups [269].

6.4.3.2 Prevention and Treatment of Common Complaints of Midlife and Aging

6.4.3.2.1 *Ginkgo (Ginkgo biloba)*

Ginkgo biloba has been approved by the German Commission E for cerebral insufficiency, vertigo and tinnitus, and peripheral vascular disease [172,270–272]. Ginkgo is thought to increase blood flow to the brain, thereby increasing uptake of glucose by brain cells and improving transmission of nerve signals [270]. A review of 40 clinical trials conducted 20 years ago in both men and women examined the effect of ginkgo on improved memory and cognition and 7 of the most rigorous trials showed a positive effect of ginkgo over placebo for memory complaints and cognitive tests [270]. A systematic review published in 2002 found benefits for ginkgo over placebo for cognition, mood, and emotional function, although there was no analysis for peri- or postmenopausal women alone. There were no differences in adverse events between placebo and control groups [273].

There have been only three studies that examined the effects of ginkgo in perimenopausal women with two of the trials having reported positive effects of ginkgo over placebo for memory and cognitive functions [274,275]. Gingko can theoretically inhibit platelet activating factor and therefore should not be used by patients on aspirin or warfarin [276].

6.4.3.2.2 *Ginseng (Panax ginseng)*

Ginseng is known as a traditional "tonic" herb that is reported to cope with stress, and boost immunity. The German Commission E lists its uses as "a tonic for invigoration and fortification in times of fatigue and debility and for declining capacity for work and concentration" [172]. Only two studies have been published examining the effects of ginseng in postmenopausal women and both showed no estrogenic effects, no improvement in vasomotor symptoms, but improvement in somatic complaints such as fatigue, insomnia, and depression compared with placebo [277,278]. It is still contraindicated in presence of breast cancer [279].

6.4.3.2.3 *Kava (Piper methysticum)*

Kava is a South Pacific herb used for treatment of anxiety and has shown significant improvement in irritability and insomnia compared with placebo in menopausal women [280]. However, because of the possible hepatotoxicity of the plant, the sale of kava has been banned in Canada, Australia, and several European countries. The exact mechanism of harm is not known but it may be that the stem peelings contain a toxic alkaloid. In response to reports of hepatotoxicity, the FDA, American Botanical Council, and various industry trade organizations have advised consumers of rare but potential risks of severe liver injury associated with the use of kava [190]. It is best to avoid this botanical completely but if kava is used, it should be limited to 6–8 weeks and extreme caution should be exercised.

6.4.3.2.4 *Motherwort (Leonurus cardiaca)*

Motherwort is another botanical historically revered as a calmative agent for the heart, especially palpitations [281]. The German Commission E has approved its use for nervousness [172]. It is also found in many menopausal formulas and was typically combined with black cohosh as a "superior antispasmodic and nervine," however, contemporary research is lacking on efficacy and safety.

6.4.3.2.5 *Valerian (Valeriana officinalis)*

Valerian has been used for centuries by Greeks, Romans, Chinese, Europeans, and American Indians. In the twentieth century, it has been approved by the German Commission E for "states of unrest and nervous sleep disturbances" [172]. Three RCTs have shown improved subjective sleep quality, although none of the studies were conducted with menopausal women [282–284]. There have been no reported drug interactions; side effects, such as nausea, headache, dizziness, and upset stomach, have been reported in less than 10% of subjects in RCTs [285].

6.4.3.2.6 *St. John's Wort (Hypericum perforatum)*

St. John's wort is one of the most heavily studied botanicals for treatment of depression. The vast majority of studies have been conducted in nonmenopausal populations. In 37 out of 39 clinical trials the herb has been shown to be superior to placebo or equivalent to antidepressant medications such as selective serotonin reuptake inhibitors (SSRIs). These studies have shown a 61%–75% improvement in mild-moderate depression, but not severe depression, with minimal side effects as compared to some of the SSRIs [286]. One non-placebo controlled clinical trial conducted in women experiencing climacteric symptoms found that 900 mg of St. John's wort taken for 12 weeks significantly improved psychological and psychosomatic symptoms and sexual well-being [287].

St. John's wort is often combined with black cohosh for treatment of menopausal symptoms (hot flashes, irritability, minor depression, mood swings, and insomnia). A multicenter drug monitoring study of 911 pre-, peri-, and postmenopausal women with psychological disorders demonstrated a synergistic effect of this combination of botanicals [288].

The adverse herb–drug interactions are well documented. St. John's wort can interact with anticoagulants, cyclosporine, digoxin, and protease inhibitors used for HIV, specifically decreasing blood concentrations of these drugs. In addition, women using oral contraceptives have reported breakthrough bleeding and in some cases, unplanned pregnancies [289].

6.5 CONCLUSIONS

Although the midlife is a time of physiologic change for women, it is also a time when good nutrition can assist in making these years the healthiest possible. Women have special nutritional requirements and these needs are best met through a healthy daily diet, enhanced with vitamins, minerals, and other dietary supplements as needed. A nutritionally balanced diet helps to maintain a healthful weight and is linked with a decrease in diseases such as cancer, diabetes, osteoporosis, and heart disease. The cornerstones of a healthy diet are fiber from whole grains, fruits, and vegetables, and a small amount of fat from n-3 fatty acids. Trans fatty acids and n-6s should be limited. Similarly, use of sugar, salt, and processed foods should be avoided or minimized.

The best way to sustain the adequate intake of nutrients is through a healthy and well-balanced diet. However, few women can consistently achieve this and careful supplementation with vitamins and minerals is important to maintain good health. In many cases, a multivitamin plus calcium supplementation may be all that is needed. Vitamins, minerals, and other dietary supplements do not replace a healthy diet but they can compensate for what is missing. Women should use supplements in consultation with their health care provider because large doses of some vitamins, minerals, and other dietary supplements may have serious side effects or may interact with other medications.

Of the botanicals reviewed in this chapter, black cohosh appears to be the most effective herb for relief of menopausal symptoms, primarily hot flashes and possibly mood disorders. Rhubarb also holds promise for relief of vasomotor and somatic complaints, but more research must be done. Phytoestrogen extracts, including soy foods and red clover appear to have at best only a minimal effect on menopausal symptoms but may have positive health effects on plasma lipid concentrations, and may reduce heart disease and improve bone health and cognition. Ginkgo may also be helpful for improvement in cognition and memory. St. John's wort has been shown to improve mild to moderate depression, but not major depression, in the general population. The other botanicals discussed have limited evidence to demonstrate safety and efficacy for relief of symptoms related to menopause or aging. Whatever decision women chose to make related to use of botanicals for relief of menopausal symptoms as well as to promote long-term health, it is critical to discuss these issues with their health care providers and so they can assist them in managing these alternative therapies through an evidence-based approach.

6.6 FUTURE RESEARCH

While there have been several observational and clinical studies examining the impact of diet, vitamins and minerals, and botanical and dietary supplements on health, rigorous double blind clinical trials are rare. Future research should focus on using large scale randomized clinical trials to assess the efficacy and safety of dietary interventions, of food sources, vitamin and mineral supplements, and botanical supplements on maintenance of health and the prevention and treatment of disease. Research should also focus on how different combinations of vitamins, mineral, and BDS products work together and the effects and safety of using several different supplements at one time, which is a common occurrence for many women [160]. Furthermore, most of the compounds discussed in this chapter have not been adequately tested for long-term safety at varying doses. These types of studies are crucial so that women can be informed of the safe dose ranges that are the most effective.

REFERENCES

1. Rosano, G.M., et al., Managing cardiovascular risk in menopausal women. *Climacteric* 9, 19–27, 2006.
2. Lindheim, S.R., et al., Comparison of estimates of insulin sensitivity in pre- and postmenopausal women using the insulin tolerance test and the frequently sampled intravenous glucose tolerance test. *J Soc Gynecol Investig* 1, 150–4, 1994.
3. Rosenthal, T.; Oparil, S., Hypertension in women. *J Hum Hypertens* 14, 691–704, 2000.
4. Behall, K.M., et al., Diets containing barley significantly reduce lipids in mildly hypercholesterolemic men and women. *Am J Clin Nutr* 80, 1185–93, 2004.
5. Behall, K.M., et al., Whole-grain diets reduce blood pressure in mildly hypercholesterolemic men and women. *J Am Diet Assoc* 106, 1445–9, 2006.
6. Erkkila, A.T., et al., Cereal fiber and whole-grain intake are associated with reduced progression of coronary-artery atherosclerosis in postmenopausal women with coronary artery disease. *Am Heart J* 150, 94–101, 2005.
7. Jacobs, D.R., Jr., et al., Whole-grain intake may reduce the risk of ischemic heart disease death in postmenopausal women: The Iowa Women's Health Study. *Am J Clin Nutr* 68, 248–57, 1998.
8. Jacobs, D.R., Jr., et al., Is whole grain intake associated with reduced total and cause-specific death rates in older women? The Iowa Women's Health Study. *Am J Public Health* 89, 322–9, 1999.
9. Jacobs, D.R., et al., Fiber from whole grains, but not refined grains, is inversely associated with all-cause mortality in older women: The Iowa Women's Health Study. *J Am Coll Nutr* 19, 326S–330S, 2000.
10. Meyer, K.A., et al., Carbohydrates, dietary fiber, and incident type 2 diabetes in older women. *Am J Clin Nutr* 71, 921–30, 2000.
11. Liu, S., et al., Whole-grain consumption and risk of coronary heart disease: Results from the Nurses' Health Study. *Am J Clin Nutr* 70, 412–9, 1999.
12. Liu, S., et al., Whole grain consumption and risk of ischemic stroke in women: A prospective study. *JAMA* 284, 1534–40, 2000.
13. Dauchet, L., et al., Fruit and vegetable consumption and risk of coronary heart disease: A meta-analysis of cohort studies. *J Nutr* 136, 2588–93, 2006.
14. He, F.J., et al., Fruit and vegetable consumption and stroke: Meta-analysis of cohort studies. *Lancet* 367, 320–6, 2006.
15. Gold, E.B., et al., Dietary factors and vasomotor symptoms in breast cancer survivors: The WHEL Study. *Menopause* 13, 423–33, 2006.
16. Geller, S.E.; Studee, L., Botanical and dietary supplements for menopausal symptoms: What works, what does not. *J Womens Health (Larchmt)* 14, 634–49, 2005.
17. Geller, S.E.; Studee, L., Soy and red clover for mid-life and aging. *Climacteric* 9, 245–63, 2006.
18. Food labelling: Health Claims; Soy Protein and Coronary Heart Disease. In *Federal Register: October 26, 1999*, ed.; 1999; Vol. 64, pp. 57699–57733.
19. Gambacciani, M., et al., Prospective evaluation of body weight and body fat distribution in early postmenopausal women with and without hormonal replacement therapy. *Maturitas* 39, 125–32, 2001.
20. Graham, S., et al., Nutritional epidemiology of postmenopausal breast cancer in western New York. *Am J Epidemiol* 134, 552–66, 1991.
21. Richardson, S., et al., The role of fat, animal protein and some vitamin consumption in breast cancer: A case control study in southern France. *Int J Cancer* 48, 1–9, 1991.

22. Barrett-Connor, E.; Friedlander, N.J., Dietary fat, calories, and the risk of breast cancer in postmenopausal women: A prospective population-based study. *J Am Coll Nutr* 12, 390–9, 1993.
23. Chlebowski, R.T., et al., Dietary fat reduction and breast cancer outcome: Interim efficacy results from the Women's Intervention Nutrition Study. *J Natl Cancer Inst* 98, 1767–76, 2006.
24. Howard, B.V., et al., Low-fat dietary pattern and weight change over 7 years: The Women's Health Initiative Dietary Modification Trial. *JAMA* 295, 39–49, 2006.
25. Howard, B.V., et al., Low-fat dietary pattern and risk of cardiovascular disease: The Women's Health Initiative Randomized Controlled Dietary Modification Trial. *JAMA* 295, 655–66, 2006.
26. Lichtenstein, A.H., et al., Diet and lifestyle recommendations revision 2006: A scientific statement from the American Heart Association Nutrition Committee. *Circulation* 114, 82–96, 2006.
27. Martin-Moreno, J.M., et al., Dietary fat, olive oil intake and breast cancer risk. *Int J Cancer* 58, 774–80, 1994.
28. Prentice, R.L., et al., Low-fat dietary pattern and risk of invasive breast cancer: The Women's Health Initiative Randomized Controlled Dietary Modification Trial. *JAMA* 295, 629–42, 2006.
29. Lueck, T.J., et al., New York Bans Most Trans Fats in Restaurants. *New York Times* December 6, 2006, pp. A1–A24.
30. Marcason, W., How many grams of trans-fat are recommended per day? *J Am Diet Assoc* 106, 1507, 2006.
31. Kromhout, D., et al., Dietary saturated and trans fatty acids and cholesterol and 25-year mortality from coronary heart disease: The Seven Countries Study. *Prev Med* 24, 308–15, 1995.
32. Ascherio, A., et al., Trans-fatty acids intake and risk of myocardial infarction. *Circulation* 89, 94–101, 1994.
33. Hu, F.B., et al., Dietary fat intake and the risk of coronary heart disease in women. *N Engl J Med* 337, 1491–9, 1997.
34. Judd, J.T., et al., Dietary trans fatty acids: Effects on plasma lipids and lipoproteins of healthy men and women. *Am J Clin Nutr* 59, 861–8, 1994.
35. Ascherio, A., et al., Trans fatty acids and coronary heart disease. *N Engl J Med* 340, 1994–8, 1999.
36. Mozaffarian, D., Trans fatty acids—Effects on systemic inflammation and endothelial function. *Atheroscler Suppl* 7, 29–32, 2006.
37. Riserus, U., Trans fatty acids and insulin resistance. *Atheroscler Suppl* 7, 37–9, 2006.
38. Lara, J.J., et al., Benefits of salmon eating on traditional and novel vascular risk factors in young, non-obese healthy subjects. *Atherosclerosis*, 2007 Jul; 193(1):213–21.
39. Pauletto, P., et al., Blood pressure and atherogenic lipoprotein profiles of fish-diet and vegetarian villagers in Tanzania: The Lugalawa study. *Lancet* 348, 784–8, 1996.
40. Saldeen, P.; Saldeen, T., Women and omega-3 fatty acids. *Obstet Gynecol Surv* 59, 722–30; quiz 745–6, 2004.
41. Hu, F.B., et al., Fish and omega-3 fatty acid intake and risk of coronary heart disease in women. *JAMA* 287, 1815–21, 2002.
42. Stark, K.D., et al., Effect of a fish-oil concentrate on serum lipids in postmenopausal women receiving and not receiving hormone replacement therapy in a placebo-controlled, double-blind trial. *Am J Clin Nutr* 72, 389–94, 2000.

43. Dietary supplementation with n-3 polyunsaturated fatty acids and vitamin E after myocardial infarction: Results of the GISSI-Prevenzione trial. Gruppo Italiano per lo Studio della Sopravvivenza nell'Infarto miocardico. *Lancet* 354, 447–55, 1999.
44. Erkkila, A.T., et al., Fish intake is associated with a reduced progression of coronary artery atherosclerosis in postmenopausal women with coronary artery disease. *Am J Clin Nutr* 80, 626–32, 2004.
45. Caygill, C.P., et al., Fat, fish, fish oil and cancer. *Br J Cancer* 74, 159–64, 1996.
46. Braga, C., et al., Intake of selected foods and nutrients and breast cancer risk: An age- and menopause-specific analysis. *Nutr Cancer* 28, 258–63, 1997.
47. Simonsen, N., et al., Adipose tissue omega-3 and omega-6 fatty acid content and breast cancer in the EURAMIC study. European Community Multicenter Study on Antioxidants, Myocardial Infarction, and Breast Cancer. *Am J Epidemiol* 147, 342–52, 1998.
48. Lu, M., et al., Prospective study of dietary fat and risk of cataract extraction among US women. *Am J Epidemiol* 161, 948–59, 2005.
49. MacLean, C., et al. *Effects of Omega-3 Fatty Acids on Lipids and Glycemic Control in Type II Diabetes and the Metabolic Syndrome and on Inflammatory Bowel Disease, Rheumatoid Arthritis, Renal Disease, Systemic Lupus Erythematosus, and Osteoporosis*; Agency for Healthcare Research and Quality: Rockville, MD, March, 2004.
50. Campagnoli, C., et al., Polyunsaturated fatty acids (PUFAs) might reduce hot flushes: An indication from two controlled trials on soy isoflavones alone and with a PUFA supplement. *Maturitas* 51, 127–34, 2005.
51. Sifton, D.W., *The PDR Family Guide to Nutrition and Health*. ed.; Medical Economics Company: Montvale, NJ, 1995; p. 782.
52. Simopoulos, A.P., Essential fatty acids in health and chronic disease. *Am J Clin Nutr* 70, 560S–569S, 1999.
53. Fairfield, K.M.; Fletcher, R.H., Vitamins for chronic disease prevention in adults: Scientific review. *JAMA* 287, 3116–26, 2002.
54. Cramer, D.W., et al., Carotenoids, antioxidants and ovarian cancer risk in pre- and postmenopausal women. *Int J Cancer* 94, 128–34, 2001.
55. Tung, K.H., et al., Association of dietary vitamin A, carotenoids, and other antioxidants with the risk of ovarian cancer. *Cancer Epidemiol Biomarkers Prev* 14, 669–76, 2005.
56. Bertone, E.R., et al., A population-based case-control study of carotenoid and vitamin A intake and ovarian cancer (United States). *Cancer Causes Control* 12, 83–90, 2001.
57. Kushi, L.H., et al., Intake of vitamins A, C, and E and postmenopausal breast cancer. The Iowa Women's Health Study. *Am J Epidemiol* 144, 165–74, 1996.
58. Bohlke, K., et al., Vitamins A, C and E and the risk of breast cancer: Results from a case-control study in Greece. *Br J Cancer* 79, 23–9, 1999.
59. Nissen, S.B., et al., Intake of vitamins A, C, and E from diet and supplements and breast cancer in postmenopausal women. *Cancer Causes Control* 14, 695–704, 2003.
60. Gaziano, J.M., et al., Dietary antioxidants and cardiovascular disease. *Ann NY Acad Sci* 669, 249–58; discussion 258–9, 1992.
61. Kardinaal, A.F., et al., Antioxidants in adipose tissue and risk of myocardial infarction: The EURAMIC Study. *Lancet* 342, 1379–84, 1993.
62. Street, D.A., et al., Serum antioxidants and myocardial infarction. Are low levels of carotenoids and α-tocopherol risk factors for myocardial infarction? *Circulation* 90, 1154–61, 1994.
63. Kushi, L.H., et al., Dietary antioxidant vitamins and death from coronary heart disease in postmenopausal women. *N Engl J Med* 334, 1156–62, 1996.

64. Palace, V.P., et al., Antioxidant potentials of vitamin A and carotenoids and their relevance to heart disease. *Free Radic Biol Med* 26, 746–61, 1999.
65. Ziegler, E.E., *Present Knowledge in Nutrition*. ed.; International Life Sciences Institute: Washington, DC, 1996.
66. Byers, T.; Guerrero, N., Epidemiologic evidence for vitamin C and vitamin E in cancer prevention. *Am J Clin Nutr* 62, 1385S–1392S, 1995.
67. Negri, E., et al., Selected micronutrients and oral and pharyngeal cancer. *Int J Cancer* 86, 122–7, 2000.
68. You, W.C., et al., Gastric dysplasia and gastric cancer: Helicobacter pylori, serum vitamin C, and other risk factors. *J Natl Cancer Inst* 92, 1607–12, 2000.
69. Howe, G.R., et al., Dietary factors and risk of breast cancer: Combined analysis of 12 case-control studies. *J Natl Cancer Inst* 82, 561–9, 1990.
70. Gandini, S., et al., Meta-analysis of studies on breast cancer risk and diet: The role of fruit and vegetable consumption and the intake of associated micronutrients. *Eur J Cancer* 36, 636–46, 2000.
71. Michels, K.B., et al., Dietary antioxidant vitamins, retinol, and breast cancer incidence in a cohort of Swedish women. *Int J Cancer* 91, 563–7, 2001.
72. Zhang, S., et al., Dietary carotenoids and vitamins A, C, and E and risk of breast cancer. *J Natl Cancer Inst* 91, 547–56, 1999.
73. Stampfer, M.J., et al., Vitamin E consumption and the risk of coronary disease in women. *N Engl J Med* 328, 1444–9, 1993.
74. Gale, C.R., et al., Vitamin C and risk of death from stroke and coronary heart disease in cohort of elderly people. *BMJ* 310, 1563–6, 1995.
75. Kritchevsky, S.B., et al., Dietary antioxidants and carotid artery wall thickness. The ARIC Study. Atherosclerosis Risk in Communities Study. *Circulation* 92, 2142–50, 1995.
76. Joshipura, K.J., et al., The effect of fruit and vegetable intake on risk for coronary heart disease. *Ann Intern Med* 134, 1106–14, 2001.
77. Miller, E.R. III, et al., Meta-analysis: High-dosage vitamin E supplementation may increase all-cause mortality. *Ann Intern Med* 142, 37–46, 2005.
78. de Gaetano, G., Low-dose aspirin and vitamin E in people at cardiovascular risk: A randomised trial in general practice. Collaborative Group of the Primary Prevention Project. *Lancet* 357, 89–95, 2001.
79. Yusuf, S., et al., Vitamin E supplementation and cardiovascular events in high-risk patients. The Heart Outcomes Prevention Evaluation Study Investigators. *N Engl J Med* 342, 154–60, 2000.
80. Lee, I.M., et al., Vitamin E in the primary prevention of cardiovascular disease and cancer: The Women's Health Study: A randomized controlled trial. *JAMA* 294, 56–65, 2005.
81. Boushey, C.J., et al., A quantitative assessment of plasma homocysteine as a risk factor for vascular disease. Probable benefits of increasing folic acid intakes. *JAMA* 274, 1049–57, 1995.
82. Eikelboom, J.W., et al., Homocyst(e)ine and cardiovascular disease: A critical review of the epidemiologic evidence. *Ann Intern Med* 131, 363–75, 1999.
83. Villa, P., et al., L-folic acid supplementation in healthy postmenopausal women: Effect on homocysteine and glycolipid metabolism. *J Clin Endocrinol Metab* 90, 4622–9, 2005.
84. De Leo, V., et al., Low-dose folic acid supplementation reduces plasma levels of the cardiovascular risk factor homocysteine in postmenopausal women. *Am J Obstet Gynecol* 183, 945–7, 2000.
85. Franken, D.G., et al., Treatment of mild hyperhomocysteinemia in vascular disease patients. *Arterioscler Thromb* 14, 465–70, 1994.

86. Morrison, H.I., et al., Serum folate and risk of fatal coronary heart disease. *JAMA* 275, 1893–6, 1996.
87. Robinson, K., et al., Low circulating folate and vitamin B6 concentrations: risk factors for stroke, peripheral vascular disease, and coronary artery disease. European COMAC Group. *Circulation* 97, 437–43, 1998.
88. Tavani, A., et al., Folate and vitamin B(6) intake and risk of acute myocardial infarction in Italy. *Eur J Clin Nutr* 58, 1266–72, 2004.
89. Lonn, E., et al., Homocysteine lowering with folic acid and B vitamins in vascular disease. *N Engl J Med* 354, 1567–77, 2006.
90. Zoungas, S., et al., Cardiovascular morbidity and mortality in the Atherosclerosis and Folic Acid Supplementation Trial (ASFAST) in chronic renal failure: a multicenter, randomized, controlled trial. *J Am Coll Cardiol* 47, 1108–16, 2006.
91. Bonaa, K.H., et al., Homocysteine lowering and cardiovascular events after acute myocardial infarction. *N Engl J Med* 354, 1578–88, 2006.
92. Ellis, J., et al., Clinical results of a cross-over treatment with pyridoxine and placebo of the carpal tunnel syndrome. *Am J Clin Nutr* 32, 2040–6, 1979.
93. Murthy, M.S., et al., Effect of pyridoxine supplementation on recurrent stone formers. *Int J Clin Pharmacol Ther Toxicol* 20, 434–7, 1982.
94. Collipp, P.J., et al., Pyridoxine treatment of childhood bronchial asthma. *Ann Allergy* 35, 93–7, 1975.
95. Foukas, M.D., An antilactogenic effect of pyridoxine. *J Obstet Gynecol Br Commonw* 80, 718–20, 1973.
96. Park, S.; Johnson, M.A., What is an adequate dose of oral vitamin B12 in older people with poor vitamin B12 status? *Nutr Rev* 64, 373–8, 2006.
97. Stabler, S.P., et al., Vitamin B-12 deficiency in the elderly: Current dilemmas. *Am J Clin Nutr* 66, 741–9, 1997.
98. Carmel, R., Subtle cobalamin deficiency. *Ann Intern Med* 124, 338–40, 1996.
99. Tang, A.M., et al., Low serum vitamin B-12 concentrations are associated with faster human immunodeficiency virus type 1 (HIV-1) disease progression. *J Nutr* 127, 345–51, 1997.
100. Werbach, M.R., *Nutritional Influences on Illness*. 2nd ed.; Third Line Press: Tarzana, CA, 1993.
101. *Dietary Guidelines for Americans 2005*, U.S. Department of Health and Human Services, U.S. Department of Agriculture.
102. Luchsinger, J.A., et al., Relation of higher folate intake to lower risk of Alzheimer disease in the elderly. *Arch Neurol* 64, 86–92, 2007.
103. Ilich, J.Z.; Kerstetter, J.E., Nutrition in bone health revisited: A story beyond calcium. *J Am Coll Nutr* 19, 715–37, 2000.
104. Gallagher, J.C., et al., Total bone calcium in normal women: Effect of age and menopause status. *J Bone Miner Res* 2, 491–6, 1987.
105. Riggs, B.L., et al., A unitary model for involutional osteoporosis: Estrogen deficiency causes both type I and type II osteoporosis in postmenopausal women and contributes to bone loss in aging men. *J Bone Miner Res* 13, 763–73, 1998.
106. Di Daniele, N., et al., Effect of supplementation of calcium and vitamin D on bone mineral density and bone mineral content in peri- and post-menopause women; A double-blind, randomized, controlled trial. *Pharmacol Res* 50, 637–41, 2004.
107. Jackson, R.D., et al., Calcium plus vitamin D supplementation and the risk of fractures. *N Engl J Med* 354, 669–83, 2006.
108. Feskanich, D., et al., Vitamin A intake and hip fractures among postmenopausal women. *JAMA* 287, 47–54, 2002.

109. NIH Consensus conference. Optimal calcium intake. NIH Consensus Development Panel on Optimal Calcium Intake. *JAMA* 272, 1942–8, 1994.
110. Maitland, T.E., et al., Associations of nationality and race with nutritional status during perimenopause: Implications for public health practice. *Ethn Dis* 16, 201–6, 2006.
111. Alaimo, K., et al., Dietary intake of vitamins, minerals, and fiber of persons ages 2 months and over in the United States: Third National Health and Nutrition Examination Survey, Phase 1, 1988–91. *Adv Data*, 1994 Nov 14; (258):1–28.
112. Siple, M.; Gordon, D., *Menopause the natural way*. Wiley: New York, NY, 2001.
113. Dawson-Hughes, B., et al., A controlled trial of the effect of calcium supplementation on bone density in postmenopausal women. *N Engl J Med* 323, 878–83, 1990.
114. Heaney, R.P., et al., Calcium absorbability from spinach. *Am J Clin Nutr* 47, 707–9, 1988.
115. Heaney, R.P., et al., Absorbability of calcium sources: The limited role of solubility. *Calcif Tissue Int* 46, 300–4, 1990.
116. The role of calcium in peri- and postmenopausal women: 2006 position statement of the North American Menopause Society. *Menopause* 13, 862–77, 2006; quiz 878–80.
117. Celotti, F.; Bignamini, A., Dietary calcium and mineral/vitamin supplementation: A controversial problem. *J Int Med Res* 27, 1–14, 1999.
118. National Institute of Diabetes and Digestive and Kidney Diseases Lactose Intolerance. http://digestive.niddk.nih.gov/ddiseases/pubs/lactoseintolerance/lactoseintolerance.pdf (December 21).
119. Lipkin, M.; Newmark, H., Calcium and the prevention of colon cancer. *J Cell Biochem Suppl* 22, 65–73, 1995.
120. Cho, E., et al., Dairy foods, calcium, and colorectal cancer: A pooled analysis of 10 cohort studies. *J Natl Cancer Inst* 96, 1015–22, 2004.
121. Terry, P., et al., Dietary calcium and vitamin D intake and risk of colorectal cancer: A prospective cohort study in women. *Nutr Cancer* 43, 39–46, 2002.
122. Baron, J.A., et al., Calcium supplements for the prevention of colorectal adenomas. Calcium Polyp Prevention Study Group. *N Engl J Med* 340, 101–7, 1999.
123. Bonithon-Kopp, C., et al., Calcium and fibre supplementation in prevention of colorectal adenoma recurrence: A randomised intervention trial. European Cancer Prevention Organisation Study Group. *Lancet* 356, 1300–6, 2000.
124. Wactawski-Wende, J., et al., Calcium plus vitamin D supplementation and the risk of colorectal cancer. *N Engl J Med* 354, 684–96, 2006.
125. Berube, S., et al., Vitamin D and calcium intakes from food or supplements and mammographic breast density. *Cancer Epidemiol Biomarkers Prev* 14, 1653–9, 2005.
126. McCullough, M.L., et al., Dairy, calcium, and vitamin D intake and postmenopausal breast cancer risk in the Cancer Prevention Study II Nutrition Cohort. *Cancer Epidemiol Biomarkers Prev* 14, 2898–904, 2005.
127. Gonzalez, A.J., et al., Calcium intake and 10-year weight change in middle-aged adults. *J Am Diet Assoc* 106, 1066–73; quiz 1082, 2006.
128. Shapses, S.A., et al., Effect of calcium supplementation on weight and fat loss in women. *J Clin Endocrinol Metab* 89, 632–7, 2004.
129. MacLaughlin, J.; Holick, M.F., Aging decreases the capacity of human skin to produce vitamin D3. *J Clin Invest* 76, 1536–8, 1985.
130. Moore, C.E., et al., Vitamin D intakes by children and adults in the United States differ among ethnic groups. *J Nutr* 135, 2478–85, 2005.
131. Malabanan, A.O.; Holick, M.F., Vitamin D and bone health in postmenopausal women. *J Womens Health (Larchmt)* 12, 151–6, 2003.

132. Harwood, R.H., et al., A randomised, controlled comparison of different calcium and vitamin D supplementation regimens in elderly women after hip fracture: The Nottingham Neck of Femur (NONOF) Study. *Age Ageing* 33, 45–51, 2004.
133. Chapuy, M.C., et al., Vitamin D3 and calcium to prevent hip fractures in the elderly women. *N Engl J Med* 327, 1637–42, 1992.
134. Chapuy, M.C., et al., Effect of calcium and cholecalciferol treatment for three years on hip fractures in elderly women. *BMJ* 308, 1081–2, 1994.
135. Dawson-Hughes, B., et al., Effect of calcium and vitamin D supplementation on bone density in men and women 65 years of age or older. *N Engl J Med* 337, 670–6, 1997.
136. Bischoff, H.A., et al., Effects of vitamin D and calcium supplementation on falls: A randomized controlled trial. *J Bone Miner Res* 18, 343–51, 2003.
137. Flicker, L., et al., Should older people in residential care receive vitamin D to prevent falls? Results of a randomized trial. *J Am Geriatr Soc* 53, 1881–8, 2005.
138. Office of Dietary Supplements Dietary Supplement Fact Sheet: Iron. http://dietary-supplements.info.nih.gov/factsheets/Iron_pf.asp#h4 (December 20).
139. Hunt, J.R., Bioavailability of iron, zinc, and other trace minerals from vegetarian diets. *Am J Clin Nutr* 78, 633S–639S, 2003.
140. Ryder, K.M., et al., Magnesium intake from food and supplements is associated with bone mineral density in healthy older white subjects. *J Am Geriatr Soc* 53, 1875–80, 2005.
141. Rude, R.K.; Gruber, H.E., Magnesium deficiency and osteoporosis: Animal and human observations. *J Nutr Biochem* 15, 710–6, 2004.
142. Sojka, J.E.; Weaver, C.M., Magnesium supplementation and osteoporosis. *Nutr Rev* 53, 71–4, 1995.
143. Laires, M.J., et al., Magnesium, insulin resistance and body composition in healthy postmenopausal women. *J Am Coll Nutr* 23, 510S–513S, 2004.
144. Nielsen, F.H.; Milne, D.B., A moderately high intake compared to a low intake of zinc depresses magnesium balance and alters indices of bone turnover in postmenopausal women. *Eur J Clin Nutr* 58, 703–10, 2004.
145. Bendich, A., The potential for dietary supplements to reduce premenstrual syndrome (PMS) symptoms. *J Am Coll Nutr* 19, 3–12, 2000.
146. Walker, A.F., et al., Magnesium supplementation alleviates premenstrual symptoms of fluid retention. *J Womens Health* 7, 1157–65, 1998.
147. Facchinetti, F., et al., Oral magnesium successfully relieves premenstrual mood changes. *Obstet Gynecol* 78, 177–81, 1991.
148. Facchinetti, F., et al., Magnesium prophylaxis of menstrual migraine: Effects on intracellular magnesium. *Headache* 31, 298–301, 1991.
149. Macdonald, H.M., et al., Low dietary potassium intakes and high dietary estimates of net endogenous acid production are associated with low bone mineral density in premenopausal women and increased markers of bone resorption in postmenopausal women. *Am J Clin Nutr* 81, 923–33, 2005.
150. New, S.A., et al., Nutritional influences on bone mineral density: A cross-sectional study in premenopausal women. *Am J Clin Nutr* 65, 1831–9, 1997.
151. Tucker, K.L., et al., Potassium, magnesium, and fruit and vegetable intakes are associated with greater bone mineral density in elderly men and women. *Am J Clin Nutr* 69, 727–36, 1999.
152. Beck, L.H., The aging kidney. Defending a delicate balance of fluid and electrolytes. *Geriatrics* 55, 26–8, 31–2, 2000.

153. Nielsen, F.H.; Milne, D.B., Some magnesium status indicators and oxidative metabolism responses to low-dietary magnesium are affected by dietary copper in postmenopausal women. *Nutrition* 19, 617–26, 2003.
154. Kolata, G., Race to fill the void in menopause drug market. *The New York Times* September 1, 2002, p 1.
155. Rossouw, J.E., et al., Risks and benefits of estrogen plus progestin in healthy postmenopausal women: Principal results from the Women's Health Initiative randomized controlled trial. *JAMA* 288, 321–33, 2002.
156. Albertazzi, P., et al., Attitudes towards and use of dietary supplementation in a sample of postmenopausal women. *Climacteric* 5, 374–82, 2002.
157. Drivdahl, C.E.; Miser, W.F., The use of alternative health care by a family practice population. *J Am Board Fam Pract* 11, 193–9, 1998.
158. Eisenberg, D.M., et al., Trends in alternative medicine use in the United States, 1990–1997: Results of a follow-up national survey. *JAMA* 280, 1569–75, 1998.
159. Kass-Annese, B., Alternative therapies for menopause. *Clin Obstet Gynecol* 43, 162–83, 2000.
160. Mahady, G.B., et al., Botanical dietary supplement use in peri- and postmenopausal women. *Menopause* 10, 65–72, 2003.
161. Botanicals and botanical preparations widely used as food supplements and related products: Coherent and comprehensive risk assessment and consumer information approaches. http://www.efsa.eu.int/science/sc_commitee/sc_documents/616_en.html (November 14, 2005).
162. Larsen, L.L.; Berry, J.A., The regulation of dietary supplements. *J Am Acad Nurse Pract* 15, 410–4, 2003.
163. Geller, S.E.; Studee, L., Contemporary alternatives to plant estrogens for menopause. *Maturitas* 55 Suppl 1, S3–S13, 2006.
164. Geller, S.E.; Studee, L., Botanical and dietary supplements for mood and anxiety in menopausal women. *Menopause* 14, 541–549, 2006.
165. Kligler, B., Black cohosh. *Am Fam Physician* 68, 114–6, 2003.
166. Dog, T.L., et al., Critical evaluation of the safety of Cimicifuga racemosa in menopause symptom relief. *Menopause* 10, 299–313, 2003.
167. Einer-Jensen, N., et al., Cimicifuga and Melbrosia lack oestrogenic effects in mice and rats. *Maturitas* 25, 149–53, 1996.
168. Freudenstein, J., et al., Lack of promotion of estrogen-dependent mammary gland tumors in vivo by an isopropanolic *Cimicifuga racemosa* extract. *Cancer Res* 62, 3448–52, 2002.
169. Seidlova-Wuttke, D., et al., Pharmacology of Cimicifuga racemosa extract BNO 1055 in rats: Bone, fat and uterus. *Maturitas* 44 Suppl 1, S39–50, 2003.
170. Burdette, J.E., et al., Black cohosh acts as a mixed competitive ligand and partial agonist of the serotonin receptor. *J Agric Food Chem* 51, 5661–70, 2003.
171. Mahady, G.B., Is black cohosh estrogenic? *Nutr Rev* 61, 183–6, 2003.
172. Blumenthal, M., *Herbal Medicine: Expanded Commission E Monographs*. ed.; Integrative Medicine Communications: Newton, MA, 2000.
173. Zava, D.T., et al., Estrogen and progestin bioactivity of foods, herbs, and spices. *Proc Soc Exp Biol Med* 217, 369–78, 1998.
174. Liu, J., et al., Evaluation of estrogenic activity of plant extracts for the potential treatment of menopausal symptoms. *J Agric Food Chem* 49, 2472–9, 2001.
175. Zierau, O., et al., Antiestrogenic activities of Cimicifuga racemosa extracts. *J Steroid Biochem Mol Biol* 80, 125–30, 2002.

176. Bodinet, C.; Freudenstein, J., Influence of Cimicifuga racemosa on the proliferation of estrogen receptor-positive human breast cancer cells. *Breast Cancer Res Treat* 76, 1–10, 2002.
177. Osmers, R., et al., Efficacy and safety of isopropanolic black cohosh extract for climacteric symptoms. *Obstet Gynecol* 105, 1074–83, 2005.
178. Frei-Kleiner, S., et al., Cimicifuga racemosa dried ethanolic extract in menopausal disorders: A double-blind placebo-controlled clinical trial. *Maturitas* 51, 397–404, 2005.
179. Wuttke, W., et al., The Cimicifuga preparation BNO 1055 vs. conjugated estrogens in a double-blind placebo-controlled study: Effects on menopause symptoms and bone markers. *Maturitas* 44 Suppl 1, S67–77, 2003.
180. Duker, E.M., et al., Effects of extracts from Cimicifuga racemosa on gonadotropin release in menopausal women and ovariectomized rats. *Planta Med* 57, 420–4, 1991.
181. Friedman-Koss, D., et al., The relationship of race/ethnicity and social class to hormone replacement therapy: Results from the Third National Health and Nutrition Examination Survey 1988–1994. *Menopause* 9, 264–72, 2002.
182. Nappi, R.E., et al., Efficacy of Cimicifuga racemosa on climacteric complaints: A randomized study versus low-dose transdermal estradiol. *Gynecol Endocrinol* 20, 30–5, 2005.
183. Liske, E., et al., Physiological investigation of a unique extract of black cohosh (Cimicifugae racemosae rhizoma): A 6-month clinical study demonstrates no systemic estrogenic effect. *J Womens Health Gend Based Med* 11, 163–74, 2002.
184. Lehmann-Willenbrock, E.; Riedel, H.H., [Clinical and endocrinologic studies of the treatment of ovarian insufficiency manifestations following hysterectomy with intact adnexa]. *Zentralbl Gynakol* 110, 611–8, 1988.
185. Vermes, G., et al., The effects of remifemin on subjective symptoms of menopause. *Adv Ther* 22, 148–54, 2005.
186. Pockaj, B.A., et al., Pilot evaluation of black cohosh for the treatment of hot flashes in women. *Cancer Invest* 22, 515–21, 2004.
187. Hernandez Munoz, G.; Pluchino, S., *Cimicifuga racemosa* for the treatment of hot flushes in women surviving breast cancer. *Maturitas* 44 Suppl 1, S59–65, 2003.
188. Jacobson, J.S., et al., Randomized trial of black cohosh for the treatment of hot flashes among women with a history of breast cancer. *J Clin Oncol* 19, 2739–45, 2001.
189. Newton, K.M., et al., Treatment of vasomotor symptoms of menopause with black cohosh, multibotanicals, soy, hormone therapy, or placebo: A randomized trial. *Ann Intern Med* 145, 869–79, 2006.
190. Blumenthal, M., Goldberg, A., Kunz, T., *The ABC Clinical Guide to Herbs*. American Botanical Council: Austin, TX, 2003.
191. Pepping, J., Black cohosh: *Cimicifuga racemosa*. *Am J Health Syst Pharm* 56, 1400–2, 1999.
192. Lontos, S., et al., Acute liver failure associated with the use of herbal preparations containing black cohosh. *Med J Aust* 179, 390–1, 2003.
193. Whiting, P.W., et al., Black cohosh and other herbal remedies associated with acute hepatitis. *Med J Aust* 177, 440–3, 2002.
194. Cohen, S.M., et al., Autoimmune hepatitis associated with the use of black cohosh: A case study. *Menopause* 11, 575–577, 2004.
195. Lynch, C.R., et al., Fulminant hepatic failure associated with the use of black cohosh: A case report. *Liver Transpl* 12, 989–92, 2006.
196. NIH *Workshop on the Safety of Black Cohosh in Clinical Studies*; National Center for Complementary and Alternative Medicine; NIH Office of Dietary Supplements: Washington, DC, 2004.

197. Halliday, J., UK herbal sector agrees black cohosh liver warning. http://www.nutraingredients.com/news/ng.asp?n=69781-uk-herbal-sector (December 22).
198. Knight, D.C.; Eden, J.A., A review of the clinical effects of phytoestrogens. *Obstet Gynecol* 87, 897–904, 1996.
199. Munro, I.C., et al., Soy isoflavones: A safety review. *Nutr Rev* 61, 1–33, 2003.
200. Beck, V., et al., Phytoestrogens derived from red clover: An alternative to estrogen replacement therapy? *J Steroid Biochem Mol Biol* 94, 499–518, 2005.
201. Piersen, C.E., et al., Chemical and biological characterization and clinical evaluation of botanical dietary supplements: A phase I red clover extract as a model. *Curr Med Chem* 11, 1361–74, 2004.
202. Piersen, C.E., Phytoestrogens in botanical dietary supplements: Implications for cancer. *Integr Cancer Ther* 2, 120–38, 2003.
203. Krebs, E.E., et al., Phytoestrogens for treatment of menopausal symptoms: A systematic review. *Obstet Gynecol* 104, 824–36, 2004.
204. Wuttke, W., et al., Phytoestrogens for hormone replacement therapy? *J Steroid Biochem Mol Biol* 83, 133–47, 2002.
205. Strong, K., et al., Preventing chronic diseases: How many lives can we save? *Lancet* 366, 1578–82, 2005.
206. Fogarty, P., et al., Epidemiology of the most frequent diseases in the European a-symptomatic post-menopausal women. Is there any difference between Ireland and the rest of Europe? *Maturitas*, 2005.
207. Anderson, J.W., et al., Meta-analysis of the effects of soy protein intake on serum lipids. *N Engl J Med* 333, 276–82, 1995.
208. Dalais, F.S., et al., The effects of soy protein containing isoflavones on lipids and indices of bone resorption in postmenopausal women. *Clin Endocrinol (Oxf)* 58, 704–9, 2003.
209. Jenkins, D.J., et al., Effects of high- and low-isoflavone soyfoods on blood lipids, oxidized LDL, homocysteine, and blood pressure in hyperlipidemic men and women. *Am J Clin Nutr* 76, 365–72, 2002.
210. Potter, S.M., et al., Soy protein and isoflavones: Their effects on blood lipids and bone density in postmenopausal women. *Am J Clin Nutr* 68, 1375S–1379S, 1998.
211. Vigna, G.B., et al., Plasma lipoproteins in soy-treated postmenopausal women: A double-blind, placebo-controlled trial. *Nutr Metab Cardiovasc Dis* 10, 315–22, 2000.
212. Wangen, K.E., et al., Soy isoflavones improve plasma lipids in normocholesterolemic and mildly hypercholesterolemic postmenopausal women. *Am J Clin Nutr* 73, 225–31, 2001.
213. Washburn, S., et al., Effect of soy protein supplementation on serum lipoproteins, blood pressure, and menopausal symptoms in perimenopausal women. *Menopause* 6, 7–13, 1999.
214. Teede, H.J., et al., Dietary soy has both beneficial and potentially adverse cardiovascular effects: A placebo-controlled study in men and postmenopausal women. *J Clin Endocrinol Metab* 86, 3053–60, 2001.
215. Engelman, H.M., et al., Blood lipid and oxidative stress responses to soy protein with isoflavones and phytic acid in postmenopausal women. *Am J Clin Nutr* 81, 590–6, 2005.
216. Mackey, R., et al., The effects of soy protein in women and men with elevated plasma lipids. *Biofactors* 12, 251–7, 2000.
217. Campbell, M.J., et al., Effect of red clover-derived isoflavone supplementation on insulin-like growth factor, lipid and antioxidant status in healthy female volunteers: A pilot study. *Eur J Clin Nutr* 58, 173–9, 2004.
218. Clifton-Bligh, P.B., et al., The effect of isoflavones extracted from red clover (Rimostil) on lipid and bone metabolism. *Menopause* 8, 259–65, 2001.

219. Schult, T.M., et al., Effect of isoflavones on lipids and bone turnover markers in menopausal women. *Maturitas* 48, 209–18, 2004.
220. Nestel, P.J., et al., Isoflavones from red clover improve systemic arterial compliance but not plasma lipids in menopausal women. *J Clin Endocrinol Metab* 84, 895–8, 1999.
221. Atkinson, C., et al., The effects of phytoestrogen isoflavones on bone density in women: A double-blind, randomized, placebo-controlled trial. *Am J Clin Nutr* 79, 326–33, 2004.
222. Howes, J.B., et al., The effects of dietary supplementation with isoflavones from red clover on the lipoprotein profiles of post menopausal women with mild to moderate hypercholesterolaemia. *Atherosclerosis* 152, 143–7, 2000.
223. Melton, L.J., III, Epidemiology worldwide. *Endocrinol Metab Clin North Am* 32, 1–13, 2003.
224. Bone Health. www.cdc.gov/nccdphp/dnpa/bonehealth (September 27).
225. Dennison, E., et al., Bone loss in Great Britain and Japan: A comparative longitudinal study. *Bone* 23, 379–82, 1998.
226. Ross, P.D., et al., A comparison of hip fracture incidence among native Japanese, Japanese Americans, and American Caucasians. *Am J Epidemiol* 133, 801–9, 1991.
227. Arjmandi, B.H., et al., One year soy protein supplementation has positive effects on bone formation markers but not bone density in postmenopausal women. *Nutr J* 4, 8, 2005.
228. Schwartz, A.V., et al., International variation in the incidence of hip fractures: Cross-national project on osteoporosis for the World Health Organization Program for Research on Aging. *Osteoporos Int* 9, 242–53, 1999.
229. Harkness, L.S., et al., Decreased bone resorption with soy isoflavone supplementation in postmenopausal women. *J Womens Health (Larchmt)* 13, 1000–7, 2004.
230. Morabito, N., et al., Effects of genistein and hormone-replacement therapy on bone loss in early postmenopausal women: A randomized double-blind placebo-controlled study. *J Bone Miner Res* 17, 1904–12, 2002.
231. Alekel, D.L., et al., Isoflavone-rich soy protein isolate attenuates bone loss in the lumbar spine of perimenopausal women. *Am J Clin Nutr* 72, 844–52, 2000.
232. Lydeking-Olsen, E., et al., Soymilk or progesterone for prevention of bone loss—a 2 year randomized, placebo-controlled trial. *Eur J Nutr* 43, 246–57, 2004.
233. Chiechi, L.M., et al., Efficacy of a soy rich diet in preventing postmenopausal osteoporosis: The Menfis randomized trial. *Maturitas* 42, 295–300, 2002.
234. Chen, Y.M., et al., Soy isoflavones have a favorable effect on bone loss in Chinese postmenopausal women with lower bone mass: A double-blind, randomized, controlled trial. *J Clin Endocrinol Metab* 88, 4740–7, 2003.
235. Chen, Y.M., et al., Beneficial effect of soy isoflavones on bone mineral content was modified by years since menopause, body weight, and calcium intake: A double-blind, randomized, controlled trial. *Menopause* 11, 246–54, 2004.
236. Uesugi, T., et al., Beneficial effects of soybean isoflavone supplementation on bone metabolism and serum lipids in postmenopausal japanese women: A four-week study. *J Am Coll Nutr* 21, 97–102, 2002.
237. Kreijkamp-Kaspers, S., et al., Effect of soy protein containing isoflavones on cognitive function, bone mineral density, and plasma lipids in postmenopausal women: A randomized controlled trial. *JAMA* 292, 65–74, 2004.
238. Gallagher, J.C., et al., The effect of soy protein isolate on bone metabolism. *Menopause* 11, 290–8, 2004.
239. Dalais, F.S., et al., Effects of dietary phytoestrogens in postmenopausal women. *Climacteric* 1, 124–9, 1998.

240. Roughead, Z.K., et al., Controlled substitution of soy protein for meat protein: Effects on calcium retention, bone, and cardiovascular health indices in postmenopausal women. *J Clin Endocrinol Metab* 90, 181–9, 2005.
241. Zhang, X., et al., Prospective cohort study of soy food consumption and risk of bone fracture among postmenopausal women. *Arch Intern Med* 165, 1890–5, 2005.
242. Ye, Y.B., et al., Soy isoflavones attenuate bone loss in early postmenopausal Chinese women: A single-blind randomized, placebo-controlled trial. *Eur J Nutr* 45, 327–34, 2006.
243. Avis, N.E., et al., Is there a menopausal syndrome? Menopausal status and symptoms across racial/ethnic groups. *Soc Sci Med* 52, 345–56, 2001.
244. Duffy, R., et al., Improved cognitive function in postmenopausal women after 12 weeks of consumption of a soya extract containing isoflavones. *Pharmacol Biochem Behav* 75, 721–9, 2003.
245. File, S.E., et al., Cognitive improvement after 6 weeks of soy supplements in postmenopausal women is limited to frontal lobe function. *Menopause* 12, 193–201, 2005.
246. Kritz-Silverstein, D., et al., Isoflavones and cognitive function in older women: The SOy and Postmenopausal Health In Aging (SOPHIA) Study. *Menopause* 10, 196–202, 2003.
247. Nachtigall, L.E.; Nachtigall, L.B., In *The Effects of Isoflavone Derived from Red Clover on Vasomotor Symptoms and Endometrial Thickness*, 9th World Congress on Menopause, Yokohama, Japan, 2000.
248. Penotti, M., et al., Effect of soy-derived isoflavones on hot flushes, endometrial thickness, and the pulsatility index of the uterine and cerebral arteries. *Fertil Steril* 79, 1112–7, 2003.
249. Nikander, E., et al., Lack of effect of isoflavonoids on the vagina and endometrium in postmenopausal women. *Fertil Steril* 83, 137–42, 2005.
250. Unfer, V., et al., Endometrial effects of long-term treatment with phytoestrogens: A randomized, double-blind, placebo-controlled study. *Fertil Steril* 82, 145–8, 2004; quiz 265.
251. Hale, G.E., et al., A double-blind randomized study on the effects of red clover isoflavones on the endometrium. *Menopause* 8, 338–46, 2001.
252. Chan, H.Y., et al., The red clover (Trifolium pratense) isoflavone biochanin A modulates the biotransformation pathways of 7,12-dimethylbenz[a]anthracene. *Br J Nutr* 90, 87–92, 2003.
253. Chinni, S.R., et al., Pleotropic effects of genistein on MCF-7 breast cancer cells. *Int J Mol Med* 12, 29–34, 2003.
254. Xiang, H., et al., A comparative study of growth-inhibitory effects of isoflavones and their metabolites on human breast and prostate cancer cell lines. *Nutr Cancer* 42, 224–32, 2002.
255. Messina, M.J.; Loprinzi, C.L., Soy for breast cancer survivors: A critical review of the literature. *J Nutr* 131, 3095S–108S, 2001.
256. Weaver, C.M.; Cheong, J.M., Soy isoflavones and bone health: The relationship is still unclear. *J Nutr* 135, 1243–7, 2005.
257. Messina, M., et al., Addressing the soy and breast cancer relationship: Review, commentary, and workshop proceedings. *J Natl Cancer Inst* 98, 1275–84, 2006.
258. de Klerk, G.J., et al., Hypokalaemia and hypertension associated with use of liquorice flavoured chewing gum. *BMJ* 314, 731–2, 1997.
259. *Radix Angelicae Sinensis*; WHO: Geneva, Switzerland, 2001.
260. Hirata, J.D., et al., Does dong quai have estrogenic effects in postmenopausal women? A double-blind, placebo-controlled trial. *Fertil Steril* 68, 981–6, 1997.
261. Kupfersztain, C., et al., The immediate effect of natural plant extract, *Angelica sinensis* and *Matricaria chamomilla* (Climex) for the treatment of hot flushes during menopause. A preliminary report. *Clin Exp Obstet Gynecol* 30, 203–6, 2003.

262. Usui, T., et al., The phytochemical lindleyin, isolated from Rhei rhizoma, mediates hormonal effects through estrogen receptors. *J Endocrinol* 175, 289–96, 2002.
263. Matsuda, H., et al., Phytoestrogens from the roots of Polygonum cuspidatum (Polygonaceae): Structure-requirement of hydroxyanthraquinones for estrogenic activity. *Bioorg Med Chem Lett* 11, 1839–42, 2001.
264. Heger, M., et al., Efficacy and safety of a special extract of *Rheum rhaponticum* (ERr 731) in perimenopausal women with climacteric complaints: A 12-week randomized, double-blind, placebo-controlled trial. *Menopause* 13, 744–59, 2006.
265. Brown, D., The use of Vitex agnus castus for hyperprolactinemia. *Quarterly Review of Natural Medicine* Spring, 1997, 19–21, 1997.
266. Lucks, B.C., et al., Vitex agnus-castus essential oil and menopausal balance: A self-care survey. *Complement Ther Nurs Midwifery* 8, 148–54, 2002.
267. Komesaroff, P.A., et al., Effects of wild yam extract on menopausal symptoms, lipids and sex hormones in healthy menopausal women. *Climacteric* 4, 144–50, 2001.
268. McMillan, T.L.; Mark, S., Complementary and alternative medicine and physical activity for menopausal symptoms. *J. Am. Med. Womens Assoc.* 59, 270–277, 2004.
269. Chenoy, R., et al., Effect of oral gamolenic acid from evening primrose oil on menopausal flushing. *BMJ* 308, 501–3, 1994.
270. Kleijnen, J.; Knipschild, P., Ginkgo biloba. *Lancet* 340, 1136–9, 1992.
271. Rudofsky, G., [Effect of Ginkgo biloba extract in arterial occlusive disease. Randomized placebo controlled crossover study]. *Fortschr Med* 105, 397–400, 1987.
272. Bauer, U., 6-Month double-blind randomised clinical trial of Ginkgo biloba extract versus placebo in two parallel groups in patients suffering from peripheral arterial insufficiency. *Arzneimittelforschung* 34, 716–20, 1984.
273. Birks, J., et al., Ginkgo biloba for cognitive impairment and dementia. *Cochrane Database Syst Rev*, CD003120, 2002.
274. Elsabagh, S., et al., Limited cognitive benefits in Stage +2 postmenopausal women after 6 weeks of treatment with Ginkgo biloba. *J Psychopharmacol* 19, 173–81, 2005.
275. Hartley, D.E., et al., Effects on cognition and mood in postmenopausal women of 1-week treatment with Ginkgo biloba. *Pharmacol Biochem Behav* 75, 711–20, 2003.
276. Fugh-Berman, A., Herb-drug interactions. *Lancet* 355, 134–8, 2000.
277. Wiklund, I.K., et al., Effects of a standardized ginseng extract on quality of life and physiological parameters in symptomatic postmenopausal women: A double-blind, placebo-controlled trial. Swedish Alternative Medicine Group. *Int J Clin Pharmacol Res* 19, 89–99, 1999.
278. Tode, T., et al., Effect of Korean red ginseng on psychological functions in patients with severe climacteric syndromes. *Int J Gynaecol Obstet* 67, 169–74, 1999.
279. Amato, P., et al., Estrogenic activity of herbs commonly used as remedies for menopausal symptoms. *Menopause* 9, 145–50, 2002.
280. Warnecke, G., [Psychosomatic dysfunctions in the female climacteric. Clinical effectiveness and tolerance of Kava Extract WS 1490]. *Fortschr Med* 109, 119–22, 1991.
281. http://Scienceviews.com/plants/motherwort.html. Last accessed on July 31, 2007.
282. Balderer, G.; Borbely, A.A., Effect of valerian on human sleep. *Psychopharmacology (Berl)* 87, 406–9, 1985.
283. Leathwood, P.D.; Chauffard, F., Aqueous extract of valerian reduces latency to fall asleep in man. *Planta Med.* 1983 Apr; 51(2):144–8.
284. Leathwood, P.D., et al., Aqueous extract of valerian root (Valeriana officinalis L.) improves sleep quality in man. *Pharmacol Biochem Behav* 17, 65–71, 1982.
285. Valeriana officinalis. *Alternative Medicine Review* 9, 438–440, 2004.

286. Linde, K., et al., St. John's wort for depression—an overview and meta-analysis of randomised clinical trials. *BMJ* 313, 253–8, 1996.
287. Grube, B., et al., St. John's Wort extract: Efficacy for menopausal symptoms of psychological origin. *Adv Ther* 16, 177–86, 1999.
288. Liske, E., Therapeutic efficacy and safety of Cimicifuga racemosa for gynecologic disorders. *Adv Ther* 15, 45–53, 1998.
289. Zhou, S., et al., Pharmacokinetic interactions of drugs with St. John's wort. *J Psychopharmacol* 18, 262–76, 2004.

Section III

Nutrition in Chronic Disease and Various Conditions

7 Obesity and Weight Management

Peter Clifton

CONTENTS

7.1 INTRODUCTION

In this chapter, we will examine whether women differ from men in their metabolic response to excess fat and whether energy restriction achieves the same outcome in men and women. Finally the very important issue of weight maintenance and whether women are more successful than men at maintaining weight will be examined.

7.2 ETIOLOGY OF OBESITY IN WOMEN

The exact etiology of obesity in either men or women is not clear and for any individual the contribution of increased energy intake or decreased activity may vary widely although most authors would accept that dietary change is probably the most significant factor. Nevertheless whatever the cause, treatment will need to include both long-term energy restriction and increased activity levels and a constant focus on weight to avoid regain.

There is a vast literature on the possible environmental causes of obesity and this section will be able to cover only a small fraction of it. There is nothing in the etiology that is unique to women. Although fat has often been the target of many interventions there probably has been little or no increase in fat intake over the last 20 years. However, it is clear that there has been an increase in carbohydrate-rich foods. For instance in Australia, in children, there has been an increase between 1985 and 1995 [1] in the consumption of energy-dense foods, such as

- Cakes and biscuits (46% increase)
- Soft drinks (30%–50% increase)
- Confectionary (40%–56% increase)
- Sugar products and dishes (60%–136% increase)

In the United States, National Health and Nutrition Examination Survey (NHANES) data (1971–2000) has shown an increase in the percentage of energy from carbohydrate by about 6.2%–6.6% (absolute), with a decrease in the percentage energy from fat and an increase in total energy intake. For men, average energy intake increased from 2450 to 2618 kcal ($p < 0.01$), and for women, from 1542 to 1877 kcal ($p > 0.01$). The increase in energy intake is attributable primarily to an increase in carbohydrate intake, with a 62.4 g increase among women ($p < 0.01$) and a 67.7 g increase among men ($p < 0.01$). Total fat intake in grams increased among women by 6.5 g ($p < 0.01$) and decreased among men by 5.3 g ($p < 0.01$) [2]. Soft drinks have been a major cause of the increase in carbohydrate in the United States, with a 135% increase in consumption from 1977 to 2001 years [3]. This increase has been associated with an increase in body mass index (BMI) in frequent consumers [4] but not all data is consistent, especially in Europe where a very large survey in 138,000 ten to sixteen year olds showed no relationship between BMI and soft drink intake [5]. A recent systematic review concluded that the association was strong enough to recommend public health action [6].

Global dietary quality in terms of high fibre, high whole grain, lower fat, and sugar is associated with weight status. The Swedish Mammography study followed 33,840 women for 9 years [7]. Normal weight and overweight women increased their weight while obese women decreased their weight. A higher score on a healthy eating scale predicted a better weight outcome in all groups and obese women lost up to 4 kg. In the Pound of Prevention study in 826 women and 214 men over 3 years, weight gain was related to the level of fat in the diet and to the level of physical activity, especially high intensity activity [8]. In the Framingham Offspring Study of 2245 men and women, a higher dietary quality (according to standard dietary guidelines) predicted a lower weight gain by about 2–5 lb over 8 years [9]. In 74,091 nurses, high fiber, whole grain foods were associated with a 1.4 kg less weight gain over 12 years. Women in the highest quintile of intake had a 50% reduction in the risk of major weight gain (>25 kg) compared with the lowest quintile. A high refined grain intake was positively associated with weight gain [10]. Similar but less dramatic findings were shown in male physicians, in whom even refined breakfast cereals were associated with protection from weight gain [11]. Breakfast cereal consumption was predictive of lower BMI in adolescent girls [12] and in the NHANES III cohort [13] although in a later NHANES cohort this was seen only in women [14]. In a large cohort from Denmark [15], protein intake, especially from animal protein, was significantly inversely associated with 5 year changes in waist circumference. In women, positive associations with the change in waist circumference were seen for carbohydrate from refined grains and potatoes and from foods with simple sugars, whereas carbohydrate from fruit and vegetables was inversely associated. Changes in men were not significant.

7.3 BODY COMPOSITION AND SEX

7.3.1 Fat

Women have a higher rate of obesity (BMI > 30) than men, but in addition, at the same BMI, the fat to lean ratio in women is about 0.9 (varying from 0.6 to 1.1) while in men it is about 0.5 (varying from 0.4 to 0.6) [16]. However, much of this additional fat, at least in premenopausal women, is subcutaneous fat in the gluteal and thigh regions, where it may exert protective effects [17,18]. At the same BMI, men have the same or an increased absolute amount of midriff fat by DEXA and thus may be more insulin resistant despite their larger lean mass [18]. This sexual dimorphism is seen already in 5–7 year olds where boys have higher waist to hip ratios due to less gluteal adiposity [19]. As women age, they have a greater increase in fat mass (26% increase per decade compared with 17% in men) and waist circumference (4% per decade compared with 2% in men) [20]. However, in Japanese subjects, males gain 2.6 times more visceral fat than premenopausal women and about the same amount as postmenopausal women. Leg fat decreased with age [21].

7.3.2 Leptin and Fat

The other major difference between men and women is in plasma leptin levels, which are significantly higher in women even after adjustment for the increased fat mass. Although plasma leptin is correlated with fat mass in men and women, the level is 3 times higher in women for a given fat mass. In response to caloric reduction and a similar decrease in percent fat mass, women have a decline in plasma leptin that is twice as great as in men [22]. In addition, in this study, the decrease in leptin per kilogram of fat mass was greater in women than in men ($-0.37 +/- 0.34$ vs. $-0.04 +/- 0.06$ ng/mL/kg; $p < 0.01$). After weight loss, the change in leptin concentrations correlated positively with the change in fat mass in men ($r = 0.60$; $p < 0.01$), but not in women ($r = 0.31$; $p = 0.17$). The loss in fat mass correlated negatively with baseline leptin levels in women ($r = -0.47$; $p < 0.05$), but not in men ($r = 0.03$). Dietary fat content has no effect on plasma leptin levels [23].

Although in men and women leptin is closely associated with BMI and percent fat equally ($r = 0.82–0.88$), hyperleptinemia is associated with insulin resistance ($r = -0.57$; $p < 0.0001$) and high waist to hip ratio (WHR) ($r = 0.75$; $p < 0.0001$) only in men [24]. On the other hand, during the hyperinsulinemic euglycemic clamp studies, hyperinsulinemia acutely increased leptin concentrations (20%) only in women. While absolute and relative reductions in body weight and body fat are similar, men mobilize more intra-abdominal fat than women, and women lose more subcutaneous fat. The greater reduction in intra-abdominal fat seen in men is accompanied by a more marked improvement in the metabolic risk profile [25]. Subcutaneous fat thickness shows a stronger association with leptin levels in males than in females, whereas no association is found with preperitoneal fat thickness (as measured by ultrasound). Leptin and the ratio of subcutaneous to preperitoneal fat are significantly related only in men.

WHR values are not correlated with leptin concentrations in either sex [26]. Leptin mRNA is expressed to a much greater degree in subcutaneous fat compared with omental fat and the ratio of expression between the two is much greater in women (5.5-fold) compared with men (1.9-fold) and a relationship could be observed in women between leptin mRNA and BMI [27]. Leptin secretion rates in women are 2–3-fold higher from subcutaneous compared with omental fat and the subcutaneous secretion rate was the major predictor of plasma leptin levels. Subcutaneous cells were ~50% bigger than those in omental fat [28]. Estrogen stimulates leptin mRNA production and leptin release [29].

7.3.3 Leptin and Energy Metabolism

Bobbioni-Harsch et al. [30] found that a high leptin level was a marker of low rates of resting energy expenditure (REE) when body weight is stable and a marker of a decrease in REE and fat oxidation during a hypocaloric diet. However, leptin, ghrelin, and adiponectin do not predict long-term weight changes in 60–91 year olds over an 18 year period [31]. Leptin was not associated with weight gain over 8 years in young men and women [32] although Savoye et al. [33] found that high basal leptin levels accounted for 18% of the variance in weight gain over 2.5 years in children aged 7–8 years and in boys and girls aged 6–9 over a 12 month period [34]. In rats, there are clear differences in physiology between males and females, with female rats increasing their food intake by 40% after a 12 h fast compared with only 10% in male rats. The increase in plasma ghrelin was 2-fold greater with fasting in female rats, suggesting this was driving the increased food intake. In response to an inflammatory stimulus (LPS), food intake was reduced equally as was ghrelin but leptin rose by 230% in female rats compared with 33% in male rats. This finding suggests again that ghrelin was a major determinant of food intake and that the changes in leptin played no role [35].

7.3.4 Fat Cell Physiology

In women, estrogen downregulates β-adrenergic receptors and upregulates α-receptors, thus reducing lipolysis rates in fat [36,37] compared with men. Differences between omental and subcutaneous fat have been conflicting but Tchernof et al. [38] clarified some of the conflict in a study in a large group of 55 women. Compared with adipocytes from the omental fat, subcutaneous adipocytes are larger, have higher LPL activity, and are more lipolytic on a per cell basis, reflecting the fact that this is the major fat storage organ in women. In contrast, omental adipocytes display greater relative responsiveness to both adrenergic receptor- and postreceptor-acting agents compared with subcutaneous adipocytes. 17-β estradiol strongly stimulates mRNA expression for Type I 11-β-hydroxysteroid dehydrogenase (HSD1) in pre-adipocytes and potentially stimulates cortisol production from cortisone but decreases P450 aromatase expression by half, thus potentially reducing estrogen production from testosterone. In men, it has no effect on HSD1 but stimulates aromatase mRNA 2.4-fold. Androgens increase the expression of mRNA for both enzymes in men by 2.5–5-fold. Leptin stimulates the expression of mRNA for both enzymes in men but decreases expression in women [39] but the physiological impact of these observations is not clear.

7.4 BODY COMPOSITION, METABOLIC SYNDROME, AND SEX

The association of obesity with the metabolic syndrome is very clear, in fact in the International Diabetes Federation definition, visceral obesity is part of the definition. Whether the metabolic syndrome is expressed differently in women is not clear. In a population of 1974 men and women in Turkey [40], 40% of women and 29% of men had the metabolic syndrome as defined by the criteria of the National Cholesterol Education Program guidelines (three or more of fasting glucose >6.1, BP > 135/85, TG > 1.7, HDL < 1.0 (M) or 1.3 (W) or waist circumference >88 or 102 cm). Women with the metabolic syndrome, regardless of the presence of obesity, were twice as likely to develop a disturbance in glucose metabolism (either impaired fasting glucose or frank diabetes) over a 4 year follow-up period compared with women without the metabolic syndrome or obesity. This relationship was not seen in men. In men, CVD events were predicted by the presence of the metabolic syndrome, regardless of the presence of obesity, but abnormal glucose metabolism was not a predictor. The converse was seen in women.

In the United States, between NHANES III (1988–1994) and NHANES 1999–2000 studies, there was a statistically significant increase in prevalence of the metabolic syndrome in women but not in men. Young women aged 20–39 years had a 76% increase in the incidence of metabolic syndrome compared with a 5% increase in men [41] driven by a marked increase in obesity in this age group. In the French MONICA (Multinational *moni*toring of trends and determinants in *ca*rdiovascular disease) cohort [42], the predictors of the metabolic syndrome were examined in 3508 men and women aged 35–64. In women, metabolic syndrome was associated more with BMI, waist girth, and low HDL cholesterol while systolic and diastolic BP and apolipoprotein B were more associated in men. Fasting insulin, glucose, triglyceride, and LDL cholesterol were not different between sexes. Thus, women need higher levels of obesity to achieve the same degree of insulin resistance and metabolic disturbance as men. The relationship of visceral and peripheral fat to the metabolic syndrome is discussed in a review by Wajchenburg in 2000 [43]. Lower intakes of carbohydrate are associated with lower rates of the metabolic syndrome in men (odds ratio of 0.44 compared with a high carbohydrate intake) but not in women while in women only a moderate alcohol intake was protective (odds ratio 0.76) [44].

In a German cohort study from Augsburg [45], elevated fasting glucose was more common in men (9.9%) compared with women (4.4%). Women in this and other studies have higher 2 h glucose levels for the same level of fasting glucose compared with men. Thus women appear to have a disturbance in insulin release while men have higher levels of insulin resistance probably related to increased visceral fat.

The development of diabetes increases the risk of cardiovascular disease in women. From eight prospective studies, the multivariate-adjusted summary odds ratio for CHD mortality due to diabetes was 2.3 (95% confidence interval, 1.9–2.8) for men and 2.9 (95% confidence interval, 2.2–3.8) for women but this difference disappeared after adjustment for classic CHD risk factors [46]. A later meta-analysis suggested the risk of fatal coronary disease in women with diabetes was 50% greater than that in men [47].

7.4.1 Polycystic Ovary Syndrome

Polycystic ovary syndrome (PCOS), a syndrome of insulin resistance, disturbed menstrual function, infertility and hyperandrogenism, is closely associated with obesity, which worsens its clinical expression [48]. There is no similar syndrome in men although obesity in men lowers testosterone, increases free estradiol, and worsens sexual and reproductive function [49,50]. Intra-abdominal fat in normal healthy women expresses Type 3 17-β-hydroxysteroid dehydrogenase (17-β-HSD), the enzyme that catalyzes the conversion of androstenedione to testosterone in the testis and exceeded the level of aromatase. The ratio of levels of 17-β-HSD mRNA to aromatase mRNA in intra-abdominal adipose tissue was positively correlated with BMI ($n = 11, r = 0.61, p < 0.05$) and waist circumference ($n = 10, r = 0.65, p < 0.05$). The converse was found in subcutaneous abdominal adipose tissue. Androstenedione *in vitro* was converted to testosterone with minimal conversion to estrone. Thus visceral fat accumulation contributes an androgenic burden in women [51]. Lifestyle modification can clearly benefit women with PCOS although there is no evidence that any one dietary strategy is beneficial [52].

7.4.2 Androgens and Cardiovascular Risk

Low sex hormone binding globulin (SHBG) and high free androgen index (FAI) are strongly related to elevated cardiovascular risk factors (higher insulin, glucose, and hemostatic and inflammatory markers and adverse lipids) even after controlling for BMI in 3297 pre- and perimenopausal women in a multiethnic sample ($p < 0.001$) [53,54]. In the Women's Health Initiative Study, lower SHBG and higher FAI levels were noted among postmenopausal women who developed CVD events, but this was not independent of BMI and other cardiovascular risk factors. Estradiol levels were not associated with risk of CVD in hormone replacement therapy users or nonusers [55].

7.4.3 C-Reactive Protein

C-reactive protein (CRP) is a sensitive inflammatory marker that predicts future cardiovascular events but is also related to obesity and falls with weight loss [56,57]. Women generally have higher levels of CRP than men, reflecting their increased fat mass. There may be a sex related difference in the relationship between CRP and the metabolic syndrome. In the Mexico City Diabetes Study of 515 men and 729 women, 14% of women and 16% of men developed the metabolic syndrome over 6 years. For women in the highest tertile of CRP, the odds ratio of developing the metabolic syndrome was 4 and diabetes was 5.5, with little effect of adjustment for BMI or the Homeostatic Model Assessment score. This relationship was not seen in men [58]. Similarly, CRP was more strongly associated with components of the metabolic syndrome in women than in men in a Japanese population [59]. In the Framingham cohort, age-adjusted CRP levels in subjects with the metabolic syndrome (24% of the population) were higher in women than in men (7.8 vs. 4.6 mg/L) [60].

7.5 WEIGHT CONTROL BEHAVIORS, DIET, AND GENDER

Women are far more likely than men to report a history of dieting (8-fold greater) and to participate in organized weight loss programs (11-fold greater than men). Exercise was the most frequently reported specific weight loss practice (66% of women and 53% of men), followed by decreasing fat intake (62% of women and 48% of men) [61]. In a large twin study in Finland, individuals who had engaged in intentional weight loss exhibited markedly more restricting, overeating, and alternating restricting or overeating than those in the no intentional weight loss group. Snacking and eating in the evening were characteristic of women with at least two weight loss attempts. Eating in response to visual and emotional cues was very pronounced in women who had attempted to lose weight but this was much less so in men. Interestingly, engaging in intentional weight loss was much more heritable in women than in men (66% vs. 38%) [62]. Female twins also have higher heritability of BMI than men (0.61 vs. 0.46 for Danish twins aged 46–59) [63]. Social status of women has an effect, with women with low employment grade in the Whitehall II study of London civil servants being twice as likely as men in this same work strata to consume unhealthy diets compared with higher status men and women [64]. High disinhibition and low restraint in female Whitehall civil servants are directly associated with BMI [65], while in US women aged 55–69, disinhibition was the major predictor of BMI and weight gain although somewhat modified by restraint [66]. In the Quebec Family Study, women had significantly higher cognitive dietary restraint and disinhibition scores than did men ($p < 0.0001$). In both genders, disinhibition and susceptibility to hunger was higher in obese subjects than in overweight and nonobese subjects ($p < 0.05$) [67].

7.5.1 Therapeutic Interventions

7.5.1.1 Low Fat Diets

Low fat diets have been advocated for weight loss for many years and have been based on several well-established principles. Low fat diets have a lower energy density than high fat diets. Since humans respond mostly to volume of food eaten rather than calories, this should lead to a lower energy intake. Lower fat diets also have higher fiber content and this may also enhance satiety. Some minor degree of faecal loss of energy occurs with high carbohydrate diets, especially those with a high fiber or high resistant starch level. In a review by Avenell et al. [68] they found that low fat diets reduced weight by an average of 3.6 kg for up to 3 years while four studies found that low fat diets are associated with lower rates of diabetes and reduced antihypertensive medication for up to 3 years. There were no sex effects in these studies.

It has been estimated that a reduction in fat by 10% of energy (without any conscious effort to reduce calories, this would occur through greater satiety and better control of food intake) would reduce weight by 16 g/day over a year with a loss of this effect beyond a year. The mechanism for the loss of this effect is not clear. So although there is good evidence that low fat diets work for some people many people cannot maintain them long term and so new and different solutions have been sought.

7.5.1.2 Very Low Carbohydrate Diets

A complete contrast to the low fat, high carbohydrate diet is the low carbohydrate diet, which has been in use for over 100 years but was popularized by Atkins many years ago. Surprisingly trials have only appeared over the last 3–4 years evaluating the effects of the Atkins diet [69]. These are very uniform in their findings, with a better weight loss of about 3.3 kg at 6 months, but no difference from low fat diets at 12 months. The diets worked by reducing caloric intake by removing a very wide range of carbohydrate-rich foods, but as compliance to this fairly severe regime drifted, so did the weight. Although triglyceride levels dropped more and HDL cholesterol levels were maintained on the Atkins diet, LDL cholesterol rose by about 2%–3%. This is a lot lower than expected and it shows that a large amount of saturated fat in the virtual absence of carbohydrate and the presence of weight loss acts differently to what is expected. There is no data beyond 12 months on Atkins diets. There are modified forms of the Atkins diet, which endeavor to replace some of the saturated fat with unsaturated fat (e.g., the South Beach Diet) but there is no trial data. One would expect similar weight loss but better LDL results compared with Atkins.

7.5.1.3 High Protein, Moderate Carbohydrate Diets

This is the compromise position diet and there are many variants, e.g., the Zone diet, the Protein Power diet, CSIRO (Commonwealth Scientific and Industrial Research Organisation) diet. It makes use of the increased satiating effect of protein with the modest reduction in carbohydrate benefiting triglyceride levels and sometimes HDL cholesterol. Fat is kept low at 30% and its composition is healthy. Only the CSIRO diet has been extensively studied in large groups of people [16,70,71] but its results have been confirmed by other investigators with smaller numbers of patients. In general, protein as a percentage of energy is doubled from 15% to 30%. People with elevated triglyceride levels gain particular benefits, at least at 3 months, with greater weight, fat, and central fat loss [70,71]. Doubling the amount of protein as a percentage of energy does not mean doubling the amount of protein. It mostly occurs by reducing the amount of fat and carbohydrate and energy with only a 10%–15% increase in the actual amount of protein. The Zone diet has a very similar composition to the CSIRO diet but it insists, with no evidence to support it, that every meal should have the correct Zone composition of 30:30:40 (protein, fat, carbohydrate).

There have now been several meta-analyses done and in one Krieger et al. [72] examined 87 short-term studies and found that protein intakes of >1.05 g/kg of actual rather than desirable body weight were associated with 0.6 kg better retention of lean mass. In studies greater than 12 weeks in duration, this increased to 1.2 kg. In studies that used a carbohydrate intake of <35%–41% there was a 2 kg greater loss of fat mass, but this was accompanied by a 0.7 kg greater loss of lean mass. In studies of 12 weeks or more in duration, this increased to 5.6 and 1.7 kg, respectively. Thus a low carbohydrate, high protein diet is associated with better fat loss and sometimes less lean mass loss. In this meta-analysis there were no sex effects. We have performed a meta-analysis (unpublished) of our published data on high protein diets for short-term weight loss and found that there were no sex effects. We found that in participants with a baseline fasting triglyceride >1.7 mmol/L, there was greater total and abdominal fat loss.

7.5.1.4 Meal Replacements

An alternative approach for weight loss is to use meal replacements like Optifast to replace 1, 2, or 3 meals. Total meal replacement can certainly lead to dramatic weight loss of 20 kg or more but in the long term the amount of weight lost is the same when more gradual approaches are taken. The best long-term data has shown that a 10% weight loss can be maintained up to 5 years with the use of 1 meal replacement/day increasing to 2 if weight regain occurs [73–75]. It is a strategy that works very well for some people. There are a relatively limited number of studies using meal replacements to achieve weight loss [76,77].

7.5.1.5 Controlled Studies

Six studies have been included in a recent meta-analysis of randomized controlled trials [78]. This meta-analysis found that a diet plan that includes meal replacements to replace 1 or more meals achieved more weight loss, ~2.5 kg more at 3 months, than a reduced energy food based diet plan. Four randomized controlled studies support the view that meal replacements may be advantageous in weight loss programs whereas two studies do not.

7.5.1.6 Adverse Outcomes from Different Diets

There is no risk from eating high fibre and high carbohydrate weight loss diets but the high protein diets have several risks attributed to them. One study suggests that women with impaired renal function have a greater decline in renal function with a greater protein intake [79]. Those with normal renal function had no such decline. Thus until evidence to the contrary is shown then care should be shown in those with renal impairment. However, as noted above, high protein weight loss diets may not actually contain an increase in the amount of protein in grams. Although high protein diets, particularly high meat diets, have been shown to increase calcium loss, high protein diets have been shown to reduce the risk of fractures [80]. High meat diets have been shown to be associated with increased colorectal cancer, but in the biggest study of all, the European Prospective Investigation into Cancer and Nutrition study from Europe, this was true only for processed meat [81]. Nevertheless, studies from the United States have also implicated red meat alone with an increased risk of colorectal cancer (but significant only in the rectosigmoid and rectum). The increased risk is of the order of 30%–40% in the highest quintile [82]. The risk can be reduced substantially by weight loss and exercise, eating chicken and fish; eating more than 28 g fiber/day removes the effect of meat altogether. So in terms of this diet, replacing processed meat with fish or chicken at lunch or ensuring fiber intake is high is the best strategy.

The Atkins diet has been portrayed as prone to many adverse outcomes but the evidence is very limited. Certainly constipation is a problem and fiber supplements may be required. Ketogenic diets can cause renal stones (about 6% incidence over 5 years) in children but not in adults. Although in theory, long-term use of the Atkins diet might lead to vitamin and mineral deficiency and possibly increased risk of GI tract cancer; this seems unlikely as a very restricted diet is actually not maintained over the long term.

Although data relating deliberate weight loss with beneficial outcomes is not clear and there is a vast and controversial literature on this subject, recent reports at the International Congress on Obesity in 2006 showed benefit on cardiovascular events and mortality from surgically induced weight loss. Certainly bariatric surgery can lead to clinical improvement or resolution in 64%–100% of patients with diabetes mellitus, 62%–69% of patients with hypertension, 85% of patients with obstructive sleep apnea, 60%–100% of patients with dyslipidemia, and up to 90% of patients with nonalcoholic fatty liver disease [83].

7.6 LEAN MASS LOSS WITH WEIGHT LOSS AND SEX

With energy restriction, both fat and lean mass loss occur but Sartorio et al. [84] demonstrated that with aerobic and resistance exercise, women appeared to be better at preventing this loss of lean mass (at least over 3 weeks). High protein weight loss diets may also be better at preserving lean mass in women [16,85]. Part of the reason may be the much greater fat free mass (FFM) in obese men compared with obese women. Thus, women have much lower limb power per unit body mass but not per unit FFM [86]. Similar findings are seen in obese adolescents [87]. However, other investigators [88] have seen no difference between men and women in loss of visceral, subcutaneous, or lean mass in response to dietary restriction although less visceral fat loss (either as an absolute amount or as a percentage) is sometimes seen in women [16,85]. Weight loss can lead to bone loss even with exercise and calcium supplementation and bone density has been inversely related to the number of times premenopausal women have been on a weight loss diet [89] and in those women with high cognitive dietary restraint and a weight of <71 kg [90].

7.6.1 Weight Maintenance

Any dietary pattern with caloric restriction can lead to weight loss but the key question is how to maintain this weight loss in the long term. The National Weight Loss register in the United States contains 4800 individuals who have lost at least 13.6 kg and maintained this loss for at least a year [91]. It was set up in 1995 to understand what behavior is required for successful weight maintenance. Approximately 20% of overweight individuals are successful at long-term weight loss when defined as losing at least 10% of initial body weight and maintaining the loss for at least 1 year. Individuals in the weight loss register maintained their body weight by a few simple strategies [92]: eating a low fat diet with very limited variety in energy-dense high calorie foods [93], eating breakfast almost every day, weighing themselves regularly and engaging in high levels of physical activity (about 1 h/day), watching little television [94], and maintaining a consistent food pattern across week days and weekends. A subset of the register ($n = 2708$, enrolled between 1995 and 2003) who had lost an average of 33 kg and maintained a 13.6 kg loss for 5.8 years before enrolment had measurements of diet and physical activity at enrolment and 1 year later. Individuals who enrolled later in the study had higher levels of fat intake (29.8%) than those who enrolled earlier, and energy from carbohydrate was proportionately decreased. Physical activity was lower in later years. The use of low carbohydrate diets had increased about 3-fold in 17% of participants in 2003. Weight regain over 1 year was related to higher levels of caloric intake, fast food consumption, and fat intake and lower levels of physical activity [95]. There were no apparent sex effects. In overfeeding studies in normal weight men and women ($n = 48$), the energy cost of the weight gain was the same in both sex at 33.7 kJ/kg, and 43.6% of the gain was lean body mass [96].

In our study of weight maintenance at 1 year after losing weight on either a high protein or a high carbohydrate diet, it was found that women who could maintain a protein intake of 90 g/day or more (about 30% of the cohort) maintained a weight loss of 4 kg more than those who had lower protein intakes [97].

Wing et al. [98] examined a self-regulation weight maintenance program delivered either face to face or over the internet in 314 participants who had lost a mean of 19.3 kg in the 2 previous years. Weight gain over 18 months was 2.5 kg in the face to face group, 4.9 kg in the control group ($p = 0.05$ for difference between these 2 groups), and 4.7 kg in the internet group. The proportion of individuals who regained 2.3 kg or more was significantly higher in the control group (72.4%) than either the face to face (45.7%) or the internet group (54.8%) ($p < 0.01$ for both). The intervention programs daily self-weighing and self-regulation.

7.7 CONCLUSION

Although body composition clearly differs between men and women, with women having more total and subcutaneous fat and men having more visceral fat and lean tissue, the response to energy restriction, regardless of macronutrient composition, is very similar in terms of percentage weight loss. There is limited evidence that women might sometimes lose less visceral fat than do men and may reduce absolute lean mass loss with exercise or high protein diets. Although leptin levels are clearly different in women and relate differently to weight loss in men and women, the implications of this finding in terms of weight maintenance are not clear. Although rates of the metabolic syndrome and diabetes are similar in men and women, diabetes probably has a greater impact in women for cardiovascular risk. Again there are well described differences in fat cell physiology between men and women but this does not appear to be of clinical relevance at present.

7.8 FUTURE RESEARCH

Whether there are weight maintenance strategies that are particularly beneficial to women is not clear and has not really been prospectively examined. It is also not clear if the health benefit of weight loss, surgical or otherwise, is different between men and women and much larger cohorts need to be studied. Thus at least 10,000 men and women who have had obesity surgery need to be examined to see if there are gender differences in the reduction in fat mass, hypertension, Type 2 diabetes, cardiovascular disease, and death over a 10 year period.

REFERENCES

1. Cook, T., Rutishauser, I., and Allsop, R. The bridging study—comparing results from the 1983, 1985 and 1995 Australian national nutrition surveys. Canberra: Australian Food and Nutrition Monitoring Unit, Commonwealth Department of Health and Aged Care, 2001.
2. Centers for Disease Control and Prevention. Trends in intake of energy and macronutrients. *MMWR Morb. Mortal. Wkly. Rep.*, 53, 80, 2004.
3. Nielsen, S.J. and Popkin, B.M. Changes in beverage intake between 1977 and 2001. *Am. J. Prev. Med.*, 27, 205, 2004.
4. Ludwig, D.S., Peterson, K.E., and Gortmaker, S.L. Relation between consumption of sugar-sweetened drinks and childhood obesity: A prospective, observational analysis. *Lancet*, 357, 505, 2001.
5. Janssen, I. et al. Behaviour in School-Aged Children Obesity Working Group. Comparison of overweight and obesity prevalence in school-aged youth from 34 countries and their relationships with physical activity and dietary patterns. *Obes. Rev.*, 6, 123, 2005.
6. Malik, V.S., Schulze, M.B., and Hu, F.B. Intake of sugar-sweetened beverages and weight gain: A systematic review. *Am. J. Clin. Nutr.*, 84, 24, 2006. Review.
7. Newby, P.K. et al. Longitudinal changes in food patterns predict changes in weight and body mass index and the effects are greatest in obese women. *J. Nutr.*, 136, 2580, 2006.
8. Sherwood, N.E. et al. Predictors of weight gain in the Pound of Prevention study. *Int. J. Obes. Relat. Metab. Disord.*, 24, 395, 2000.
9. Quatromoni, P.A. et al. Dietary quality predicts adult weight gain: Findings from the Framingham Offspring Study. *Obesity (Silver Spring)*, 14, 1383, 2006.
10. Liu, S. et al. Relation between changes in intakes of dietary fiber and grain products and changes in weight and development of obesity among middle-aged women. *Am. J. Clin. Nutr.*, 78, 920, 2003.
11. Bazzano, L.A. et al. Dietary intake of whole and refined grain breakfast cereals and weight gain in men. *Obes. Res.*, 13, 1952, 2005.
12. Barton, B.A. et al. The relationship of breakfast and cereal consumption to nutrient intake and body mass index: The National Heart, Lung, and Blood Institute Growth and Health Study. *J. Am. Diet. Assoc.*, 105, 1383, 2005.

13. Cho, S. et al. The effect of breakfast type on total daily energy intake and body mass index: Results from the Third National Health and Nutrition Examination Survey (NHANES III). *J. Am. Coll. Nutr.*, 22, 296, 2003.
14. Song, W.O. et al. Is consumption of breakfast associated with body mass index in US adults? *J. Am. Diet. Assoc.*, 105, 1373, 2005.
15. Halkjaer, J. et al. Intake of macronutrients as predictors of 5-y changes in waist circumference. *Am. J. Clin. Nutr.*, 84, 789, 2006.
16. Farnsworth, E. et al. Effect of a high-protein, energy-restricted diet on body composition, glycemic control, and lipid concentrations in overweight and obese hyperinsulinemic men and women. *Am. J. Clin. Nutr.*, 78, 31, 2003.
17. Snijder, M.B. et al. Regional body composition as a determinant of arterial stiffness in the elderly: The Hoorn Study. *J. Hypertens.*, 22, 2339, 2004.
18. Ferreira, I. et al. Central fat mass versus peripheral fat and lean mass: Opposite (adverse versus favorable) associations with arterial stiffness? The Amsterdam Growth and Health Longitudinal Study. *J. Clin. Endocrinol. Metab.*, 89, 2632, 2004.
19. Webster-Gandy, J., Warren, J., and Henry, C.J. Sexual dimorphism in fat patterning in a sample of 5 to 7-year-old children in Oxford. *Int. J. Food. Sci. Nutr.*, 54, 467, 2003.
20. Poehlman, E.T. et al. Physiological predictors of increasing total and central adiposity in aging men and women. *Arch. Intern. Med.*, 155, 2443, 1995.
21. Kotani, K. et al. Sexual dimorphism of age-related changes in whole-body fat distribution in the obese. *Int. J. Obes. Relat. Metab. Disord.*, 18, 207, 1994.
22. Nicklas, B.J. et al. Gender differences in the response of plasma leptin concentrations to weight loss in obese older individuals. *Obes. Res.*, 5, 62, 1997.
23. Havel, P.J. et al. Relationship of plasma leptin to plasma insulin and adiposity in normal weight and overweight women: Effects of dietary fat content and sustained weight loss. *J. Clin. Endocrinol. Metab.*, 81, 4406, 1996.
24. Kennedy, A. et al. The metabolic significance of leptin in humans: Gender-based differences in relationship to adiposity, insulin sensitivity, and energy expenditure. *J. Clin. Endocrinol. Metab.*, 82, 1293, 1997.
25. Wirth, A. and Steinmetz, B. Gender differences in changes in subcutaneous and intra-abdominal fat during weight reduction: An ultrasound study. *Obes. Res.*, 6, 393, 1998.
26. Minocci, A. et al. Leptin plasma concentrations are dependent on body fat distribution in obese patients. *Int. J. Obes. Relat. Metab. Disord.*, 24, 1139, 2000.
27. Montague, C.T. et al. Depot- and sex-specific differences in human leptin mRNA expression: Implications for the control of regional fat distribution. *Diabetes*, 46, 342, 1997.
28. Van Harmelen, V. et al. Leptin secretion from subcutaneous and visceral adipose tissue in women. *Diabetes*, 47, 913, 1998.
29. Machinal-Quelin, F. et al. Direct in vitro effects of androgens and estrogens on ob gene expression and leptin secretion in human adipose tissue. *Endocrine*, 18, 179, 2002.
30. Bobbioni-Harsch, E. et al. Leptin plasma levels as a marker of sparing-energy mechanisms in obese women. *Int. J. Obes. Relat. Metab. Disord.*, 23, 470, 1995.
31. Langenberg, C. et al. Ghrelin, adiponectin, and leptin do not predict long-term changes in weight and body mass index in older adults: Longitudinal analysis of the Rancho Bernardo cohort. *Am. J. Epidemiol.*, 162, 1189, 2005.
32. Folsom, A.R. et al. Serum leptin and weight gain over 8 years in African American and Caucasian young adults. *Obes. Res.*, 7, 1, 1999.
33. Savoye, M. et al. Importance of plasma leptin in predicting future weight gain in obese children: A two-and-a-half-year longitudinal study. *Int. J. Obes. Relat. Metab. Disord.*, 26, 942, 2002.

34. Byrnes, S.E. et al. Leptin and total cholesterol are predictors of weight gain in pre-pubertal children. *Int. J. Obes. Relat. Metab. Disord.*, 23, 146, 1999.
35. Gayle, D.A. et al. Gender-specific orexigenic and anorexigenic mechanisms in rats. *Life Sci.*, 79, 1531, 2006.
36. Lonnqvist, F. et al. Sex differences in visceral fat lipolysis and metabolic complications of obesity. *Arterioscler. Thromb. Vasc. Biol.*, 17, 1472, 1997.
37. Pedersen, S.B. et al. Estrogen controls lipolysis by up-regulating α2A-adrenergic receptors directly in human adipose tissue through the estrogen receptor-α. Implications for the female fat distribution. *J. Clin. Endocrinol. Metab.*, 89, 1869, 2004.
38. Tchernof, A. et al. Regional differences in adipose tissue metabolism in women: Minor effect of obesity and body fat distribution. *Diabetes*, 55, 1353, 2006.
39. Dieudonne, M.N. et al. Sex steroids and leptin regulate 11β-hydroxysteroid dehydrogenase I and P450 aromatase expressions in human preadipocytes: Sex specificities. *J. Steroid. Biochem. Mol. Biol.*, 99, 189, 2006.
40. Onat, A. et al. Sex difference in development of diabetes and cardiovascular disease on the way from obesity and metabolic syndrome. *Metabolism*, 54, 800, 2005.
41. Ford, E.S., Giles, W.H., and Mokdad, A.H. Increasing prevalence of the metabolic syndrome among U.S. adults. *Diabetes Care*, 27, 2444, 2004.
42. Dallongeville, J. et al. The association of metabolic disorders with the metabolic syndrome is different in men and women. *Ann. Nutr. Metab.*, 48, 43, 2004.
43. Wajchenberg, B.L. Subcutaneous and visceral adipose tissue: Their relation to the metabolic syndrome. *Endocr. Rev.*, 21, 697, 2000.
44. Zhu, S. et al. Lifestyle behaviors associated with lower risk of having the metabolic syndrome. *Metabolism*, 53, 1503, 2004.
45. Rathmann, W. et al. High prevalence of undiagnosed diabetes mellitus in Southern Germany: Target populations for efficient screening. The KORA survey 2000. *Diabetologia*, 46, 182, 2003.
46. Kanaya, A.M., Grady, D., and Barrett-Connor, E. Explaining the sex difference in coronary heart disease mortality among patients with type 2 diabetes mellitus: A meta-analysis. *Arch. Intern. Med.*, 162, 1737, 2002.
47. Huxley, R., Barzi, F., and Woodward, M. Excess risk of fatal coronary heart disease associated with diabetes in men and women: Meta-analysis of 37 prospective cohort studies. *Brit. Med. J.*, 332, 73, 2006.
48. Norman, R.J., Wu, R., and Stankiewicz, M.T. Polycystic ovary syndrome. *Med. J. Aust.*, 180, 132, 2004.
49. Jarow, J.P. et al. Effect of obesity and fertility status on sex steroid levels in men. *Urology*, 42, 171, 1993.
50. Sallmen, M. et al. Reduced fertility among overweight and obese men. *Epidemiology*, 17, 520, 2006.
51. Corbould, A.M. et al. The effect of obesity on the ratio of type 3 17β-hydroxysteroid dehydrogenase mRNA to cytochrome P450 aromatase mRNA in subcutaneous abdominal and intra-abdominal adipose tissue of women. *Int. J. Obes. Relat. Metab. Disord.*, 26, 165, 2002.
52. Moran, L.J. et al. Effects of lifestyle modification in polycystic ovarian syndrome. *Reprod. Biomed. Online*, 12, 569, 2006.
53. Sutton-Tyrrell, K. et al. SWAN Investigators. Sex-hormone-binding globulin and the free androgen index are related to cardiovascular risk factors in multiethnic premenopausal and perimenopausal women enrolled in the Study of Women Across the Nation (SWAN). *Circulation*, 111, 1242, 2005.

54. Sowers, M.R. et al. Androgens are associated with hemostatic and inflammatory factors among women at the mid-life. *J. Clin. Endocrinol. Metab.*, 90, 6064, 2005.
55. Rexrode, K.M. et al. Sex hormone levels and risk of cardiovascular events in postmenopausal women. *Circulation*, 108, 1688, 2003.
56. Heilbronn, L.K., Noakes, M., and Clifton, P.M. Energy restriction and weight loss on very-low-fat diets reduce C-reactive protein concentrations in obese, healthy women. *Arterioscler. Thromb. Vasc. Biol.*, 21, 968, 2001.
57. Heilbronn, L.K. and Clifton, P.M. C-reactive protein and coronary artery disease: Influence of obesity, caloric restriction and weight loss. *J. Nutr. Biochem.*, 13, 316, 2002.
58. Han, T.S. et al. Prospective study of C-reactive protein in relation to the development of diabetes and metabolic syndrome in the Mexico City Diabetes Study. *Diabetes Care*, 25, 2016, 2002.
59. Nakanishi, N., Shiraishi, T., and Wada, M. C-reactive protein concentration is more strongly related to metabolic syndrome in women than in men: The Minoh Study. *Circ. J.*, 69, 386, 2005.
60. Rutter, M.K. et al. C-reactive protein, the metabolic syndrome, and prediction of cardiovascular events in the Framingham Offspring Study. *Circulation*, 110, 380, 2004.
61. Neumark-Sztainer, D. et al. Weight control behaviors among adult men and women: Cause for concern? *Obes. Res.*, 7, 179, 1999.
62. Keski-Rahkonen, A. et al. Intentional weight loss in young adults: Sex-specific genetic and environmental effects. *Obes. Res.*, 13, 745, 2005.
63. Herskind, A.M. et al. Sex and age specific assessment of genetic and environmental influences on body mass index in twins. *Int. J. Obes. Relat. Metab. Disord.*, 20, 106, 1996.
64. Martikainen, P., Brunner, E., and Marmot, M. Socioeconomic differences in dietary patterns among middle-aged men and women. *Soc. Sci. Med.*, 56, 1397, 2003.
65. Dykes, J. et al. Socioeconomic gradient in body size and obesity among women: The role of dietary restraint, disinhibition and hunger in the Whitehall II study. *Int. J. Obes. Relat. Metab. Disord.*, 28, 262, 2004.
66. Hays, N.P. et al. Eating behavior correlates of adult weight gain and obesity in healthy women aged 55–65 y. *Am. J. Clin. Nutr.*, 75, 476, 2002.
67. Provencher, V. et al. Eating behaviors and indexes of body composition in men and women from the Quebec Family Study. *Obes. Res.*, 11, 783, 2003.
68. Avenell, A. et al. What are the long-term benefits of weight reducing diets in adults? A systematic review of randomized controlled trials. *J. Hum. Nutr. Diet.*, 17, 317, 2004.
69. Nordmann, A.J. et al. Effects of low-carbohydrate vs. low-fat diets on weight loss and cardiovascular risk factors: A meta-analysis of randomized controlled trials. *Arch. Intern. Med.*, 166, 285, 2006. Review.
70. Noakes, M. et al. Effect of an energy-restricted, high-protein, low-fat diet relative to a conventional high-carbohydrate, low-fat diet on weight loss, body composition, nutritional status, and markers of cardiovascular health in obese women. *Am. J. Clin. Nutr.*, 81, 1298, 2005.
71. Parker, B. et al. Effect of a high-protein, high-monounsaturated fat weight loss diet on glycemic control and lipid levels in type 2 diabetes. *Diabetes Care*, 25, 425, 2002.
72. Krieger, J.W. et al. Effects of variation in protein and carbohydrate intake on body mass and composition during energy restriction: A meta-regression 1. *Am. J. Clin. Nutr.*, 83, 260, 2006.
73. Ditschuneit, H.H. et al. Metabolic and weight-loss effects of a long-term dietary intervention in obese patients. *Am. J. Clin. Nutr.*, 69, 198, 1999.

74. Flechtner-Mors, M. et al. Metabolic and weight loss effects of long-term dietary intervention in obese patients: Four-year results. *Obes. Res.*, 8, 399, 2000.
75. Ditschuneit, H.H. and Flechtner-Mors, M. Value of structured meals for weight management: Risk factors and long-term weight maintenance. *Obes. Res.*, 9 (Suppl 4), 284S, 2001.
76. Ryan, D.H. et al. Look AHEAD Research Group. Look AHEAD (Action for Health in Diabetes): Design and methods for a clinical trial of weight loss for the prevention of cardiovascular disease in type 2 diabetes. *Cont. Clin. Trial*, 24, 610, 2003.
77. Heber, D. et al. Clinical evaluation of a minimal intervention meal replacement regimen for weight reduction. *J. Am. Coll. Nutr.*, 13, 608, 1994.
78. Heymsfield, S.B. et al. Weight management using a meal replacement strategy: Meta and pooling analysis from six studies. *Int. J. Obes. Relat. Metab. Disord.*, 5, 537, 2003.
79. Knight, E.L. et al. The impact of protein intake on renal function decline in women with normal renal function or mild renal insufficiency. *Ann. Intern. Med.*, 138, 460, 2003.
80. Munger, R.G., Cerhan, J.R., and Chiu, B.C. Prospective study of dietary protein intake and risk of hip fracture in postmenopausal women. *Am. J. Clin. Nutr.*, 69, 147, 1999.
81. Norat, T. et al. Meat, fish, and colorectal cancer risk: The European Prospective Investigation into cancer and nutrition. *J. Natl. Cancer Inst.*, 97, 906, 2005.
82. Chao, A. et al. Meat consumption and risk of colorectal cancer. *JAMA*, 293, 172, 2005.
83. Kushner, R.F. and Noble, C.A. Long-term outcome of bariatric surgery: An interim analysis. *Mayo Clin. Proc.*, 81, S46, 2006.
84. Sartorio, A. et al. Gender-related changes in body composition, muscle strength and power output after a short-term multidisciplinary weight loss intervention in morbid obesity. *J. Endocrinol. Invest.*, 28, 494, 2005.
85. Bowen, J., Noakes, M., and Clifton, P.M. Effect of calcium and dairy foods in high protein, energy-restricted diets on weight loss and metabolic parameters in overweight adults. *Int. J. Obes. (Lond.)*, 29, 957, 2005.
86. Sartorio, A. et al. Influence of gender, age and BMI on lower limb muscular power output in a large population of obese men and women. *Int. J. Obes. Relat. Metab. Disord.*, 28, 91, 2004.
87. Sartorio, A. et al. Age- and gender-related variations of leg power output and body composition in severely obese children and adolescents. *J. Endocrinol. Invest.*, 29, 48, 2006.
88. Janssen, I. and Ross, R. Effects of sex on the change in visceral, subcutaneous adipose tissue and skeletal muscle in response to weight loss. *Int. J. Obes. Relat. Metab. Disord.*, 23, 1035, 1999.
89. Bacon, L. et al. Low bone mass in premenopausal chronic dieting obese women. *Eur. J. Clin. Nutr.*, 58, 966, 2004.
90. Van Loan, M.D. and Keim, N.L. Influence of cognitive eating restraint on total-body measurements of bone mineral density and bone mineral content in premenopausal women aged 18–45 y: A cross-sectional study. *Am. J. Clin. Nutr.*, 72, 837, 2000.
91. Hill, J.O. et al. The National Weight Control Registry: Is it useful in helping deal with our obesity epidemic? *J. Nutr. Educ. Behav.*, 37, 206, 2005.
92. Wing, R.R. and Phelan, S. Long-term weight loss maintenance. *Am. J. Clin. Nutr.*, 82, 222S, 2005.
93. Raynor, H.A. et al. Amount of food group variety consumed in the diet and long-term weight loss maintenance. *Obes. Res.*, 13, 883, 2005.
94. Raynor, D.A. et al. Television viewing and long-term weight maintenance: Results from the national weight control registry. *Obesity (Silver Spring)*, 14, 1816, 2006.
95. Phelan, S. et al. Are the eating and exercise habits of successful weight losers changing? *Obesity (Silver Spring)*,14, 710, 2006.

96. Forbes, G.B. et al. Deliberate overfeeding in women and men: Energy cost and composition of the weight gain. *Br. J. Nutr.*, 56, 1, 1986.
97. Clifton, P.M. et al. Effect of an energy reduced high protein red meat diet on weight loss and metabolic parameters in obese women. *Asia Pac. J. Clin. Nutr.*, 12, S10, 2003.
98. Wing, R.R. et al. A self-regulation program for maintenance of weight loss. *N. Engl. J. Med.*, 355, 1563, 2006.

8 The Metabolic Syndrome and Type 2 Diabetes Mellitus

Janet A. Vogt and Thomas M.S. Wolever

CONTENTS

8.1 INTRODUCTION

This chapter examines the evidence for sex-specific dietary recommendations for the prevention and treatment of the metabolic syndrome (MetS) and type 2 diabetes mellitus (T2DM) in women. Women with the MetS are at an increased risk for developing T2DM [1,2], so rather than discussing all forms of diabetes, we have chosen to focus in particular on T2DM. A central feature of the MetS, which has also been linked to increased incidence of T2DM, is abdominal obesity. While this is briefly discussed in the section on the etiology of the MetS and T2DM, it was not the purpose of this chapter to review the literature on women, nutrition, and abdominal obesity. The reader is referred to Chapter 7 for this discussion. This chapter discusses present nutrition knowledge pertaining to the MetS and T2DM, with an emphasis on findings relevant to women.

8.2 DEFINITIONS

8.2.1 THE METABOLIC SYNDROME (METS)

The MetS is characterized by a group of metabolic risk factors in the individual. The following six risk factors have been identified by the National Cholesterol Education Program's Adult Treatment Panel III (ATP III) [1]:

- Abdominal obesity (reflected in increased waist circumference)
- Atherogenic dyslipidemia (elevated triglycerides (TG), small low-density lipoprotein (LDL) particles, decreased high-density lipoprotein (HDL)-cholesterol levels)
- Elevated blood pressure
- Insulin resistance (with or without glucose intolerance)
- Prothrombotic state (elevated plasma plasminogen activator inhibitor and fibrinogen)
- Proinflammatory state (elevated C-reactive protein)

Between 1998 and 2005, a number of organizations put forward lists of simple criteria for the diagnosis of the MetS [3]. The clinical criteria proposed by ATP III in 2001 include the following: triglycerides $\geq$150 mg/dL ($\geq$1.7 mmol/L); blood pressure $\geq$130/$\geq$85 mm Hg; fasting glucose $\geq$110 mg/dL ($\geq$6.16 mmol/L); waist circumference >102 cm (>40 in.) in men and >88 cm (>35 in.) in women; and HDL-cholesterol <40 mg/dL (<1.03 mmol/L) in men, and <50 mg/dL (<1.29 mmol/L) in women. A diagnosis of the MetS can be made based on the presence of three of these five criteria.

In 2005, the International Diabetes Federation (IDF) published a new set of criteria that slightly modified the ATP III set of risk factors [4]. First, they made the presence of abdominal obesity a prerequisite risk factor for diagnosis. In its presence, two additional risk factors listed by ATP III were necessary for diagnosis. They specified criteria for abdominal obesity by nationality or ethnicity, and lowered the threshold of waist circumference for men and women of European origin to >94 cm (>37 in.) and >80 cm (>32 in.), respectively. The second modification made by the IDF was the lowering of the fasting glucose cut-off to 100 mg/dL (5.6 mmol/L) in keeping with the recently modified American Diabetes Association criteria for impaired fasting glucose (IFG) [5]. The IDF definition of the MetS has a high concordance with the ATP III definition and identifies similar proportions of subjects with the MetS [6].

8.2.2 INSULIN RESISTANCE

Insulin resistance (IR) is a generalized metabolic disorder in which insulin is unable to exert a normal physiological effect in target tissue [7], resulting in a decrease in insulin-mediated glucose uptake, especially in skeletal muscle and the liver [8]. Although excess body fat (particularly abdominal obesity) and physical inactivity promote the development of IR, some individuals are genetically predisposed to it [1]. The IR that manifests itself in individuals with only mild-to-moderate overweight can be referred to as "primary insulin resistance" [9].

8.2.3 Impaired Fasting Glucose

Impaired Fasting Glucose (IFG) is a condition wherein fasting blood glucose is above normal (between 5.6 and 6.9 mmol/L), but below the diabetic criterion of 7.0 mmol/L [10].

8.2.4 Impaired Glucose Tolerance

Impaired Glucose Tolerance (IGT) is a condition wherein blood glucose, 2 h following an oral glucose tolerance test, is between 7.8 and 11.0 mmol/L, the criterion for diabetes being ≥11.1 mmol/L [10,11]. Between 4% and 8% of people with IGT develop diabetes each year, depending on the population in question [12,13].

8.2.5 Diabetes Mellitus

Diabetes mellitus comprises a heterogeneous group of disorders characterized by an elevation in blood sugar due to defective insulin secretion, insulin action, or both. The chronic blood sugar elevation of diabetes can result in many long-term complications, particularly damage, dysfunction, and failure of various organs such as the kidneys, eyes, nerves, heart, and blood vessels. The threshold for diagnosis of diabetes is ≥7.0 mmol/L for fasting plasma glucose (FPG), and ≥11.1 mmol/L for 2 h plasma glucose in a 75 g oral glucose tolerance test [10,11,14].

8.2.5.1 Type 1 Diabetes Mellitus

Also known as insulin-dependent diabetes mellitus, this refers to diabetes that is primarily caused by pancreatic β-cell destruction, usually leading to absolute insulin deficiency [10,11,14].

8.2.5.2 Type 2 Diabetes Mellitus (T2DM)

Also known as non-insulin-dependent diabetes mellitus, this form of diabetes results from a progressive insulin secretory defect in the context of insulin resistance (IR), and ranges from predominant IR with relative insulin deficiency to a predominant secretory defect with IR [10,11,14].

8.2.5.3 Gestational Diabetes

Gestational diabetes refers to glucose intolerance with first onset or recognition during pregnancy [11]. Approximately 2%–5% of all nondiabetic pregnant women develop gestational diabetes. Women who develop gestational diabetes have up to a 45% higher risk of recurrence with the next pregnancy and as much as a 63% risk of developing T2DM later in life [15].

8.2.6 Glycosylated Hemoglobin (HbA1c)

Glycosylated hemoglobin (HbA1c) is a function of both fasting blood glucose and postprandial blood glucose levels, and is used as a measure of glycemic control over a 2–3 month period. The typical HbA1c level found in normal individuals is <6%, and levels greater than 7% are associated with increased risk of both microvascular and macrovascular complications in people with diabetes [10,11].

8.3 PREVALENCE RATES OF THE MetS AND DIABETES

Based on data from NHANES III (1988–1994), it was estimated that approximately 22% of US adults had the MetS, according to the ATP III criteria [16]. The prevalence was shown to increase with age and was similar for men and women overall, although within the African-American and Mexican-American populations women had higher prevalence rates than men. The percentage of Mexican-American women with the MetS (27.2%) was significantly higher than that of black women and white women (20.9% and 22.9%, respectively). In 1999–2000, the prevalence of the MetS in American women was estimated to be ~29% [17].

It has been suggested that as many as 78% of nondiabetic, overweight, and obese people with the MetS may have IR [18], which in turn confers increased risk for T2DM [9]. In 2004, the incidence of newly diagnosed diabetes among US adults between 18 and 79 years of age was 7.0 per 1000 population per year, representing a 43% increase in incidence since 1997. After adjustment for age, the increase in incidence was still 41%, suggesting that the majority of the change was not due to the aging of the population [19]. Figure 8.1 shows the age-adjusted prevalence rates of diagnosed diabetes in the US population, including children, from 1980 to 2004 [19].

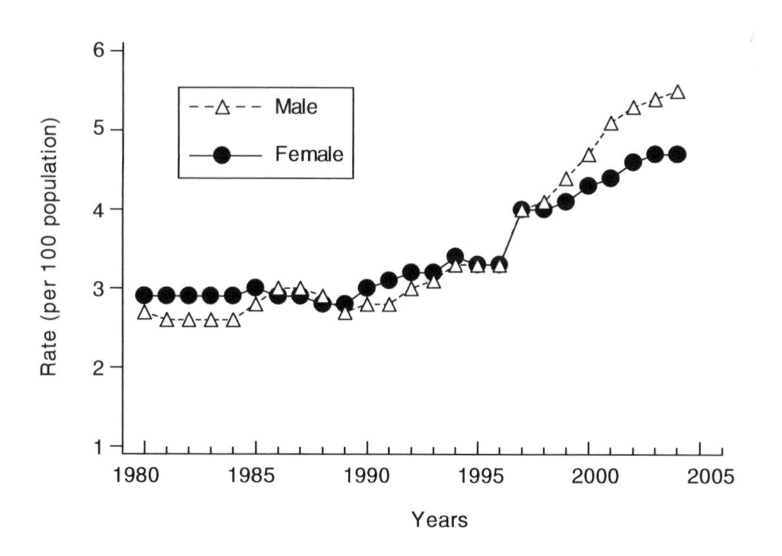

FIGURE 8.1 Age-adjusted prevalence of diagnosed diabetes per 100 population by sex, the United States, 1980–2004. (From http://www.cdc.gov/diabetes/statistics/.)

The prevalence rates reflect the increase in incidence observed between 1997 and 2004, and the increase in prevalence is greater for males than for females. The total prevalence of diabetes among people aged 20 years or older in the United States was 9.6% in 2005 and was slightly higher in men (10.5%) than in women (8.8%) [20].

In 2000 to 2001, approximately 1.1 million Canadians, aged 18 years and older, reported that they were diabetic. The prevalence of diabetes for the population in that age range was 4.5% and was slightly higher in men (4.8%), compared with women (4.2%) [21]. In 2005, the prevalence reported for the population aged 12 years and over was 4.8% and was also slightly higher in men (5.4%) compared with women (4.4%) [22].

8.4 ETIOLOGY OF THE METS AND T2DM

The etiology of the MetS is not well understood and no single pathogenesis for the syndrome has been identified [3]. Two underlying conditions, abdominal obesity [23] and IR [8,24], contribute to the pathogenesis of the MetS. The strong correlation between abdominal obesity and IR [3] may be due to the unusually high release of nonesterified fatty acids (NEFA) from the visceral fat compartment. High levels of intraportal NEFA [25] cause a decrease in hepatic insulin extraction [26], resulting in higher peripheral insulin levels and, ultimately, IR. The NEFA can also contribute to accumulation of lipid in sites other than adipose tissue. Such lipid accumulation in muscle and liver tissue may be a predisposing factor for IR and dyslipidemia [27,28].

Insulin resistance, whether of genetic origin, acquired, or both, can progress toward T2DM. As long as the pancreatic β-cells function normally, IR will result in compensatory hyperinsulinemia and glucose metabolism will remain relatively normal. Individuals can exist in a "compensated insulin-resistant state," having either normal glucose tolerance or impaired glucose tolerance (IGT), but not diabetes [29]. However, if the pancreas is unable to produce enough insulin to compensate for the IR, blood glucose levels will increase. Chronic hyperglycemia leads to a condition of glucotoxicity, resulting in the glycation of insulin and other proteins (such as hemoglobin), and their release into the circulation [30]. The decrease in β-cell function is accompanied by an increase in hepatic glucose output and further worsening of the IR. Ultimately, the individual develops T2DM [3]. In an 8 year follow-up study of middle-aged adults from the Framingham Offspring (FOS) cohort, the presence of the MetS at baseline accounted for over half of the population-attributable risk for T2DM [2]. The age-adjusted relative risk of T2DM for women was 6.90, and was 6.92 for men.

A person with a family history of diabetes is 2–3 times as likely to develop IR as someone with no family history of the disease. Maternal and paternal heredity of T2DM similarly influences the risk of early abnormalities of glucose metabolism in both sexes. On the other hand, while both maternal and paternal heredity of T2DM influence the risk of T2DM in men, only maternal heredity influences this risk in women [31].

The female sex hormones may play a major role in preventing IR and the development of T2DM. The incidence of metabolic abnormalities increases with menopause, but these can be improved by certain types of hormone replacement therapy (HRT) [32]. Even after adjusting for confounding variables, being postmenopausal is associated with a 60% increased risk of the MetS [33].

Estrogen promotes accumulation of fat in the gluteo-femoral region [34] and, independent of the effects of age and total body fat, the loss of estrogen with menopause is associated with a preferential increase in abdominal fat, as shown by both cross-sectional [35] and longitudinal studies [36,37]. It is unclear whether this is caused directly by estrogen deficiency, or indirectly, through its effect on central fat redistribution [38]. Alternatively, it can be argued that the change in fat distribution may be due to increased levels of testosterone after menopause [39]. Abdominal fat accumulation can be predicted by the free androgen index [39], and both a high free androgen index and low plasma estradiol concentrations have been associated with IR [40,41]. However, the fact that prepubescent girls are intrinsically more insulin resistant than boys [42], but that this situation reverses itself in adulthood, supports the protective effects of female sex hormones with respect to IR [43].

The strong link between abdominal obesity and metabolic risk factors associated with the MetS led ATP III to define the syndrome as a clustering of metabolic complications resulting from obesity [9]. People with abdominal obesity have higher insulin levels and are more insulin resistant than people of similar weight that have a peripheral obesity [44]. In a study of adults of varied glucose tolerance status who were carefully matched for BMI and total body fat, IR was most strongly associated with intra-abdominal fat in women, whereas in men it was associated with total abdominal fat [45]. In a study in older hypertensive adults, women had a higher percentage of total body fat, more abdominal subcutaneous, and less visceral fat than men. However, insulin sensitivity (IS) in women was negatively correlated with BMI and all fat measurements (including visceral), whereas a negative correlation with total and abdominal body fat, but not visceral fat, was observed in men [46].

Modest weight loss has been shown to improve visceral adiposity and IR in women. There is a preferential loss of abdominal fat with aerobic exercise, as visceral adipocytes seem to respond more quickly to exercise-induced weight loss than subcutaneous adipocytes [47]. However, women appear to be at a disadvantage when it comes to the relationship between abdominal obesity and the MetS. Weight loss-induced mobilization of intra-abdominal, or visceral fat is higher in men than women, whether interventions achieve similar decreases in body fat and body weight in both sexes [48], or greater decreases in body weight in men [49]. Losses of subcutaneous fat have been greater in women [48], or similar between the sexes [49]. In one study, where diet-induced weight loss was ~15% of initial weight in both men and women, men achieved a 44% reduction in visceral adipose tissue, and their postweight loss levels were not significantly different from the male lean controls, whereas women achieved a 30% reduction in visceral adipose tissue and had postweight loss levels of visceral adipose tissue twofold greater than in female lean controls [49]. As a result of their greater mobilization of intra-abdominal fat, weight loss is associated with greater improvement in the metabolic risk profile for men, compared to women. In particular, men experience more pronounced decreases in triglyceride (TG) levels and increases in HDL-cholesterol levels [48]. This is particularly critical, given that a meta-analysis of prospective studies has shown that for every mmol/L increase in TG, the risk for cardiovascular disease increases 37% for women, as opposed to 14% for men, independently of HDL-cholesterol [50].

Before discussing the epidemiologic findings on dietary intake in women and the associated risks of the MetS and T2DM, a few points warrant consideration. Associations between diet and disease suggested by such studies are dependent on how well dietary intake is assessed. It is apparent that actual food choices [51] and accuracy [52] of dietary assessment may vary by sex. Men and women may rate differently on scales that measure social desirability and social approval, and the relationships between these ratings and self-reported dietary intake are influenced by sex [53,54]. In addition, the associations may be confounded by other alterations in dietary and lifestyle patterns that have not, or cannot, be measured. Furthermore, in most prospective studies cited in this review, a food frequency questionnaire (FFQ) was used to assess dietary intake. The validity of a FFQ for measuring carbohydrate intake cannot be taken for granted, and we are not aware of any published information indicating the validity of any FFQ for determining diet GI. Therefore, the results of studies demonstrating, or failing to demonstrate links between health outcomes and diet GI, diet GL, or carbohydrate intake, assessed by FFQ, should be interpreted with caution. Nonetheless, epidemiologic studies, especially prospective ones, are critical for identifying dietary components and nutrients that may have potential for treatment and intervention in these diseases.

8.5 NUTRITION AND THE MetS

8.5.1 Diet and Risk

8.5.1.1 Concept of the Glycemic Index and Glycemic Load

There has been a great deal of interest in the relation of dietary carbohydrate to the development of IR and the MetS. Total carbohydrate is a rather crude measure, and the quality of dietary carbohydrate must be taken into consideration. A key quality of dietary carbohydrate is the degree to which it influences blood glucose levels. In order to quantify glycemic responses induced by different carbohydrate-containing foods, the glycemic index (GI) was developed [55]. It is based on the increase in blood glucose concentration, and is defined as the incremental area under the glycemic response curve (measured over 2 h) that is elicited by 50 g of available carbohydrate from a test food, and expressed as a percentage of the response after 50 g of glucose, as ingested by the same subject [56]. Differences in the GI values of foods reflect, in part, differences in carbohydrate digestion and absorption in the gut, which in turn are affected by the structure of the food [57,58]. Blood glucose and insulin responses are dependent on both the quantity and quality of carbohydrate consumed. Hence, the amount of carbohydrate in a food can be multiplied by its GI to calculate the glycemic load (GL) [59]. To calculate the total dietary GL, the GL scores from all foods consumed are added.

8.5.1.2 Diet GI, Diet GL, and Fiber Intake

Cross-sectional studies in men and women have yielded conflicting findings for the role of diet GI and GL in the development of the MetS or IR. Although a positive association with IR was found in the FOS [60], no association with IS, and no interaction with sex were found in the Insulin Resistance Atherosclerosis Study

(IRAS) [61]. However, both studies found significant associations for dietary fiber; a positive association with IS [61], and negative associations with fasting insulin [61] and IR [60]. Similar associations were found for whole-grain intake [60,62]. One study also reported negative associations between IR and both cereal fiber and fruit fiber [60]. In this study, the association with whole-grain intake was largely explained by cereal fiber intake. The prevalence of the MetS was 38% and 33% lower in subjects in the highest quintile of intake for cereal fiber and whole grains, respectively. The data were not analyzed by sex. The Hoorn Study, a cross-sectional study, has confirmed the inverse association between dietary fiber intake and fasting plasma insulin (FPI) in older women, but not older men [63], while the Coronary Artery Risk Development in Young Adults (CARDIA) Study, a prospective study [64], has confirmed the inverse association between dietary fiber intake and IR, but found no significant interaction with sex [64]. Thus, there is insufficient evidence to suggest that the apparent inverse association between IR and the intake of whole grains and dietary fiber differs between men and women.

Although cross-sectional studies in men and women have yielded conflicting findings for the role of diet GI and GL in the development of the MetS, within a sample of healthy postmenopausal women from the Nurses' Health Study (NHS), total carbohydrate intake, total diet GI, and total diet GL were each positively associated with fasting TG levels. This association was strongest for GL [65]. There was nearly a twofold difference in TG concentrations between extreme quintiles of GL, especially in overweight and obese, compared to lean women. Given the particular importance of elevated TG levels as a risk factor for cardiovascular disease in women [50], this association warrants more research.

8.5.1.3 Dietary Fat

In cross-sectional studies, total dietary fat intake has been positively associated with FPI levels in healthy women [66], and with insulin levels 2 h after an oral glucose challenge in healthy women, but not men [63]. However, the IRAS Study in men and women found no association between dietary fats and IS for the cohort as a whole [67], although among obese participants, polyunsaturated fat (PUFA) intake was inversely associated with IS, with no significant interaction between sex and this association. Of two studies that reported associations for PUFA in men, the Zutphen Elderly Study reported an inverse association with FPI [68], whereas the Hoorn Study reported a positive association with 2 h plasma glucose [69]. In the Hoorn Study, no associations were found between dietary fats and 2 h plasma glucose in women. A positive association between saturated fat and FPI has been reported in the Zutphen Elderly Study and the Normative Aging Study, both cross-sectional studies in healthy men [68,70], and the San Luis Valley Diabetes Study, a prospective study in healthy men and women [71]. There was no analysis by sex in the latter study. A cross-sectional study in healthy Italian adults found positive associations for butter (predominantly saturated fat), and negative associations for olive (predominantly MUFA) and vegetable oil (predominantly PUFA), with fasting glucose levels for both men and women [72]. Taken together, these data do not suggest a sex-based difference in the effect of dietary fat intake on indices of IR.

There is some evidence of an interaction between dietary fat and genes in Singaporean women. Perilipin (PLIN) is a protein that plays a critical role in the regulation of adipocyte lipid storage and body fat accumulation. Significant associations between PLIN genetic variants and body weight have been demonstrated [73,74]. Using data from the Singapore National Health Survey, one study reported that women with saturated fat intakes between 11.8% and 19% of energy had a 48% increase in the prevalence of IR, compared to women with saturated fat intakes between 3.1% and 9.4%, only if they were homozygous for the PLIN minor alleles, 11,482G→A or 14,995A→T [75]. In contrast, IR decreased as carbohydrate intake increased. This gene–diet interaction was found to be homogeneous across the three major ethnic groups (Chinese, Malays, and Indians) for women, but no significant interactions were found among men in this study.

8.5.1.4 Dairy Intake

Dairy intake has been inversely associated with the MetS in a cross-sectional study in men and women, the Tehran Lipid and Glucose Study (TLGS) [76], and a prospective study in women, the Women's Health Study (WHS) [77]. Dairy intake has also been inversely associated with IR in men and women participating in the CARDIA Study [64]. The TLGS and WHS also found inverse associations between calcium intake and risk of the MetS. In the WHS, the odds of having the MetS decreased by ~36% for women in the highest quintile of total calcium intake, compared to women in the lowest quintile [77]. In the CARDIA Study, the association with IR was in overweight and obese individuals but not those with BMI <25 and there was no significant interaction with sex, although the higher dairy consumers were somewhat more likely to be women. It should also be noted that all three of these studies found positive associations between dairy consumption and dietary fiber intake. These data do not suggest a sex-based difference in the effect of dairy or calcium intake on IR and risk of the MetS.

8.5.1.5 Overall Dietary Patterns

Analysis of dietary patterns in relation to the MetS has yielded some interesting associations. Two papers based on data from women in the Framingham Offspring-Spouse Study, a prospective study, have reported low dietary fiber and high dietary fat intakes as common components of dietary patterns associated with increased risks of abdominal obesity and the MetS [78,79]. Data from two cross-sectional investigations in men and women, the DESIR Study (Data from an Epidemiological Study on the Insulin Resistance Syndrome) [80] and the Malmö Diet and Cancer Study [81] have yielded conflicting results for bread consumption, but similar associations for dairy consumption. The Malmö Study found that a food intake pattern characterized by high intakes of white bread was associated with a higher risk of hyperinsulinemia in women than an intake pattern that obtained the majority of calories from a dairy spread [81]. The white bread pattern was also associated with a higher risk of dyslipidemia in both women and men. The DESIR Study found that consumption of bread was inversely associated with fasting glucose levels and HDL-cholesterol levels in women, while it was inversely associated with fasting glucose and TG levels in men [80]. In this study, consumption of dairy products was inversely associated with all measured components of the MetS in men, but only with diastolic blood pressure in women. The frequency of an aggregate measure representing the MetS (serum TG, diastolic blood pressure, HDL-cholesterol, and fasting glucose) was inversely associated with bread and dairy intake in men, but not in women. The contradictory results for bread intake are most likely due to differences in degree of grain refinement and fiber content between the breads typically consumed in the two study populations. These latter two studies seem to suggest a stronger protective effect of dairy intake in men than women, but care must be taken in drawing conclusions from these data. Whereas our earlier conclusion of no sex-based differences in the effects of dairy intake was based on associations between dairy intake and disease risk, the latter two studies are reporting overall dietary patterns for which dairy intake is simply a marker. It is possible that the reported sex-based difference may be due to another unmeasured dietary or lifestyle factor that is related to this dietary pattern.

8.5.2 Dietary Intervention

8.5.2.1 Overall Diet Guidelines and Approaches

Current guidelines for the management of the MetS do not distinguish between men and women [82,83]. Long-term lifestyle management involving modification of diet and physical activity levels is recommended, and long-term maintenance of the dietary regimen is critical. This prompts the suggestion that dietary approaches must be somewhat individualized in order to enhance adherence. It has been argued that a hypocaloric diet with moderately high fat levels (~35% of energy from fat) can enhance long-term compliance, leading to better weight maintenance than a typical low-fat diet [84]. Based on the dietary associations reported in prospective studies, it has also been suggested that dietary fat sources should stress nonhydrogenated vegetable oils, fish, avocado, and nuts; dietary carbohydrates should stress whole grains and legumes to increase fiber intake and decrease refined carbohydrate intake; and protein intake should contribute 20%–25% of energy intake, emphasizing poultry, fish, soy, and nuts, as opposed to red meat [82]. A summary of these suggestions is presented in Table 8.1.

TABLE 8.1
Overall Diet Guidelines for Treating the Metabolic Syndrome in Adults

- The primary focus should be on weight reduction
- Emphasize long-term lifestyle management involving modification of diet and physical activity levels
- Dietary approaches should be somewhat individualized in order to enhance adherence and long-term maintenance
- Dietary fat sources should stress nonhydrogenated vegetable oils, fish, avocado, and nuts
- Dietary carbohydrates should stress whole grains and legumes to increase fiber intake and decrease refined carbohydrate intake
- Dietary protein intake should contribute 20% to 25% of energy intake, emphasizing poultry, fish, soy, and nuts, as opposed to red meat

A 6 month intervention trial in men and women with the MetS who were randomized to the Dietary Approaches to Stop Hypertension (DASH) diet, a weight-reducing diet emphasizing healthy food choices compared to a control diet (consisting of their usual food intake), reported improvements in HDL-cholesterol, TG, blood pressure (systolic and diastolic), body weight, and fasting blood glucose on the DASH diet [85]. Results were better on the DASH diet than on the weight-reducing diet, and were similar for men and women. The main differences between diets were that saturated fat and dietary fiber ranged from 7% and 29 g/day, respectively, in the DASH diet, to 14% and 10 g/day in the control diet, largely due to increased fruit, whole-grain, and low-fat dairy intake and decreased intake of fats, oils, and sweets on the DASH diet.

8.5.2.2 Weight Loss Strategies and the MetS

Overweight and obesity are commonly associated with the MetS, and are major risk factors for the development of T2DM [86]. Thus, dietary treatment of the MetS should focus primarily on weight reduction [87]. A recent review and meta-analysis of long-term nonpharmacological weight loss interventions in adults with IGT or IFG concluded that strategies using dietary, physical activity, or behavioral interventions yielded significant improvements in weight [88]. Five of the studies included in the meta-analysis looked at T2DM incidence as an outcome, and three of these—the Diabetes Prevention Program Study (DPP) [89], the Da Qing Study [90], and the Finnish Diabetes Prevention Study (FDP) [91]—reported that T2DM incidence was significantly lower in the intervention versus control groups at 3–6 years follow-up, and was associated with weight loss. The interventions in these three trials included both dietary and exercise components, and resulted in modest reductions in body weight of ~5%–6%, accompanied by reductions in T2DM incidence of ~40%–60%. The DPP Study found no difference in outcome between men and women [89] and, although the FDP Study reported a slightly larger reduction in risk of T2DM for men (63%) than for women (54%), these estimates were not significantly different [91]. The number of intervention contacts with subjects was significantly correlated with weight loss, confirming that frequency of contact is an essential component of successful individualized weight loss strategies [92]. Those studies that looked at glycemic control, blood pressure, or lipid concentrations noted modest improvements. Thus, lifestyle strategies aimed at weight reduction in IFG and IGT seem effective for both men and women with respect to both weight loss success and its effect on the risk of T2DM.

To compare the relative merits of four popular weight-loss diets, 160 overweight and obese adults, with hypertension, dyslipidemia, or fasting hyperglycemia, were randomized to one of the following four diets for a year: Atkins (carbohydrate restriction), Zone (macronutrient balance), Weight Watchers (calorie restriction), or Ornish (fat restriction) [93]. Subjects received standardized recommendations pertaining to supplements, exercise, and external support. Weight loss and waist size reduction were modest and did not differ between women and men. Each diet reduced the LDL to HDL ratio by ~10%, with no significant effects on blood pressure or glucose, and the amount of weight loss was associated with self-reported dietary adherence level, but not with diet group. Women in the top tertile of adherence lost, on average, 7% of their initial body weight. Thus, the results of this study suggest that as long as people can adhere to a diet that promotes a negative energy balance, in the absence of an exercise intervention, weight loss success appears to be similar for men and women.

Contrary to the results reported above, a more intensive dietary weight-loss strategy yielded sex-related differences in the amount of weight loss and in insulin-stimulated glucose disposal. A 13 week very low calorie diet (VLCD), consisting of 10 weeks at 800 kcal/day, followed by 3 weeks at 1200 kcal/day, in sedentary, normoglycemic individuals induced a 15.8% loss of initial body weight in men and a 13.3% loss in women, and also improved glucose disposal in both sexes [49]. Although improvement in IS did not significantly differ between men and women, glucose utilization in weight-reduced obese men was similar to that of lean male controls, whereas in weight-reduced obese women it remained lower than in lean female controls. It is unclear whether glucose utilization would have further improved in women with a longer intervention, or whether a VLCD alone is more effective for men than for women.

Although it has been suggested that an individual's metabolic status may determine the most appropriate choice of dietary macronutrient balance [94], studies in women have yielded conflicting evidence. In obese nondiabetic women, categorized as insulin sensitive or insulin resistant at baseline, insulin sensitive women had more success with a 16 week weight-loss diet that had percent energy from carbohydrate and fat of 60% and 20%, respectively, whereas insulin resistant women had more success with a diet that had equal percentages of dietary energy from carbohydrate and fat (both 40%) [95]. Insulin sensitive women lost 13.5% of their initial body weight on the low-fat diet, as opposed to 6.8% on the low-carbohydrate diet, whereas insulin resistant women lost 13.4% of their initial body weight on the low-carbohydrate diet, as opposed to 8.5% on the low-fat diet. Overall, increased IS was directly correlated with the degree of weight loss. Conversely, a different study reported that when obese nondiabetic women followed a hypocaloric 43% carbohydrate 42% fat diet, the ability to lose weight over 1–2 months did not vary as a function of hyperinsulinemia or IR [96]. Although the differences in the duration of the two studies may have contributed to the lack of agreement in outcomes, more research is needed to determine if a weight-loss diet with a lower carbohydrate-to-fat ratio is more effective in obese nondiabetic women with IR.

8.5.2.3 Dietary Carbohydrate

Some groups have promoted carbohydrate restriction as a dietary intervention in the MetS [97]. They have argued that this approach may improve fasting glucose and insulin, plasma TG, HDL-cholesterol and blood pressure, and cause a spontaneous reduction in caloric intake, thus enhancing weight loss [98,99]. Even in the absence of weight loss, when compared to a low fat (less than 30% of energy) diet, a very low carbohydrate (less than 10% of energy) diet increased fasting HDL-cholesterol, and decreased fasting TG and the total/HDL-cholesterol ratio in healthy normolipidemic women [100]. Similar results, although smaller in magnitude, were found in men [101]. However, serum total and LDL-cholesterol were also increased with the very low carbohydrate diet. In addition, the women studied were relatively young and healthy [100], making extrapolation of the results to older individuals with the MetS rather difficult.

People with the MetS are also at increased risk for coronary heart disease (CHD). A recent review and meta-analysis of 15 randomized controlled trials of low GI diets in CHD found weak evidence of a relationship between low GI diets and slightly lower total cholesterol, compared with higher GI diets, and a small reduction in HbA1c after 12 weeks on low GI diets (but not at 4–5 weeks). There was no evidence that low GI diets have an effect on LDL- or HDL-cholesterol, TG, fasting glucose, or fasting insulin levels [102]. However, randomized intervention trials in people at risk for, or diagnosed with, CHD has examined the effects of low-GI diets on insulin-stimulated glucose uptake in isolated fat cells and suggest beneficial effects of this dietary approach, especially in women with a parental history of CHD. In a 4 week trial in men and women with CHD, the postprandial insulin response to an OGTT was significantly lower, and insulin-stimulated glucose uptake was significantly greater, in the low-GI diet group, compared to the high-GI diet group [103]. There was no subanalysis by sex. In a 3 week trial in 28 premenopausal women, parental history of CHD influenced the effect of a low-GI versus a high-GI diet on glucose uptake [104]. Among women with no parental history of CHD, there was no effect of diet on insulin-stimulated glucose uptake, whereas in those with a parental history, the percent increase in insulin-stimulated glucose uptake was significantly higher after the low-GI intervention. Whole-body IS, on the other hand, was significantly higher following a low-GI versus a high-GI diet, regardless of parental history of heart disease.

To study the effects of dietary advice aimed at reducing the amount or altering the source of dietary carbohydrate on IR in subjects with IGT, we randomly assigned them to high-carbohydrate-high-GI, high-carbohydrate-low-GI, or low-carbohydrate-high-MUFA diets [105]. After 4 months, the glucose disposition index, a measure of the ability of β-cells to overcome IR, was increased on the low-GI diet (+0.17) compared to the high-GI diet (−0.03) and the high-MUFA diet (−0.09). We did not have enough data to compare men and women. A 12 week study in overweight or obese adults with the MetS found a greater increase in acute insulin secretion (33.2%) following a diet that emphasized rye bread and pasta, compared to that (5.5%) following a diet that emphasized oat and wheat bread and potatoes as the primary carbohydrates [106]. Although the GI was not reported for these two diets, they are similar to the low-GI and high-GI diets, respectively, in our study. Women in the latter study were associated with a greater increase in IS than were males. Enhancement of the acute insulin response has also been shown with 8 weeks of high-fiber rye bread consumption in normoglycemic postmenopausal women [107]. More studies are needed to determine whether the increase in IS following the low-GI interventions is actually greater for women than for men.

A 6 week crossover trial in overweight or obese hyperinsulinemic adults showed that IS improved after consumption of a whole-grain diet, as compared to a refined grain diet, independent of body weight and sex [108]. Some authors have argued that, through its effect on satiety, dietary fiber can enhance control of body weight and thereby play a significant role in the management of the MetS [109,110]. In a 12 year prospective study in healthy women, those who consumed more whole grains consistently weighed less than those who consumed less [111]. In addition, dietary fiber intake was associated with a 49% lower risk of major weight gain when extreme quintiles of intake were compared, whereas there was a positive association between weight gain and the intake of refined-grain foods [111]. Long-term effects of increased fiber and low GI foods on body weight regulation, such as those seen in the study cited above, may be mediated indirectly by altered IS or gut hormone secretion [110].

Glucagon-like peptide-1 (GLP-1) is a gut hormone that enhances insulin secretion stimulated by oral, as opposed to intravenous, glucose administration [112]. Intravenous infusions of GLP-1 promote satiety and decrease energy intake in humans [113]. When a preload of galactose (a monosaccharide) and guar gum (a soluble dietary fiber) was consumed along with a standard breakfast, the GLP-1 release due to breakfast was increased and extended, and the area under the curve for GLP-1 release was positively related to percent body fat in women, but not in men. The increased GLP-1 response in women was also related to a significant increase in satiety [114]. Conversely, another study showed a pronounced attenuation of plasma GLP-1 secretion in response to oral carbohydrate in obese women, compared to lean women, in the absence of such a difference in response to oral fat [115], suggesting that reduced GLP-1 secretion in response to nutrients could be involved in the pathogenesis of obesity and diabetes in women.

As mentioned earlier, the prevalence of the MetS is inversely associated with cereal fiber intake [60]. Insoluble fiber is the predominant fraction of cereal fiber. Seventeen normoglycemic overweight and obese women participated in a crossover study wherein they consumed nine portions of bread that had been enriched with a highly purified insoluble fiber (or white bread in the control phase) over 72 h [116]. Whole-body IS, measured by euglycemic-hyperinsulinemic clamp, was improved after fiber consumption. The same group examined acute and delayed responses in glucose, insulin, glucose-dependent insulinotropic polypeptide (GIP), and glucagon-like polypeptide 1 (GLP-1) using short-term dietary intervention with purified insoluble fibers in 14 normoglycemic young women [117]. The results showed an accelerated insulin response directly after ingestion of insoluble fibers, associated with an earlier response of GIP, suggesting that GIP may mediate the insulin response. Ingestion of the fiber-enriched bread was also associated with a significant reduction of postprandial glucose the following day. It has been suggested that development of T2DM is preceded by a reduced insulinotropic effect of GIP [118] and therefore, the acceleration of GIP response elicited by insoluble fiber in this study may provide a mechanistic explanation for the association between dietary fiber and lowered risk of T2DM in women.

Two studies have shown an effect of dietary fiber, incorporated in baked products, on postprandial insulin response in women. An acute study in normal weight and overweight women showed that, compared with muffins that were low in both β-glucan and resistant starch, the areas under the curve (AUC) for both glucose and insulin decreased when β-glucan (17% and 33%, respectively) or when resistant starch (24% and 38%, respectively) content was increased. The largest decrease in

AUC for both glucose and insulin occurred following meals containing high amounts of both β-glucan and resistant starch (33% and 59% for glucose and insulin, respectively) [119]. In a 3 week intervention study in overweight women with IGT, the serum insulin response elicited by an intravenous glucose challenge was reduced by 35%, after a diet containing low-GI–high-fiber, compared to high-GI–low-fiber, bread products and there were no changes in either fasting glucose or insulin [120].

8.5.2.4 Dietary Fat

A couple of studies comparing the effects of different types of dietary fat on glucose metabolism in men and women with IGT suggest a beneficial effect of monounsaturated fat (MUFA). In one study, people who were either normoglycemic or had IGT were randomized to a controlled isoenergetic diet, high in either saturated (SFA) or MUFA for 3 months [121]. IS was impaired on the high-SFA diet, but did not change on the high-MUFA diet. Beneficial effects of substituting MUFA for SFA were only seen at fat intakes up to 37% of dietary energy, emphasizing the importance of total fat intake when assessing the effects of fat quality. In another study, following a 3 week run-in diet high in saturated fat, men and postmenopausal women with IGT who were moderately obese were randomized to either a high MUFA (40% fat, 19% MUFA) or high PUFA (34% fat, 10% PUFA) diet for 8 weeks [122]. There was a tendency toward a greater reduction in FPG, and glucose effectiveness was significantly higher, after the MUFA diet, compared to the PUFA diet. Neither of these studies included a subanalysis by sex, so they do not inform us as to whether or not differences exist between men and women in the effects of MUFA on glucose metabolism and IS.

8.5.2.5 Isoflavone Supplementation

Soy isoflavones are a type of phytoestrogen and have many effects which are similar to those of estrogen. Hence, they have become popular among postmenopausal women as an alternative for hormone replacement therapy (HRT). Acceptance of HRT is relatively low in Taiwanese women and phytoestrogen supplementation is one of the more popular alternative therapies [123]. Two studies in postmenopausal women provide weak evidence of beneficial effects of isoflavone supplementation on glucose and insulin responses. To compare the effects on glucose and insulin profiles of soy isoflavones, as opposed to estrogen replacement therapy (ERT), 30 postmenopausal women were randomized to either 100 mg isoflavones and 300 mg calcium or 0.625 mg conjugated estrogen and 300 mg calcium [123]. After 6 months of treatment, fasting blood glucose was reduced by 17% and 15%, and insulin was reduced by 44% and 33%, respectively, in the isoflavone and ERT groups. Although the authors concluded that isoflavones and ERT were equally effective in reducing fasting glucose and insulin levels in postmenopausal women, others have argued that the study is inconclusive due to the lack of a proper placebo group [124].

In a 12 week crossover trial in postmenopausal women, a dietary supplement with 30 g/day soy protein and 132 mg/day isoflavones significantly lowered mean values of fasting insulin and HbA1c, when compared to 12 weeks on the control trial [125]. However, because the dietary supplement contained both protein and isoflavones from soy, it is not possible to attribute these effects to one or the other component. Furthermore, the control trial used 30 g cellulose/day, so it is possible that the effects seen in the dietary supplement trial were due to a higher dietary protein level.

8.6 NUTRITION AND TYPE 2 DIABETES

8.6.1 Diet and Risk

8.6.1.1 Lifestyle and Food Intake Patterns

As discussed earlier, interventions employing lifestyle modifications in individuals with IGT have demonstrated modest weight loss accompanied by significant reductions in risk of T2DM. Similarly, the NHS found evidence to support the hypothesis that the risk for T2DM could be reduced by a combination of diet and lifestyle changes [126]. The diet associated with lower risk of T2DM was characterized by high intakes of cereal fiber and PUFA, low intake of trans fat, a low GL, and moderate alcohol consumption. Compared with the rest of the cohort, the 3.4% of women who were in the low-risk group had a 91% reduced risk of developing T2DM. However, the relatively low number of women in this group suggests that this regimen may not be easily adhered to.

Examination of food intake patterns in relation to T2DM risk has revealed associations for a number of foods and food categories. Data from the NHS in women [127], and the Health Professionals Follow-up Study (HPFS) in men [128], found that a consumption pattern high in vegetables, fruit, fish, poultry, and whole grains was associated with a modest nonsignificant risk reduction. Conversely, a pattern typified by high consumption of red meat, processed meats, french fries, high-fat dairy products, refined grains, sweets, and desserts was associated with relative risks of T2DM of 1.49 in women and 1.59 in men, when comparing extreme quintiles of intake. Another prospective study, the WHS, confirmed these findings [129]. Thus, there is no suggestion of a significant difference in risk of T2DM between sexes, based on these patterns of intake.

In men and women examined in the Finnish Mobile Clinic Health Examination Survey (FMCHES), a food intake pattern typified by higher intake of fruits and vegetables was associated with a relative risk, between extreme quartiles of dietary pattern scores, of 0.72 for T2DM, whereas a pattern typified by higher intake of butter, potatoes, and whole milk was associated with a relative risk of 1.49 [130]. No significant interaction was found for sex, but the authors noted that the associations appeared to be more pronounced for women. Conversely, the WHS reported no association between total intake of fruits and vegetables and risk of T2DM, although a high intake of green leafy or dark yellow vegetables was associated with reduced risk among women with a BMI $\geq$25, compared to those with a BMI $<$25 [131]. Both the NHS [59] and the HPFS [132] have examined the relation between T2DM risk and fiber from fruits and vegetables and have found no evidence of a protective effect.

8.6.1.2 Dietary Carbohydrate

Epidemiological studies indicate that the risk of T2DM is not predicted by intake of either total carbohydrate or simple sugars [133]. Data from the NHS [59,134], the Iowa Women's Health Study (IWHS) [135], and the HPFS [132] have not found any association between total carbohydrate and T2DM risk. Likewise, neither the NHS [134,135] nor the WHS [136] have found evidence of an association between sucrose and risk of T2DM for women. On the other hand, in the Nurses' Health Study II (NHS II), sugar-sweetened beverages, which are high in high-fructose corn syrup, have been associated with weight gain and an increased risk of T2DM in young and middle-aged women [137].

The relationship between intake of refined grains and T2DM risk is unclear. In the NHS, a relative risk of 1.31, when comparing extreme quintiles of refined grain intake, increased to 1.57 when the ratio of refined to whole grains was examined [138]. Furthermore, both the NHS [127] and the HPFS [128] found that a high intake of refined grains was one component of a dietary pattern associated with increased T2DM risk. However, the IWHS reported no association [135]. In men and women participating in the FMCHES, the risk of T2DM was reduced by ~40%, when extreme quintiles of intake were compared [139], whereas FOS reported no cross-sectional associations between refined grain intake and either fasting insulin or HbA1c in men and women [140].

Cereal fiber intake is associated with a decreased risk of developing T2DM [141]. This inverse association has been demonstrated for women in the NHS [59,126], the NHS II [142], and the IWHS [135]; for men in the HPFS [131]; and both women and men in the FMCHES [139]. In women, intake of ~7.5–9.5 g/day of cereal fiber is associated with a 30%–35% reduction in T2DM risk [59,135,142]. Similarly, a 30% reduction in T2DM risk is associated with an increase from 2.5 to 10 g/day cereal fiber intake in men [131]. The FMCHES included both women and men and reported a 60% decrease in risk of T2DM, when extreme quartiles of cereal fiber intake were compared, but did not find an interaction with sex [139]. Therefore, there is nothing to suggest that associations between cereal fiber intake and T2DM risk differ by sex. In addition, an inverse association between fasting C-peptide concentrations and cereal fiber intake was reported for a subsample of women from the NHS and NHS II [143].

There is reasonably strong evidence of a relationship between diet GI and T2DM risk, based on the prospective data. The NHS [59] and NHS II [142] in women and the HPFS in men [132] have shown a 40%–60% increase in risk of T2DM associated with an increase in GI of ~11–14 units. The IRAS Study in both men and women found that a high-GI diet predicted T2DM risks among nonabdominally obese people and people who experienced an increase in waist circumference, but not among abdominally obese people. However, there was no analysis by sex [144]. Conversely, the IWHS found no association in women [135]. The data are less convincing for diet GL. The NHS reported a 47% increase in T2DM risk with an increase of 67 GL units [59], and identified a diet low in GL as one component of a lifestyle associated with a lower risk of T2DM in women [126], and a positive association between fasting C-peptide concentrations and GL was reported for the subsample of women from the NHS and NHS II [143]. In contrast, other reports from the NHS II [142], the HPFS [132], and IRAS [144] have found no evidence of an association between GL and T2DM risk.

Whole-grain consumption is a way of looking at the quality of carbohydrate that reflects both GI and cereal fiber content [145]. A recent review of the role of cereal grains and legumes in the etiology and management of diabetes identified the importance of whole-grain structure when considering effects on carbohydrate metabolism [146]. The reduction in postprandial glucose excursion resulting from consumption of whole-grain products, as opposed to their refined grain counterparts, places less demand for insulin on the pancreatic β-cells [147]. An inverse association between whole-grain intake and T2DM risk has been demonstrated in the NHS [127,138], the IWHS [135], the HPFS [128,148], and the FMCHES [139]. In the NHS [138], the IWHS [135], and the HPFS [148], intake of approximately three daily servings of whole-grain products was associated with a 20%–40% reduction in T2DM risk, compared with consumption of one or less servings per day. The FMCHES also found this association, for men and women, but found no significant interaction with sex [139], and the FOS found a significant association between whole-grain intake and fasting insulin levels, but no interaction with sex [140]. Thus, there is no evidence of sex-based differences in the inverse association between whole-grain intake and T2DM risk.

8.6.1.3 Dietary Magnesium

Whole grains, along with nuts and green leafy vegetables, are major food sources of magnesium. A 33% decrease in T2DM risk has been associated with an increase in magnesium intake, from a level of 220–250 mg/day to a level of 360–430 mg/day, in the NHS [134], the IWHS [135], and cohorts from both the NHS and the HPFS [149]. The WHS also found a modest inverse association, significant only for women with a BMI $\geq$25, and this was accompanied by an inverse association between magnesium intake and fasting insulin levels in a random subsample of overweight women [150]. The NHS also reported that higher consumption of nuts and peanut butter was associated with a lower risk of T2DM [151]. These data suggest an inverse association between magnesium intake and T2DM risk for both men and women.

8.6.1.4 Dietary Fat

The NHS [59,152], IWHS [153], HPFS [131], and the Norfolk arm of the European Prospective Investigation of Cancer (EPIC-Norfolk) Study in both women and men [154] have failed to find an association between total dietary fat intake and T2DM risk, although the San Luis Valley Diabetes Study (SVLD) in men and women found that every 40 g/day increase in total fat intake was associated with a 3.4-fold increase in T2DM risk [155]. However, the SVLD used 24 h dietary recalls which can be a poor indicator of an individual's usual intake. Moreover, there was no analysis by sex in the SVLD. While neither the NHS [152] nor the IWHS [153] have found associations for either MUFA or SFA with T2DM risk, there is some evidence of an inverse association between PUFA and T2DM risk in women. The NHS found inverse associations for PUFA and vegetable fat, such that replacing 2% of energy from trans fat with an isoenergetic amount of PUFA would result in a 40% lower risk of T2DM [152]. The study also reported a positive association for trans fatty acids, but no evidence of associations for total, saturated, or MUFA. The IWHS found that substitution of PUFA for saturated fat appeared to reduce the T2DM risk for women [153], and the NHS identified dietary PUFA as a key component of a healthy lifestyle associated with a lower T2DM risk in women [126]. The evidence for an association between PUFA and risk of T2DM in men, on the other hand, is inconsistent [156].

Data from the NHS [134,152] and the IWHS [153] suggest that the risk of T2DM is decreased by 20%–40% with increases in vegetable fat intake from ~18 to 42 g/day. Another report from the NHS [59] and one from the HPFS [132] have both shown a similar reduction in risk, although it was not found to be significant in these studies. The EPIC-Norfolk study reported an inverse association between the energy-adjusted ratio of dietary PUFA to saturated fat (P:S ratio) and T2DM risk, and found processed and other meats among the dietary items that typified the lowest quintile of the P:S ratio, while fish, fruit, vegetables, bread, breakfast cereal, and nuts were among the foods that typified the highest quintile. There was no evidence of an interaction between sex and the P:S ratio [154].

The relationship between intake of trans fatty acids and risk of T2DM remains unclear for both women and men. The NHS has reported a direct association between a high intake of trans fat and an increased risk of T2DM [126,152], but the IWHS reported an inverse association [153], and the HPFS reported no association [157].

8.6.1.5 Dairy and Calcium Intake

Intake of dairy products has been associated with a 20% reduction in the risk of T2DM in both the WHS [158] and the HPFS [159], when extreme quintiles of intake are compared. The risk reduction was mainly attributable to low-fat dairy products. In the NHS, women who consumed at least three daily servings of dairy foods had an 11% lower risk of T2DM than those who consumed less than one daily serving, but this was not significant after adjustment for total vitamin D and calcium intake. In this study, the relative risks of T2DM, between extreme quintiles of intake, were 0.87, 0.79, and 0.82 for supplemental vitamin D, total calcium intake, and supplemental calcium intake, respectively [160].

8.6.1.6 Antioxidant Intake

The FMCHES in women and men found dietary intakes of a number of antioxidants were significantly associated with a reduced risk of T2DM [161]. Among the antioxidants thus identified were vitamin E, α-tocopherol, γ-tocopherol, δ-tocopherol, and β-tocotrienol, and β-cryptoxanthin. There was a borderline interaction between sex and the association between α-carotene intake and risk, but this was thought to be due to chance. A cross-sectional analysis of screening and baseline data from postmenopausal women who were enrolled in the Soy Health Effects (SHE) Study, and not taking HRT, found a trend toward lower fasting insulin for women with moderate and high genistein consumption, compared with those who did not consume genistein, but women with a high genistein intake also had a significantly lower BMI and waist circumference than those with no daily genistein consumption. After adjustment for BMI and other factors, insulin concentrations 2 h after an oral glucose tolerance test were inversely associated with genistein, daidzen, and total isoflavone intake [162]. The authors suggested that these associations may be explained by alterations in sex hormone-binding globulin observed with soy intake in other studies [163,164], but the mechanisms by which phytoestrogens may exert beneficial effects on diabetes risk are still unclear [165].

8.6.1.7 Coffee Intake

An inverse association between coffee consumption and T2DM risk has been found in women of the Göteborg BEDA study [166] and the NHS [167,168], in men of the HPFS [168], and in two large population-based cohorts of Dutch [169] and Finnish [170] men and women. For women, the reduction in risk associated with consumption of four or more cups/day was found to range from 30% [168,170] to approximately 50% [166,167]. The Finnish study tested for an interaction with sex but found none, although the association appeared stronger in women, who had a relative risk of 0.21, compared with a relative risk of 0.45 in men, associated with ten or more cups per day [170]. In the Göteborg BEDA study, after adjustment for serum TG, which were nonsignificantly higher in women with low coffee intake, the association was attenuated, suggesting that a protective effect of coffee may be mediated by effects on TG [166]. When decaffeinated coffee was examined in the NHS and HPFS cohorts, it was associated with relative risks of T2DM of 0.74 for men and 0.85 for women, comparing intake of four cups per day with nondrinkers [168]. There was also an inverse association between total caffeine intake and T2DM risk in these cohorts.

Coffee is a major dietary source of caffeine and contains significant amounts of magnesium and other micronutrients. In fact, coffee may contain over 100 active chemical compounds, dependent on the brewing method [166]. It is unclear which components of coffee may be responsible for the association with reduced T2DM risk. In women, caffeine may be positively associated with plasma levels of estrogen, estradiol, and sex hormone-binding globulin, and inversely associated with testosterone levels [171,172]. Thus, the effects of caffeine and those of phytoestrogens, also present in coffee, may explain the effects of coffee on the risk of T2DM in women.

8.6.1.8 Dietary Iron Intake

Both the IWHS [173] and the NHS [174] have found an increase in T2DM risk of ~30% across increasing quintiles of heme iron intake. In the NHS, there were no associations between total, dietary, supplemental, or nonheme iron and risk of T2DM, and multivariate modeling suggested that women who consumed $\geq$2.25 mg/day of heme iron were 52% more likely to develop T2DM, compared with women who consumed $<$0.75 mg/day. However, the studies differed with respect to an interaction between alcohol intake and the association between dietary iron intake and risk of T2DM. In the IWHS, this association appeared to be stronger among women who consumed more alcohol, whereas the NHS found no interaction between alcohol intake and this association.

8.6.1.9 Alcohol Intake

One review of diet composition and T2DM risk found moderate alcohol consumption, defined as one to two drinks per day, was associated with a 30%–40% lower risk of T2DM, compared with abstainers [133]. This conclusion was based on findings from seven prospective cohort studies, only one of which was in women, and one of which included both men and women. A meta-analysis based on 15 prospective cohort studies, 4 of which included both men and women [175–178], and 3 of which included only women [126, 173, 179], reported a U-shaped relationship between alcohol consumption and risk of T2DM, with the lowest relative risks of 0.70, 0.69, and 0.72 found at intake ranges of 6–12, 12–24, and 24–48 g/day, respectively [180]. These intake ranges were defined as "moderate" by the study authors. The meta-analysis revealed nonsignificant trends for larger relative risk reduction associated with moderate alcohol consumption in women, compared with men, but the four studies that reported results for both men and women did not find this trend [175–178]. However, the Atherosclerosis Risk in Communities Study (ARIC) found a relative T2DM risk of 1.5 for men who drank more than 21 drinks per week, compared to those who drank one or less. This association was not apparent in women [175].

An inverse association between moderate alcohol intake and risk of T2DM in women has also been reported by one of the Dutch Prospect EPIC (EPIC-Dutch) cohorts [181], and in a study of women in Gothenburg, Sweden [182]. However, the term moderate was not clearly defined in these reports. The EPIC-Dutch study also found lifetime alcohol consumption, when corrected for current alcohol consumption, was associated with risk of T2DM in a U-shaped fashion [181]. The NHS II reported a linear inverse association up to 29.9 g/day of alcohol, beyond which risk of T2DM increased, compared with light to moderate (5.0–29.9 g/day) drinkers [179]. It seems clear that some moderate level of alcohol consumption, above 5–6 g/day, is associated with a lower risk of T2DM in women, but the upper limit of moderate intake remains somewhat obscure. It is possible that the beneficial effects of moderate alcohol consumption on risk of T2DM may be mediated by dietary exposures and other aspects of lifestyle associated with moderate drinking. There is insufficient evidence to suggest that the beneficial effect is greater in women than in men.

8.6.1.10 Diet, Inflammation, and T2DM

Type 2 diabetes is associated with low-grade systemic inflammation which, in turn, is implicated in the pathogenesis of atherosclerosis and suggested to be responsible for the increased cardiovascular complications in diabetic patients [183–185]. To investigate the relation between a dietary pattern associated with biomarkers of inflammation and the incidence of T2DM in women, a nested case-control study was conducted in women with T2DM and controls from the NHS [186]. As well, two large cohorts from the NHS and NHS II were followed for incident diabetes [186]. In the nested study, a dietary pattern that was high in sugar-sweetened soft drinks, refined grains, diet soft drinks, and processed meat, but low in wine, coffee, and both cruciferous and yellow vegetables, was directly related to inflammatory markers, and associated with a relative risk of 3.09 for developing T2DM, comparing extreme quintiles. This result was confirmed in the two prospective cohorts with relative risks of 2.56 and 2.93, respectively.

Adiponectin is a protein, secreted by adipose tissue, that is associated with improved IS [187,188], and is also purported to have anti-inflammatory and anti-atherosclerotic effects on the cells lining the walls of blood vessels [189]. Its concentration in plasma decreases with increasing obesity, an effect that is greater in men than in women [190]. Plasma adiponectin concentration has been associated with better glycemic control in a sample of women with T2DM in the NHS [191]. In a cross-sectional study of men and postmenopausal women, some with T2DM and some with normal glucose tolerance, the presence of T2DM and coronary artery disease was significantly associated with decreased plasma adiponectin, independent of BMI, in women [192]. In men, the presence of coronary artery disease, but not of T2DM, was significantly associated with decreased plasma adiponectin. It is possible that women with low adiponectin levels may be predisposed to IR and the development of T2DM. Thus, the association between dietary patterns and risk of T2DM in women may be mediated in part by inflammation and endothelial dysfunction.

An investigation of the link between diet and plasma adiponectin levels in T2DM, in a cross-sectional sample of women from the NHS, reported plasma adiponectin concentrations that were 24% higher in women in the highest, compared to the lowest, quintile of cereal fiber intake [193]. Dietary GL and GI, on the other hand, were significantly inversely associated with plasma adiponectin concentrations. These associations were consistent across lean, overweight, and obese women. Data from an analogous cohort of diabetic men support these findings, although in men, there was a trend for the association between cereal fiber and plasma adiponectin to be stronger in those with lower BMI [194].

8.6.2 Dietary Intervention

Table 8.2 presents a summary of the recent guidelines for medical nutrition therapy in diabetes, issued by the American Diabetes Association [10].

8.6.2.1 Rationale for Review of Dietary Interventions in T2DM

This section is not intended to be an exhaustive review of the literature on dietary interventions in T2DM. Instead, we have focused primarily on those included in two relevant, and recent, Cochrane Reviews [195,196]. We have examined all studies deemed eligible for inclusion in these reviews, identified those in which a subanalysis by sex was included, and presented the findings of these subanalyses in the following discussion. In addition to these studies, we have included intervention studies identified as relating to specific topics raised in the previous section on diet and the risk of T2DM.

TABLE 8.2
Medical Nutrition Therapy for Treating Type 2 Diabetes Mellitus in Adults

- Medical nutrition therapy for people with T2DM should be individualized
- Monitoring total grams of carbohydrate is a critical strategy in achieving glycemic control. The use of the GI/GL may provide additional benefit
- Saturated fat intake should contribute <7% of total energy intake, and intake of trans fat should be minimized
- If chronic kidney disease is present, protein intake should be limited to the recommended dietary allowance
- The primary focus for all overweight or obese adults with T2DM should be on weight reduction
- The primary approach to weight loss should emphasize therapeutic lifestyle change, involving modification of diet and physical activity levels

8.6.2.2 Weight Loss in T2DM

One of the primary components of diabetes care for overweight and obese patients is weight loss, as it has been associated with improvements in IS and glycemic control [197]. In addition, moderate, intentional weight loss has been associated with decreased mortality in people with T2DM [198]. A recent review and meta-analysis of long-term nonpharmacological weight loss interventions in adults with T2DM considered 22 randomized controlled trials with follow-up periods of at least 1 year, and with weight loss or weight control as one of the primary stated goals. All participants were overweight or obese, with a mean age of 55 years. The authors concluded that strategies using dietary, physical activity, or behavioral interventions produced small between-group improvements in weight, and multicomponent interventions including VLCD or low-calorie diets (LCD) may be a promising approach to weight loss in this population [196]. Five of the studies included a subanalysis by sex, and are described in the following paragraphs.

The review included two studies that compared VLCD with LCD, and the pooled between-group change in weight for these two studies was a nonsignificant reduction of 3.0 kg, or 1.6% of baseline weight, at 72 weeks [199] and 104 weeks [200] of follow-up. One study included a subanalysis by sex, and evaluated a year-long behavioral weight control intervention in 93 T2DM patients, randomized to either a balanced LCD of 1000–1200 kcal/day throughout, or the LCD in alternation with two 12 week periods of a 400–500 kcal/day VLCD [200]. At the end of the intervention period, there was a trend for patients in the VLCD group to lose more weight (14.2 kg) than those in the LCD group (10.5 kg), and patients in the VLCD group remained off medication significantly longer. Women in the VLCD group lost significantly more (14.1 kg) than those in the LCD group (8.6 kg) at 1 year, whereas men experienced similar losses between the VLCD group (15.4 kg) and the LCD group (15.5 kg). Improvements were also seen in HbA1c, FPG, FPI, total and HDL-cholesterol, and TG for both diet groups at 1 year. At the 2 year follow-up, in spite of weight regain in both groups, weight loss from baseline was still significant for both diets (~6.5 kg), but improvements in FPG, HbA1c, and

FPI were not maintained. In the other study, patients either consumed a 1000–1500 kcal LCD, with recommendations to increase intake of complex carbohydrate and decrease fat intake, throughout the 20 week intervention, or they were put on a VLCD (400 kcal/day) for Weeks 4–12, and the LCD for Weeks 0–4 and 12–20 [199]. Initial weight loss was greater in the VLCD group (18.6 kg) than in the LCD group (10.1 kg), as was weight regain during the 1 year follow-up, so although long-term weight loss was significant for both groups, they did not differ at 72 weeks (8.6 kg versus 6.8 kg, respectively). However, the VLCD group achieved greater improvements in glycemic control than the LCD group at 20 weeks and 72 weeks, and HDL-cholesterol increased significantly at both 20 and 72 weeks, with a trend toward a greater effect in the VLCD group. Total cholesterol and TG both decreased significantly at 20 weeks, but rebounded. There was no subanalysis by sex in this study. Together, these studies suggest that although intermittent use of a VLCD, alternating with an LCD, may enhance short-term weight loss in women, the long-term effects of this approach on weight loss and lipid levels are not better than those achieved with an LCD alone. However, use of a VLCD may be effective in improving long-term glycemic control.

To compare a "low-carbohydrate" (LC) diet to a "modified fat" (MF) diet, 93 overweight or obese T2DM patients were randomized to receive dietary advice to consume either a 1500 kcal diet obtaining 40% of energy from fat and 40% from carbohydrate with a P:S ratio of 0.5 (LC), or a 1500 kcal diet with 54% carbohydrate, 26% fat, and a P:S ratio of 1.7 (MF) [201]. Both groups reported a 3 kg weight loss at 1 month, and a 4 kg loss at 1 year, and achieved significant reductions in FPG at 1 month and 1 year, with no changes seen in insulin. Triglycerides were significantly reduced in both groups at 1 month, but had returned to baseline levels at 1 year. The transient reduction in TG in the MF group was experienced in men but not in women. Otherwise, trends for men and women did not differ. Patients in the MF group also experienced a sustained decrease in plasma cholesterol. Under the conditions of this study, the MF diet seems to confer an advantage in lowering plasma cholesterol, with no disadvantage as far as fasting glucose control is concerned. However, there do not appear to be any sex-based differences in the long-term effects of these diets.

In a study that compared weight reduction in obese T2DM patients receiving either individual dietary instructions delivered by a nurse, or a short, written leaflet given by a doctor, both modes of delivery resulted in significant weight loss for both men and women at 3 months (~3.5 kg) and at 1 year (~4 kg) [202]. The dietary instructions stressed the importance of weight reduction, and encouraged reduced consumption of saturated fats and increased consumption of complex carbohydrates and vegetables. There were no significant differences between either treatment groups or sex with respect to the changes in body weight. Fasting plasma glucose decreased significantly in both treatment groups. However, HbA1c was significantly decreased only in women who were given the leaflet and in men that received individual counseling from the nurse. When data were analyzed for men and women together, better diabetic control and increased HDL-cholesterol were observed with weight loss of more than 5 kg, as opposed to 5 kg or less. These results do not have any clear implications for sex-based treatment of T2DM.

Fifty obese T2DM patients participated in a 4 month intervention that compared behavior modification (BM) to basic nutrition education (NE) and standard care (SC), with follow-up at 16 months [203]. During the intervention, the BM and NE groups had weekly group meetings with staff, whereas the SC group had only monthly contact. Patients in both the NE and SC groups were given a caloric goal and asked to follow an Exchange Diet Eating Plan, but specific dietary goals were not prescribed. Those in the BM group were instructed to record their caloric intake and, later in the program, to monitor intake of high-sugar foods and increase fiber intake. In addition, an exercise component was included in the weekly meetings for the BM group. Overall, participants reported reduced consumption of foods high in fat and in sugar, and reduced poor food choices, with none of these dietary improvements differing significantly between treatment groups. The BM group achieved a significantly greater weight loss than the other groups at 4 months, but there were no significant differences between groups at 16 months, and no significant treatment effects on any other outcomes. Overall, FPG, HbA1c, postprandial glucose, FPI and total cholesterol decreased, and HDL-cholesterol increased over the 4 month intervention. However, only FPI and HDL-cholesterol remained significant at 16 months. No differences were observed in TG levels. Only those patients that lost at least 4.6 kg showed significant improvements in FPG and HbA1c. Men lost significantly more weight than women (4.4 kg compared to 1.7 kg) from 0–16 months, and had a greater decrease in HbA1c and postprandial glucose from 0–4 months. However, these differences were not sustained at 16 months. Women had slightly greater increases in HDL-cholesterol at both 4 and 16 months and although changes in HDL-cholesterol were strongly correlated with changes in weight in men, no such correlation was found for women. These findings do not have clear implications for sex-based recommendations to improve long-term control in T2DM.

Forty-nine obese patients with obese spouses were randomly assigned to participate, either by themselves (alone) or along with their spouse (together), in a 20 week behavioral weight control program [204]. They were instructed to consume between 1200 and 1500 kcal/day, to increase their intake of complex carbohydrate and fiber, decrease their intake of fat and simple carbohydrate, and to expend at least 1000 kcal/week in an exercise program. Participants in both groups achieved a caloric intake of 1300–1400 kcal/day and a fat intake between 33% and 34% by the end of the 20 week program. Overall, the 43 patients who completed the study showed significant improvements in BMI, FPG, and HbA1c, with no differences found between treatment groups. Weight loss at 20 weeks was ~9.5 kg, and ~9.3 kg at 72 weeks. There was a significant interaction between time and sex, indicating that women did better when treated with their spouses, and men did better when treated alone. These findings suggest that the degree of spousal involvement in a behavioral modification weight loss program may be an important consideration when treating women with T2DM.

In a review of dietary advice for treatment of T2DM in adults, 18 randomized controlled trials with follow-up periods of at least 6 months were considered [195]. The authors concluded that there is a lack of high-quality data and an urgent need for well-designed studies that examine a range of interventions. However, there is some evidence that addition of an exercise component can improve metabolic control, as reflected by HbA1c levels, at 6 and 12 weeks of follow-up. Of nine studies that compared two types of dietary advice, three included a sub-analysis by sex [200,201,205]. Two of these have already been discussed in this chapter [200,201], and the other is discussed below [205].

To evaluate a weight loss and exercise program in older African-Americans, 64 participants were randomized to either a "usual care" (UC) group or a "diet and exercise" (DE) group, and followed for 6 months [205]. The UC group attended a class that discussed methods of glycemic control and received two mailings of nutrition information. Patients in the DE group were prescribed a diet with 55%–60% carbohydrate, 12%–20% protein, and less than 30% fat, aimed at weight loss of $\leq$2 lb/week, and encouraged to participate in moderate physical activity 3 times/week. Significant net differences in the DE versus UC were observed for nutrition knowledge, physical activity, and dietary intake of fat, saturated fat, and cholesterol at 3 months, and for weight and HbA1c at 3 months (−2.0 kg and −1.6%, respectively) and at 6 months (−2.4 kg and −2.4%, respectively). There was no interaction between sex and treatment on HbA1c changes, but the overall net weight loss from baseline was significant in women at 3 months (−2.2 kg) and 6 months (−2.8 kg), whereas it was nonsignificant for men at 3 months (−1.0 kg) and 6 months (−2.0 kg). However, this modest sex-based difference does not suggest sex-based differences for treatment.

Five studies discussed in the review of diet advice for T2DM compared a low-fat diet to either a modified fat or a low-carbohydrate diet [201,206–209]. In general, weight loss was greater in the low-fat diet groups, but only marginal changes were observed in HbA1c, making it difficult to draw conclusions regarding long-term glycemic control. As discussed earlier, the only one of these studies to include a subanalysis by sex reported a transient reduction in TG on the low-fat diet in men, but not in women [201], and no sex-based differences in long-term treatment effects. One study employed a 16 week weight loss strategy involving diet, exercise, and behavior modification to compare the effects of calorie restriction alone (LC) versus calorie plus fat restriction (LF) on weight loss and glycemic control in obese women, 44 with T2DM and 46 with a family history of T2DM [208]. The prescribed diets were 1000–1500 kcal/day, and the LF group was to keep fat intake below 20% of energy. Overall, the women assigned to the LF diet reported a fat intake of ~22% of energy, compared to ~30% for the women on the LC diet. Among women with T2DM, the LF diet resulted in a significantly greater weight loss over 16 weeks (7.7 versus 4.6 kg), and at one-year follow-up (5.2 versus 1.0 kg), compared to the LC group. Significant decreases in glucose, and HDL- and total cholesterol were seen in women with T2DM for both dietary groups, but only HDL-cholesterol remained significantly decreased after 1 year. There was no effect of dietary treatment on weight loss or physiological changes in women with a family history of T2DM. Although this study suggests that diets low in both total energy and fat may be effective in achieving weight loss in women with T2DM, studies employing measured intake may be necessary to determine whether or not long-term improvements in glycemic control could also be achieved with this dietary approach.

8.6.2.3 Dietary Fiber

As mentioned in the previous section, cereal fiber intake is inversely associated with T2DM risk for both men and women. In short-term intervention trials, many different dietary fiber supplements have shown modest beneficial effects on blood glucose control in older overweight and obese adults with T2DM. Some of the fibers that have been studied are β-glucan [210], locust bean gum [211], psyllium [212], arabinoxylan [213], and oat bran flour [214]. All the fibers significantly reduced postprandial glucose, and all except locust bean gum lowered postprandial insulin levels. Although women were included in these studies, the sample sizes were typically too small to perform a subanalysis by sex.

Intervention trials of a longer duration examining the effect of dietary fiber supplementation on blood glucose control in adults with T2DM have yielded mixed results. In 13 older obese adults (including one woman), improvements were observed in glycemic control and plasma insulin levels after 6 weeks of 50 g/day total fiber (25 g insoluble), compared to 24 g total fiber (16 g insoluble) [215]. In a group of overweight and obese older adults, randomized to consume three 5 g premeal doses per day of either psyllium (as Metamucil) or a placebo that contained an inert fiber, for 6 weeks, a significant reduction in FPG was observed on the psyllium arm, with no treatment differences observed between men and women [216]. In contrast, FPG and HbA1C were not significantly affected after 3 months in 16 older overweight adults (seven women) on a diet supplemented with 19 g/day compared to 5 g/day, additional wheat bran cereal fiber [217]. No differences were found between men and women. When we randomly assigned 91 adults with T2DM to receive ~10% of energy from a low-GI/high-fiber breakfast cereal, a high-GI/low-fiber cereal, or oil or margarine containing MUFA for 6 months, the patients in the low-GI/high-fiber group consumed ~50 g/day of dietary fiber, as opposed to ~23 g/day in the other two diet groups [209]. After 6 months on the diets there were no significant differences in fasting glucose and HbA1c levels between the low-GI/high-fiber and high-GI/low-fiber diets. Thus, interventions lasting 3 months or more are needed to determine whether effects of dietary fiber on glycemic control, seen at 6 weeks, are sustained over a longer time period. At present, there is nothing to suggest that the acute effects are sustained, and no evidence that these effects differ between men and women.

8.6.2.4 Dietary GI

A modest beneficial effect of low-GI diets, in comparison to high-GI diets, on blood glucose control in men and women with T2DM has been demonstrated in a number of small, short-term randomized crossover trials [218–221]. The difference between the low- and high-GI diets consumed in these studies ranged from 12 to 41 GI units, and the duration of the studies ranged from 2 to 12 weeks. In some studies, the observed effect of the low-GI diet may have been confounded by a higher fiber content than that of the high-fiber diets [218,221]. None of the studies included analysis by sex. A study in six healthy men has also demonstrated improvements in glycemic control after 2 weeks on a low-GI diet (GI = 63 compared with 104) [222]. As discussed above, when 91 adults with T2DM were randomized to receive ~10%

of energy from a low-GI breakfast cereal, a high-GI breakfast cereal, or oil or margarine containing MUFA for 6 months, there were no significant differences between the effects of the two cereal treatments on fasting serum glucose and HbA1c [209]. However, the difference in GI between the two diet treatments was only ~10 GI units, compared with differences of ~12–28 GI units achieved in most other studies in which glycemic control was improved [223]. More studies are needed that are of longer duration, achieve greater differences in GI between groups, and include a subanalysis by sex.

8.6.2.5 Dietary Fat

When compared to saturated fat, PUFA appears to cause a transient increase in IS, but has no effect on long-term glycemic control in either men or women. In a 5 week randomized crossover study in 17 adults (6 with T2DM, 6 nonobese nondiabetic, and 5 obese nondiabetic without T2DM), IS increased after a diet rich in PUFA, and abdominal subcutaneous fat area decreased overall following the PUFA diet, compared with a diet rich in saturated fat [224]. However, there were no changes in FPG, FPI, or HbA1c. Analysis by sex revealed that the change in abdominal subcutaneous fat was significant only in women. When the data were analyzed by subject group, this change was significant in both the obese and nonobese groups without T2DM but there was no effect of diet on abdominal subcutaneous fat in the group with T2DM. In a 30 week randomized crossover trial in adults with well-controlled T2DM, no effects were seen on glycemic control, or on postprandial blood glucose, plasma insulin, and C-peptide after consuming a diet with a moderately high ratio of PUFA to saturated fat (P:S 1.0), compared to a low ratio (P:S 0.3) [225]. This was in spite of increased insulin receptor binding capacity on the high P:S diet. However, lower total and LDL-cholesterol levels were observed with the high P:S diet. A subanalysis by sex found no significant differences between men and women for lipid and IS outcomes.

When compared with the effect of MUFA, PUFA appears to have no effect on long-term glycemic control. Although a parallel trial in overweight and obese adults with T2DM and hypertension found significant increases in FPG after 6 weeks of dietary supplementation with 4 g/day of either purified eicosapentaenoic acid (EPA) or purified docosahexaenoic acid (DHA), compared to olive oil, neither EPA nor DHA had significant effects on HbA1c, fasting plasma insulin and C-peptide, or IS at 6 weeks [226]. There was no subanalysis by sex. In a 2 week randomized crossover trial in older overweight and obese men with T2DM, although FPG and FPI were significantly higher after consuming a diet high in linoleic acid, compared with a diet high in oleic acid, this study was not of long enough duration to assess dietary effects on long-term glycemic control [227]. There is no sufficient evidence to comment on the possibility of sex-based differences.

Although trans fatty acids appear to have deleterious effects on blood glucose control in T2DM, it is unclear whether these effects differ between men and women. In a 6-week randomized crossover study in obese middle-aged men and women with T2DM, diets high (20% of energy) in trans-MUFA or saturated fat were associated with higher postprandial insulin responses than a diet high in cis-MUFA [228]. In an

8 week parallel trial in overweight and obese adults with T2DM, comparing the effects of supplementation with 3.0 g/day of conjugated linoleic acid (CLA) to a placebo representative of the fat content of a habitual Western diet, fasting glucose concentrations were increased, and IS was decreased, by the CLA [229]. Neither of these studies included a subanalysis by sex. On the other hand, in a randomized crossover study in young, nondiabetic women, a 4 week diet with a lower trans fat content (5.1% of energy) did not result in differences in glucose or insulin responses, when compared to a diet obtaining the same amount of energy from oleic acid (cis-MUFA) [230]. It is unclear whether the differences in postprandial insulin responses between these two studies were due to the much higher level of trans fatty acids in the first study, the difference in health status and age of subjects between the two studies, or the sex of the subjects.

8.6.2.6 Nuts

As mentioned in the previous section, a higher intake of nuts has been associated with a lower risk of T2DM in women [151]. When 20 young healthy men and women supplemented their diets with 100 g/day almonds for 4 weeks, there was no main effect of time or sex on either the IS index or glucose effectiveness, but there was a significant time × sex interaction on both indices, such that they increased in women (almost significantly), but tended to decrease in men (not significantly) [231]. It is unclear whether these trends would have resulted in significant differences with a longer intervention, a higher dose of almonds, or in subjects with impaired glycemic control. The investigators then tested the effects of four diets on oral glucose tolerance in a 4 week randomized crossover trial in 17 women (14 of whom were postmenopausal) and 13 men. All subjects were older, obese, and had T2DM. The four diets were: high-fat/high-almond (HFA; 37% total fat, 10% from almonds); low-fat/high almond (LFA; 25% total fat, 10% from almonds); high-fat/control (HFC; 37% total fat, 10% from olive or canola oil); and low-fat/control (LFC; 25% total fat, 10% from olive or canola oil). There was no main effect of fat source (almond versus oil) or fat level on any insulin or glucose index, but the almond-enriched diets significantly decreased HDL-cholesterol, although there was no effect of fat source on the ratios of LDL- to HDL-cholesterol or total- to HDL-cholesterol. They did not report an effect of sex on these results. A 6 month randomized parallel study in 41 older, overweight, and obese adults with T2DM, looked at the effect of 30 g/day walnuts, in addition to a low-fat diet (30% of energy as fat) that included fish [232]. There were improvements in both the HDL-concentration and the ratio of HDL to total cholesterol on the walnut-diet, with no deleterious effect on HbA1c levels. The data were not analyzed by sex. Although the study in young adults is suggestive of a possible sex-based difference in the effect of almonds on IS, there is not enough evidence to evaluate this in adults with T2DM.

8.6.2.7 Milk Protein

Milk proteins appear to induce the rapid release of insulinotropic amino acids and incretin hormones [233]. Whey protein, in particular, appears to be a strong stimulus for GLP-1 release. In a randomized crossover study in six women and eight men with

T2DM, supplementation of both breakfast and lunch (both high-GI) with 27.6 g whey powder resulted in increases in postprandial insulin responses of 31% and 57% for breakfast and lunch, respectively [234]. After lunch, the blood glucose response was significantly reduced by 21%, and GIP levels were significantly increased with the whey supplement, although there was no effect of treatment on GLP-1 levels. There was no subanalysis by sex.

8.6.2.8 Alcohol Intake

To investigate the effect of moderate alcohol consumption on IS and glycemic control, a group of nondiabetic postmenopausal women participated in a randomized crossover trial [235]. Consumption of 30 g/day (2 drinks/day) of alcohol, over an 8 week period, had beneficial effects on insulin and TG concentrations and IS. Although this finding is compatible with those studies showing an association between moderate alcohol intake and reduced risk of T2DM in women, it is not known if this level of consumption would result in similar benefits for diabetic women.

8.6.2.9 Diet and Inflammation in T2DM

In a 14 week intervention study designed to assess the effects of different weight loss regimens on adipocytokine and inflammatory cytokine levels, 33 obese postmenopausal women with T2DM were randomized to one of three treatments: a weight-loss diet (40% fat; 30% MUFA) designed to achieve a caloric deficit of ~600 kcal/day (D); an exercise program designed to achieve a caloric deficit of ~250 to 300 kcal/day (3–4 days/week) (E); or a combination of the diet and exercise programs (D + E) [236]. Plasma C-reactive protein decreased on all three treatments, whereas leptin levels decreased only on the D and D + E interventions, with no differences between treatments. No differences were found for plasma resistin, tumor necrosis factor-α, or adiponectin, although there was a trend for adiponectin to increase on the D and D + E interventions. As noted earlier, increased plasma adiponectin concentration has been associated with better glycemic control in women with T2DM [191]. More studies are needed to clarify the relationship between plasma adiponectin, inflammation, and T2DM.

8.7 CONCLUSION AND SUMMARY OF MAIN FINDINGS

Based on our review of the literature, there do not appear to be striking interactions between sex and the effects of various nutrients and dietary components on either risk for, or treatment of, the MetS or T2DM.

8.7.1 Diet and Risk of the MetS

A diet high in whole grains, fiber, PUFA, and low-fat dairy products, and low in saturated fat appears to be associated with a decreased risk of the MetS in both men and women. There is some evidence of an interaction between dietary fat, variants of the PLIN gene, and IR in Singaporean women, but not Singaporean men.

8.7.2 Dietary Intervention in the MetS

Both lifestyle interventions and dietary interventions aimed at weight loss appear to be equally effective in men and women with the MetS. However, weight loss induced by a VLCD, in the absence of an exercise component, may be more effective for men than women with respect to improvements in insulin-stimulated glucose disposal. Low GI interventions have been shown to improve insulin-stimulated glucose uptake in isolated fat cells, the glucose disposition index, and acute insulin secretion, with one study demonstrating a greater increase in IS for women than for men. Low GI diets are often high in fiber which has also been shown to improve IS in women. Beneficial effects of MUFA, compared to either saturated fat or PUFA, are observed on glucose metabolism in both women and men.

8.7.3 Diet and Risk of T2DM

A diet high in whole grains, cereal fiber, magnesium, calcium, and low-fat dairy products, with moderate alcohol consumption (2 or less drinks/day) and low in GI is associated with a lower risk of T2DM in both men and women. The relationship between intake of refined grains and T2DM risk is unclear, and there is no evidence of a sex-based difference. There is some evidence of an inverse association between PUFA intake and T2DM risk in women, but the evidence for men is inconsistent. The protective effect of coffee consumption, however, is relevant for both women and men. Heme iron intake is associated with an increased risk of T2DM in women.

8.7.4 Dietary Intervention in T2DM

Multicomponent interventions including VLCD or LCD may be a promising approach to weight loss in men and women with T2DM. Intermittent use of a VLCD, alternating with an LCD, may enhance short-term weight loss in women, as opposed to men, although this difference does not seem to be sustained. A low-fat LCD may be more effective than a moderate-fat LCD in achieving weight loss in women with T2DM, although this does not appear to be accompanied by sustained improvements in glucose control. There is some evidence that women with T2DM may achieve better results from behavioral weight control programs if their spouse participates with them, although the same cannot be said for men. Both low GI diets and dietary fiber have been shown to have modest beneficial short-term effects on blood glucose control in men and women with T2DM. However, intervention trials of longer duration in men and women have yielded mixed results. Compared to saturated fat, PUFA has a transient positive effect on IS, but no effect on long-term glycemic control in either women or men. It is not clear whether the deleterious effects of trans fatty acids on blood glucose control differ between women and men.

8.8 FUTURE RESEARCH

8.8.1 General Recommendations

To determine whether an association found in a prospective trial in women is of relevance to women in particular, or whether it applies to both sexes, one has to be able to compare the data for women to an analogous sample of men. There is a need for more large-scale epidemiologic trials that include enough women and men to support a subanalysis by sex. Regardless of whether or not a statistically significant effect of sex is found, the results of such an analysis should be reported [237]. The same applies to the assessment of outcomes in intervention trials. A recent survey of research published in four major medical journals in selected years found that only 25%–33% of the studies that included men and women analyzed the data by sex [238]. It has been argued that understanding sex differences will enable researchers to design more effective interventions for both men and women, and that subanalysis by sex can be planned for and conducted without compromising the quality of the research or making the study too costly [237].

Much of the prospective data on the relationships between dietary intake and risks of the MetS and T2DM in women have been provided by the NHS. While this is a very well designed ongoing study, the participants are predominantly Caucasian, well-educated, professionals working in the health system, and therefore having ready access to health information. Given that the rate of diabetes is significantly higher in non-Hispanic, African-American, and Mexican-American, compared to Caucasian women, especially in those older than 60 years of age, there is an argument for more trials of this scope targeting women in these communities. It has also been argued that management of the MetS is complex, and will require consideration of a patient's racial background and sex [239].

8.8.2 Specific Recommendations

There is a need for more research to determine if visceral fat is more predictive of IS in women than men, and whether the lesser weight loss-induced mobilization of visceral fat observed in women, and its associated attenuation in blood lipid improvements, has implications for risk of CHD in women. This is of particular importance in women with the MetS or T2DM.

Since VLCD-induced weight loss may be less effective for women than men with respect to improvements in IS, and there seem to be beneficial effects of low-GI diets on insulin-stimulated glucose uptake in isolated fat cells in women, more research is needed on the effects of low-GI weight loss interventions, such as those cited involving rye bread, on IS in women with the MetS.

Intervention trials in women who are homozygous for the PLIN minor alleles are needed to determine whether diets with less than 10% of dietary energy from saturated fat can prevent or reverse the development of IR.

There is a need for more research examining the impact of metabolic status (especially IR and T2DM) on the choice of macronutrient balance for weight-loss diets in women. Research on the role of low-carbohydrate diets in women with IR has yielded conflicting results. The increase in total and LDL-cholesterol in young healthy women consuming a very low carbohydrate diet (<10% of energy) suggests more research is necessary before this approach can be promoted as an intervention for women with IR. Conversely, women with T2DM may benefit more from a low-fat weight loss intervention, but there is insufficient evidence of improvement in long-term glycemic control to support recommendation of this approach at present.

There is a need for more research examining the relationship between plasma adiponectin levels, IS, and T2DM in both men and women, and to determine if the attenuation of plasma GLP-1 secretion in response to oral carbohydrate in obese women is involved in the pathogenesis of obesity and diabetes in women.

In order to determine whether the beneficial effects of coffee on T2DM risk are greater in women than in men, intervention studies are needed that standardize the coffee source, method of preparation, and size of serving. Particular attention should be paid to the relationship between coffee intake, levels of sex hormones and sex hormone-binding globulin, and TG levels in women.

REFERENCES

1. NCEP Expert Panel on the Detection, Evaluation, and Treatment of High Blood Pressure in Adults. Executive Summary of the Third Report of the National Cholesterol Education Program (NCEP) Expert Panel on the Detection, Evaluation, and Treatment of High Blood Pressure in Adults (Adult Treatment Panel III). *J. Am. Med. Assoc.*, 285, 2486, 2001.
2. Wilson, P.W.F., et al., Metabolic syndrome as a precursor of cardiovascular disease and type 2 diabetes mellitus. *Circulation*, 112, 3066, 2005.
3. Grundy, S.M., et al., Diagnosis and management of the metabolic syndrome: an American Heart Association/National Heart, Lung, and Blood Institute scientific statement. *Circulation*, 112, 2735, 2005.
4. International Diabetes Federation (IDF) Task Force on Epidemiology and Prevention. The IDF consensus worldwide definitions of the metabolic syndrome. Published in 2005. Last accessed on July 31, 2007. http://www.idf.org/webdata/docs/Mets_def_update2006.pdf
5. Expert Committee on the Diagnosis and Classification of Diabetes Mellitus. Follow-up report on the diagnosis of diabetes mellitus. *Diabetes Care*, 26, 3160, 2003.
6. Guerrero-Romero, F. and Rodríguez-Moran, M., Concordance between the 2005 International Diabetes Federation definition for diagnosing metabolic syndrome with the National Cholesterol Education Program Adult Treatment Panel III and the World Health Organization definitions. *Diabetes Care*, 28, 2588, 2005.
7. Sheppard, P.R. and Kahn, B.B., Glucose transporters and insulin action. *N. Engl. J. Med.*, 341, 248, 1999.
8. Reaven, G.M., Banting Lecture 1988. Role of insulin resistance in human disease. *Diabetes*, 37, 1595, 1988.
9. Grundy, S.M., et al., Definition of Metabolic Syndrome: Report of the National Heart, Lung, and Blood Institute/American Heart Association Conference on Scientific Issues Related to Definition. *Circulation*, 109, 433, 2004.
10. American Diabetes Association. Standards of medical care in diabetes—2006. *Diabetes Care*, 29, S4, 2006.
11. Canadian Diabetes Association Clinical Practice Guidelines Expert Committee. Canadian Diabetes Association 2003 Clinical Practice Guidelines for the Prevention and Management of Diabetes in Canada. *Can. J. Diabetes*, 27 (suppl 2), 2003.
12. Edelstein, S.L., et al., Predictors of progression from impaired glucose tolerance to NIDDM: an analysis of six prospective studies. *Diabetes*, 46, 701, 1997.
13. DeVegt, F., et al., Relation of impaired fasting and postload glucose with incident type 2 diabetes in a Dutch population: the Hoorn Study. *J. Am. Med. Assoc.*, 285, 2109, 2001.

14. Hux, J.E., et al., Eds., *Diabetes in Ontario: An ICES Practice Atlas*, Institute for Clinical Evaluative Sciences, Toronto, 2003 (glossary).
15. CDC Diabetes Program. United States Department of Health and Human Services, Centers for Disease Control and Prevention. Diabetes and women's health across the life stages: a public health perspective. Published in 2001. Atlanta, GA. Last accessed on July 31, 2007. http://www.cdc.gov/diabetes/pubs/pdf/womenshort.pdf
16. Ford, E.S., Giles, W.H., and Dietz, W.H., Prevalence of the metabolic syndrome among US adults: findings from the third national health and nutrition examination survey. *J. Am. Med. Assoc.*, 287, 356, 2002.
17. Ford, E.S., Giles, W.H., and Mokdad, A.H., Increasing prevalence of the metabolic syndrome among U.S. adults. *Diabetes Care*, 27, 2444, 2004.
18. McLaughlin, T., et al., Use of metabolic markers to identify overweight individuals who are insulin resistant. *Ann. Intern. Med.*, 139, 802, 2003.
19. United States Department of Health and Human Services, Centers for Disease Control and Prevention, National Center for Chronic Disease Prevention and Health Promotion, Division of Diabetes Translation. Last accessed on July 31, 2007. http://www.cdc.gov/diabetes/statistics/
20. National Diabetes Information Clearinghouse. National Institute of Diabetes and Digestive and Kidney Diseases, National Institutes of Health. Last accessed on July 31, 2007. http://diabetes.niddk.nih.gov/dm/pubs/statistics/index.htm#7
21. Millar, W.J. and Young, T.K., Tracking diabetes: prevalence, incidence and risk factors. Health Reports (Statistics Canada, Catalogue 82–003) 2003; 14(3): 35–47. Last accessed on July 31, 2007. http://www.statcan.ca
22. Statistics Canada. Smoking and diabetes care: results from the CCHS cycle 3.1 (2005), Catalogue 82–621–002, 2006. Last accessed on July 31, 2007. http://www.statcan.ca
23. Carr, D.B., et al., Intra-abdominal fat is a major determinant of the National Cholesterol Education Program Adult Treatment Panel III criteria for the metabolic syndrome. *Diabetes*, 53, 2087, 2004.
24. Ferrannini, E., et al., Hyperinsulinemia: the key feature of a cardiovascular and metabolic syndrome. *Diabetologia*, 34, 416, 1991.
25. Rebuffé-Scrive, M., et al., Metabolism of adipose tissue in intra-abdominal depots in severely obese men and women. *Metabolism*, 39, 1021, 1990.
26. Strömblad, G. and Björntorp, P., Reduced hepatic insulin clearance in rats with dietary induced obesity. *Metabolism*, 35, 323, 1986.
27. Petersen, K.F. and Shulman, G.I., Pathogenesis of skeletal muscle insulin resistance in type 2 diabetes mellitus. *Am. J. Cardiol.*, 90, 11, 2002.
28. Browning, J.D., et al., Prevalence of hepatic steatosis in an urban population in the United States: impact of ethnicity. *Hepatology*, 40, 1387, 2004.
29. Olefsky, J.M. and Nolan, J.J., Insulin resistance and non-insulin-dependent diabetes mellitus: cellular and molecular mechanisms. *Am. J. Clin. Nutr.*, 61, 980S, 1995.
30. McClenaghan, N.H., Determining the relationship between dietary carbohydrate intake and insulin resistance. *Nutr. Res. Rev.*, 18, 222, 2005.
31. Kuhl, J., et al., Characterisation of subjects with early abnormalities of glucose tolerance in the Stockholm Diabetes Prevention Programme: the impact of sex and type 2 diabetes heredity. *Diabetologia*, 48, 35, 2005.
32. Dallongeville, J., et al., Multiple coronary heart disease risk factors are associated with menopause and influenced by substitutive hormonal therapy in a cohort of French women. *Atherosclerosis*, 118, 123, 1995.

33. Park, Y.-W., et al., The metabolic syndrome: prevalence and associated risk factor findings in the US population from the Third National Health and Nutrition Examination Survey, 1988–1994. *Arch. Intern. Med.*, 163, 427, 2003.
34. Krotkiewski, M., et al., Impact of obesity on metabolism in men and women. Importance of regional adipose tissue distribution. *J. Clin. Invest.*, 72, 1150, 1983.
35. Zamboni, M., et al., Body fat distribution in pre- and post-menopausal women: metabolic and anthropometric variables and their inter-relationships. *Int. J. Obes. Relat. Metab. Disord.*, 16, 495, 1992.
36. Poehlman, E.T., Toth, M.J., and Gardner, A.W., Changes in energy balance and body composition at menopause: a controlled longitudinal study. *Ann. Intern. Med.*, 123, 673, 1995.
37. Björkelund, C., et al., Reproductive history in relation to relative weight and fat distribution. *Int. J. Obes. Relat. Metab. Disord.*, 20, 213, 1996.
38. Carr, M.C., The emergence of the metabolic syndrome with menopause. *J. Clin. Endocrinol. Metab.*, 88, 2404, 2003.
39. Tufano, A., et al., Anthropometric, hormonal and biochemical differences in lean and obese women before and after menopause. *J. Endocrinol. Invest.*, 27, 648, 2004.
40. Lee, C.C., Kasa-Vubu, J.Z., and Supiano, M.A., Androgenicity and obesity are independently associated with insulin sensitivity in postmenopausal women. *Metabolism*, 53, 507, 2004.
41. Golden, S.H., et al., Glucose and insulin components of the metabolic syndrome are associated with hyperandrogenism in postmenopausal women: the Atherosclerosis Risk in Communities Study. *Am. J. Epidemiol.*, 160, 540, 2004.
42. Murphy, M.J., et al., Girls at five are intrinsically more insulin resistant than boys: the programming hypotheses revisited—the EarlyBird Study (EarlyBird 6). *Pediatrics*, 113, 82, 2004.
43. Mittendorfer, B., Insulin resistance: sex matters. *Curr. Opin. Clin. Nutr. Metab. Care*, 8, 367, 2005.
44. Laaksonen, D.E., et al., Relationships between changes in abdominal fat distribution and insulin sensitivity during a very low calorie diet in abdominally obese men and women. *Nutr. Metab. Cardiovasc. Dis.*, 13, 349, 2003.
45. Rattarasarn, C., et al., Gender differences of regional abdominal fat distribution and their relationships with insulin sensitivity in healthy and glucose-intolerant Thais. *J. Clin. Endocrinol. Metab.*, 89, 6266, 2004.
46. Ouyang, P., et al., Relationships of insulin sensitivity with fatness and fitness and in older men and women. *J. Womens Health*, 13, 177, 2004.
47. Despres, J.P., et al., Loss of abdominal fat and metabolic response to exercise training in obese women. *Am. J. Physiol.*, 261, E159, 1991.
48. Wirth, A. and Steinmetz, B., Gender differences in changes in subcutaneous and intra-abdominal fat during weight reduction: an ultrasound study. *Obes. Res.*, 6, 393, 1998.
49. Goodpaster, B.H., et al., Effects of weight loss on regional fat distribution and insulin sensitivity in obesity. *Diabetes*, 48, 839, 1999.
50. Hokanson, J.E. and Austin, M.A., Plasma triglyceride level is a risk factor for cardiovascular disease independent of high-density lipoprotein cholesterol level: a meta-analysis of population-based prospective studies. *J. Cardiovasc. Risk*, 3, 213, 1996.
51. Beer-Borst, S., et al., Dietary patterns in six European populations: results from EURALIM, a collaborative European data harmonization and information campaign. *Eur. J. Clin. Nutr.*, 54, 253, 2000.
52. Liu, K., et al., A study of the reliability and comparative validity of the CARDIA dietary history. *Ethn. Dis.*, 4, 15, 1994.

53. Hebert, J.R., et al., Social desirability bias in dietary self-report may compromise the validity of dietary intake measures. *Int. J. Epidemiol.*, 24, 389, 1995.
54. Hebert, J.R., et al., Gender differences in social desirability and social approval bias in dietary self-report. *Am. J. Epidemiol.*, 146, 1046, 1997.
55. Jenkins, D.J.A., et al., Glycemic index of foods: a physiological basis for carbohydrate exchange. *Am. J. Clin. Nutr.*, 34, 362, 1981.
56. Wolever, T.M.S., et al., Determination of the glycaemic index of foods: interlaboratory study. *Eur. J. Clin. Nutr.*, 57, 475, 2003.
57. Jenkins, D.J.A., et al., Dietary fibre, lente carbohydrates and the insulin-resistant diseases. *Brit. J. Nutr.*, 83 (suppl 1), S157, 2000.
58. Wolever, T.M.S., *The Glycaemic Index: A Physiological Classification of Dietary Carbohydrate*, CAB International, Cambridge, 2006.
59. Salmerón, J., et al., Dietary fiber, glycemic load, and risk of non-insulin-dependent diabetes mellitus in women. *J. Am. Med. Assoc.*, 277, 472, 1997.
60. McKeown, N.M., et al., Carbohydrate nutrition, insulin resistance, and the prevalence of the metabolic syndrome in the Framingham Offspring Cohort. *Diabetes Care*, 27, 538, 2004.
61. Liese, A.D., et al., Dietary glycemic index and glycemic load, carbohydrate and fiber intake, and measures of insulin sensitivity, secretion, and adiposity in the Insulin Resistance Atherosclerosis Study. *Diabetes Care*, 28, 2832, 2005.
62. Liese, A.D., et al., Whole-grain intake and insulin sensitivity: the Insulin Resistance Atherosclerosis Study. *Am. J. Clin. Nutr.*, 78, 965, 2003.
63. Mooy, J.M., et al., Determinants of specific serum insulin concentrations in a general Caucasian population aged 50 to 74 years (the Hoorn Study). *Diabetic Medicine*, 15, 45, 1998.
64. Pereira, M.A., et al., Dairy consumption, obesity, and the insulin resistance syndrome in young adults: the CARDIA Study. *J. Am. Med. Assoc.*, 287, 2081, 2002.
65. Liu, S., et al., Dietary glycemic load assessed by food-frequency questionnaire in relation to plasma high-density-lipoprotein cholesterol and fasting plasma triacylglycerols in postmenopausal women. *Am. J. Clin. Nutr.*, 73, 560, 2001.
66. Mayer, E.J., et al., Usual dietary fat intake and insulin concentrations in healthy women twins. *Diabetes Care*, 16, 1459, 1993.
67. Mayer-Davis, E.J., et al., Dietary fat and insulin sensitivity in a triethnic population: the role of obesity. The Insulin Resistance Atherosclerosis Study (IRAS). *Am. J. Clin. Nutr.*, 65, 79, 1997.
68. Feskens, E.J., Loeber, J.G., and Kromhout, D., Diet and physical activity as determinants of hyperinsulinemia: the Zutphen Elderly Study. *Am. J. Epidemiol.*, 140, 350, 1994.
69. Mooy, J.M., et al., Prevalence and determinants of glucose intolerance in a Dutch Caucasian population: The Hoorn Study. *Diabetes Care*, 18, 1270, 1995.
70. Parker, D.R., et al., Relationship of dietary saturated fatty acids and body habitus to serum insulin concentrations: the Normative Aging Study. *Am. J. Clin. Nutr.*, 58, 129, 1993.
71. Marshall, J.A., Bessesen, D.H., and Hamman, R.F., High saturated fat and low starch and fibre are associated with hyperinsulinaemia in a non-diabetic population: the San Luis Valley Diabetes Study. *Diabetologia*, 40, 430, 1997.
72. Trevisan, M., et al., Consumption of olive oil, butter, and vegetable oils and coronary heart disease risk factors. *J. Am. Med. Assoc.*, 263, 688, 1990.
73. Qi, L., et al., Genetic variation at the perilipin (PLIN) locus is associated with obesity-related phenotypes in White women. *Clin. Genet.*, 66, 299, 2004.

74. Qi, L., et al., Intragenic linkage disequilibrium structure of the human perilipin gene (PLIN) and haplotype association with increased obesity risk in a multiethnic Asian population. *J. Mol. Med.*, 83, 448, 2005.
75. Corella, D., et al., Perilipin gene variation determines higher susceptibility to insulin resistance in Asian women when consuming a high-saturated fat, low-carbohydrate diet. *Diabetes Care*, 29, 1313, 2006.
76. Azadbakht, L., et al., Dairy consumption is inversely associated with the prevalence of the metabolic syndrome in Tehranian adults. *Am. J. Clin. Nutr.*, 82, 523, 2005.
77. Liu, S., et al., Dietary calcium, vitamin D, and the prevalence of metabolic syndrome in middle-aged and older U.S. women. *Diabetes Care*, 28, 2926, 2005.
78. Sonnenberg, L., et al., Dietary patterns and the metabolic syndrome in obese and non-obese Framingham women. *Obes. Res.*, 13, 153, 2005.
79. Millen, B.E., et al., Nutritional risk and the metabolic syndrome in women: opportunities for preventive intervention from the Framingham Nutrition Study. *Am. J. Clin. Nutr.*, 84, 434, 2006.
80. Mennen, L.I., et al., Possible protective effect of bread and dairy products on the risk of the metabolic syndrome. *Nutr. Res.*, 20, 335, 2000.
81. Wirfält, E., et al., Food patterns and components of the metabolic syndrome in men and women: a cross-sectional study within the Malmö diet and cancer cohort. *Am. J. Epidemiol.*, 154, 1150, 2001.
82. Meisler, J.G., Toward optimal health: the experts discuss the metabolic syndrome. *J. Womens Health*, 12, 717, 2003.
83. Godfrey, J.R., Toward optimal health: Scott Grundy, MD, PhD discusses metabolic syndrome. *J. Womens Health*, 14, 883, 2005.
84. McManus, K., Antinoro, L., and Sacks, F., A randomized controlled trial of a moderate-fat, low-energy diet compared with a low-fat, low-energy diet for weight loss in overweight adults. *Int. J. Obes.*, 25, 1503, 2001.
85. Azadbakht, L., et al., Beneficial effects of a dietary approaches to stop hypertension eating plan on features of the metabolic syndrome. *Diabetes Care*, 28, 2823, 2005.
86. Stoeckli, R. and Keller, U., Nutritional fats and the risk of type 2 diabetes and cancer. *Physiol. Behav.*, 83, 611, 2004.
87. Riccardi, G. and Rivellese, A.A., Dietary treatment of the metabolic syndrome—the optimal diet. *Brit. J. Nutr.*, 83 (suppl 1), S143, 2000.
88. Norris, S.L., et al., Long-term non-pharmacological weight loss interventions for adults with prediabetes. *Cochrane Database Syst. Rev.*, 2, CD005270, 2005.
89. Knowler, W.C., et al., Reduction in the incidence of type 2 diabetes with lifestyle intervention or metformin. *N. Engl. J. Med.*, 346, 393, 2002.
90. Pan, X.-R., et al., Effects of diet and exercise in preventing NIDDM in people with impaired glucose tolerance: the Da Qing IGT and Diabetes Study. *Diabetes Care*, 20, 537, 1997.
91. Tuomilehto, J., et al., Prevention of type 2 diabetes mellitus by changes in lifestyle among subjects with impaired glucose tolerance. *N. Engl. J. Med.* 344, 1343, 2001.
92. Mann, J.I., Can dietary intervention produce long-term reduction in insulin resistance? *Brit. J. Nutr.*, 83 (suppl 1), S169, 2000.
93. Dansinger, M.L., et al., Comparison of the Atkins, Ornish, Weight Watchers, and Zone diets for weight loss and heart disease risk reduction. *J. Am. Med. Assoc.*, 293, 43, 2005.
94. Reaven, G.M., The insulin resistance syndrome: definition and dietary approaches to treatment. *Annu. Rev. Nutr.*, 25, 391, 2005.
95. Cornier, M.A., et al., Insulin sensitivity determines the effectiveness of dietary macronutrient composition on weight loss in obese women. *Obesity Res.*, 13, 703, 2005.

96. McLaughlin, T., et al., Differences in insulin resistance do not predict weight loss in response to hypocaloric diets in healthy obese women. *J. Clin. Endocrinol. Metab.*, 84, 578, 1999.
97. Volek, J.S. and Feinman, R.D., Carbohydrate restriction improves the features of metabolic syndrome. Metabolic syndrome may be defined by the response to carbohydrate restriction. *Nutr. Metab.*, 2, 31, 2005.
98. Boden, G., et al., Effect of a low-carbohydrate diet on appetite, blood glucose levels, and insulin resistance in obese patients with type 2 diabetes. *Ann. Intern. Med.*, 142, 403, 2005.
99. Miller, B.V., et al., An evaluation of the Atkins' diet. *Metabolic Syndrome and Related Disorders*, 1, 299, 2003.
100. Volek, J.S., et al., An isoenergetic very low carbohydrate diet improves serum HDL cholestrol and triacylglycerol concentrations, the total cholestrol to HDL cholesterol ratio and postprandial lipemic responses compared with a low fat diet in normal weight, normolipidemic women. *J. Nutr.*, 133, 2756, 2003.
101. Sharman, M.J., et al., A ketogenic diet favorably affects serum biomarkers for cardiovascular disease in normal-weight men. *J. Nutr.*, 132, 1879, 2002.
102. Kelly, S., et al., Low glycaemic index diets for coronary heart disease. *Cochrane Database Syst. Rev.*, 4, CD004467, 2004.
103. Frost, G., et al., The effect of low-glycemic carbohydrate on insulin and glucose response in vivo and in vitro in patients with coronary heart disease. *Metabolism*, 45, 669, 1996.
104. Frost, G., et al., Insulin sensitivity in women at risk of coronary heart disease and the effect of a low glycemic diet. *Metabolism*, 47, 1245, 1998.
105. Wolever, T.M.S. and Mehling, C., High-carbohydrate-low-glycaemic index dietary advice improves glucose disposition index in subjects with impaired glucose tolerance. *Brit. J. Nutr.*, 87, 477, 2002.
106. Laaksonen, D.E., et al., Dietary carbohydrate modification enhances insulin secretion in persons with the metabolic syndrome. *Am. J. Clin. Nutr.*, 82, 1218, 2005.
107. Juntunen, K.S., et al., High-fiber rye bread and insulin secretion and sensitivity in healthy postmenopausal women. *Am. J. Clin. Nutr.*, 77, 385, 2003.
108. Pereira, M.A., et al., Effect of whole grains on insulin sensitivity in overweight hyperinsulinemic adults. *Am. J. Clin. Nutr.*, 75, 848, 2002.
109. Delzenne, N.M. and Cani, P.D., A place for dietary fibre in the management of the metabolic syndrome. *Curr. Opin. Clin. Nutr. Metab. Care.*, 8, 636, 2005.
110. Wolever, T.M.S., Role of dietary fibre in obesity and the metabolic syndrome. *Metab. Synd. Rounds.*, 3, 1, 2005.
111. Liu, S., et al., Relation between changes in intakes of dietary fiber and grain products and changes in weight and development of obesity among middle-aged women. *Am. J. Clin. Nutr.*, 78, 920, 2003.
112. Kreymann, B., et al., Glucagon-like peptide-1 (7–36): a physiological incretin in man. *Lancet*, 2, 1300, 1987.
113. Flint, A., et al., Glucagon-like peptide 1 promotes satiety and suppresses energy intake in humans. *J. Clin. Invest.*, 101, 515, 1998.
114. Adam, T.C. and Westerterp-Plantenga, M.S., Nutrient-stimulated GLP-1 release in normal-weight men and women. *Horm. Metab. Res.*, 37, 111, 2005.
115. Ranganath, L.R., et al., Attenuated GLP-1 secretion in obesity: cause or consequence? *Gut*, 38, 916, 1996.
116. Weickert, M.O., et al., Cereal fiber improves whole-body insulin sensitivity in overweight and obese women. *Diabetes Care*, 29, 775, 2006.

117. Weickert, M.O., et al., Impact of cereal fibre on glucose-regulating factors. *Diabetologia*, 48, 2343, 2005.
118. Meier, J.J., et al., Reduced insulinotropic effect of gastric inhibitory polypeptide in first-degree relatives of patients with type 2 diabetes. *Diabetes*, 50, 2497, 2001.
119. Behall, K.M., et al., Consumption of both resistant starch and β-glucan improves postprandial plasma glucose and insulin in women. *Diabetes Care*, 29, 976, 2006.
120. Östman, E.M., et al., A dietary exchange of common bread for tailored bread of low glycaemic index and rich in dietary fibre improved insulin economy in young women with impaired glucose tolerance. *Eur. J. Clin. Nutr.*, 60, 334, 2006.
121. Vessby, B., et al., Substituting dietary saturated for monounsaturated fat impairs insulin sensitivity in healthy men and women: the KANWU study. *Diabetologia*, 44, 312, 2001.
122. Louheranta, A.M., et al., Association of the fatty acid profile of serum lipids with glucose and insulin metabolism during 2 fat-modified diets in subjects with impaired glucose tolerance. *Am. J. Clin. Nutr.*, 76, 331, 2002.
123. Cheng, S.-Y., et al., The hypoglycemic effects of soy isoflavones on postmenopausal women. *J. Womens Health*, 13, 1080, 2004.
124. Messina, M., Hypoglycemic effects of isoflavones unproven. *J. Womens Health*, 14, 468, 2005.
125. Jayagopal, V., et al., Beneficial effects of soy phytoestrogen intake in postmenopausal women with type 2 diabetes. *Diabetes Care*, 25, 1709, 2002.
126. Hu, F.B., et al., Diet, lifestyle, and the risk of type 2 diabetes mellitus in women. *N. Engl. J. Med.*, 345, 790, 2001.
127. Fung, T.T., et al., Dietary patterns, meat intake, and the risk of type 2 diabetes in women. *Arch. Intern. Med.*, 164, 2235, 2004.
128. Van Dam, R.M., et al., Dietary patterns and risk for type 2 diabetes mellitus in U.S. men. *Ann. Intern. Med.*, 136, 201, 2002.
129. Song, Y., et al., A prospective study of red meat consumption and type 2 diabetes in middle-aged and elderly women: the women's Health Study. *Diabetes Care*, 27, 2108, 2004.
130. Montonen, J., et al., Dietary patterns and the incidence of type 2 diabetes. *Am. J. Epidemiol.*, 161, 219, 2005.
131. Liu, S., et al., A prospective study of fruit and vegetable intake and the risk of type 2 diabetes in women. *Diabetes Care*, 27, 2993, 2004.
132. Salmerón, J., et al., Dietary fiber, glycemic load, and risk of NIDDM in men. *Diabetes Care*, 20, 545, 1997.
133. Parillo, M. and Riccardi, G., Diet composition and the risk of type 2 diabetes: epidemiological and clinical evidence. *Brit. J. Nutr.*, 92, 7, 2004.
134. Colditz, G.A., et al., Diet and risk of clinical diabetes in women. *Am. J. Clin. Nutr.*, 55, 1018, 1992.
135. Meyer, K.A., et al., Carbohydrates, dietary fiber, and incident Type II diabetes in older women. *Am. J. Clin. Nutr.*, 71, 921, 2000.
136. Janket, S.-J., et al., A prospective study of sugar intake and risk of type 2 diabetes in women. *Diabetes Care*, 26, 1008, 2003.
137. Schulze, M.B., et al., Sugar-sweetened beverages, weight gain, and incidence of type 2 diabetes in young and middle-aged women. *J. Am. Med. Assoc.*, 292, 927, 2004.
138. Liu, S., et al., A prospective study of whole-grain intake and risk of type 2 diabetes mellitus in U.S. women. *Am. J. Public Health*, 90, 1409, 2000.
139. Montonen, J., et al., Whole-grain and fiber intake and the incidence of type 2 diabetes. *Am. J. Clin. Nutr.*, 77, 622, 2003.

140. McKeown, N.M., et al., Whole-grain intake is favorably associated with metabolic risk factors for type 2 diabetes and cardiovascular disease in the Framingham Offspring Study. *Am. J. Clin. Nutr.*, 76, 390, 2002.
141. Jenkins, D.J.A., et al., Viscous and nonviscous fibres, nonabsorbable and low glycaemic index carbohydrates, blood lipids and coronary heart disease. *Curr. Opin. Lipid.*, 11, 49, 2000.
142. Schulze, M.B., et al., Glycemic index, glycemic load, and dietary fiber intake and incidence of type 2 diabetes in younger and middle-aged women. *Am. J. Clin. Nutr.*, 80, 348, 2004.
143. Wu, T., et al., Fructose, glycemic load, and quantity and quality of carbohydrate in relation to plasma C-peptide concentrations in US women. *Am. J. Clin. Nutr.*, 80, 1043, 2004.
144. Schulz, M., et al., Is the association between dietary glycemic index and type 2 diabetes modified by waist circumference? *Diabetes Care*, 29, 1102, 2006.
145. Willett, W.C., Manson, J.E., and Liu, S., Glycemic index, glycemic load, and risk of type 2 diabetes. *Am. J. Clin. Nutr.*, 76, S274, 2002.
146. Venn, B.J. and Mann, J.I., Cereal grains, legumes and diabetes. *Eur. J. Clin. Nutr.*, 58, 1443, 2004.
147. Jenkins, D.J.A., et al., Wholemeal versus wholegrain breads: proportion of whole or cracked grain and the glycaemic response. *Brit. Med. J.*, 297, 958, 1988.
148. Fung, T.T., et al., Whole-grain intake and the risk of Type 2 diabetes: a prospective study in men. *Am. J. Clin. Nutr.*, 76, 535, 2002.
149. Lopez-Ridaura, R., et al., Magnesium intake and risk of type 2 diabetes in men and women. *Diabetes Care*, 27, 134, 2004.
150. Song, Y., et al., Dietary magnesium intake in relation to plasma insulin levels and risk of type 2 diabetes in women. *Diabetes Care*, 27, 59, 2004.
151. Jiang, R., et al., Nut and peanut butter consumption and risk of type 2 diabetes in women. *J. Am. Med. Assoc.*, 288, 2554, 2002.
152. Salmerón, J., et al., Dietary fat intake and risk of type 2 diabetes in women. *Am. J. Clin. Nutr.*, 73, 1019, 2001.
153. Meyer, K.A., et al., Dietary fat and incidence of type 2 diabetes in older Iowa women. *Diabetes Care*, 24, 1528, 2001.
154. Harding, A.-H., et al., Dietary fat and the risk of clinical type 2 diabetes: the European prospective Investigation of Cancer-Norfolk Study. *Am. J. Epidemiol.*, 159, 73, 2004.
155. Marshall, J.A., et al., Dietary fat predicts conversion from impaired glucose tolerance to NIDDM. The San Luis Valley Diabetes Study. *Diabetes Care*, 17, 50, 1994.
156. Hu, F.B., Van Dam, R.M., and Liu, S., Diet and risk of type 2 diabetes: the role of types of fat and carbohydrate. *Diabetologia*, 44, 805, 2001.
157. Van Dam, R.M., et al., Dietary fat and meat intake in relation to risk of type 2 diabetes in men. *Diabetes Care*, 25, 417, 2002.
158. Liu, S., et al., A prospective study of dairy intake and the risk of type 2 diabetes in women. *Diabetes Care*, 29, 1579, 2006.
159. Choi, H.K., et al., Dairy consumption and risk of type 2 diabetes mellitus in men. *Arch. Intern. Med.*, 165, 997, 2005.
160. Pittas, A.G., et al., Vitamin D and calcium intake in relation to type 2 diabetes in women. *Diabetes Care*, 29, 650, 2006.
161. Montonen, J., et al., Dietary antioxidant intake and risk of type 2 diabetes. *Diabetes Care*, 27, 362, 2004.
162. Goodman-Gruen, D. and Kritz-Silverstein, D., Usual dietary isoflavone intake is associated with cardiovascular disease risk factors in postmenopausal women. *J. Nutr.*, 131, 1202, 2001.

163. Duncan, A.M., et al., Modest hormonal effects of soy isoflavones in postmenopausal women. *J. Clin. Endocrinol. Metab.*, 84, 3479, 1999.
164. Pino, A.M., et al., Dietary isoflavones affect sex hormone-binding globulin levels in postmenopausal women. *J. Clin. Endocrinol. Metab.*, 85, 2797, 2000.
165. Bhathena, S.J. and Velasquez, M.T., Beneficial role of dietary phytoestrogens in obesity and diabetes. *Am. J. Clin. Nutr.*, 76, 1191, 2002.
166. Rosengren, A., et al., Coffee and incidence of diabetes in Swedish women: a prospective 18-year follow-up study. *J. Intern. Med.*, 255, 89, 2004.
167. Van Dam, R.M., et al., Coffee, caffeine, and risk of type 2 diabetes. *Diabetes Care*, 29, 398, 2006.
168. Salazar-Martinez, E., et al., Coffee consumption and risk for type 2 diabetes mellitus. *Ann. Intern. Med.*, 140, 1, 2004.
169. Van Dam, R.M. and Feskens, E.J.M., Coffee consumption and risk of type 2 diabetes mellitus. *Lancet*, 360, 1477, 2002.
170. Tuomilehto, J., et al., Coffee consumption and risk of type 2 diabetes mellitus among middle-aged Finnish men and women. *J. Am. Med. Assoc.*, 291, 1213, 2004.
171. Ferrini, R.L. and Barrett-Connor, E., Caffeine intake and endogenous sex steroid levels in postmenopausal women: the Rancho Bernardo Study. *Am. J. Epidemiol.*, 144, 642, 1996.
172. Nagata, C., Kabuto, M., and Shimizu, H., Association of coffee, green tea, and caffeine intakes with serum concentrations of estradiol and sex hormone-binding globulin in premenopausal Japanese women. *Nutr. Cancer.*, 30, 21, 1998.
173. Lee, D.-H., Folsom, A.R., and Jacobs, D.R. Jr., Dietary iron intake and type 2 diabetes incidence in postmenopausal women: the Iowa Women's Health Study. *Diabetologia*, 47, 185, 2004.
174. Rajpathak, S., et al., Iron intake and the risk of type 2 diabetes in women. *Diabetes Care*, 29, 1370, 2006.
175. Kao, W.H.L., et al., Alcohol consumption and the risk of type 2 diabetes mellitus: Atherosclerosis Risk in Communities Study. *Am. J. Epidemiol.*, 154, 748, 2001.
176. DeVegt, F., et al., Moderate alcohol consumption is associated with lower risk for incident diabetes and mortality: the Hoorn Study. *Diabetes Res. Clin. Pract.*, 57, 53, 2002.
177. Meisinger, C., et al., Sex differences in risk factors for incident type 2 diabetes mellitus: the MONICA Augsburg cohort study. *Arch. Intern. Med.*, 162, 82, 2002.
178. Carlsson, S., et al., Alcohol consumption and the incidence of type 2 diabetes: a 20-year follow-up of the Finnish Twin Cohort Study. *Diabetes Care*, 26, 2785, 2003.
179. Wannamethee, S.G., et al., Alcohol drinking patterns and risk of type 2 diabetes mellitus among younger women. *Arch. Intern. Med.*, 163, 1329, 2003.
180. Koppes, L.L.J., Moderate alcohol consumption lowers the risk of type 2 diabetes: a meta-analysis of prospective observational studies. *Diabetes Care*, 28, 719, 2005.
181. Beulens, J.W.J., et al., Alcohol consumption and risk of type 2 diabetes among older women. *Diabetes Care*, 28, 2933, 2005.
182. Lapidus, L., et al., Alcohol intake among women and its relationship to diabetes incidence and all-cause mortality. *Diabetes Care*, 28, 2230, 2005.
183. Pradhan, A.D., et al., C-reactive protein, interleukin 6, and risk of developing type 2 diabetes mellitus. *J. Am. Med. Assoc.*, 286, 327, 2001.
184. Libby, P., Ridker, P.M., and Maseri, A., Inflammation and atherosclerosis. *Circulation*, 105, 1135, 2002.
185. Natarajan, R. and Nadler, J.L., Lipid inflammatory mediators in diabetic vascular disease. *Arterioscler. Thromb. Vasc. Biol.*, 24, 1542, 2004.

186. Schulze, M.B., et al., Dietary pattern, inflammation, and incidence of type 2 diabetes in women. *Am. J. Clin. Nutr.*, 82, 675, 2005.
187. Berg, A.H., et al., The adipocyte-secreted protein Acrp30 enhances hepatic insulin action. *Nat. Med.*, 7, 947, 2001.
188. Fruebis, J., et al., Proteolytic cleavage product of 30-kDa adipocyte complement-related protein increases fatty acid oxidation in muscle and causes weight loss in mice. *Proc. Natl. Acad. Sci. USA.*, 98, 2005, 2001.
189. Goldstein, B.J. and Scalia, R., Adiponectin: a novel adipokine linking adipocytes and vascular function. *J. Clin. Endocrinol. Metab.*, 89, 2563, 2004.
190. Arita, Y., et al., Paradoxical decrease of an adipose-specific protein, adiponectin, in obesity. *Biochem. Biophys. Res. Commun.*, 257, 79, 1999.
191. Mantzoros, C.S., et al., Circulating adiponectin levels are associated with better glycemic control, more favorable lipid profile, and reduced inflammation in women with type 2 diabetes. *J. Clin. Endocrinol. Metab.*, 90, 4542, 2005.
192. Hotta, K., et al., Plasma concentrations of a novel, adipose-specific protein, adiponectin, in type 2 diabetic patients. *Arterioscler. Thromb. Vasc. Biol.*, 20, 1595, 2000.
193. Qi, L., et al., Whole-grain, bran, and cereal fiber intakes and markers of systemic inflammation in diabetic women. *Diabetes Care*, 29, 207, 2006.
194. Qi, L., et al., Dietary glycemic index, glycemic load, cereal fiber, and plasma adiponectin concentration in diabetic men. *Diabetes Care*, 28, 1022, 2005.
195. Moore, H., et al., Dietary advice for treatment of type 2 diabetes mellitus in adults. *Cochrane Database Syst. Rev.*, 2, CD004097, 2004.
196. Norris, S.L., et al., Long-term non-pharmacological weight loss interventions for adults with type 2 diabetes mellitus. *Cochrane Database Syst. Rev.*, 2, CD004095, 2005.
197. Pi-Sunyer, F.X., Weight loss and mortality in type 2 diabetes. *Diabetes Care*, 23, 1451, 2000.
198. Williamson, D.F., et al., Intentional weight loss and mortality among overweight individuals with diabetes. *Diabetes Care*, 23, 1499, 2000.
199. Wing, R.R., et al., Effects of a very-low-calorie diet on long-term glycemic control in obese type 2 diabetic subjects. *Arch. Intern. Med.*, 151, 1334, 1991.
200. Wing, R.R., et al., Year-long weight loss treatment for obese patients with type II diabetes: does including an intermittent very-low-calorie diet improve outcome? *Am. J. Med.*, 97, 354, 1994.
201. Hockaday, T.D.R., et al., Prospective comparison of modified-fat-high-carbohydrate with standard low-carbohydrate dietary advice in the treatment of diabetes: one year follow-up study. *Brit. J. Nutr.*, 39, 357, 1978.
202. Korhonen, T., et al., Efficacy of dietary instructions in newly diagnosed non-insulin-dependent diabetic patients. *Acta. Med. Scand.*, 222, 323, 1987.
203. Wing, R.R., et al., Behavior change, weight loss, and physiological improvements in type II diabetic patients. *J. Consult. Clin. Psych.*, 53, 111, 1985.
204. Wing, R.R., et al., A "family-based" approach to the treatment of obese type II diabetic patients. *J. Consult. Clin. Psych.*, 59, 156, 1991.
205. Agurs-Collins, T.D., et al., A randomized controlled trial of weight reduction and exercise for diabetes management in older African-American subjects. *Diabetes Care*, 20, 1503, 1997.
206. DeBont, A.J., et al., A randomized controlled trial of the effect of low fat diet advice on dietary response in insulin independent diabetic women. *Diabetologia*, 21, 529, 1981.
207. Milne, R.M., et al., Long-term comparison of three dietary prescriptions in the treatment of NIDDM. *Diabetes Care*, 17, 74, 1994.

208. Pascale, R.W., et al., Effects of a behavioral weight loss program stressing calorie restriction versus calorie plus fat restriction in obese individuals with NIDDM or a family history of diabetes. *Diabetes Care*, 18, 1241, 1995.
209. Tsihlias, E.B., et al., Comparison of high- and low-glycemic-index breakfast cereals with monounsaturated fat in the long-term dietary management of type 2 diabetes. *Am. J. Clin. Nutr.*, 72, 439, 2000.
210. Tappy, L., Gugolz, E., and Wursch, P., Effects of breakfast cereals containing various amounts of β-glucan fibers on plasma glucose and insulin responses in NIDDM subjects. *Diabetes Care*, 19, 831, 1996.
211. Feldman, N., et al., Enrichment of an Israeli ethnic food with fibres and their effects on the glycaemic and insulinaemic responses in subjects with non-insulin-dependent diabetes mellitus. *Brit. J. Nutr.*, 74, 681, 1995.
212. Pastors, J.G., et al., Psyllium fiber reduces rise in postprandial glucose and insulin concentrations in patients with non-insulin-dependent diabetes. *Am. J. Clin. Nutr.*, 53, 1431, 1991.
213. Lu, Z., et al., Arabinoxylan fibre improves metabolic control in people with type 2 diabetes. *Eur. J. Clin. Nutr.*, 58, 621, 2004.
214. Tapola, N., et al., Glycemic responses of oat bran products in type 2 diabetic patients. *Nutr. Metab. Cardiovasc. Dis.*, 15, 255, 2005.
215. Chandalia, M., et al., Beneficial effects of high dietary fiber intake in patients with T2DM. *N. Engl. J. Med.*, 342, 1392, 2000.
216. Rodríguez-Morán, M., Guerrero-Romero, F., and Lazcano-Burciaga, G., Lipid- and glucose-lowering efficacy of *Plantago psyllium* in type 2 diabetes. *J. Diabet. Complications*, 12, 273, 1998.
217. Jenkins, D.J.A., et al., Effect of wheat bran on glycemic control and risk factors for cardiovascular disease in type 2 diabetes. *Diabetes Care*, 25, 1522, 2002.
218. Jenkins, D.J.A., et al., Low-glycemic-index starchy foods in the diabetic diet. *Am. J. Clin. Nutr.*, 48, 248, 1988.
219. Brand, J.C., et al., Low-glycemic index foods improve long-term glycemic control in NIDDM. *Diabetes Care*, 14, 95, 1991.
220. Wolever, T.M.S., et al., Beneficial effect of low-glycemic index diet in overweight NIDDM subjects. *Diabetes Care*, 15, 562, 1992.
221. Jimenez-Cruz, A., et al., A flexible, low-glycemic index Mexican-style diet in overweight and obese subjects with type 2 diabetes improves metabolic parameters during a 6-week treatment period. *Diabetes Care*, 26, 1967, 2003.
222. Jenkins, D.J.A., et al., Metabolic effects of a low-glycemic-index diet. *Am. J. Clin. Nutr.*, 46, 968, 1987.
223. Wolever, T.M.S., The glycemic index: flogging a dead horse? *Diabetes Care*, 20, 452, 1997.
224. Summers, L.K.M., et al., Substituting dietary saturated fat with polyunsaturated fat changes abdominal fat distribution and improves insulin sensitivity. *Diabetologia*, 45, 369, 2002.
225. Heine, R.J., et al., Linoleic-acid-enriched diet: long-term effects on serum lipoprotein and apolipoprotein concentrations and insulin sensitivity in noninsulin-dependent diabetic patients. *Am. J. Clin. Nutr.*, 49, 448, 1989.
226. Woodman, R.J., et al., Effects of purified eicosapentaenoic and docosahexaenoic acids on glycemic control, blood pressure, and serum lipids in type 2 diabetic patients with treated hypertension. *Am. J. Clin. Nutr.*, 76, 1007, 2002.
227. Madigan, C., et al., Dietary unsaturated fatty acids in type 2 diabetes: higher levels of postprandial lipoprotein on a linoleic acid-rich sunflower oil diet compared with an oleic acid-rich olive oil diet. *Diabetes Care*, 23, 1472, 2000.

228. Christiansen, E., et al., Intake of a diet high in trans monounsaturated fatty acids or saturated fatty acids. *Diabetes Care*, 20, 881, 1997.
229. Moloney, F., et al., Conjugated linoleic acid supplementation, insulin sensitivity, and lipoprotein metabolism in patients with type 2 diabetes mellitus. *Am. J. Clin. Nutr.*, 80, 887, 2004.
230. Louheranta, A.M., et al., A high-trans fatty acid diet and insulin sensitivity in young healthy women. *Metabolism*, 48, 870, 1999.
231. Lovejoy, J.C., et al., Effect of diets enriched in almonds on insulin action and serum lipids in adults with normal glucose tolerance or type 2 diabetes. *Am. J. Clin. Nutr.* 76, 1000, 2002.
232. Tapsell, L.C., et al., Including walnuts in a low-fat/modified-fat diet improves HDL cholesterol-to-total cholesterol ratios in patients with type 2 diabetes. *Diabetes Care*, 27, 2777, 2004.
233. King, J.C., The milk debate. *Arch. Intern. Med.*, 165, 975, 2005.
234. Frid, A.H., et al., Effect of whey on blood glucose and insulin responses to composite breakfast and lunch meals in type 2 diabetic subjects. *Am. J. Clin. Nutr.*, 82, 69, 2005.
235. Davies, M.J., et al., Effects of moderate alcohol intake on fasting insulin and glucose concentrations and insulin sensitivity in postmenopausal women. *J. Am. Med. Assoc.*, 287, 2559, 2002.
236. Giannopoulou, I., et al., Effects of diet and/or exercise on the adipocytokine and inflammatory cytokine levels of postmenopausal women with type 2 diabetes. *Metabolism*, 54, 866, 2005.
237. Keitt, S.K., et al., Understanding the biology of sex and gender differences: using subgroup analysis and statistical design to detect sex differences in clinical trials. *MedGenMed.*, 5, 39, 2003. (ejournal at www.medscape.com).
238. Vidaver, R.M., et al., Women subjects in NIH-funded clinical research literature: lack of progress in both representation and analysis by sex. *J. Womens Health Gend. Based Med.*, 9, 495, 2000.
239. Bell-Anderson, K. and Samman, S., Nutrition and metabolism: race, sex and the metabolic syndrome. *Curr. Opin. Lipid.*, 17, 82, 2006.

9 Cardiovascular Disease

Alice H. Lichtenstein and Nirupa R. Matthan

CONTENTS

9.1 INTRODUCTION

Since the turn of the century, interest in cardiovascular diseases (CVDs), among women in particular, has increased dramatically in the United States. In 2002, the American Heart Association (AHA) and the National Heart, Lung, and Blood Institute (NHLBI) of the National Institutes of Health (NIH) both began campaigns to draw much needed attention to CVD risk factors in women. The AHA titled its campaign "Go Red for Women," issuing a "national call for women to take charge of their heart health and live stronger, longer lives;" and the NHLBI titled its campaign "The Heart Truth: A National Awareness Campaign on Women and

Heart Disease." Both programs stress nonpharmacological interventions as a means to reduce women's CVD risk, primarily emphasizing dietary modification, physical activity, and smoking cessation. Concomitant with these efforts has been evidence-based guideline development, specifically for CVD prevention and treatment in women [1]. These guidelines are particularly important in light of the recent findings indicating that hormone replacement therapy does not appear to be effective at preventing CVD in women [2,3].

There are a number of common myths associated with CVD as it relates to women. The first is that heart disease is predominantly a man's disease, and that chest pain in women is likely attributable to causes other than heart disease [4]. In truth, more women than men die of heart disease. Research has shown that although the majority of women have heard heart disease is the leading cause of death among women, they do not internalize this information, as evidenced by their failure to adopt heart-healthy lifestyles [5,6]. Fortunately, this may be changing. In 1997, only 30% of women identified CVD as the lead cause of female mortality, compared with 46% of women in 2003 [7].

The second myth is that most women consider the risk of cancer greater than the risk of heart disease [7]; however, heart disease claims nearly twice as many women's lives as does cancer. This misconception may be the result of women's greater exposure to and reliance on the mass media rather than on their health care providers for information on heart disease [5].

The third myth is that doctors are aware of the level of heart disease risk in women and treat women accordingly. In reality, undertreatment and underdiagnosis of heart disease in women likely contributes to the poorer prognosis in women than in men. Public health efforts, such as the aforementioned instituted by the NIH and AHA, are changing this situation.

9.2 BASICS ABOUT CVD

CVD is the leading cause of death and disability in developed countries [8], and more recently in many developing countries [9]. The disorder is characterized by thickening of the artery wall, referred to as atherosclerosis. Etymologically, this term comes from a combination of the Greek words *athere*, gruel and *skleros*, hardening, and it describes a subgroup of arteriosclerotic disorders distinguished by the presence of fatty plaque (atheromas) within the intima and media of medium and large arteries (Figure 9.1).

Evidence suggests that multiple factors independently contribute to progression of lesions [10], including both fatty streaks and atherosclerotic plaques (Figure 9.2). Atherosclerotic plaques are raised lesions that can impede blood flow and potentially rupture, thereby setting off a cascade of adverse events. They are characterized by the accumulation of cholesteryl ester in the arterial wall. The cholesteryl ester is derived from monocytes that penetrate the endothelial layer, convert to macrophages and take up lipid via scavenger receptors, and secrete factors that result in the recruitment of smooth-muscle cells from the medial layer of the vessel wall. These smooth-muscle cells take up low density lipoprotein (LDL) particles that have traversed the endothelial layer via an LDL-specific receptor-mediated pathway.

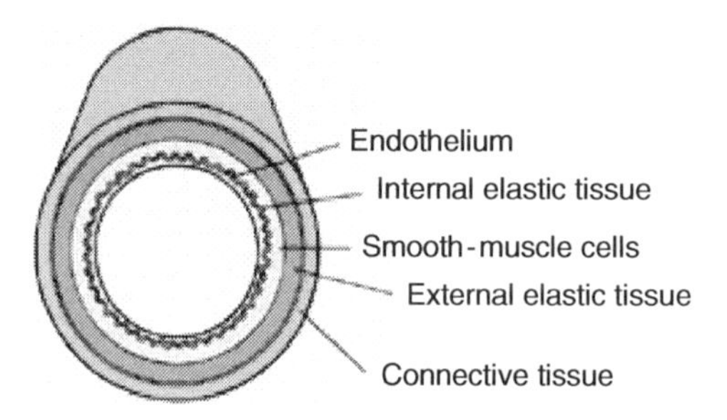

FIGURE 9.1 Cross-section of an Artery. (From Beers, M.H. ed., *Atherosclerosis*, The Merck Manual of Medical Information, 2nd Home ed., Merck & Co., Inc., Whitehouse Station, NJ, p. 196, 2003. http://www.merck.com/mmhe/sec03/ch032/ch032a.html. With permission.)

As the cells accumulate cholesteryl ester they are referred to as foam cells because of their pearly white, vacuolated appearance. Atherosclerotic plaque can be further classified by the fibrous cap that forms over the cholesteryl ester core. Lesions with relatively thick fibrous caps are more stable than those with thin caps. Lesions with thin caps tend to have an unstable surface prone to rupturing, setting off a cascade of events frequently leading to a cardiovascular event.

In contrast, fatty streaks are flat or slightly raised accumulations of lipid-rich macrophages and smooth-muscle cells, ubiquitous in humans, and appearing early-on in life [11–13]. They rarely impede blood flow, and their presence largely goes unnoticed. Although evidence suggests that some fatty streaks can progress to fibrous plaque, their distribution in the vessel walls is not similar to atherosclerotic plaque, suggesting this is not always the case.

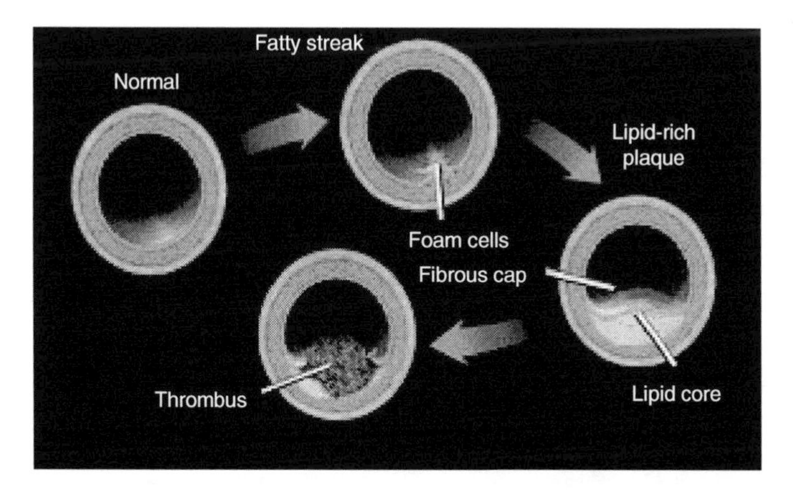

FIGURE 9.2 Development of atherosclerotic plaques. (From *Diabetes Roundtable* in *PUFA Newsletter*, http://www.fatsoflife.com/pufa/article.asp?nid=1&edition=this&id=394. With permission.)

A number of factors accelerate atherogenesis, the formation and progression of atherosclerotic plaque. These factors include elevated LDL cholesterol levels, low high density lipoprotein (HDL) cholesterol levels, use of tobacco products, hypertension, diabetes mellitus, family history of CVD, and advancing age. Each contributes to endothelial cell activation, recruitment of monocytes in the intima, and infiltration of the epithelial and smooth-muscle cells [10]. These events not only lead to cholesterol accumulation in the vessel wall, but also activate protein growth factors that stimulate smooth-muscle cell proliferation. This can have adverse consequences because smooth-muscle cells have LDL receptors, paving the pathway for cholesteryl ester deposition in the arterial wall.

In addition, response to mechanical injury, such as chronic hypercholesterolemia, exposure to toxins or viruses, or immunological activity can lead to monocyte aggregation and adherence at the site of injury, resulting in impeded blood flow. Infiltration of monocytes into the vessel wall can produce reactive oxygen species such as superoxide anion, hydrogen peroxide, and peroxynitrite. These compounds increase oxidative stress and activate proinflammatory and proatherogenic genes, including those that encode for adhesion molecules and chemokines [10]. These events can further promote the recruitment of monocytes. The increased oxidative stress favors differentiation of monocytes into macrophages in the arterial wall and uptake of oxidized LDL by scavenger receptors in a nonsaturable fashion; the result is foam cell formation.

9.3 ISSUES UNIQUE TO WOMEN

9.3.1 Symptoms and Physiological Differences in CVD Manifestation

CVD mortality in men has consistently declined since 1984 whereas rates in women, for the most part, have remained steady or increased (Figure 9.3) [8,14,15]. One reason may be that heart attack warning signs and symptoms are sex-specific,

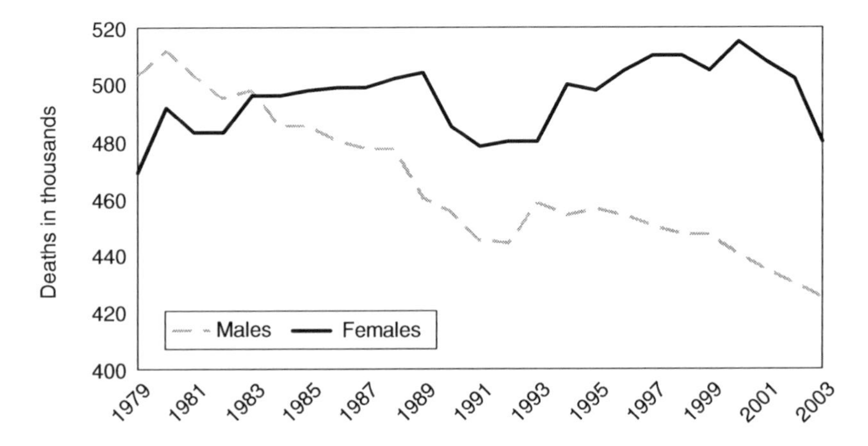

FIGURE 9.3 CVD mortality trends (1979–2003). (From Women and Cardiovascular Diseases—Statistics, American Heart Association, 2007. With permission.)

TABLE 9.1
Gender Differences in Chest Pain and Nonchest Pain Symptoms

Symptoms	Women (%)	Men (%)
No chest pain	30	29
Chest symptoms		
Pain in center or left chest	57	70
Chest heaviness, pressure, or tightness or squeezing	43	30
Nonchest pain symptoms		
Midback pain	13	2
Nausea or vomiting	30	16
Dyspnea	50	35
Palpitations	10	3
Indigestion	22	12
Fatigue	18	9
Arm or shoulder pain	38	27
Sweating	30	23
Jaw pain	4	7
Dizziness or fainting	21	18
Neck or throat pain	10	8

Source: From Milner, K.A., Funk, M., Richards, S., Wilmes, R.M., Vaccarino, V., and Krumholz, H.M., *Am. J. Cardiol.*, 84, 396, 1999.

and that symptoms in women are more likely to be underrecognized. Rather than the classic distinct pain, tightening or squeezing in the chest upon exertion, women more commonly report shortness of breath or unusual fatigue when engaging in normal activities of daily life, diffuse chest pain, nausea or vomiting, dizziness, or mild indigestion (Table 9.1) [16]. In one female cohort, 43% reported not experiencing any chest discomfort prior to their heart attack, and 95% reported relatively vague symptoms, such as fatigue and sleeplessness up to a month before their event occurred [17]. Additionally, direct measures of vessel narrowing (stenosis) and atherosclerotic plaque area demonstrate sex differences in disease manifestation. Over a 5 year period, women have more stenosis but less plaque development than men [18]. Observations such as this suggest sex differences in atherosclerotic lesion development, which may necessitate sex-specific approaches to diagnosis and treatment.

9.3.2 Diagnosis and Treatment

CVD has caused more deaths among women than among men since 1984 [8]. Nevertheless, CVD in women is still underrecognized, both by health care providers [19] and by women themselves [7]. Recent surveys found that fewer than 1 in 5 physicians knew that more women than men died of CVD [19], and less than half of women identified CVD as the leading cause of mortality in women (Figure 9.4) [7].

Even when women are screened for hypercholesterolemia and are aware of their diagnosis, a lower percentage of women receive medication for the disorder and have it under control [20]. This apparent disparity in diagnosis and treatment for heart disease between women and men is likely due to lack of information, differences in symptoms, less aggressive treatment regimens, and paucity of research data on CVD among women. Nevertheless, an AHA consensus statement [21] concluded that,

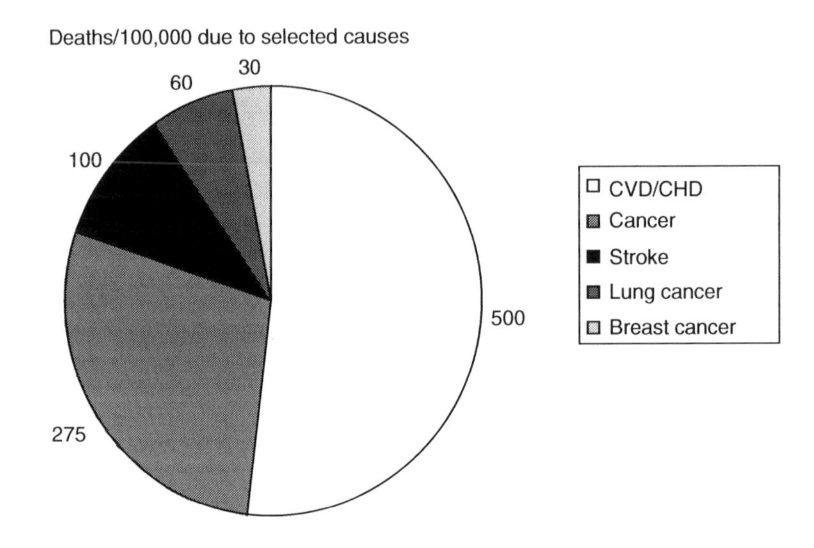

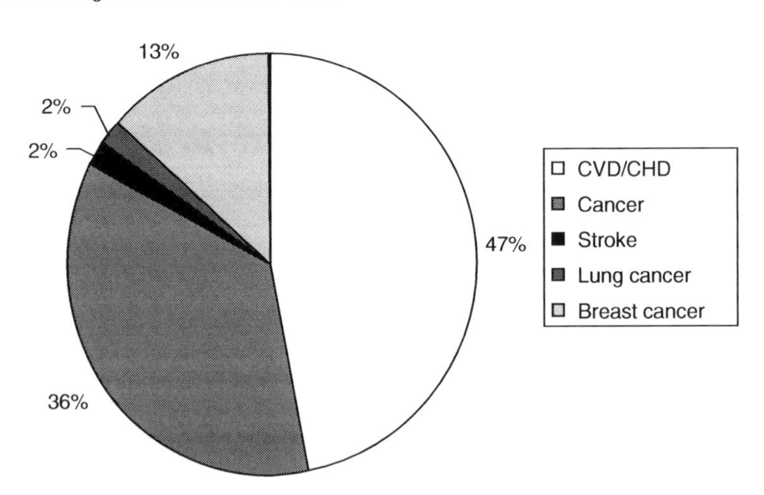

FIGURE 9.4 Actual leading cause of death for women (top) vs. perceived leading causes of death for women (bottom). (From Mosca, L., Jones, W.K., King, K.B., Ouyang, P., Redberg, R.F., and Hill, M.N., *Arch. Fam. Med.*, 9, 506, 2000.)

to-date, noninvasive diagnostic and prognostic testing, as well as preventive and therapeutic interventions, are equally effective at reducing risk of CVD in both women and men. Specific recommendations for prevention and treatment of CVD in women have recently been reviewed and summarized (Table 9.2) [1].

9.3.3 Survival Prognosis

Once CVD is diagnosed in a woman, their prognosis for survival is less favorable than that of men on account of numerous factors, including later age of onset, greater

TABLE 9.2
Evidence-Based Guidelines for CVD Prevention in Women

Lifestyle interventions

Cigarette smoking

Women should not smoke and should avoid environmental tobacco smoke. Provide counseling, nicotine replacement, and other pharmacotherapy as indicated in conjunction with a behavioral program or formal smoking cessation program (Class I, Level B)

Physical activity

Women should accumulate a minimum of 30 min of moderate-intensity physical activity (e.g., brisk walking) on most, and preferably all, days of the week (Class I, Level B)

Women who need to lose weight or sustain weight loss should accumulate a minimum of 60–90 min of moderate-intensity physical activity (e.g., brisk walking) on most, and preferably all, days of the week (Class I, Level C)

Rehabilitation

A comprehensive risk-reduction regimen, such as cardiovascular or stroke rehabilitation or a physician-guided home- or community-based exercise training program, should be recommended to women with a recent acute coronary syndrome or coronary intervention, new-onset or chronic angina, recent cerebrovascular event, peripheral arterial disease (Class I, Level A), or current or prior symptoms of heart failure and an LVEF <40% (Class I, Level B)

Dietary intake

Women should consume a diet rich in fruits and vegetables; choose whole-grain, high-fiber foods; consume fish, especially oily fish,[a] at least twice a week; limit intake of saturated fat to <10% of energy, and if possible to <7%, cholesterol to <300 mg/day, alcohol intake to no more than 1 drink per day,[b] and sodium intake to <2.3 g/day (~1 tsp salt). Consumption of trans-fatty acids should be as low as possible (e.g., <1% of energy) (Class I, Level B)

Weight maintenance or reduction

Women should maintain or lose weight through an appropriate balance of physical activity, caloric intake, and formal behavioral programs when indicated to maintain or achieve a BMI between 18.5 and 24.9 kg/m^2 and a waist circumference ≤35 in. (Class I, Level B)

Omega-3 fatty acids

As an adjunct to diet, omega-3 fatty acids in capsule form (~850–1000 mg of EPA and DHA) may be considered in women with CHD, and higher doses (2–4 g) may be used for treatment of women with high triglyceride levels (Class IIb, Level B)

Depression

Consider screening women with CHD for depression and refer or treat when indicated (Class IIa, Level B)

(*continued*)

TABLE 9.2 (Continued)
Evidence-Based Guidelines for CVD Prevention in Women

Major risk factor interventions
Blood pressure—optimal level and lifestyle
Encourage an optimal blood pressure of <120/80 mm Hg through lifestyle approaches such as weight control, increased physical activity, alcohol moderation, sodium restriction, and increased consumption of fresh fruits, vegetables, and low-fat dairy products (Class I, Level B)
Blood pressure—pharmacotherapy
Pharmacotherapy is indicated when blood pressure is ≥140/90 mm Hg or at an even lower blood pressure in the setting of chronic kidney disease or diabetes (≥130/80 mm Hg). Thiazide diuretics should be part of the drug regimen for most patients unless contraindicated or if there are compelling indications for other agents in specific vascular diseases. Initial treatment of high-risk women[b] should be with β-blockers or ACE inhibitors (or ARBs) or both, with addition of other drugs such as thiazides as needed to achieve goal blood pressure (Class I, Level A)
Lipid and lipoprotein levels—optimal levels and lifestyle
The following levels of lipids and lipoproteins in women should be encouraged through lifestyle approaches: LDL-C <100 mg/dL, HDL-C >50 mg/dL, triglycerides <150 mg/dL, and non–HDL-C (total cholesterol−HDL cholesterol) <130 mg/dL (Class I, Level B). If a woman is at high risk[c] or has hypercholesterolemia, intake of saturated fat should be <7% and cholesterol intake <200 mg/day) (Class I, Level B)
Lipids—pharmacotherapy for LDL lowering, high-risk women
Utilize LDL-C–lowering drug therapy simultaneously with lifestyle therapy in women with CHD to achieve an LDL-C <100 mg/dL (Class I, Level A) and similarly in women with other atherosclerotic CVD or diabetes mellitus or 10-year absolute risk >20% (Class I, Level B)
A reduction to <70 mg/dL is reasonable in very-high-risk women[d] with CHD and may require an LDL-lowering drug combination (Class IIa, Level B)
Lipids—pharmacotherapy for LDL lowering, other at-risk women
Utilize LDL-C–lowering therapy if LDL-C level is ≥130 mg/dL with lifestyle therapy and there are multiple risk factors and 10-year absolute risk 10%–20% (Class I, Level B)
Utilize LDL-C–lowering therapy if LDL-C level is ≥160 mg/dL with lifestyle therapy and multiple risk factors even if 10-year absolute risk is <10% (Class I, Level B)
Utilize LDL-C–lowering therapy if LDL ≥190 mg/dL regardless of the presence or absence of other risk factors or CVD on lifestyle therapy (Class I, Level B)
Lipids—pharmacotherapy for low HDL or elevated non–HDL, high-risk women
Utilize niacin[e] or fibrate therapy when HDL-C is low or non–HDL-C is elevated in high-risk women[e] after LDL-C goal is reached (Class IIa, Level B)
Lipids—pharmacotherapy for low HDL or elevated non–HDL, other at-risk women
Consider niacin[e] or fibrate therapy when HDL-C is low or non–HDL-C is elevated after LDL-C goal is reached in women with multiple risk factors and a 10-year absolute risk 10%–20% (Class IIb, Level B)
Diabetes mellitus
Lifestyle and pharmacotherapy should be used as indicated in women with diabetes (Class I, Level B) to achieve an HbA_{1C} <7% if this can be accomplished without significant hypoglycemia (Class I, Level C)

TABLE 9.2 (Continued)
Evidence-Based Guidelines for CVD Prevention in Women

Preventive drug interventions

Aspirin, high risk

Aspirin therapy (75–325 mg/day)[f] should be used in high-risk[c] women unless contraindicated (Class I, Level A)

If a high-risk[c] woman is intolerant of aspirin therapy, clopidogrel should be substituted (Class I, Level B)

Aspirin—other at-risk or healthy women

In women ≥65 years, consider aspirin therapy (81 mg daily or 100 mg every other day) if blood pressure is controlled and benefit for ischemic stroke and MI prevention is likely to outweigh risk of gastrointestinal bleeding and hemorrhagic stroke (Class IIa, Level B) and in women <65 years when benefit for ischemic stroke prevention is likely to outweigh adverse effects of therapy (Class IIb, Level B)

β-Blockers

β-Blockers should be used indefinitely in all women after MI, acute coronary syndrome, or left ventricular dysfunction with or without heart failure symptoms, unless contraindicated (Class I, Level A)

ACE inhibitors/ARBs

ACE inhibitors should be used (unless contraindicated) in women after MI and in those with clinical evidence of heart failure or an LVEF ≤40% or with diabetes mellitus (Class I, Level A). In women after MI and in those with clinical evidence of heart failure or an LVEF ≤40% or with diabetes mellitus who are intolerant of ACE inhibitors, ARBs should be used instead (Class I, Level B)

Aldosterone blockade

Use aldosterone blockade after MI in women who do not have significant renal dysfunction or hyperkalemia who are already receiving therapeutic doses of an ACE inhibitor and β-blocker, and have LVEF ≤40% with symptomatic heart failure (Class I, Level B)

Source: From Mosca, L. et al., *Circulation*, 115, 1481, 2007.

LVEF indicates left ventricular ejection fraction; BMI, body mass index; EPA, eicosapentaenoic acid; DHA, docosahexaenoic acid; CHD, coronary heart disease; ACE, angiotensin-converting enzyme; ARB, angiotensin receptor blocker; LDL-C, low-density lipoprotein cholesterol; HDL-C, high-density lipoprotein cholesterol; CVD, cardiovascular disease; and MI, myocardial infarction.

[a] Pregnant and lactating women should avoid eating fish potentially high in methylmercury (e.g., shark, swordfish, king mackerel, or tile fish) and should eat up to 12 oz/wk of a variety of fish and shellfish low in mercury and check the Environmental Protection Agency and the U.S. Food and Drug Administration's Web sites for updates and local advisories about safety of local catch.

[b] A drink equivalent is equal to a 12-oz bottle of beer, a 5-oz glass of wine, or a 1.5-oz shot of 80-proof spirit.

[c] Criteria for high risk include established CHD, cerebrovascular disease, peripheral arterial disease, abdominal aortic aneurysm, end-stage or chronic renal disease, diabetes mellitus, and 10-year Framingham risk >20%.

[d] Criteria for very high risk include established CVD plus any of the following: multiple major risk factors, severe and poorly controlled risk factors, or diabetes mellitus.

[e] Dietary supplement niacin should not be used as a substitute for prescription niacin.

[f] After percutaneous intervention with stent placement or coronary artery bypass grafting within previous year and in women with noncoronary forms of CVD, use current guidelines for aspirin and clopidogrel.

prevalence of comorbid diseases, more advanced stage of disease upon diagnosis, and higher complication rates of postrevascularization [22,23]. Estimates indicate that 38% of women compared with 25% of men die within one year after their first heart attack. Thirty-five percent of female heart attack survivors experience a second heart attack within 6 years compared with half that number, 18%, of men [8]. In addition, women are nearly two times as likely as men to die after undergoing bypass surgery and half as likely to get an angioplasty to open a narrowed blood vessel [24].

9.3.4 Risk Factors

Although the traditional risk factors for CVD, such as high cholesterol, high blood pressure and obesity, have detrimental effects in both women and men, certain factors have a greater impact in women. For instance, women with diabetes are at higher risk of developing CVD than either men with or without diabetes or women without diabetes [25]. This has been attributed to higher prevalence of hypertension, dyslipidemia (high triglyceride, low HDL cholesterol), elevated LDL cholesterol, obesity, microalbuminuria, platelet hyperaggregability, and endothelial dysfunction among these women.

A women's risk of developing coronary heart disease (CHD) increases two- to threefold after menopause onset [8], and rates of CVD continue to increase with age. Among women aged 55–64, each additional year of life brings an additional 0.8%–1.3% risk of experiencing a new or recurrent myocardial infarction. By age 65–74, the rates increases to about 1.8%–2.1% per year, and by age 80, the rate increases to about 1.4%–2.4% per year. Furthermore, risk factors for CVD are more prevalent than clinically overt disease in the peri- and postmenopausal age group. Of women aged 55–64 years, it has been estimated that about 44% have hypertension, 37% have high total cholesterol (>240 mg/dL), 36% have borderline high total cholesterol (200–240 mg/dL), 51% have elevated LDL cholesterol (based on individual degree of cardiac risk), 3% have reduced HDL cholesterol (<35 mg/dL), and 23% smoke cigarettes [8].

Consensus panels convened by the NHLBI or NIH periodically recommend cholesterol screening guidelines for American adults and disseminate them through the National Cholesterol Education Panel (NCEP) [26]. Current NCEP guidelines for adults over the age of 20 years without established CVD recommend screening nonfasting total cholesterol and HDL cholesterol levels. If these values are normal (i.e., total cholesterol <200 mg/dL and HDL cholesterol >35 mg/dL), repeat screening is recommended in 5 years. Because cholesterol levels can change more rapidly among perimenopausal women than among the general population, such women should be screened yearly.

If total cholesterol is in the borderline high range (200–239 mg/dL) and HDL <35 mg/dL, or if total cholesterol is >240 mg/dL, NCEP guidelines recommend obtaining a fasting lipid profile, and calculating LDL values using the Friedwald formula: LDL = total cholesterol − HDL cholesterol − (triglyceride/5), assuming triglyceride levels are below 400 mg/dL. Based on the value of this calculated LDL, dietary or drug therapy is recommended. The NCEP recommendations correlate the patient's extent of cardiac risk with the intensity of treatment (the target LDL level); thus, patients with established CVD receive the most intensive therapy. Dietary

TABLE 9.3
Adult Treatment Panel III Classification of LDL, Total, and HDL Cholesterol (mg/dL)[a]

LDL cholesterol	
<100	Optimal
100–129	Near or above optimal
130–159	Borderline high
160–189	High
≥190	Very high
Total cholesterol	
<200	Desirable
200–239	Borderline high
≥240	High
HDL cholesterol	
<40	Low
≥60	High

Source: From Expert Panel on Detection Evaluation and Treatment of High Blood Cholesterol in Adults, *J. Am. Med. Assoc.*, 285, 2486, 2001.

[a] LDL, low-density lipoprotein; HDL, high-density lipoprotein

therapy should be initiated when LDL cholesterol levels are ≥160 mg/dL for individuals without CVD and with fewer than two CVD risk factors, when LDL cholesterol levels are ≥130 mg/dL for individuals without CVD, and with two or more risk factors, and when LDL cholesterol levels are ≥100 mg/dL for individuals with CVD. Drug therapy should commence when LDL cholesterol levels are ≥190 mg/dL for individuals without CVD and with fewer than two risk factors, when LDL cholesterol levels are ≥160 mg/dL for individuals without CVD and two or more risk factors, and when LDL cholesterol levels are ≥130 mg/dL for individuals with CVD [26]. More recent recommendations suggest that target LDL cholesterol levels should be 70 mg/dL for individuals in the highest risk category [27].

The NCEP has also defined specific risk factors for CVD in women [26]. In addition to elevated LDL cholesterol (cutoffs for high value depend on number of other risk factors) (Table 9.3), they include age ≥55 years or premature menopause without estrogen replacement therapy (in contrast to age ≥45 for men); cigarette smoking; diabetes mellitus; family history of CVD, defined as having a mother or other female first-degree relative who has experienced a myocardial infarction or sudden death before age 65 or a father or other male first-degree relative who has experienced a myocardial infarction or sudden death before age 55; hypertension, defined as blood pressure ≥140/90 mm Hg or taking antihypertensive medication; and low HDL cholesterol levels (<35 mg/dL) (Table 9.4). A negative risk factor associated with decreased CVD risk is HDL cholesterol levels above ≥60 mg/dL. High HDL cholesterol levels are more prevalent in women than men.

TABLE 9.4
Major Risk Factors (Exclusive of LDL Cholesterol) that Modify LDL Goals[a]

Cigarette smoking
Hypertension (blood pressure ≥140/90 mm Hg or on antihypertensive medication)
Low HDL cholesterol (<40 mg/dL)[b]
Family history of premature CHD
CHD in male first-degree relative <55 years
CHD in female first-degree relative >65 years
Age (men ≥45 years; women ≥55 years)

Source: From Expert Panel on Detection Evaluation and Treatment of High Blood Cholesterol in Adults, *J. Am. Med. Assoc.*, 285, 2486, 2001. With permission.

[a] Diabetes is regarded as a coronary heart disease (CHD) risk equivalent. LDL, low-density lipoprotein; HDL, high-density lipoprotein.

[b] HDL cholesterol ≥60 mg/dL counts as a "negative" risk factor; its presence removes one risk factor from the total count.

Global risk scores, scores that account for multiple risk factors, can be used to assess the risk of suffering a fatal or severe CVD event in the next 10 years [28]. One such tool that is frequently used to estimate CVD risk is the Framingham Risk Score, which considers sex, age, total cholesterol, HDL cholesterol, and systolic blood pressure (Table 9.5). The total number of points accrued as determined by answers to the risk factor assessments is used to estimate 10 year risk, which is expressed as a percentage (see bottom of Table 9.5). The 10 year risk is used to set LDL cholesterol level treatment goals, including the LDL cholesterol level at which to initiate diet therapy and the LDL cholesterol level at which drug therapy should be considered (Table 9.6). As useful as this score might be, a recent report suggested that among women classified as low risk by Framingham Risk Score, one-third had significant subclinical atherosclerosis [29]. In addition, the sisters of the women with premature heart disease appeared to be at increased risk themselves. Aggressive primary prevention therapy over and above that currently recommended may be warranted for this group of women [29].

9.4 APPROACHES TO THE PREVENTION AND MANAGEMENT OF CVD

9.4.1 Diet

9.4.1.1 Dietary Fat

The relationship between type of dietary fat, atherosclerotic vascular disease risk, and lipid or lipoprotein profiles has been studied since the early 1900s [30].

TABLE 9.5
Framingham Point Score Estimate of 10 Year Risk for Women

Age	Points
20–34	−7
35–39	−3
40–44	0
45–49	3
50–54	6
55–59	8
60–64	10
65–69	12
70–74	14
75–69	16

	Points				
Total Cholesterol (mg/dL) Ages	20–39	40–49	50–59	60–69	70–79
<160	0	0	0	0	0
160–199	4	3	2	1	1
200–239	8	6	4	2	1
240–279	11	8	5	3	2
≥280	13	10	7	4	2
Smoking					
Nonsmoker	0	0	0	0	0
Smoker	9	7	4	3	1

HDL (mg/dL)	Points
≥60	−1
50–59	0
40–49	1
<40	2

Systolic BP (mm Hg)	Treated	Untreated
<120	0	0
120–129	1	3
130–139	2	4
140–159	3	5
≥160	4	6

Point Total	10 Year Risk	Point Total	10 Year Risk	Point Total	10 Year Risk
<9	<1	14	2	20	11
9	1	15	3	21	14
10	1	16	4	22	17
11	1	17	5	23	22
12	1	18	6	24	27
13	2	19	8	≥25	≥30

Source: From Expert Panel on Detection Evaluation and Treatment of High Blood Cholesterol in Adults, *J. Am. Med. Assoc.*, 285, 2486, 2001. With permission.

TABLE 9.6
LDL Cholesterol Goals and Cutoff Points for Therapeutic Lifestyle Changes and Drug Therapy by Risk Category[a]

	LDL Cholesterol		
Risk Category	**LDL Goal (mg/dL)**	**Level at Which to Initiate TLC (mg/dL)**	**LDL Level at Which to Consider Drug Therapy**
CHD or CHD risk equivalents (10 year risk >20%)	<100	≥100	≥130 (100–129: drug optional)
2+ Risk factors			
(10 year risk 10%–20%)	<130	>130	≥130
(10 year risk <10%)	<130	>130	≥160
0–1 Risk factor	<160	>160	≥190 (160–189: LDL-lowering drug optional)

Source: From Expert Panel on Detection Evaluation and Treatment of High Blood Cholesterol in Adults, *J. Am. Med. Assoc.*, 285, 2486, 2001.

[a] LDL, low-density lipoprotein; CHD, coronary heart disease.

Most observational data from international comparisons and migration studies have identified a positive relationship between saturated fatty acid (SFA) intake and CVD [31–33]. Prospective observational studies have reported a higher relative risk of CHD with higher SFA intakes, after adjusting for diet and lifestyle factors associated with CHD [34,35]. This association is often attenuated and in some cases becomes nonsignificant after adjusting for other dietary factors, such as unsaturated fatty acids, fiber, and fruits and vegetables. However, the negative association of CHD with the intake of polyunsaturated fatty acids (PUFAs), linoleic and α-linolenic acid or the ratio PUFA or SFA (P/S), and the positive association with trans fatty acids (TFAs) remained significant in most cases [34]. Data from large scale primary and secondary intervention studies support a positive relationship between CHD and dietary SFA intake and a negative relationship with the dietary P/S ratio, although the magnitude of the effect was not always statistically significant [36–44].

The vast majority of the data are limited to male subjects, the exceptions being the Nurses Health Study [34], the Minnesota Coronary Survey [45], and the Finnish Mental Hospital Study [39]. Recently, an association was found between high SFA and low PUFA intake and decreased coronary atherosclerosis progression among postmenopausal females with established CHD [46]. These observations were unexpected in light of prior reports with regard to the relationship between dietary fat type and CVD risk [26,47]; one potential explanation is that women respond to dietary factors affecting CVD progression differently than do men. However, Boniface and Tefft [48] reported that dietary SFA intake was associated with a significantly higher risk of CHD in healthy female but not male subjects. Similarly, Jakobsen et al. [49]

observed that dietary SFA was positively associated with CHD risk in younger females but not in older females or males. And a recent review of currently available clinical intervention data concluded that women and men respond similarly to dietary fat modification and lipid and lipoprotein levels [50].

9.4.1.1.1 Level of Dietary Fat

Dietary fat serves as a major energy source for humans. One gram of fat contributes 9 calories, a little more than twice that contributed by protein or carbohydrate, 4 cal/g, and somewhat more than that contributed by alcohol, 7 cal/g. When considering the importance of the level of dietary fat with respect to CVD prevention and management there are two major factors to consider, the impact on plasma lipoprotein profiles and body weight. The potential relationship with body weight is important to consider because of secondary effects on plasma lipids, blood pressure, dyslipidemia, and Type 2 diabetes, all potential risk factors for CVD.

When considering the effect of the level of dietary fat on plasma lipoprotein profiles, the focus is usually on triglyceride and HDL cholesterol levels or total cholesterol to HDL cholesterol ratios. Relatively consistent evidence indicates that when body weight is maintained at a constant level, decreasing the total fat content of the diet, expressed as a percent of total energy, and replacing it with carbohydrate, results in an increase in triglyceride levels, decrease in HDL cholesterol levels, and less favorable (higher) total cholesterol to HDL cholesterol ratio [51–53]. Low HDL cholesterol levels are an independent risk factor for CVD [26]. Low fat diets are of particular concern in diabetic or overweight individuals who tend to have low HDL cholesterol levels [54].

With respect to the effect of the level of dietary fat on body weight, two published reviews of long-term data have concluded that even a relatively large downward shift in dietary fat intake, ~10% of energy, resulted in only modest weight loss, 1.0 kg over a 12 month period in normal weight subjects and 3 kg in overweight or obese subjects [55,56]. Some evidence suggests that dietary fiber content may be a mitigating factor. That is, substituting fruits, vegetables, and whole grains for fat instead of fat-free cookies, cakes, and snack foods may be more efficacious in promoting weight loss within the context of low fat diets.

9.4.1.1.2 Type of Dietary Fat

Studies done in the mid-1960s demonstrated that changes in the dietary fatty acid profiles altered plasma total cholesterol levels in most individuals [57–59]. As analytical techniques became more sophisticated, data on lipid, lipoprotein, and apolipoprotein levels routinely became available.

9.4.1.1.2.1 Saturated Fatty Acids

Early evidence demonstrated that the consumption of foods relatively high in SFA increased plasma total cholesterol levels and that not all SFA had identical effects [57–59]. Subsequent work confirmed the hypercholesterolemic effect of SFA, demonstrating that SFA intake results in an increase in both LDL and HDL cholesterol levels [60]. Short-chain fatty acids (6:0 to 10:0) and stearic acid (18:0) produce little or no change in blood cholesterol levels, whereas SFA with intermediate chain lengths, lauric (12:0) to palmitic (16:0) acids, appears to be the most potent in

TABLE 9.7
Major Dietary Fatty Acids

Code	Common Name	Formula
Saturated		
12:00	Lauric acid	$CH_3(CH_2)_{10}COOH$
14:00	Myristic acid	$CH_3(CH_2)_{12}COOH$
16:00	Palmitic acid	$CH_3(CH_2)_{14}COOH$
18:00	Stearic acid	$CH_3(CH_2)_{16}COOH$
Monounsaturated		
16:1 n-7 cis	Palmitoleic acid	$CH_3(CH_2)_5CH{=}(c)CH(CH_2)_7COOH$
18:1 n-9 cis	Oleic acid	$CH_3(CH_2)_7CH{=}(c)CH(CH_2)_7COOH$
18:1 n-9 trans	Elaidic acid	$CH_3(CH_2)_7CH{=}(t)CH(CH_2)_7COOH$
Polyunsaturated		
18:2 n-6,9 all cis	Linoleic acid	$CH_3(CH_2)_4CH{=}(c)CHCH_2CH{=}(c)CH(CH_2)_7COOH$
18:3 n-3,6,9 all cis	α-Linoleic acid	$CH_3CH_2CH{=}(c)CHCH_2CH{=}(c)CHCH_2CH{=}(c)CH(CH_2)_7COOH$
18:3 n-6,9,12 all cis	γ-Linoleic acid	$CH_3(CH_2)_4CH{=}(c)CHCH_2CH{=}(c)CHCH_2CH{=}(c)CH(CH_2)_4COOH$
20:4 n-6,9,12,15 all cis	Arachidonic acid	$CH_3(CH_2)_4CH{=}(c)CHCH_2CH{=}(c)CHCH_2CH{=}(c)CHCH_2CH{=}(c)CH(CH_2)_3COOH$
20:5 n-3,6,9,12,15 all cis	Eicosapentaenoic acid	$CH_3(CH_2CH{=}(c)CH)_5(CH_2)_3COOH$
22:6 n-3,6,9,12,15,18 all cis	Docosahexaenoic acid	$CH_3(CH_2CH{=}(c)CH)_6(CH_2)_2COOH$

increasing blood cholesterol levels [57,61] (Table 9.7). The minimal effect of the shorter chain fatty acids is attributed to their being absorbed directly into the portal circulation and of 18:0 to its high rate of conversion to18:1, a monounsaturated fatty acid (MUFA) [62,63]. The LDL cholesterol raising effect of the intermediate chain length saturated fat is attributed to a decreased fractional catabolic rate of plasma LDL, with little effect on production rate [64,65].

SFA tends to be solid at room temperature. Notable exceptions are the tropical oils (palm, palm kernel, and coconut) that are liquid at room temperature because they have high levels of short-chain SFA. Efforts to reduce dietary SFA intakes should include use of lean meat, the trimming of excess fat and skin from poultry, limiting portion size, and the substituting nonfat and low-fat dairy products for their full fat counterparts. The judicious use of ingredient listings and nutrient labels on processed foods will also help achieve the goal of reducing the SFA intakes.

9.4.1.1.2.2 Unsaturated Fatty Acids

Unsaturated fatty acids are fatty acids that contain one or more double bonds in the acyl chain. As the name implies, MUFAs have one double bond and PUFAs have two or more double bonds. The majority of double bonds in fatty acids occurring in food are in the cis configuration, that is, the hydrogen atoms attached to the carbons forming the double bond are on the same side of the acyl chain. Alternatively, some double bonds occur in the trans configuration, that is, the hydrogen atoms attached to the carbons forming the double bond are on the opposite side of the acyl chain. Relative to SFA, both MUFA and PUFA lower both LDL and HDL cholesterol levels. The absolute magnitude of the change is greater for LDL cholesterol than HDL cholesterol. The data suggests that MUFA has a slightly smaller effect than PUFA in lowering both LDL and HDL cholesterol levels so that the change in the total cholesterol or HDL cholesterol ratio (decrease) is similar [66]. Because of the changes in plasma lipids and lipoproteins caused when unsaturated fat displaces SFA from the diet such a shift should be encouraged in the prevention and management of CVD.

9.4.1.1.2.3 Monounsaturated Fatty Acids

The major MUFA in the diet is oleic acid (18:1) (Table 9.7). Vegetable oils high in MUFA include canola (rapeseed) and olive oil. Fats from meats also are relatively high in MUFA but unlike vegetable oils, they also contain relatively high levels of SFA, hence would not be recommended as good source of MUFA. When MUFAs displace carbohydrate in the diet, CHD risk moderately decreases [66] (Figure 9.5). When MUFAs displace SFA in the diet, CHD risk decreases.

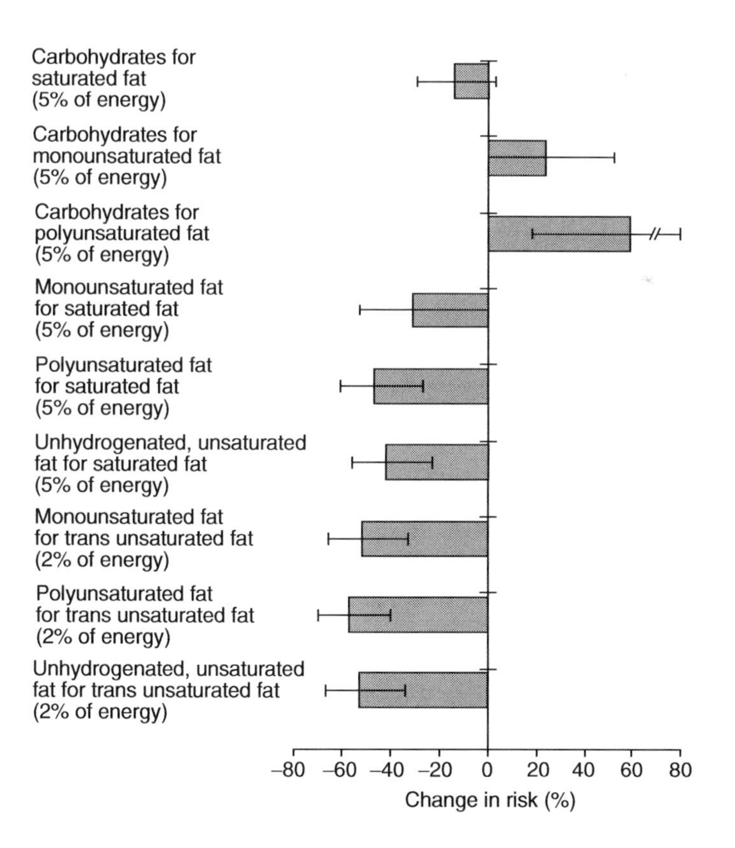

FIGURE 9.5 Dietary fat intake and the risk of coronary heart disease in women. (From Hu, F.B., et al., *N. Engl. J. Med.*, 337, 1491, 1997. With permission.)

9.4.1.1.2.4 Polyunsaturated Fatty Acids

There is a wider range of PUFA than MUFA in the diet. Dietary PUFA vary on the basis of chain length, degree of saturation (number of double bonds), and position of the double bond(s) (positional isomers). Two positional isomers of interest with respect to diet and CVD risk are n-6 and n-3 (Table 9.7). The distinction is made on the basis of the location of the first double bond counting from the methyl end of the fatty acyl chain (as opposed to the carboxyl end). If the first double bond is six carbons from the methyl end, the fatty acid is classified as an n-6 fatty acid. If the first double bond is three carbons from the methyl end the fatty acid is classified as an n-3 fatty acid. When PUFA displaces carbohydrate in the diet, CHD risk decreases [66] (Figure 9.5). Vegetable oils high in PUFA include soybean, corn, sunflower, and safflower oils. The major n-6 PUFA in the diet is linoleic acid (18:2 n-6). However, other n-6 PUFAs, such as γ-linolenic acid (18:3 n-6) and arachidonic acid (20:4 n-6), occur in smaller amounts but are important biologically.

9.4.1.1.2.5 n-3 Fatty Acids

Quantitatively, the major n-3 PUFA in the diet is α-linolenic acid (18:3 n-3). Major dietary sources include flaxseed, soybean, and canola oils. Two other n-3 PUFAs, eicosapentaenoic acid (EPA, 20:5 n-3) and docosahexaenoic acid (DHA, 22:6 n-3), are sometimes referred to as very long chain n-3 fatty acids (Table 9.7). The major source of these fatty acids is marine oils or in fish. Dietary intakes of EPA and DHA are associated with decreased risk of heart disease and stroke [67–70]. Intervention studies have substantiated these findings [71]. The beneficial effects of EPA and DHA are attributed to decreased arrhythmias, lower triglyceride concentrations in hypertriglyceridemic individuals, lower blood pressure, and decreased platelet aggregation [72–74]. In individuals with elevated triglyceride levels, n-3 fatty acids decrease plasma concentrations by decreasing hepatic production rates of very low density lipoprotein with little effect on fractional catabolic rates [75,76]. α-linolenic acid can be converted to EPA, albeit at very low rates (~5%) [77]. α-linolenic acid does not have the cardioprotective effects of EPA and DHA [71]. For this reason current recommendations are to consume two fish meals per week to ensure adequate intakes of EPA and DHA [74].

9.4.1.1.2.6 Trans Fatty Acids

TFAs, by definition, contain at least one double bond in the trans configuration. Dietary TFAs occur naturally in meat and dairy products as a result of anaerobic bacterial fermentation in ruminant animals. TFAs are also introduced into the diet as a result of the consumption of hydrogenated vegetable or fish oils [78]. Hydrogenation results in a number of changes in the fatty acyl chain: the conversion of cis to trans double bonds (geometric isomers), the saturation of double bonds, and the migration of double bonds along the acyl chain, resulting in multiple positional isomers. Oils are primarily hydrogenated to increase viscosity (change a liquid oil into a semiliquid or solid) and extend shelf life (decrease susceptibility to oxidation).

Since the early 1990s attention has been focused on the effects of TFAs on specific lipoprotein fractions [79]. The findings of this work have suggested that similar to SFAs, TFAs result in increased LDL cholesterol levels. In contrast to SFAs, they do not raise HDL cholesterol levels. These changes result in a less favorable LDL cholesterol:HDL cholesterol ratio, with respect to CVD risk [80,81]. Relative to unsaturated fat, both saturated fat and partially-hydrogenated fat result in higher LDL cholesterol concentrations attributable to lower fractional catabolic rates, with little change in production rates [65]. When trans fatty acids displace MUFA or PUFA in the diet, CHD risk increases [66] (Figure 9.5).

The major source of dietary TFAs is from hydrogenated fat, primarily in products made thereof, such as commercially fried foods and baked goods. On January 1, 2006, the US Food and Drug Administration required the Nutrients Facts Panel of packaged food to include information on the amount of TFAs in the product. This has resulted in a reformulation and decrease in the level of TFAs in many foods covered by this legislation. There are currently efforts by a number of large cities in the United States to require restaurants to phase hydrogenated fat out of the foods they prepare. All these efforts should result in a decrease in TFA intakes.

9.4.1.2 Dietary Cholesterol

The observation that dietary cholesterol increased blood cholesterol levels and was associated with the development of CVD was originally made early in the twentieth century in rabbits [30]. In humans, a positive correlation has been repeatedly observed between dietary cholesterol and both blood cholesterol levels and CVD risk [82,83]. Whether the increase in plasma cholesterol levels induced by dietary cholesterol is linear or curvilinear, or whether there is a break point or threshold or ceiling relationship beyond which individuals are no longer responsive, remains to be determined. However, it is important to note that the effect of dietary cholesterol is less than that of SFA and as such receives less emphasis with respect to dietary recommendations [84]. This may be due, in part, to the high level of variability in response to dietary cholesterol [85]. With few exceptions, dietary cholesterol is present in foods of animal origin. Therefore, restricting saturated fat intake is likely to result in a decrease in dietary cholesterol intake.

9.4.1.3 Fiber

Dietary soluble fiber, primarily β-glucan, has been reported to have a modest independent effect on decreasing blood total and LDL cholesterol levels. A meta-analysis concluded that 3 g of soluble fiber (equivalent of three servings of oatmeal) reduced both total and LDL cholesterol levels by ~5 mg/dL [86]. Most evidence suggests that soluble fiber exerts its hypocholesterolaemic effect by binding bile acids and cholesterol in the intestine, resulting in an increased fecal loss and altered colonic metabolism of bile acids [87]. The fermentation of fiber polysaccharides in the colon yields short-chain fatty acids. Some evidence suggests that these compounds may have hypocholesterolaemic effects via alterations in hepatic metabolism. However, recent work indicates that in women, dietary insoluble fiber, from cereal products, is associated with decreased CVD risk and slower progression of atherosclerotic lesions than soluble fiber from fruits and vegetables [88,89]. For this reason, it is prudent to recommend diets rich in both whole grains, and fruits and vegetables to reduce CVD risk.

9.4.1.4 Soy Protein

The potential relationship between soy protein and the risk of developing CVD has a long history dating back to the 1940s [90]. Despite the relatively protracted lead-time attempts to more precisely define this relationship, it has been slow in coming and somewhat inconsistent [91]. Reinvigorated interest developed in the relationship between soy protein and blood lipid levels after a meta-analysis was published in the mid-1990s suggesting that soy protein resulted in significant reductions in total and LDL cholesterol levels, with the most pronounced effect in hypercholesterolemic individuals [92]. Changes in HDL cholesterol levels were not significant. It was unclear whether the effect on total and LDL cholesterol levels was attributable to the soy protein, per se, or other soybean derived factor(s), the most likely of which the constitutive isoflavones. Since that time a number of well-controlled studies have reexamined the effect of soy protein and isoflavones on blood lipid levels in humans. The results of more recent studies are variable [93–95]. Declines in LDL cholesterol levels attributable to the substitution of 25–50 g of soy protein for animal protein range from a null to small (3%–6%) in normocholesterolemic and hypercholesterolemic individuals. Changes in HDL cholesterol levels were highly variable, ranging from −15% to +7%. Soy derived isoflavones do not appear to have an independent effect on blood lipid levels [93,96]. On the basis of the most recent data it can be concluded that there is little effect of soy protein on plasma lipid levels. Nevertheless, consumption of soy protein rich foods may indirectly reduce CVD risk if they displace animal and full fat dairy products that contain saturated fat and cholesterol from the diet.

9.4.1.5 Phytosterols (Plant Sterols or Stanols)

Sterols are the designation for a group of compounds that are essential constituents of cell membranes in animals and plants. Cholesterol is the major sterol of mammalian cells. Phytosterols, frequently referred to as plant sterol or stenol such as β-sitosterol, campesterol, and stigmasterol, are the major sterols of plant cells. Plant stanols are saturated versions of plant sterols. Plant stanol esters, the form incorporated into some foods, contain a fatty acid. In humans, phytosterols are not synthesized, are poorly absorbed and hinder cholesterol absorption [97]. It is this later property that has been exploited in the use of these compounds as blood cholesterol lowering agents. Maximal LDL cholesterol lowering attributable to phytosterols occurs at a dose of about 2 g/day [98] and results in about 10% lower LDL cholesterol concentrations. There is a wide range of phytosterol containing foods and capsules that are currently available. Few side effects of plant sterols have been reported with the exception of decreased levels of circulating carotenoids. The long-term effect of this is unclear at this time and should continue to be monitored carefully.

9.4.1.6 Antioxidant Nutrients

Considerable interest had been generated on the potential benefit of dietary supplementation with vitamin E and other antioxidant nutrients in reducing CVD risk [99]. Support from this hypothesis came from two sources. First, epidemiological observations suggested that vitamin E supplement use was associated with decreased risk of CVD [100,101]. Second, from the in vitro work demonstrating that vitamin E in LDL was correlated with decreased susceptibility of the lipoprotein particle to oxidation and that in cell culture oxidized LDL resulted in foam cell formation [102,103]. A number of recent intervention studies have failed to demonstrate a benefit of vitamin E or other antioxidant vitamins. At this time the data do not support a recommendation to use antioxidant vitamins for the prevention or management of CVD [103,104].

9.4.2 Physical Activity

Often sidelined when issues related to women and CVD prevention are addressed is the importance of regular physical activity. Physical activity, such as walking, has been shown to have positive effects on body weight, dyslipidemia, hypertensions, and diabetes in women [105–107]. Importantly, substantial reductions in CVD have been reported in women regardless of whether the physical activity is vigorous or less strenuous, such as walking [108]. Encouragingly, the benefits of regular physical activity are consistent and irrespective of race or ethnic group, age, and body weight [108].

9.4.3 Smoking Cessation

As many as 30% of all CHD deaths in the United States each year are attributable to cigarette smoking, with the risk being strongly dose-related [8]. Cigarette smoking independently increases the risk of CHD by increasing blood pressure, decreasing exercise tolerance, decreasing HDL cholesterol, increasing the tendency for blood to clot, and introducing potentially toxic compounds into the circulation. Smoking also increases the risk of recurrent CHD after bypass surgery. Women who smoke and use oral contraceptives greatly increase their risk for CHD and stroke compared with women who do not smoke but use oral contraceptives.

Numerous prospective investigations have demonstrated a substantial decrease in CHD mortality for former smokers compared with continuing smokers. This decrease in risk occurs relatively soon after smoking cessation, and increasing intervals since the last cigarette smoked are associated with progressively lower mortality rates from CHD [109].

9.5 CURRENT RECOMMENDATIONS TO PREVENT AND TREAT CVD

There are a number of recommendations for the prevention and treatment of CVD. Those that focus on diet and lifestyle modification include NCEP [26] and the AHA [84]. The dietary components are summarized in Table 9.8 and Table 9.9, respectively.

9.6 BARRIERS TO CVD PREVENTION IN WOMEN

There are some unique characteristics of women that can impede efforts to initiate lifestyle modifications to decrease CVD risk. In some cases it is their own lack of awareness or internalization that CVD is a major health risk [5,7] or their physician's

TABLE 9.8
National Cholesterol Education Program Adult Treatment Panel III Therapeutic Lifestyle Change Diet (TLC)

SFA	<7%
PUFA	up to 10%
MUFA	up to 20%
Total fat	25%–35%
CHO	50%–60%
Fiber	20–30 g/day
Protein	~15% E
Cholesterol	<200 mg/day
Total Calories	Balance E intake and expenditure

Source: From Expert Panel on Detection Evaluation and Treatment of High Blood Cholesterol in Adults, *J. Am. Med. Assoc.*, 285, 2486, 2001. With permission.

awareness that CVD is a major health risk in women [19,22] and use of diagnostic techniques tailored to women's unique needs [23]. Women may also feel reluctant to raise questions about their own health concerns [5] or lack of adequate treatment of mitigating factors that alter CVD risk outcomes, such as depression [110]. Other

TABLE 9.9
American Heart Association Diet and Lifestyle Recommendations

Balance calorie intake and physical activity to achieve or maintain a healthy body weight
Consume a diet rich in vegetables and fruits
Choose whole-grain, high-fiber foods
Consume fish, especially oily fish, at least twice a week
Limit your intake of saturated fat to <7% energy, trans fat to <1% energy, and cholesterol to <300 mg/day by
- choosing lean meats and vegetable alternatives
- selecting fat-free (skim), 1% fat, and low-fat dairy products
- minimizing intake of partially hydrogenated fat

Minimize beverages and foods with added sugars
Choose and prepare foods with little or no salt
If you consume alcohol, do so in moderation
When you eat food that is prepared outside home, follow AHA Diet and Lifestyle Recommendations

Source: From Lichtenstein, A.H., et al., *Circulation*, 114, 82, 2006.

factors identified that could contribute to delayed intervention in women include lower psychosocial factors such as low self-esteem, competing priorities, and multiple care-giving responsibilities [22,111]. Until these and similar issues are addressed the efficacy of interventions cannot be maximized in women.

9.7 CONCLUSION

CVD, particularly CHD and stroke, remains the leading causes of death of women in America and most developed countries. Recent statistics show that the rate of heart disease has declined in men but not in women. This is, in part, because of lack of awareness by healthcare providers, the public and women themselves, as well as sex differences in risk factors, symptoms, and diagnosis accuracy that impact on treatment. Until recently, women have been underrepresented in many studies that have set the standard for detection and treatment of heart disease. The good news is that CVD is largely preventable; therefore, prevention of risk factors for CVD is an important practical solution for women. Additionally, scientific and media attention is now being directed toward a better appreciation of the influence of sex on heart disease risk and management. Regarding CVD risk assessment, the NCEP has now defined specific risk factors for CVD in women [26]. In addition to the traditional risk factors such as high cholesterol, high blood pressure, and obesity, which have detrimental effects in both men and women, factors that have a greater impact in women than in men include diabetes, hypertriglyceridemia, and low HDL cholesterol. Similarly, in terms of dietary and lifestyle recommendations, the AHA has released evidence-based guidelines for CVD prevention in women [1,84]. On the basis of available data, the AHA recommends a heart-healthy diet, defined as an eating pattern that includes intake of a variety of vegetables, fruits, whole grains, low-fat, or nonfat dairy products, fish, legumes, and sources of protein low in SFA (e.g., poultry, lean meats, plant sources). In addition, intake of SFA should be $<7\%$ of calories, cholesterol <300 mg/day, and TFAs $<1\%$ of calories.

Furthermore, the recently launched campaigns by the AHA and NIH to create awareness of heart disease in women, which emphasize dietary modification, physical activity, and smoking cessation; the initiation of studies focused primarily on women, such as the Women's Health Initiative, an extensive 14 year study of 140,000 postmenopausal women; and the increase in proportion of women participating in clinical trials should provide valuable information on the unique features of heart disease in women, which will undoubtedly have a significant impact on prevention, clinical care, and outcomes of women and provide direction for future work.

9.8 FUTURE RESEARCH

Future research is needed to develop biomarkers of dietary patterns, which will allow for a better assessment of how this lifestyle variable predicts CVD risk in women. More consistent monitoring needs to be in place to assess the best pharmacological and surgical approaches to treating established CHD and decreasing CVD risk in women. Underassessed to date is the value of the current public health programs to increase awareness and decrease CVD risk in women.

REFERENCES

1. Mosca, L. et al., Evidence-based guidelines for cardiovascular disease prevention in women, 2007 update, *Circulation*, 115, 1481, 2007.
2. Raza, J.A., Reinhart, R.A., and Movahed, A., Ischemic heart disease in women and the role of hormone therapy, *Int. J. Cardiol.*, 96, 7, 2004.
3. ESHRE Capri Workshop Group, Hormones and cardiovascular health in women, *Human Reprod. Update*, 12, 483, 2006.
4. Mieres, J.H. et al., American Society of Nuclear Cardiology consensus statement: Task Force on Women and Coronary Artery Disease—the role of myocardial perfusion imaging in the clinical evaluation of coronary artery disease in women, *J. Nucl. Cardiol.*, 10, 95, 2003.
5. Mosca, L. et al., Awareness, perception, and knowledge of heart disease risk and prevention among women in the United States. American Heart Association Women's Heart Disease and Stroke Campaign Task Force, *Arch. Fam. Med.*, 9, 506, 2000.
6. Hardesty, P. and Trupp, R.J., Prevention: The key to reducing cardiovascular disease risk in women, *J. Cardiov. Nurs.*, 20, 433, 2005.
7. Mosca, L. et al., Tracking women's awareness of heart disease: An American Heart Association national study, *Circulation*, 109, 573, 2004.
8. American Heart Association, http://www.americanheart.org/presenter.jhtml?identifier = 3000941, 2006.
9. World Health Organization, Diet, nutrition and the prevention of chronic diseases, *World Health Organ. Tech. Rep. Ser.*, 916: i–viii, 2003.
10. Libby, P. and Theroux, P., Pathophysiology of coronary artery disease, *Circulation*, 111, 3481, 2005.
11. McGill, H.C., Jr. et al., Origin of atherosclerosis in childhood and adolescence, *Am. J. Clin. Nutr.*, 72, 1307S, 2000.
12. Raitakari, O.T. et al., Cardiovascular risk factors in childhood and carotid artery intima-media thickness in adulthood: The Cardiovascular Risk in Young Finns Study, *J. Am. Med. Assoc.*, 290, 2277, 2003.
13. Li, S. et al., Childhood cardiovascular risk factors and carotid vascular changes in adulthood: The Bogalusa Heart Study, *J. Am. Med. Assoc.*, 290, 2271, 2003.
14. Champney, K.P. and Wenger, N.K., Recognition and prevention of cardiovascular disease in women, *Compr. Ther.*, 31, 255, 2005.
15. Cooper, R. et al., Trends and disparities in coronary heart disease, stroke, and other cardiovascular diseases in the United States: Findings of the national conference on cardiovascular disease prevention, *Circulation*, 102, 3137, 2000.
16. Milner, K.A. et al., Gender differences in symptom presentation associated with coronary heart disease, *Am. J. Cardiol.*, 84, 396, 1999.
17. McSweeney, J.C. et al., Women's early warning symptoms of acute myocardial infarction, *Circulation*, 108, 2619, 2003.
18. Iemolo, F. et al., Sex differences in carotid plaque and stenosis, *Stroke*, 35, 477, 2004.
19. Mosca, L. et al., National study of physician awareness and adherence to cardiovascular disease prevention guidelines, *Circulation*, 111, 499, 2005.
20. Ford, E.S. et al., Serum total cholesterol concentrations and awareness, treatment, and control of hypercholesterolemia among US adults: Findings from the National Health and Nutrition Examination Survey, 1999 to 2000., *Circulation*, 107, 2185, 2003.
21. Mieres, J.H. et al., Role of noninvasive testing in the clinical evaluation of women with suspected coronary artery disease: Consensus statement from the Cardiac Imaging Committee, Council on Clinical Cardiology, and the Cardiovascular Imaging and

Intervention Committee, Council on Cardiovascular Radiology and Intervention, American Heart Association, *Circulation*, 111, 682, 2005.

22. Bello, N. and Mosca, L., Epidemiology of coronary heart disease in women, *Prog. Cardiovasc. Dis.*, 46, 287, 2004.
23. Polk, D.M. and Naqvi, T.Z., Cardiovascular disease in women: Sex differences in presentation, risk factors, and evaluation, *Curr. Cardiol. Rep.*, 7, 166, 2005.
24. Ayanian, J.Z. and Epstein, A.M., Differences in the use of procedures between women and men hospitalized for coronary heart disease, *N. Engl. J. Med.*, 325, 221, 1991.
25. Allende-Vigo, M.Z., Cardiovascular disease in women with diabetes mellitus: A review, *Puerto Rico Health Sci. J.*, 23, 193, 2004.
26. Expert Panel on Detection Evaluation and Treatment of High Blood Cholesterol in Adults, Executive Summary of The Third Report of The National Cholesterol Education Program (NCEP) Expert Panel on Detection, Evaluation, And Treatment of High Blood Cholesterol In Adults (Adult Treatment Panel III), *J. Am. Med. Assoc.*, 285, 2486, 2001.
27. Grundy, S.M. et al., Implications of recent clinical trials for the National Cholesterol Education Program Adult Treatment Panel III guidelines, *Circulation*, 110, 227, 2004.
28. Ferrer, J., Neyro, J.L., and Estevez, A., Identification of risk factors for prevention and early diagnosis of a-symptomatic post-menopausal women, *Maturitas*, 52 (Suppl 1), S7, 2005.
29. Michos, E.D. et al., Women with a low Framingham risk score and a family history of premature coronary heart disease have a high prevalence of subclinical coronary atherosclerosis, *Am. Heart J.*, 150, 1276, 2005.
30. Finking, G. and Hanke, H., Nikolaj Nikolajewitsch Anitschkow (1885–1964) established the cholesterol-fed rabbit as a model for atherosclerosis research, *Atherosclerosis*, 135, 1, 1997.
31. Kromhout, D. et al., Dietary saturated and trans fatty acids and cholesterol and 25-year mortality from coronary heart disease: The Seven Countries Study, *Prev. Med.*, 24, 308, 1995.
32. Kushi, L.H. et al., Diet and 20-year mortality from coronary heart disease. The Ireland–Boston Diet-Heart Study, *N. Engl. J. Med.*, 312, 811, 1985.
33. Kato, H. et al., Epidemiologic studies of coronary heart disease and stroke in Japanese men living in Japan, Hawaii and California, *Am. J. Epidemiol.*, 97, 372, 1973.
34. Oh, K. et al., Dietary fat intake and risk of coronary heart disease in women: 20 years of follow-up of the nurses' health study, *Am. J. Epidemiol.*, 161, 672, 2005.
35. Ascherio, A. et al., Dietary fat and risk of coronary heart disease in men: Cohort follow up study in the United States, *BMJ*, 313, 84, 1996.
36. MRFIT Research Group, Mortality after $10\frac{1}{2}$ years for hypertensive participants in the Multiple Risk Factor Intervention Trial., *Circulation*, 82, 1616, 1990.
37. World Health Organization European Collaborative Group, European collaborative trial of multifactorial prevention of coronary heart disease: Final report on the 6-year results, *Lancet*, 1, 869, 1986.
38. Frantz, I.D., Jr. et al., Test of effect of lipid lowering by diet on cardiovascular risk. The Minnesota Coronary Survey, *Arteriosclerosis*, 9, 129, 1989.
39. Miettinen, M. et al., Dietary prevention of coronary heart disease in women: The Finnish Mental Hospital Study, *Int. J. Epidemiol.*, 12, 17, 1983.
40. Hjermann, I. et al., Effect of diet and smoking intervention on the incidence of coronary heart disease. Report from the Oslo Study Group of a randomised trial in healthy men, *Lancet*, 2, 1303, 1981.
41. Turpeinen, O. et al., Dietary prevention of coronary heart disease: The Finnish Mental Hospital Study, *Int. J. Epidemiol.*, 8, 99, 1979.

42. Woodhill, J.M. et al., Low fat, low cholesterol diet in secondary prevention of coronary heart disease, *Adv. Exp. Med. Biol.*, 109, 317, 1978.
43. Dayton, S. et al., Controlled trial of a diet high in unsaturated fat for prevention of atherosclerotic complications, *Lancet*, 2, 1060, 1968.
44. Leren, P., The Oslo diet-heart study. Eleven-year report, *Circulation*, 42, 935, 1970.
45. Luepker, R.V., Current status of cholesterol treatment in the community: The Minnesota Heart Survey, *Am. J. Med.*, 102, 37, 1997.
46. Mozaffarian, D., Rimm, E.B., and Herrington, D.M., Dietary fats, carbohydrate, and progression of coronary atherosclerosis in postmenopausal women, *Am. J. Clin. Nutr.*, 80, 1175, 2004.
47. Krauss, R.M. et al., American Heart Association Dietary Guidelines: Revision 2000: A statement for healthcare professionals from the Nutrition Committee of the American Heart Association, *Circulation*, 102, 2284, 2000.
48. Boniface, D.R. and Tefft, M.E., Dietary fats and 16-year coronary heart disease mortality in a cohort of men and women in Great Britain, *Eur. J. Clin. Nutr.*, 56, 786, 2002.
49. Jakobsen, M.U. et al., Dietary fat and risk of coronary heart disease: Possible effect modification by gender and age, *Am. J. Epidemiol.*, 160, 141, 2004.
50. Lapointe, A., Balk, E.M., and Lichtenstein, A.H., Gender differences in plasma lipid response to dietary fat, *Nutr. Rev.*, 64, 234, 2006.
51. Lichtenstein, A.H. et al., Short-term consumption of a low-fat diet beneficially affects plasma lipid concentrations only when accompanied by weight loss, hypercholesterolemia, low-fat diet, and plasma lipids, *Arterioscler. Thromb.*, 14, 1751, 1994.
52. Schaefer, E.J. et al., Body weight and low-density lipoprotein cholesterol changes after consumption of a low-fat ad libitum diet., *J. Am. Med. Assoc.*, 274, 1450, 1995.
53. Kasim-Karakas, S.E. et al., Changes in plasma lipoproteins during low-fat, high-carbohydrate diets: Effects of energy intake, *Am. J. Clin. Nutr.*, 71, 1439, 2000.
54. Bantle, J.P. et al., Nutrition recommendations and interventions for diabetes, *Diab. Care*, 29, 2140, 2006.
55. Yao, M. and Roberts, S.B., Dietary energy density and weight regulation, *Nutr. Rev.*, 59, 247, 2001.
56. Willett, W.C. and Leibel, R.L., Dietary fat is not a major determinant of body fat, *Am. J. Med.*, 113 (Suppl 9B), 47S, 2002.
57. Keys, A., Anderson, J.T., and Grande, F., Serum cholesterol response to changes in the diet, *Metab. Clin. Exp.*, 14, 747, 1965.
58. Keys, A. et al., The relation in man between cholesterol levels in the diet and in the blood, *Science*, 112, 79, 1950.
59. Hegsted, D.M. et al., Interrelations between the kind and amount of dietary fat and dietary cholesterol in experimental hypercholesterolemia, *Am. J. Clin. Nutr.*, 7, 5, 1959.
60. Kris-Etherton, P.M. and Yu, S., Individual fatty acid effects on plasma lipids and lipoproteins: Human studies, *Am. J. Clin. Nutr.*, 65, 1628S, 1997.
61. McGandy, R.B. et al., Use of semisynthetic fats in determining effects of specific dietary fatty acids on serum lipids in man, *Am. J. Clin. Nutr.*, 23, 1288, 1970.
62. Bonanome, A. and Grundy, S.M., Effect of dietary stearic acid on plasma cholesterol and lipoprotein levels, *N. Engl. J. Med.*, 318, 1244, 1988.
63. Denke, M.A., Cholesterol-lowering diets. A review of the evidence, *Arch. Int. Med.*, 155, 17, 1995.
64. Shepherd, J. et al., Effects of saturated and polyunsaturated fat diets on the chemical composition and metabolism of low density lipoproteins in man, *J. Lipid Res.*, 21, 91, 1980.

65. Matthan, N.R. et al., Dietary hydrogenated fat increases high-density lipoprotein apoA-I catabolism and decreases low-density lipoprotein apoB-100 catabolism in hypercholesterolemic women, *Arterioscler. Thromb. Vasc. Biol.*, 24, 1092, 2004.
66. Hu, F.B. et al., Dietary fat intake and the risk of coronary heart disease in women., *N. Engl. J. Med.*, 337, 1491, 1997.
67. Albert, C.M. et al., Blood levels of long-chain n-3 fatty acids and the risk of sudden death, *N. Engl. J. Med.*, 346, 1113, 2002.
68. Albert, C.M. et al., Fish consumption and risk of sudden cardiac death, *J. Am. Med. Assoc.*, 279, 23, 1998.
69. Erkkilä, A.T. et al., Fish intake is associated with a reduced progression of coronary artery atherosclerosis in postmenopausal women with coronary artery disease, *Am. J. Clin. Nutr.*, 80, 626, 2004.
70. Balk, E. et al., Effects of omega-3 fatty acids on cardiovascular risk factors and intermediate markers of cardiovascular disease, *Evid. Rep. Technol. Assess.*, 93, 2004.
71. Wang, C.H. et al., Omega-3 fatty acids from fish or fish oil supplements, but not α-linolenic acid, benfit cardiovascular disease outcomes in primary and secondary prevention studies: A systematic review, *Am. J. Clin. Nutr.*, 84, 5, 2006.
72. Nair, S.S. et al., Prevention of cardiac arrhythmia by dietary (n-3) polyunsaturated fatty acids and their mechanism of action, *J. Nutr.*, 127, 383, 1997.
73. Appel, L.J. et al., Does supplementation of diet with 'fish oil' reduce blood pressure? A meta-analysis of controlled clinical trials., *Arch. Int. Med.*, 153, 1429, 1993.
74. Kris-Etherton, P.M. et al., Fish consumption, fish oil, omega-3 fatty acids, and cardiovascular disease, *Circulation*, 106, 2747, 2002.
75. Chan, D.C. et al., Randomized controlled trial of the effect of n-3 fatty acid supplementation on the metabolism of apolipoprotein B-100 and chylomicron remnants in men with visceral obesity, *Am. J. Clin. Nutr.*, 77, 300, 2003.
76. Nestel, P.J. et al., Suppression by diets rich in fish oil of very low density lipoprotein production in man, *J. Clin. Invest.*, 74, 82, 1984.
77. Brenna, J.T., Efficiency of conversion of alpha-linolenic acid to long chain n-3 fatty acids in man, *Curr. Opin. Clin. Nutr. Metab. Care.*, 5, 127, 2002.
78. Lichtenstein, A.H., Trans fatty acids, plasma lipid levels, and risk of developing cardiovascular disease. A statement for healthcare professionals from the American Heart Association, *Circulation*, 95, 2588, 1997.
79. Mensink, R.P. and Katan, M.B., Effect of dietary trans fatty acids on high-density and low-density lipoprotein cholesterol levels in healthy subjects., *N. Engl. J. Med.*, 323, 439, 1990.
80. Lichtenstein, A.H. et al. Comparison of different forms of hydrogenated fats on serum lipid levels in moderately hypercholesterolemic female and male subjects., *N. Engl. J. Med.*, 340, 1933, 1999.
81. Ascherio, A. et al., Trans fatty acids and coronary heart disease, *N. Engl. J. Med.*, 340, 1994, 1999.
82. Stamler, J. and Shekelle, R., Dietary cholesterol and human coronary heart disease. The epidemiologic evidence, *Arch. Pathol. Lab. Med.*, 112, 1032, 1988.
83. Clarke, R. et al., Dietary lipids and blood cholesterol: Quantitative meta-analysis of metabolic ward studies, *BMJ*, 314, 112, 1997.
84. Lichtenstein, A.H. et al., Diet and lifestyle recommendations revision 2006: A scientific statement from the American Heart Association Nutrition Committee., *Circulation*, 114, 82, 2006.
85. Katan, M.B. and Beynen, A.C., Characteristics of human hypo- and hyperresponders to dietary cholesterol, *Am. J. Epidemiol.*, 125, 387, 1987.

86. Brown, L. et al., Cholesterol-lowering effects of dietary fiber: A meta-analysis, *Am. J. Clin. Nutr.*, 69, 30, 1999.
87. Lipsky, H., Gloger, M., and Frishman, W.H., Dietary fiber for reducing blood cholesterol, *J. Clin. Pharmacol.*, 30, 699, 1990.
88. Erkkilä, A.T. et al., Cereal fiber and whole-grain intake are associated with reduced progression of coronary-artery atherosclerosis in postmenopausal women with coronary artery disease, *Am. Heart J.*, 150, 94, 2005.
89. Steffen, L.M. et al., Associations of whole-grain, refined-grain, and fruit and vegetable consumption with risks of all-cause mortality and incident coronary artery disease and ischemic stroke: The Atherosclerosis Risk in Communities (ARIC) Study, *Am. J. Clin. Nutr.*, 78, 383, 2003.
90. Carroll, K.K. and Kurowska, E.M., Soy consumption and cholesterol reduction: Review of animal and human studies, *J. Nutr.*, 125, 594S, 1995.
91. Vega-Lopez, S. and Lichtenstein, A.H., Dietary protein type and cardiovascular disease risk factors, *Prev. Cardiol.*, 8, 31, 2005.
92. Anderson, J.W., Johnstone, B.M., and Cook-Newell, M.E., Meta-analysis of the effects of soy protein intake on serum lipids., *N. Engl. J. Med.*, 333, 276, 1995.
93. Balk, E. et al., Effects of soy on health outcomes, *Evid. Rep.: Technol. Assess. (Summ.)*, 126, 1, 2005.
94. Kreijkamp-Kaspers, S. et al., Effect of soy protein containing isoflavones on cognitive function, bone mineral density, and plasma lipids in postmenopausal women: A randomized controlled trial, *J. Am. Med. Assoc.*, 292, 65, 2004.
95. Sacks, F.M. et al., Soy protein, isoflavones, and cardiovascular health: An American Heart Association Science Advisory for professionals from the Nutrition Committee, *Circulation*, 113, 1034, 2006.
96. Lichtenstein, A.H. et al., Lipoprotein response to diets high in soy or animal protein with and without isoflavones in moderately hypercholesterolemic subjects, *Arterioscler. Thromb. Vasc. Biol.*, 22, 1852, 2002.
97. Lichtenstein, A.H., Plant sterols and blood lipid levels, *Curr. Opin. Nutr. Metab. Care*, 5, 147, 2002.
98. Katan, M.B. et al., Efficacy and safety of plant stanols and sterols in the management of blood cholesterol levels, *Mayo Clin. Proc.*, 78, 965, 2003.
99. Lichtenstein, A.H. and Russell, R.M., Essential nutrients: Food or supplements? Where should the emphasis be? *J. Am. Med. Assoc.*, 294, 351, 2005.
100. Stampfer, M.J. et al., Vitamin E consumption and the risk of coronary disease in women, *N. Engl. J. Med.*, 328, 1444, 1993.
101. Rimm, E.B. et al., Vitamin E consumption and the risk of coronary heart disease in men, *N. Engl. J. Med.*, 328, 1450, 1993.
102. Reaven, P.D. et al. Effect of dietary antioxidant combinations in humans. Protection of LDL by vitamin E but not by β-carotene, *Arterioscler. Thromb.*, 13, 590, 1993.
103. Kris-Etherton, P. et al., Antioxidant vitamin supplements and cardiovascular disease, *Circulation*, 110, 637, 2004.
104. Gibbons, R. J. et al., ACC/AHA 2002 guideline update for the management of patients with chronic stable angina—summary article: A report of the American College of Cardiology/American Heart Association Task Force on Practice Guidelines (Committee on the Management of Patients With Chronic Stable Angina), *Circulation*, 107, 149, 2003.
105. Manson, J.E. et al., A prospective study of walking as compared with vigorous exercise in the prevention of coronary heart disease in women, *N. Engl. J. Med.*, 341, 650, 1999.
106. Albright, C. and Thompson, D.L., The effectiveness of walking in preventing cardiovascular disease in women: A review of the current literature, *J. Women's Health*, 15, 271, 2006.

107. Kelley, G.A., Kelley, K.S., and Tran, Z.V., Aerobic exercise and lipids and lipoproteins in women: A meta-analysis of randomized controlled trials. *J. Women's Health*, 13, 1148, 2004.
108. Manson, J.E. et al., Walking compared with vigorous exercise for the prevention of cardiovascular events in women, *N. Engl. J. Med.*, 347, 716, 2002.
109. Ockene, I.S. and Miller, N.H., Cigarette smoking, cardiovascular disease, and stroke: A statement for healthcare professionals from the American Heart Association. American Heart Association Task Force on Risk Reduction, *Circulation*, 96, 3243, 1997.
110. Naqvi, T.Z., Naqvi, S.S., and Merz, C.N., Gender differences in the link between depression and cardiovascular disease, *Psychosom. Med.*, 67 (Suppl 1), S15, 2005.
111. Mosca, L., McGillen, C., and Rubenfire, M., Gender differences in barriers to lifestyle change for cardiovascular disease prevention, *J. Women's Health*, 7, 711, 1998.

10 Breast and Ovarian Cancer

Bette J. Caan and Cynthia A. Thomson

CONTENTS

10.1 THE CANCER BURDEN

Cancer, a spectrum of diseases that are all characterized by loss of regulation over cell growth and differentiation and acquisition of the ability to metastasize to distant parts of the body, is the second leading cause of death in the United States, accounting for approximately 565,000 deaths, or about 25% of all deaths, each year [1]. In addition to the individual and social burden of the disease, the yearly direct medical costs of cancer are estimated at $60.9 billion and indirect morbidity costs at $15.5 billion [2].

Women are diagnosed with cancer more frequently than men, likely related to their prolonged lifespan and the fact that age is a major predictor of cancer risk [3]. Over 660,000 new cases of cancer are diagnosed annually in women. While for the majority of cancers the burden is equivalent across genders, certainly this is not always true. For example, while colorectal cancer and non-Hodgkin lymphomas are diagnosed in males and females at relatively equal rates, women appear to be at a greater risk for breast and thyroid cancer and are diagnosed with bladder cancers less frequently (Figure 10.1). For lung cancer the secular trend that showed a substantial increase in risk among males starting in the mid-1940s did

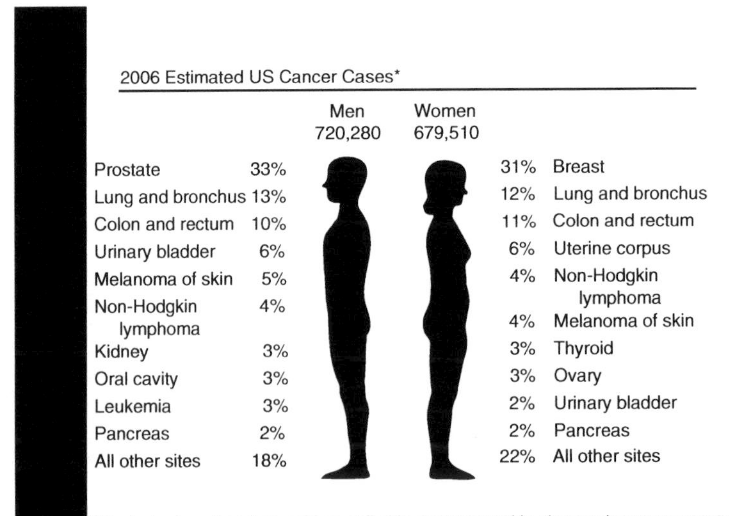

FIGURE 10.1 2006 Estimated US cancer cases. American Cancer Society, 2006.

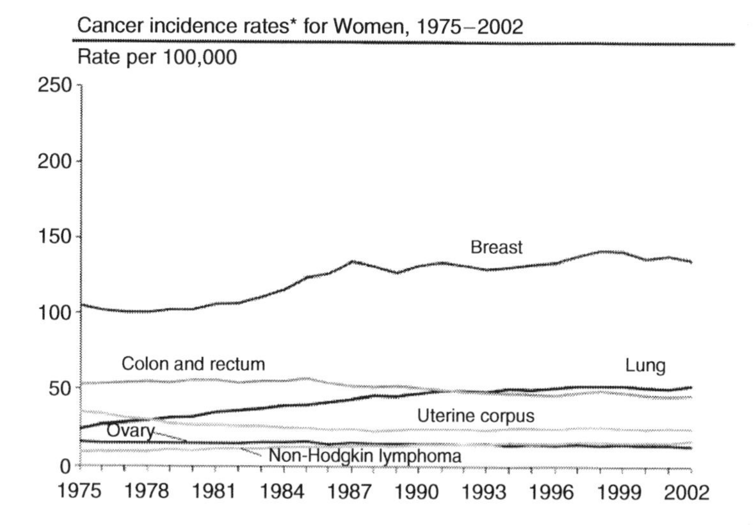

FIGURE 10.2 Cancer incidence rates for women 1975–2002.

not demonstrate a significant rise in incidence until the mid-1970s for females. This pattern is supported by trends in tobacco use by gender since the early 1900s.

Two cancers that are of particular concern for females are breast and ovarian cancer. Among women, breast cancer occurs most commonly, representing about one-third of all new cases; and has an age-adjusted incidence rate of 129.1 per 100,000 (Figure 10.2). Although in women, lung cancer and colorectal cancer are the second and third most commonly occurring cancers, respectively, ovarian cancer is associated with an especially high morbidity and mortality (Figure 10.3). Trends in breast and ovarian cancer diagnosis suggest that incidence, while increasing for breast cancer in recent years, is slightly reduced for ovarian cancer, with rates down a modest 0.7% annually for the past two decades (Figure 10.3).

It is important to note that second to lung cancer, breast cancer is the leading cause of cancer death worldwide among women [4] (Table 10.1). However, especially in North America, survival rates for breast cancer have improved substantially such that just under 100% of women with ductal carcinoma in situ, 98% of women with stage I, 88% of women diagnosed with stage IIA, and 76% of women with stage IIB disease will be alive 5 years after their diagnosis [3].

Survival after a diagnosis of ovarian cancer is much lower than for breast cancer, related primarily to the fact that less than 20% of cases are diagnosed before the disease is regionally invasive. Only 76% of women diagnosed with ovarian cancer survive even 12 months and less than 50% are alive at 5 year postdiagnosis [3].

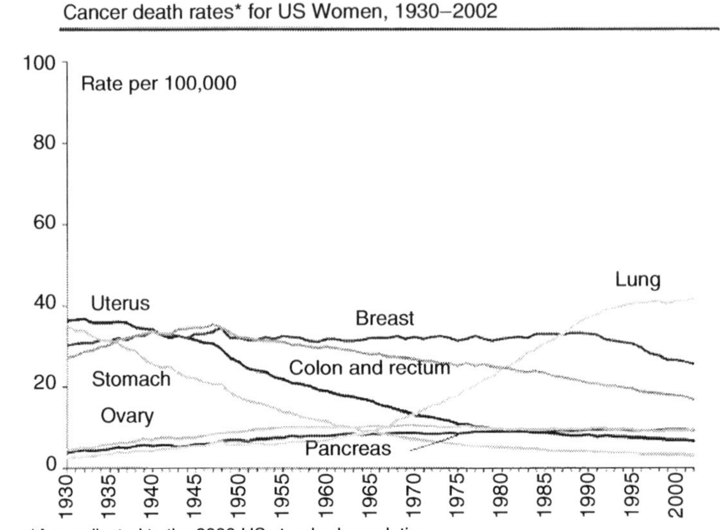

FIGURE 10.3 Cancer death rates for US women, 1930–2002.

The mean age at which a woman is diagnosed with breast cancer worldwide is estimated to be 61 years and for ovarian cancer 63 years [5], ages at which most women remain productive members of society, suggesting that the economic impact in lost work is likely significant.

10.2 BREAST AND OVARIAN CANCER: ETIOLOGY AND RISK FACTORS

10.2.1 Introduction

While genetic susceptibility plays a role in cancer etiology, environmental factors are considered more important, and may explain as much as 80%–90% of the variability in disease occurrence [6]. Among the environmental influences, lifestyle factors, specifically: diet, obesity, physical inactivity and tobacco use, account for about a third of all cancers [1]. This is especially true for breast and ovarian cancer. A comprehensive review of the literature regarding the role of nutrition and physical activity in the prevention of cancer has been discussed in detail recently in the American Cancer Society Guidelines on Nutrition and Physical Activity for Cancer Prevention [7] and, in 1997, and will be updated in 2007 by an expert panel convened by the American Institute for Cancer Research and the World Cancer Research Fund in Food Nutrition and the Prevention of Cancer: a global prospective [8].

TABLE 10.1
Estimated Breast Cancer Cases/Deaths Worldwide

Region	New Cases (2000)	Deaths (2000)
Eastern Africa	13,615	6,119
Middle Africa	3,902	1,775
Northern Africa	18,724	8,388
Southern Africa	5,537	2,504
Western Africa	17,389	7,830
Caribbean	6,210	2,310
Central America	18,663	5,888
South America	69,924	22,735
Northern America	202,044	51,184
Eastern Asia	142,656	38,826
South-Eastern Asia	55,907	24,961
South Central Asia	129,620	62,212
Western Asia	20,155	8,459
Eastern Europe	110,975	43,058
Northern Europe	54,551	20,992
Southern Europe	65,284	25,205
Western Europe	115,308	40,443
Australia/New Zealand	12,748	3,427
Melanesia	470	209
Micronesia	62	28
Polynesia	127	58

Source: From Ferlay, J., Bray, F., Pisani, P., and Parkin, D.M. in *GLOBOCAN 2000: Cancer Incidence, Mortality and Prevalence Worldwide, Version 1.0,* IARC Press, Lyon, 2001, IARC CancerBase No. 5. With permission.

In addition, the role of lifestyle in cancer prevention has been the subject of study in numerous ecological and epidemiological studies, as well as in some meta-analyses, pooled projects, and clinical trials [9,10].

This chapter will review data on the associations between nutritional factors and the development of breast and ovarian cancer. Both of these cancers will be discussed with regard to dietary fat intake and fruit and vegetable intake as well as body size and physical activity. Common underlying mechanisms that have been suggested to contribute to risk or protection for these cancers will be described and a review of risk factors will be offered. Additionally, nutrients of particular relevance and a brief discussion of nonnutrient risk factors specific to each cancer site will be provided. Since the majority of data come from epidemiologic studies, the observed associations will be considered in terms of generally accepted criteria for inference of causality. Those criteria include (1) strength of the association; (2) consistency of the association across different studies in different populations; (3) existence of appropriate temporal relations; and (4) existence of a dose–response relation. In the cases where meta-analyses or pooled studies or even randomized clinical trials have been performed, considerable weight will be given to those types of analyses. This chapter will utilize the expert consensus from the aforementioned comprehensive reports and review more recent work that has not been included in these documents to help draw conclusions about associations. Additionally, the chapter will consider dietary guidelines for following a healthy lifestyle and potentially reducing the risk of breast and ovarian cancer given our current knowledge. Finally, suggestions for future research will be given both throughout and at the conclusion of the chapter.

10.2.2 Overview

Numerous risk factors for breast and ovarian cancer have been described, many of which are associated with both cancers. Generally, these factors can be categorized as genetic/demographic, nutritional/behavioral as well as hormonal. Table 10.2 summarizes established and suspected risk factors for these two more common cancers diagnosed among women.

10.2.3 Nonnutrient Risk Factors

10.2.3.1 Breast Cancer

Breast cancer risk increases with advancing age and both incidence and mortality rates for non-Hispanic white and black women are considerably higher than for other ethnic groups [5]. A family history of breast cancer is a well-established risk factor for disease with an approximate twofold increase in incidence [8], but an even greater increase in risk if a first degree relative is affected [11]. Mammographic density, hypothesized to be marker of cell proliferation in the breast, is also associated with increased risk [11].

A number of reproductive, related risk factors for breast cancer have been established. Risk is increased by early onset of menarche, nulliparity, late age at first birth, and late natural menopause [8,12]. Menarche represents the onset of monthly cycling of hormones that induce ovulation, menstruation, and cell proliferation within the breast and endometrium. Breast cancer risk usually decreases by 10%–24% with each 1 year delay in menarche [13]. Nulliparous women are at higher risk than nonparous women and a higher number of births have been associated with reduced lifetime risk. In addition to number, closer spaced births may also confer benefit, giving the breast less time to accumulate DNA damage between pregnancies [11]. A younger age at first full-term pregnancy predicts a lower lifetime risk of breast cancer, reflecting the final maturation of the breast with hormonal exposures during first pregnancy and preparation for lactation [11].

Menopause marks the end of monthly cycling of hormones that induce regular breast cell proliferation; each year of delay is associated with a 3% increase in breast cancer risk [14]. In short, an increase in reproductive lifetime that starts at an early age and ends later in life and has few interruptions for pregnancy and lactation is related to an increased risk in breast cancer. This points to a role for endogenous hormones, specifically estrogen, as playing a major role in the underlying mechanisms attributed to increased breast cancer incidence [8].

TABLE 10.2
Established and Suspected Risk Factors for Breast and Ovarian Cancer

Cancer Type	Genetic/Demographic	Type of Association	Nutritional/Behavioral	Type of Association	Hormonal/Reproductive	Type of Association
Breast	Family history of breast cancer	+	Premenopausal obesity	−	Early menarche	+
	Non-Hispanic White and Black women	+	Postmenopausal obesity/	+	Short cycle length	+
			substantial adult weight gain	−	Low parity	+
	Mamographic density/benign breast disease	+	Regular physical activity		Young age at first full-term pregnancy	−
			Diet	?−		
	High socioeconomic status	+	Low total fat	?−	Lactation (>1 yr)	−
	Increasing age	+	Omega-3 fatty acids/fish	?−	Late age at menopause	−
			High fruit and vegetables	?−	Oral contraceptive use	+
			Carotenoids	+	Recent or long-term HRT use; estrogen plus progestin and to a lesser degree unopposed estrogen	+
			Alcohol			

(*continued*)

TABLE 10.2 (Continued)
Established and Suspected Risk Factors for Breast and Ovarian Cancer

Cancer Type	Genetic/Demographic	Type of Association	Nutritional/Behavioral	Type of Association	Hormonal/Reproductive	Type of Association
Ovarian	Family history of breast or ovarian cancer	+	Obesity/higher BMI	+	Low parity	+
			Perimenopausal weight gain	?+	Oral contraceptive agents	–
	European/Asian ethnicity	+	Increased lean body mass in early life	?–	Tubal ligation	–
					HRT use; unopposed estrogen	+
			Height	+	Postmenopausal	+
			Diet		No history of lactation	+
			High in total fat	?+		
			High in cholesterol	?+		
			High in carotenoids	–		
			High in vegetables	?–		
			High cruciferous vegetable	?–		
			Supplemental Vitamin C, E	?–		
			Physical activity			
			Inadequate	?+		
			Excessive	?+		
			Regular, moderate level	–		
			Alcohol (wine)	?–		
			Greater pack-years of smoking	?+		

+ indicates a positive association.
– indicates a negative association.
? indicates a suspected, but not sufficiently investigated association.

Exogenous hormones play a role in breast cancer risk as well. Current use of oral contraceptives has been associated with a small increase in risk at a time when absolute risk of breast cancer is low [11]. Hormone therapy (HT), in contrast, is associated with an increase in breast cancer risk that has a much larger attributable risk because HT is used at a time when breast cancer risk is substantially higher. The risk for breast cancer associated with HT appears to be strongest for those using a combination of estrogen plus progestin rather than those using unopposed estrogen [15–18] and is probably confined to current users or users of long duration [19].

10.2.3.2 Ovarian Cancer

Family history of cancer, and specifically hormone-related cancer, appears to increase the risk for ovarian cancer. Further, an earlier diagnosis of breast cancer has been associated with increased risk for ovarian cancer, particularly among BRCA carriers [20]. The evidence associating reproductive factors with breast cancer is more complete than for ovarian cancer. In the case of ovarian cancer, a greater number of live births as well as oral contraceptive use and tubal ligation are associated with a reduction in risk, while other factors such as HT use show inconsistent associations [21,22]. This may be related to duration of use or type of HT used in that unopposed estrogen use appears to increase risk while combined estrogen–progesterone therapy may not. Further, age at first pregnancy and age at menopause, while considered important factors in the development of breast cancer, have not been reported to be significant risk factors for ovarian cancer, suggesting that either these relationships have not been fully explored in the context of ovarian cancer or that other reproductive factors influence risk to a much greater extent than age-specificity of these biological events.

10.2.4 Body Size: Obesity and Weight Gain

10.2.4.1 Breast Cancer

While there is a general acceptance that adult body mass is related to breast cancer risk, the association between these two factors is dependent on several things. There appears to be an interaction between body size and breast cancer risk. Menopausal status and body size are generally weakly related to postmenopausal breast cancer, but inversely related to premenopausal breast cancer [8]. This interaction has been demonstrated in a number of studies and most convincingly in two pooled projects with large sample sizes. A pooled analysis published in 2000 [23] which included data from seven cohort studies comprised of 337,819 women and 4385 incident breast cancers found that obese premenopausal women had a reduced risk of breast cancer (BMI >31 kg/m^2 compared to <21 kg/m^2 RR 0.54; 95% CI 0.34, 0.85) and overweight and obese postmenopausal women had an increased risk of breast cancer (BMI >28 kg/m^2 compared to <21 kg/m^2 RR 1.26; 95% CI 1.09, 1.46). A more recent pooled analysis of 176,886 women and 1879 incident breast cancer cases from the European Prospective Investigation into Cancer (EPIC) study consisting of cohorts from nine countries [24] found an increased risk in postmenopausal women who were not hormone users and an inverse relationship in premenopausal women.

The most prevailing theory to explain the inverse relationship in premenopausal women is that younger women who are significantly overweight are more likely to be anovulatory [25], which in and of itself is associated with decreased estradiol and progesterone levels that may explain lower breast cancer rates [26]. It also has been suggested that because heavier women have less dense breasts. It is breast density that is related to breast cancer risk, since when breast density is controlled for, the association between BMI and breast cancer risk in premenopausal women becomes positive [27].

For postmenopausal women, obesity may increase breast cancer risk by affecting levels of endogenous estrogens, through the conversion of androstendione to estrogens in adipose tissue. As mentioned above, the relationship, while relatively consistent across studies, [8] has been weak in terms of magnitude. Further, it may be obscured among women using exogenous hormones who are already at elevated risk of breast cancer [24,28].

There is accumulating evidence that adult weight gain is related to breast cancer risk [29–31], but this relationship may be dependent on menopausal status and may be more pronounced in women who do not use hormones. It is also unclear if this relationship is independent of obesity at the time of diagnosis or if certain periods of weight gain in the lifespan are more critical than others and if subsequent weight loss modifies risk, particularly in relation to the menopausal transition period.

The Nurses' Health Study [30], the EPIC cohort [29], and the American Cancer Society Cancer Prevention Study II Nutrition Cohort [28], all large prospective cohorts, report an ~50% increase (RR 1.45, 1.50, and 1.54, respectively) in risk of postmenopausal breast cancer in relation to adult weight gain that becomes apparent at gains in the range of 20 or more kilograms. This relationship was either more pronounced [30] or only evident [29,32] in women not using menopausal hormone therapy. Several studies have suggested that preventing weight gain from age 30 to menopause [31] or from the first pregnancy to menopause [33] may be most clinically relevant and others have suggested that substantial weight loss postmenopause can modify this increased risk [30]. While adult weight gain and adult obesity may be closely related, understanding critical periods of risk warrants further investigation and may help disentangle these relationships and clarify underlying mechanisms.

10.2.4.2 Ovarian Cancer

The evidence for an effect of body size on ovarian cancer risk (as compared to breast cancer) is less extensive, but expanding. Obesity and higher body mass index (BMI) have been associated with increased risk for ovarian cancer in several, but not all, case-control and cohort studies conducted in the United States and internationally [34–38]. Data from the Iowa Women's Health Study indicate increased risk of ovarian cancer development among women with higher waist-to-hip ratio [39], a likely manifestation of insulin resistance. The Western New York Diet Study suggested that BMI was not associated with an increased risk for ovarian cancer, building on earlier data from this same cohort published in 1983 by Byers et al. that presented data from a study of 274 women diagnosed with ovarian cancer and 1034 hospital controls which suggested that, among women over age 50 years, obesity might reduce risk for ovarian cancer ($p < 0.10$) [22]. Of interest, but insufficiently explored, is the notion that body weight may be differentially associated with various histologic types of epithelial ovarian cancer as suggested by a pooled analysis conducted by Kurian which showed an inverse association between serous-type cancer and body mass index, but not other histological types [40].

As has been suggested for breast cancer, another factor that may influence the relationship between body weight and ovarian cancer risk is timing of weight gain over one's lifespan. The England study conducted in Norway showed a significant increased risk for ovarian cancer among women reporting BMIs in the overweight or obesity ranges during adolescence and early adulthood, but not when BMI was increased in later life [41]. In a Chinese cohort study, BMI at age 21 years was not associated with increased risk for or survival from ovarian cancer even among obese women [38].

10.2.5 Body Size: Height

10.2.5.1 Breast Cancer

Attention to the relationship of breast cancer with height has increased in recent years due to increased interest in the effects of early diet on breast cancer risk in later life. Early nutritional factors affect both rate of growth and adult height within a range of genetic potential [8]. It has been hypothesized that growth factors that contribute to skeletal growth also contribute to the proliferation of mammary cell stems and increase mammary mass [42], as well as promote the early onset of puberty, which itself is a risk factor for breast cancer. The American Institute for Cancer Research (AICR) panel report concluded that the evidence that rapid growth is a risk factor for breast cancer is convincing [8]. Since the AICR report findings, several large pooled analyses have corroborated these findings. In two separate pooled analyses, the first consisting of 337,819 women across seven prospective cohort studies [23], and the EPIC study of cohorts from nine different European countries including 200,000 women [24], the pooled RR for a 5 cm increment in height were 1.02 (95% CI 0.96, 1.10) and 1.05 (95% CI 1.00–1.16), respectively in premenopausal women and 1.07 (95% CI 1.03, 1.12) and 1.10 (95% CI 1.05–1.16) in postmenopausal women, supporting a role of growth, as assessed by adult height, and breast cancer risk.

10.2.5.2 Ovarian Cancer

Consistent with the breast cancer studies, greater adult height has also been associated with increased risk for ovarian cancer, although fewer studies assessing this relationship have been conducted. For example, the Netherlands cohort study showed a greater than twofold increased risk for developing ovarian cancer among women whose height measured at least 175 cm vs. women with heights below 160 cm [43]. Further, a Norwegian cohort study suggested that risk was increased most significantly for ovarian cancer in relation to greater adult height [41].The American Cancer Society cohort study of over 300,000 adults residing in the United States reported 1511 deaths due to ovarian cancer, and risk for ovarian cancer was significantly increased among women with adult height of greater than 177 cm [44].

10.2.6 Body Size: Birthweight

10.2.6.1 Breast Cancer

The relationship between birthweight, a proxy for in utero growth, and breast cancer risk has been studied for the past decade. It has been postulated [45] that high levels of estrogens and of the insulin-like growth factor-1 system during the prenatal period are associated with higher birthweight and a higher number of mammary-tissue specific stems cells. In addition to increasing mammary mass, the higher number of stems cells may increase susceptibility to DNA mutations, one possible mechanism proposed for increasing adult breast cancer risk. This association has been studied by many authors and most, but not all, studies have found support for an association between birthweight and breast cancer [46]. Michels and Xue [47] in their review of 26 papers examining the association between birthweight and subsequent breast cancer risk found a combined relative risk of 1.23 (95% CI 1.13–1.34) comparing women with high birthweight to these with low birthweight, with more support for effect on premenopausal than postmenopausal breast cancer risk. A recent Swedish cohort study of 38,566 women confirmed this finding of an effect in premenopausal, but not postmenopausal women [48]. Future investigation is needed to identify whether growth patterns occurring later in childhood and adulthood may modify this relationship. No studies reporting the association between birthweight and ovarian cancer risk are currently available, but given other overlapping risk factors this association should be explored.

10.2.7 Physical Activity

10.2.7.1 Breast Cancer

The role of physical activity in preventing the development of breast cancer has been studied extensively, particularly over the past decade [49,51]. The studies of physical activity and breast cancer have considered both recreational and occupational physical activity, usually by means of self-report, but with widely differing methods of ascertainment ranging from a single, global question [51,52] to quantitative questionnaires asking for details regarding type, intensity, frequency, and duration of different activities [53,54]. Activity at some point in adulthood has been most frequently assessed, and some studies have examined activity around the time of puberty or young adulthood, while still others have attempted to assess lifetime activity or activity at various times of life.

The findings for breast cancer suggest a reasonably clear, modest reduction of about 20%–30% in risk of breast cancer for active women compared to sedentary women [50,55] and a meta-analysis concluded that the increased relative risk associated with inactivity was 1.25 (95% CI 1.20–1.30) for women age 15–44 years, but 1.34 (95% CI 1.29–1.39) for women age 45–69 years [56].

The inverse relation between physical activity and breast cancer appears to be modified by menopausal status, and perhaps, by other factors. The risk reduction is larger among postmenopausal women [49,50], and, in at least some studies, is not even evident among premenopausal women [54,57,58]. In the Norwegian–Swedish

Women's Lifestyle and Health cohort study, where 99,504 women aged 30 and 49 years were followed for an average of 9.1 years, no association was observed between breast cancer incidence and physical activity at ages 14, 30, or enrollment [59]. This finding raises the possibility that the risk of breast cancer occurring during the perimenopausal years may also be less affected by physical activity.

The evidence regarding effect modification of the physical activity–breast cancer relation by other factors, such as BMI and hormone use, is inconsistent [50]. For instance, the risk reduction with physical activity was essentially limited to the leanest women in the Women's Health Initiative (WHI) Cohort [60], as well as in a large Norwegian cohort [61], but in a population-based case-control study, the risk reduction was greatest in the women who were heaviest at age 18 [62]. Although no overall relation between physical activity and breast cancer was observed in the Nurses' Health Study II, stratification by oral contraceptive use revealed a nonsignificant inverse association in current users [58]. In contrast, a nonsignificant interaction ($p = 0.09$) between physical activity and hormone therapy was observed in the American Cancer Society Cancer Prevention Study II Nutrition Cohort that suggested a marginally greater decrease in risk with physical activity among women who were not current hormone users [63].

An important question about the relation between physical activity and breast cancer occurrence is the appropriate time frame of exposure. However, studies that have focused on physical activity around the time of puberty or in young adulthood [64–66] have generally observed weaker associations than those focusing on current activity. A number of studies have found strong inverse associations between lifetime activity and breast cancer risk [67–71], suggesting that consistent participation in physical activity throughout adulthood may influence breast cancer risk more than activity at any specific point in time.

10.2.7.2 Ovarian Cancer

In contrast to breast cancer, the data on physical activity and ovarian cancer risk are suggestive, but far less convincing, that engagement in regular physical activity will reduce the risk of ovarian cancer. In the population-based case-control study conducted in the context of the Canadian Cancer Registries Epidemiological Research Group [72], which included 442 epithelial ovarian cancer cases, frequency of total recreational physical activity was associated with a significant reduction in ovarian cancer risk (OR 0.73; 95% CI 0.58–0.93).

However, in the Iowa Women's Health Study, among women with the highest levels of physical activity, ovarian cancer risk was actually increased, suggesting that extremes in activity (nonactive and excessively active) could enhance risk while a moderate level of physical activity will reduce risk [39]. This "U-shape" response curve is also theorized by research from Bertone [73] and colleagues using data from the Nurses' Health Study that suggested that frequent vigorous activity in contrast to moderate activity may actually increase ovarian cancer risk, although the trend was not statistically significant [73]. The Netherlands cohort study also supports this hypothesis showing an inverse association between moderate physical activity and ovarian cancer risk [74].

Several plausible biological mechanisms exist that suggest a protective effect of physical activity on both breast and ovarian cancer. The hypothesized mechanisms include modulating hormone levels, control of body weight and fatness, and enhanced immune function [50]. The most recent guidelines from the American Cancer Society [7] suggest that the best nutritional advice is to engage in moderate to vigorous exercise on a regular basis to reduce cancer risk.

10.2.8 Diet and Cancer Overview

10.2.8.1 Breast Cancer

There have been several decades of research on diet and breast cancer risk and while the literature is voluminous from individual studies, the evidence for individual dietary components on risk of breast cancer remains inconsistent. Table 10.3 summarizes the evidence from select research, including only meta-analyses or pooled analyses for those food groups where there is either considerable controversy, such as fat or fruits and vegetables, or a demonstrated effect such as alcohol. The recent ACS report also suggests that in addition to engaging in moderate physical activity, women also minimize lifetime weight gain through caloric restriction and physical activity and avoid or limit intake of alcoholic beverages to reduce cancer risk.

10.2.8.2 Ovarian Cancer

The relationship between dietary factors and ovarian cancer risk has been explored for several decades, yet no consistent protective dietary pattern has been identified. Table 10.4 summarizes the evidence from several larger cohort and case-control studies. Generally it has been suggested, consistent with other cancer preventive dietary recommendations, that women reduce their intake of dietary fat, total calories, and cholesterol while increasing intake of vegetables in an effort to reduce ovarian cancer risk. Further, maintaining a healthy body weight throughout adulthood will likely also reduce risk.

10.2.9 Dietary Fat

10.2.9.1 Breast Cancer

The relationship between fat intake and breast cancer has been the subject of considerable controversy over the last several decades. The hypothesis that diets high in dietary fat increase breast cancer risk was generated originally by ecological data demonstrating that per capita availability of fat consumption was highly correlated with both breast cancer incidence and mortality rates [75]. Animal data supported this theory by demonstrating that high fat diets increased the occurrence of mammary tumors in rodents [76].

Observational data, in contrast, have not demonstrated a clear relationship between fat intake and breast cancer risk. Data from case-control studies have generally shown a positive relationship while those from prospective studies have not. In 1990, meta-analyses of 12 case-control studies [77], based upon 4312 cases and 5978 controls examining the relationship of total fat to breast cancer incidence, demonstrated a significant increased risk for breast cancer with higher intakes of fat

TABLE 10.3
Dietary Factors and Breast Cancer Risk

Study	Sample Size	Fat Variable	Outcome	Comments
Dietary Fat				
Howe, 1990 Meta-analyses Case-control studies	4,312 cases/5,978 controls	Total fat per 100 gm increase	Overall OR 1.3	Significant for postmenopausal but not premenopausal women
Hunter, 1996 Meta-analyses Cohort studies	337,819 4,980 breast cancer cases	Total fat Highest quintile compared to lowest	RR 1.05 (CI 0.94–1.16)	No significant association for total fat or for saturated, mono, or poly-unsaturated fat
Boyd, 2003 Meta-analyses, Case-control and cohort studies	45 studies	Total fat Highest vs. lowest level	RR 1.13 (CI 1.03–1.25) RR 1.11 (CI 0.99–1.25) RR 1.14 (CI 0.99–1.32)	Overall 14 cohort studies 31 case-control studies significant increased risk for saturated fat
Prentice, 2006 Randomized clinical trial	48,835 women	Low fat diet pattern ≤20% kcal from fat compared to control	HR 0.91 (CI 0.83–1.01)	Women with diets high in fat intially had a sign 22% reduction in risk of breast cancer
Maclean, 2006 Systematic review	11 different studies	Omega-3 fatty acids	RR 1.47 (CI 1.10–1.98) RR range 0.68–0.72	1 increased risk 3 decreased risk 7 no significant association

(continued)

TABLE 10.3 (Continued)
Dietary Factors and Breast Cancer Risk

Study	Sample Size	Fat Variable	Outcome	Comments
Fruits and vegetables		**Fruits and vegetables variable**		
Gandini, 2000 Meta-analyses Case-control and cohort	17 studies	High consumption vs. low consumption	RR 0.75 (CI 0.66–0.85) RR 0.94 (CI 0.79–1.11)	Vegetables, 17 studies Fruits, 12 studies Significant decreased risk for β-carotene and Vit C
Smith–Warner, 2000 Meta-analyses	351,825 women 7377 BC cases	Highest vs. lowest quintile	RR 0.96 (CI 0.89–1.04) RR 0.93 (CI 0.86–1.00)	Vegetables Fruits Weak assoc. for fruits but not vegetables
Riboli, 2003 Meta-analyses Case-control and cohort	25 studies	Per 100g/d increase	RR 0.91 (CI 0.86–0.97) RR 0.94 (CI 0.94–0.99)	Vegetables Fruits Both vegetables and fruits were significant for case-control but not cohort studies
Gills, 2006 Multi-country cohort study	285,526 women 3659 BC cases	Highest vs. lowest quintile	RR 0.98 (CI 0.84–1.14) RR 1.09 (CI 0.94–1.25)	Vegetables

				Fruit No significant association for fruits, veg., or any of six specific vegetable subgroups
Alcohol		**Alcohol variable**		
Smith-Warner 1998	322,647 women	Per 10g/day of alcohol	RR 1.09 (CI 1.04–1.13)	Specific type of alcohol did not influence risk
Meta-analyses of Cohort studies	4335 BC cases	2–5 drinks/day vs. none	RR 1.41 (CI 1.18–1.69)	
Collaborative Group on Hormonal Factors in BC (Hamajima N, 2002)	53 studies	Per 10g/day of alcohol	RR 1.07 (CI 1.06–1.09)	
Meta-analyses Case-control and cohort studies	58,515 BC cases	3–4 drinks/day vs. none	RR 1.46 (CI 1.33–1.61)	
Key J, 2006 Meta-analyses Case-control and cohort	98 studies 75,728 BC cases	Per 10 g/day of alcohol	RR 1.10 (CI 1.05–1.15)	Specific type of alcohol did not influence risk
Soy intake		**Soy variable**		
Trock, 2006 Meta-analyses Case-control and cohort	18 studies	High vs. low soy intake	RR 0.86 (CI 0.75–0.99)	Stronger for premenopausal than for postmenopausal but significant in both

TABLE 10.4
Dietary Factors and Ovarian Cancer Risk

Study	Sample Size Case/Controls	Vegetables	Alcohol	Fat/Cholesterol	Milk/Dairy
Case-Control					
Webb, 2004	696/786		0.49 (0.3–0.81) (wine)		
Kuper, 2000	549/516		No significant association		
Pan, 2004	442/2135	Total vegetables—No significant association; Cruciferous—0.76 (CI 0.56–0.99)	No significant association	Total fat—no significant association; Cholesterol—1.42 (1.03–1.97)	No significant association
Nagel, 2003 (recurrence)	609	HR 0.75, 95% CI 0.57–0.99, *p* for trend, 0.01			
Tung, 2005	558/607	β-carotene 0.66 (CI 0.45–0.97)			
Cohort					
Iowa Women's Health Kushi, 1999	208 cases	RR 0.44–1.00, *p* for trend, 0.01			
Swedish mammography Li, 2003	285 cases	RR 0.61 for 3 srvg/day vs. <1 (CI 0.38–0.97)			
Meta-analysis					
Koushik, 2005	Cohort studies w/2012 cases	No significant association			

(OR 1.35, $p < 0.0001$ for 100 g daily increase in fat intake) and the association was significant for postmenopausal breast cancer (OR 1.48, $p < 0.0001$), but not premenopausal breast cancer (OR 1.1 ns). In contrast, using only prospective studies [78], a meta-analyses of seven studies investigating the relationship of total fat to breast cancer incidence that included 4980 cases from studies involving 337,819 women, did not find a statistically significant risk (RR 1.1; CI 0.9–1.2) in breast cancer with greater intake of fat. Another meta-analyses including studies published up until July 2003 including 45 risk estimates [79], but including a combination of case-control and cohort studies of dietary fat and breast cancer had a summary relative risk of 1.13 (95% CI 1.03–1.25) comparing the highest and lowest level intakes of fat with no apparent differences seen between estimates from case-control compared to cohort studies.

Some have speculated that the failure to find a fat–breast cancer association in prospective observational studies is due in part to measurement error in reporting dietary fat intake using food frequency questionnaires (FFQ) [80,81]. Large cohort studies often rely on the self-administered FFQ because of cost and logistics, while case-control studies, smaller in size, often use a more detailed diet history that is frequently interviewer-administered. To try and better understand the effect of FFQ measurement error on the association of dietary fat to breast cancer incidence two recent cohort studies compared the association using two different dietary instruments, a FFQ and a food record. Of interest, when dietary fat is measured using food records, there was a positive significant relationship identified between total fat and breast cancer risk, but no relationship was seen when the FFQ is used to estimate fat intake [82,83].

The WHI, a randomized clinical trial designed to test whether a low fat diet could reduce the risk of breast cancer incidence in postmenopausal women has recently been completed [9] and is the largest randomized trial to test the effect of a low fat dietary pattern on breast cancer risk. A total of 48,835 women were randomized to either a low fat dietary pattern or control with an aim to reduce fat intake to 20% of calories from fat in the intervention group. After ~8 years of follow-up the intervention group had a marginally significant 9% lower risk of breast cancer incidence (HR 0.91; CI 0.83–1.01). Women whose diets were highest in fat initially (>37% calories from fat) and randomized to the low fat (<20% caloric intake) intervention had a statistically significant 22% reduction in risk of breast cancer (HR 0.77; CI 0.64–0.95).

While the results from WHI are not conclusive, they do suggest that certain subgroups, such as those with current high fat diets, may benefit from a reduction in dietary fat intake. In addition, since the majority of women did not reach the 20% target of percent energy from fat, but reached only about two-third of the targeted reduction, it is possible that larger reductions in fat or longer follow-up will result in more conclusive results. Follow up is underway.

Some animal studies have found effects of specific dietary fats on mammary tumor growth, but the evidence from human studies is not convincing for any fat subtype. Most recently, select studies have suggested that fish intake may be associated with a decrease in risk of breast cancer [84,85]. However, a recent systematic review from 11 prospective studies of omega-3 fatty acids (for which marine oils are the main source) on breast cancer risk did not strongly support this association: one showed a statistically significant increased risk (RR 1.47), three showed a statistically significant decreased risk (RR 0.68–0.72) and seven showed no significant association [86].

Considering results from WHI and data reported from ecological [74], case-control studies [77] and the few cohort studies that have used food records to measure dietary intake [82,83] the evidence for the fat–breast cancer hypothesis, while far from convincing, suggests a weak association that still deserves further investigation. It is also possible that a reduction in fat may not by itself be adequate and that changes in other lifestyle factors such as weight gain prevention and increases in physical activity must accompany dietary changes to demonstrate larger effects on breast cancer risk.

Data from large cohort studies using methodology other than food frequencies, data examining diet at periods earlier in a woman's life, periods not so proximal to breast cancer events, and longer follow-up on the WHI should all continue to be explored. Additionally, more understanding of the underlying mechanisms by which diets high in fat may increase breast cancer risk may help identify particular subpopulations, tumor subtypes, or periods of risk that are most likely to benefit from dietary fat reduction.

10.2.9.2 Ovarian Cancer

Similar to breast cancer, much of the interest relating dietary fat intake to risk for ovarian cancer is grounded in mechanistic evidence that dietary fat modulates immunity (including inflammatory response), alters hormone levels/exposure, contributes to body weight and adiposity when consumed in excess, and thus indirectly promotes elevation in insulin-like growth factors.

As early as 1986, Rose et al. was able to determine a positive association between dietary fat intake and ovarian cancer risk [87]. Adoption of a Western diet, which is higher in dietary fat, has been identified as a plausible explanation for the increase in ovarian cancer among Japanese women immigrating to the United States [88] and has also been associated with increased ovarian cancer mortality in Japan [89]. Other studies have indicated that high fat intake, high animal protein intake, and higher total energy intake all are associated with an increased risk for ovarian cancer. For example, evidence from several epidemiological studies as well as a large meta-analysis showed that diets high in saturated fat, red meat, and animal fat were associated with a significant increase in risk for ovarian cancer [90]. Higher red meat consumption was associated with increased risk for ovarian cancer in an Italian case-control study (OR 1.3; 95% CI 1.1–1.5) [91]. Most recently the WHI trial found that, compared to controls, those randomized to a low fat dietary pattern had a lower risk (HR 0.83; 95% CI 0.60–1.14; weighted p-value 0.3) of ovarian cancer (Ross Prentice, personal communication). Yet, other evidence suggests no significant relationship between dietary fat intake and ovarian cancer risk [92,93]. Monounsaturated fat intake has been suggested to be protective [94,95].

A prospective analysis among women participating in the Iowa Women's Health Study suggested that epithelial ovarian cancer was associated with greater cholesterol intake (RR 1.00–1.55, p for trend, 0.06) particularly among women who consumed greater than four eggs/week (RR 1.00–1.81, p for trend, 0.04) [96], an association that appears to be independent of dietary fat intake. The increased risk associated with egg intake was corroborated in a case-control study among Australian women [97], but not in a more recent analysis from the Swedish Mammography cohort [98].

Thus, while the evidence is not convincing, most researchers and clinicians recognize the potential beneficial role of a low fat diet in reducing ovarian cancer risk. Further studies specifically addressing various types of fat including monounsaturated vs. saturated fat as well as exposure to trans fatty acids are needed to provide more conclusive evidence of the role of dietary fat in ovarian cancer prevention. In addition, more definitive information as to the protective or detrimental "dose" of specific fatty acids is required.

10.2.10 Fruits, Vegetables, and Carotenoids

10.2.10.1 Breast Cancer

Fruits and vegetables are foods that contain any number of the following food/nutrient components that may protect against cancer initiation and progress: vitamins, minerals, fiber, carotenoids, and other bioactive substances, such as flavonoids, lignans, terpenes, sterols, indoles, and phenols.

In 1997 the AICR report [8], based on articles published up until 1996, concluded that, "Almost all data from epidemiological studies on fruit and vegetable intake and breast cancer risk show either decreased risk with higher intakes or no relationship: the evidence is more abundant and consistent for vegetables, particularly green vegetables, than for fruits. Diets high in vegetables and fruits probably decrease the risk of breast cancer." Among the particular nutrients present in fruits and vegetables, they concluded that the evidence was strongest for carotenoids and Vitamin C. This statement is unlikely to change substantially in the 2007 report.

Since then, there have been four large meta-analyses or pooled projects [99–102] examining the relationship of fruit and vegetable intake to breast cancer risk. The first, a meta-analysis of both case-control studies and cohort studies done in 2000 [100] utilizing studies conducted between 1982 and 1997 found a 25% significant reduction in breast cancer risk with a high consumption of vegetables, but no significant reduction with fruit intake. At the nutrient level both Vitamin C (RR = 0.80; 95% CI 0.68–0.95) and β-carotene (RR = 0.82; 95% CI 0.76–0.91) were associated with a significant reduction of risk in breast cancer incidence. In another meta-analysis combining 15 case-control and 10 cohort studies [101], again vegetables, but not fruit, were associated with a reduced risk of breast cancer; however, most of the association was attributed to a reduced risk in the case-control, not the cohort studies. A pooled analysis of nine cohort studies [99], all of which were in the aforementioned meta-analyses found a slightly different result; marginally significant and modest reduced risk for fruits (pooled RR 0.93; 95% CI 0.86–1.00, *p* for trend, 0.08), but no association with vegetables. The latest of the pooled studies [102] comes from the EPIC study. This analysis draws upon 285,526 women from eight of the ten countries and includes 3659 invasive breast cancers. Advantages of this large study are that the cohorts represent a wide range of dietary patterns across countries from both northern and southern Europe to allow for adequate variation in fruit and vegetable intake. In this study, no significant associations were found for total vegetables or for total fruits or for each of six specific vegetable subgroups (leafy vegetables, fruiting vegetables, root vegetables, cabbages, mushrooms, garlic/onions).

While the addition of this newer evidence does not strongly support the former AICR conclusion, a newer panel of experts from the International Agency for Research on Cancer [103] convened a working group in 2003 to review the literature on fruit and vegetables and breast cancer and concluded that, "they could not exclude the possibility that fruit and vegetable intake was associated with a slight decreased risk in breast cancer." The effects of fruits and vegetables on breast cancer risk still remain inconclusive.

Again as with dietary fat, measurement errors associated with FFQs may be obscuring the ability to observe stronger associations. More precise dietary assessment methods should be used to measure fruit and vegetable intake to see if these more recent findings are confirmed. It is also possible that certain constituents found in fruits and vegetables such as antioxidants, isothiocyanates, polyphenols, monoterpenes, may demonstrate stronger protective relationships that are undetectable when whole food groups are examined, particularly when all vegetables and fruits including fruit juices are combined. Future studies should examine specific bioactive food components and should explore variability in genetic susceptibility to possible benefits of fruits and vegetables. Further, life-long exposure at sufficient levels may be essential in order for protective effects to be demonstrated.

10.2.10.2 Ovarian Cancer

Among the dietary factors that hold the greatest promise for protection against ovarian cancer are the carotenoids, bioactive compounds found in fruits and vegetables and known to be responsible for the broad spectrum of colors present in these foods (Table 10.4). While there are over 400 known carotenoids in the human diet, 5 are considered to be of greatest importance in terms of both relative quantities in the diet as well as cancer preventive biological activity. These five carotenoids include α-carotene, β-carotene, lutein, lycopene, and β-cryptoxanthin. Studies assessing the association between carotenoids and cancer generally evaluate total intake as well as intake of these five specific carotenoids. Intake of vegetables tends to correlate with intake of carotenoids, suggesting that protective effects of vegetable intake may reflect exposure to higher amounts of carotenoids. It is important to note that the correlation between vegetable intake and plasma carotenoid levels (as a biomarker of carotenoid intake) is highly dependent on the vegetables consumed in that vegetables with minimal color such as russet potatoes, corn, and iceberg lettuce will not produce an increase in plasma carotenoid levels. Thus, studies that include vegetables of low color are less likely to "test" the relationship between carotenoids and cancer risk.

The New York Women's cohort study suggested that total dietary carotenoid intake was associated with an estimated 67% reduction in ovarian cancer risk (OR 0.33; 95%

CI 0.16–0.68) [104]. This protective relationship was also demonstrated in a case-control study in Italy, where β-carotene intake was associated with a significant 20% reduction in risk and lutein was associated with a 40% reduction in risk [105]. A case-control study from the United States which included dietary data collected from 558 cases and 607 matched-controls [106] suggested that while β-carotene intake was protective (OR 0.66; 95% CI 0.45–0.99) no other carotenoids were shown to be protective, although the inverse association with lutein intake was borderline significant (0.58; 95% CI 0.34–0.97; $p = 0.06$). Green leafy vegetables which are known to be high in lutein, were also protective against ovarian cancer in the Iowa Women's Health Study [96]. In a study by Bertone et al. [107], women with the highest dietary intake of lutein/zeaxanthin experienced a 40% reduction in ovarian cancer risk (multivariate RR 0.6; 95% CI 0.36–0.99) while the Bosetti study [108] showed an inverse association with β-carotene (OR 0.8) as well as lutein/zeaxanthin intake (OR 0.6). In a US case-control study by Cramer et al. [109] the protective association among those consuming high levels of carotenoids was strongest among postmenopausal women (OR 0.55; 95% CI 0.36–0.84). The Adventist Health Study found reduced risk of ovarian cancer among women with higher intake of tomato (RR 0.32) [110] while carotenoid intake as well as vitamins A, C, and E intake were not shown to protect against ovarian cancer among women participating in the Canadian National Breast Cancer Screening Study [111].

Cruciferous vegetables, which include vegetables such as broccoli, cabbage, cauliflower, collards and condiments including mustards and horseradish, are a significant source of carotenoids as well as isothiocyanates, additional cancer-protective bioactive chemicals which have been shown to be protective against ovarian cancer [112]. Further, the Nagel study, which assessed the role of cruciferous vegetables in relation to survival of ovarian cancer, also supported a protective role of these vegetables (HR 0.75; 95% CI 0.57–0.98).

Prospective data from the Nurses' Health Study did not show a protective association with total vegetable intake or diet plus supplemental β-carotene intake; however, greater reported intake of vegetables during adolescence was suggested to be protective against the development of ovarian cancer later in life (RR 0.54; 95% CI 0.29–1.03; p for trend; 0.04). A more recent pooled analysis which included 12 international cohort studies also found no significant protective relationship between vegetable intake and ovarian cancer risk [113] even when individual vegetables were evaluated. However, the likelihood that intake of any one specific vegetable would be great enough to modify ovarian cancer risk is low. Of interest, the Pan study [112] showed that among Canadian women participating in the NECSS project who reported taking supplemental β-carotene for over 10 years, a 69% reduction in ovarian cancer risk was identified.

Again, common biological mechanisms of cancer-preventive activity have been identified and suggest a protective effect of vegetables, fruits, and carotenoids in reducing both breast and ovarian cancer risk. These protective mechanisms range from enhancement of immune function, to modulation of apoptosis, to antioxidant as well as anti-inflammatory activity to reduction in DNA damage.

10.2.11 Alcohol

10.2.11.1 Breast Cancer

In studies that span over three decades and number well over 100 investigations, excessive evidence implicates alcohol consumption as a cause of cancer of the breast [7,114,115]. Many of these studies have found a modest increased risk of about 30%–50% from moderate alcohol consumption (~1–2 drinks/day) [116–119], [120,121]. Women with low folate intakes may in particular be susceptible to the increased risk associated with alcohol consumption and risk does not appear to be related to particular types of alcohol, but rather overall intake [122].

In the 1997 AICR report [8] the expert panel concluded that among the many hypothesized relationships between food or nutrients and breast cancer risk, the association with alcohol is the most consistent and that high alcohol intake probably increases the risk for breast cancer.

Since then, a pooled analysis, collaborative reanalysis, and a meta-analyses have all supported this conclusion. In a pooled analysis of 322,647 women and 4335 breast cancer cases who were followed for up to 11 years [114], risk increased linearly with increasing alcohol intake; the pooled multivariate relative risk for an increment of 10 g/day (approximately one alcoholic beverage) was 1.09 (95% CI 1.04–1.13). The increased risk for 2–5 drinks/day vs. none was ~40% (RR 1.41; 95% CI 1.18–1.69). Specific alcohol type did not alter risk. In the collaborative reanalysis [115] of data from 53 studies that included 58,515 breast cancer cases the increased risk ranged between 32% and 46% for greater than 3 drinks/day compared with none and a 7.1% (95% CI 5.5%–8.7%) increase for each 10 g/day intake of alcohol. In the meta-analyses including between 60,653 and 75,728 breast cancer cases [123], depending on the specific analyses, the excess risk associated with alcohol drinking was 22% (95% CI 9%–37%) and similar to the aforementioned pooled analysis, each 10 g/day increase of alcohol was associated with a 10% higher risk (95% CI 5%–15%).

Several possible mechanisms have been proposed for alcohol acting as a modifier of breast cancer risk including a direct effect on circulating estradiol levels [124] and alterations in other hormones as well, through mutagenesis by acetaldehyde, a metabolite of ethanol, by inducing oxidative damage or by affecting folate absorption and one-carbon metabolism pathways [125]. The latter mechanism is supported by a number of studies that have demonstrated that an adequate folate intake might attenuate the increased risk of breast cancer associated with alcohol consumption [126–129].

Despite the consistency in the overall association, several important questions remain including whether the association between alcohol intake and breast cancer risk is affected by the timing of alcohol exposure, modified by other risk factors such as body size, menopausal status, and HT, or more pronounced among women diagnosed with hormone receptor positive tumors. Understanding these issues will help provide information on the underlying pathways that may link alcohol use to breast cancer risk.

10.2.11.2 Ovarian Cancer

Alcohol intake has been shown to modulate sex hormone levels and in this role has been suggested as an important dietary factor to assess in terms of ovarian cancer risk. A large case-control study from Australia which included 696 epithelial ovarian cancer cases [130] showed that wine intake at the uppermost quartile (>1 glass/day) was associated with a 44% reduction in ovarian cancer risk, while intake of beer and spirits showed no significant relationship with ovarian cancer. In an Italian cohort who reported relatively frequent wine consumption no significant protective effect of wine intake in relation to ovarian cancer risk was demonstrated [131]. The unique potentially protective association with wine intake suggests that the antioxidant effects of wine intake may be of importance to ovarian cancer risk reduction. A U.S. case-control trial of similar sample size did not support a protective effect of wine and, in addition, did show a significant rise in risk for ovarian cancer among women reporting greater beer intake from age 20 to 30 years [34]. A pooled analysis of ten studies further supports these null associations [132] as did the Netherlands cohort study [133]. In examining the interaction between folate status, alcohol intake, and ovarian cancer risk, the Swedish Mammography Cohort showed, similar to the breast cancer research that folate intake was associated with reduced risk among high alcohol consumers [134].

10.2.12 Additional Nutrients of Interest

10.2.12.1 Breast Cancer: Soy and Phytoestrogens

Phytoestrogens such as the isoflavones found in most soy products, and lignans, also found in most plant foods including various seeds, wholegrain products, fruits and vegetables but are the richest in flaxseed, have generated interest as they may decrease the risk of breast cancer. One potentially anticarcinogenic preventive action of these compounds is by binding to estrogen receptors in the breast; they act as weak estrogens without much effect, but block the binding of more potent endogenous estrogens. Nonhormonal mechanisms associated with the inhibition of cancer cell growth have been proposed as well. While soy isoflavones have been shown to exert beneficial hormonal effects in both cell culture systems and laboratory animal models [135], in recent years, data from in vitro and animal studies also suggest that under certain circumstances such as prolonged exposure [136,137] some isoflavonoids, particularly genistein, may actually be harmful and stimulate the growth of estrogen sensitive tumors. In addition, data from human feeding studies on nipple aspirate fluid, which itself is a possible marker for breast cancer risk, suggest that consumption of soy products may have effects that potentially increase the risk of breast cancer [138].

The ecological literature supports a relationship between soy and breast cancer risk in that populations that consume greater amounts of soy such as in Japan and China have lower rates of death from breast cancer than seen in the United States and most European countries [139]. Clinical evidence from feeding studies in humans on the effect of soy on serum hormone concentrations is inconsistent in premenopausal women [135,140], but demonstrates a modest estrogenic effect in response to soy feeding in postmenopausal women [135]. While results from individual case-control and cohort studies have been inconsistent, a recently completed meta-analyses of soy intake and breast cancer risk that included 12 case-control and 6 cohort or nested case-control studies [141] found that soy was associated with a modest risk reduction (pooled OR 0.86; 95% CI 0.75–0.99) and was somewhat stronger in premenopausal women (pooled OR 0.77; 95% CI 0.60–0.98). The large heterogeneity across studies in terms of soy "exposures," however, limits the interpretation of these data. Additionally, the Shanghai Breast Cancer study including 1459 breast cancer cases and 1556 controls, examined intakes of soy during adolescence [142], a period when breast tissue is particularly sensitive to environmental stimuli, and found a 50% risk reduction for the lowest quintile of intake compared to the highest. However, the authors recognize that they could not disentangle the effects of soy foods during adolescence from that of prepubertal or cumulative lifetime exposure to soy.

The epidemiological literature on lignans is inconsistent as well. Several studies have assessed either dietary lignan intake or urinary or serum lignans and breast cancer risk [136]. The majority of these studies showed a negative association [136], and in those where they were able to examine effect modification by menopausal status, the protective effect appeared to be stronger for premenopausal women than for postmenopausal women [143,144].

The existing literature on either soy or lignans does not allow definitive conclusions to be drawn about the effect of these food components on breast cancer risk. Data from meta-analyses are hard to interpret since there is a great deal of heterogeneity between studies and the possibility for exposure misclassification is high. Before recommendations on their use for the prevention of breast cancer can be made, more research is needed. The recommendation from a recent workshop addressing the soy and breast cancer relationship suggests that the potential impact of soy foods on breast cancer risk be studied in interventions of high-risk women using cancer risk markers (e.g., cell proliferation, apoptosis) in breast tissue samples and using standardized soy products [137]. Clinically, breast cancer survivors with ER + tumor types are suggested to exercise precaution with soy intake until more is known regarding the association with breast cancer recurrence.

10.2.12.2 Ovarian Cancer: Antioxidants

Several antioxidant micronutrients have also been investigated to determine if they are protective against ovarian cancer. A large case-control study from Australia which included over 600 cases of invasive epithelial ovarian cancer as well as a second case-control study from Canada showed that vitamin E intake was inversely and significantly associated with both ovarian cancer survival and risk [112]. These findings are similar to those of Zhang et al. who also demonstrated a significant reduction in ovarian cancer risk with higher dietary intakes of vitamins A and C [38] as well as the report of McCann et al. which showed vitamin E intake was inversely and significantly associated with ovarian cancer risk (OR 0.58; 95% CI 0.38–0.88) [145].

10.2.12.3 Ovarian Cancer: Lactose

Increased intake of milk and dairy as well as lactose and galactose has specifically been identified to increase ovarian cancer risk in select populations [146], but not according to a recent meta-analysis of the literature [147]. The increased risk was identified among women consuming greater than four servings of dairy each day and was specific to serous type ovarian cancer.

10.3 CONCLUSION

There have been decades of research on the role of a broad range of dietary components on the risk of both breast and ovarian cancer. This chapter has presented the pertinent literature on nutritional factors where there is broad interest, controversy or where the dietary risk factor is fairly well established. Many additional nutrients or food groups have been widely studied, but are not included in this review because the evidence for their benefit is either negative, lacking, or inadequately studied. For a more comprehensive review of the role of diet in cancer prevention, the reader is directed to the American Cancer Society Guidelines on Nutrition and Physical Activity for Cancer Prevention (2006) or the forthcoming revision of the American Institute for Cancer Research and the World Cancer Research Fund in Food Nutrition and the Prevention of Cancer: A Global Prospective [8]. At present, no one nutrient, food group, or dietary pattern has convincingly been shown to reduce the risk of either breast or ovarian cancer. There is general consensus that engaging in moderate to vigorous physical activity on a regular basis, minimizing lifetime weight gain, and limiting alcohol may all reduce the risk of breast cancer. Less evidence is available regarding ovarian cancer risk, but avoidance of overweight or obesity, moderate physical activity and higher intake of vegetables and fruit is advised. However, cancer researchers and clinicians alike agree that supporting efforts toward a healthier lifestyle are justified and should be promoted. Table 10.5 summarizes some specific behavior-related suggestions to promote healthy behavior in hopes of modifying individual risk for female-related cancers.

10.4 FUTURE RESEARCH

Ideas for future research for specific food components and breast and ovarian cancer are incorporated into individual sections of this chapter. While the evidence suggesting a relationship between certain dietary factors and the prevention of breast and ovarian cancer is still inconclusive, there is a need for expanded research in an effort to develop more evidence-based guidelines for clinical practice.

There are several general issues that need to be addressed, including:

- Expansion of research beyond case-control and cohort studies to randomized, controlled clinical trials in order to advance beyond associations to defining causation
- Study of the efficacy of whole diet, food interventions to advance understanding beyond the reductionism of interventions focusing on a single nutrient or bioactive food component
- Inclusion of mechanistic-based research in the context of dietary intervention trials
- Continued efforts to establish relevant surrogate endpoint biomarkers of breast and ovarian cancers (beyond breast density) that can support the implementation of shorter duration studies with reduced sample size, approaches that are significantly more cost-effective
- Longitudinal studies of diet and dietary interventions to reduce cancer risk via modification of in utero or prepubescent exposures

TABLE 10.5
Dietary Guidelines to Promote Healthy Behaviors

Health Behaviors to Reduce Disease Risk
Increase emphasis on a plant-based diet
Increase vegetable intake
Select a wide variety of vegetables — color
Reduce cooking and processing of plant foods
Make vegetables the main course with meat as a side dish
Reduce fat intake
Select healthy fats
Olive, almond, sunflower, canola oils
Nuts and seeds
High n-3 fatty acids
Fish such as salmon, mackerel
Flaxseed
Control animal fat intake
Select lean cuts of meat, poultry
Use low or no-fat dairy products
Nonfat salad dressings, sauces, etc
Eat more fish
Avoid trans fats — read food labels
Increase fiber
Whole grains — breads >3 grams fiber/serving
Cereal with >6 grams fiber/serving and <8 grams sugars
Beans — low cost, high fiber
Vegetables at each meal and snack
Control body weight
Monitor for even small increases in body weight after adolescence
Be physically active
Consume small, frequent meals
Eat at home — avoiding processed and "fast" foods
Drink plenty of water
Limit alcohol intake to no more than 2 drinks per day

- Prospective hypotheses of subgroups of relevance in the translation of science related to diet intervention effects on breast and ovarian cancer risk (i.e., pre vs. postmenopasual breast cancers, ER+ vs. ER− tumor types, variable ovarian cancer histopathologies, obese vs. nonobese, etc);
- Studies of the potential synergistic and health-promoting effects of combined diet and medical therapies for breast and ovarian cancer (e.g., Aromatase inhibitors plus garlic and Mediterranean diet to reduce hyperlipidemia associated with AI use)
- Targeted weight control interventions that focus on increasing lean mass and reducing android adiposity independent of a net reduction in body weight to increase survival of female cancers
- Application of genetic variance to hypotheses testing of food–cancer associations

Clearly, while the epidemiological evidence has expanded significantly over the past several decades, there are still many gaps in our understanding of how diet relates to breast and ovarian cancer. Cancer is a complex disease and the need for more refined and focused hypotheses testing is real. Only when more targeted diet interventions are tested will we have the evidence-base to develop specific recommendations for clinical practice.

REFERENCES

1. American Cancer Society *Breast Cancer Facts and Figures 2005–2006*; American Cancer Society, Inc.: Atlanta, 2006.
2. Chang, S., et al., Estimating the cost of cancer: Results on the basis of claims data analyses for cancer patients diagnosed with seven types of cancer during 1999 to 2000, *J. Clin. Oncol., 22*, 3524, 2004.
3. American Cancer Society, *Cancer Facts & Figures 2005*; American Cancer Society: Atlanta, 2005.
4. Parkin, D.M., et al., Estimating the world cancer burden: Globocan 2000, *Int. J .Cancer, 94*, 153, 2001.
5. Ries, L., et al., *Cancer Statistics Review, 1975–2003*; National Cancer Institute, editor, Bethesda, MD, 2005.
6. Lichtenstein, P., et al., Environmental and heritable factors in the causation of cancer–analyses of cohorts of twins from Sweden, Denmark, and Finland, *N. Engl. J. Med., 343*, 78, 2000.
7. Kushi, L.H., et al., American Cancer Society Guidelines on Nutrition and Physical Activity for cancer prevention: reducing the risk of cancer with healthy food choices and physical activity, *CA Cancer J. Clin., 56*, 254, 2006.
8. World Cancer Research Fund, A.I.C.R. *Food, Nutrition and the Prevention of Cancer: A.I.C.R. a Global Perspective*; American Institute for Cancer Research: Washington, DC, 1997.
9. Prentice, R.L., et al., Low-fat dietary pattern and risk of invasive breast cancer: The Women's Health Initiative Randomized Controlled Dietary Modification Trial, *JAMA, 295*, 629, 2006.
10. Schatzkin, A., et al., Lack of effect of a low-fat, high-fiber diet on the recurrence of colorectal adenomas, *N. Engl. J. Med., 342*, 1148, 2000.
11. Colditz, G., Baer, H., and Tamimi, R., Breast Cancer, in *Cancer Epidemiology and Prevention*, Schottenfeld, D.; Fraumeni, J.F.J., editors; 2006; Chapter 51, pp. 995–1012.
12. Kelsey, J.L., Gammon, M.D., and John, E.M., Reproductive factors and breast cancer, *Epidemiol. Rev., 15*, 36, 1993.
13. Bernstein, L., Epidemiology of endocrine-related risk factors for breast cancer, *J. Mammary Gland Biol. Neoplasia., 7*, 3, 2002.
14. Colditz, G.A. and Rosner, B., Cumulative risk of breast cancer to age 70 years according to risk factor status: Data from the Nurses' Health Study, *Am. J. Epidemiol., 152*, 950,2000.
15. Rossouw, J., et al., Risks and benefits of estrogen plus progestin in healthy postmenopausal women: Principal results from the Women's Health Initiative randomized controlled trial, *JAMA, 288*, 321,2003.
16. Anderson, G.L., et al., Effects of conjugated equine estrogen in postmenopausal women with hysterectomy: The Women's Health Initiative randomized controlled trial, *JAMA, 291*, 1701, 2004.

17. Beral, V., Breast cancer and hormone-replacement therapy in the Million Women Study, *Lancet, 362*, 419, 2003.
18. Schairer, C., et al., Menopausal estrogen and estrogen–progestin replacement therapy and breast cancer risk, *JAMA, 283*, 485, 2000.
19. Collaborative Group on Hormonal Factors in Breast Cancer, Breast cancer and hormone replacement therapy: Collaborative reanalysis of data from 51 epidemiological studies of 52,705 women with breast cancer and 108,411 women without breast cancer, *Lancet, 350*, 1047, 1997.
20. Sogaard, M., Kjaer, S.K., and Gayther, S., Ovarian cancer and genetic susceptibility in relation to the BRCA1 and BRCA2 genes. Occurrence, clinical importance and intervention, *Acta Obstet. Gynecol. Scand., 85*, 93, 2006.
21. Weiderpass, E., et al., Prospective study of physical activity in different periods of life and the risk of ovarian cancer, *Int. J. Cancer, 118*, 3153, 2006.
22. Byers, T., et al., A case-control study of dietary and nondietary factors in ovarian cancer, *J. Natl. Cancer Inst., 71*, 681, 1983.
23. van den Brandt, P.A., et al., Pooled analysis of prospective cohort studies on height, weight, and breast cancer risk, *Am. J. Epidemiol., 152*, 514, 2000.
24. Lahmann, P.H., et al., Body size and breast cancer risk: Findings from the European Prospective Investigation into Cancer and Nutrition (EPIC), *Int. J. Cancer, 111*, 762, 2004.
25. Sherman, B., et al., Relationship of body weight to menarcheal and menopausal age: Implications for breast cancer risk, *J. Clin. Endocrinol. Metab., 52*, 488, 1981.
26. Pike, M.C., Reducing cancer risk in women through lifestyle-mediated changes in hormone levels, *Cancer Detect. Prev., 14*, 595, 1990.
27. Boyd, N.F., et al., Body size, mammographic density, and breast cancer risk, *Cancer Epidemiol. Biomarkers Prev., 15*, 2086, 2006.
28. Feigelson, H.S., et al., Weight gain, body mass index, hormone replacement therapy, and postmenopausal breast cancer in a large prospective study, *Cancer Epidemiol. Biomarkers Prev., 13*, 220, 2004.
29. Lahmann, P.H., et al., Long-term weight change and breast cancer risk: The European prospective investigation into cancer and nutrition (EPIC), *Br. J. Cancer, 93*, 582, 2005.
30. Eliassen, A.H., et al., Adult weight change and risk of postmenopausal breast cancer, *JAMA, 296*, 193, 2006.
31. Harvie, M., et al., Association of gain and loss of weight before and after menopause with risk of postmenopausal breast cancer in the Iowa women's health study, *Cancer Epidemiol. Biomarkers Prev., 14*, 656, 2005.
32. Feigelson, H.S., et al., Adult weight gain and histopathologic characteristics of breast cancer among postmenopausal women, *Cancer, 107*, 12, 2006.
33. Han, D., et al., Lifetime adult weight gain, central adiposity, and the risk of pre- and postmenopausal breast cancer in the Western New York exposures and breast cancer study, *Int. J. Cancer, 119*, 2931, 2006.
34. Peterson, N.B., et al., Alcohol consumption and ovarian cancer risk in a population-based case-control study, *Int. J. Cancer, 119*, 2423, 2006.
35. Rossing, M.A., et al., Body size and risk of epithelial ovarian cancer (United States), *Cancer Causes Control, 17*, 713, 2006.
36. Wright, J.D., et al., Relationship of ovarian neoplasms and body mass index, *J. Reprod. Med., 50*, 595, 2005.
37. Niwa, Y., et al., Relationship between body mass index and the risk of ovarian cancer in the Japanese population: Findings from the Japanese Collaborate Cohort (JACC) study, *J. Obstet. Gynaecol. Res., 31*, 452, 2005.

38. Zhang, M., Lee, A.H., and Binns, C.W., Reproductive and dietary risk factors for epithelial ovarian cancer in China, *Gynecol. Oncol., 92*, 320, 2004.
39. Anderson, J.P., Ross, J.A., and Folsom, A.R., Anthropometric variables, physical activity, and incidence of ovarian cancer: The Iowa Women's Health Study, *Cancer, 100*, 1515, 2004.
40. Kurian, A.W., et. al., Histologic types of epithelial ovarian cancer: Have they different risk factors? *Gynecol. Oncol., 96*, 520, 2005.
41. Engeland, A., Tretli, S., and Bjorge, T., Height, body mass index, and ovarian cancer: A follow-up of 1.1 million Norwegian women, *J. Natl. Cancer Inst., 95*, 1244, 2003.
42. Clinton, S.K., Diet, anthropometry and breast cancer: Integration of experimental and epidemiologic approaches, *J. Nutr., 127*(5 Suppl), 916S, 1997.
43. Schouten, L.J., Goldbohm, R.A., and van den Brandt, P.A., Height, weight, weight change, and ovarian cancer risk in the Netherlands cohort study on diet and cancer, *Am. J. Epidemiol., 157*, 424, 2003.
44. Rodriguez, C., et. al., Body mass index, height, and the risk of ovarian cancer mortality in a prospective cohort of postmenopausal women, *Cancer Epidemiol. Biomarkers Prev. 11*, 822, 2002.
45. Trichopoulos, D., Lagiou, P., and Adami, H.O., Towards an integrated model for breast cancer etiology: The crucial role of the number of mammary tissue-specific stem cells, *Breast Cancer Res., 7*, 13, 2005.
46. Ahlgren, M., et. al., Growth patterns and the risk of breast cancer in women, *N. Engl. J. Med., 351*, 1619, 2004.
47. Michels, K.B. and Xue, F., Role of birthweight in the etiology of breast cancer, *Int. J. Cancer, 119*, 2007, 2006.
48. Lof, M., et. al., Birth weight in relation to endometrial and breast cancer risks in Swedish women, *Br. J. Cancer, 96*, 134, 2007.
49. Thune, I. and Furberg, A.S., Physical activity and cancer risk: Dose–response and cancer, all sites and site-specific, *Med. Sci. Sports Exerc., 33*(6 Suppl), S530, 2001.
50. Lee, I.-M. and Oguma, Y. Physical Activity, in *cancer Epidemiol. and Prevention*, 3rd ed.; Schottenfeld, D.; Fraumeni, J.F.J., editors; 2006; Chapter 23, pp. 449–467.
51. Sternfield, B. and Lee, I.-M. Physical activity and cancer: the evidence, the issues, and the challenges, In Physical Activity and Health: Epidemiologic Methods and Studies; Lee, I.-M., editor; Oxford University Press: New York, N.Y. In press.
52. Albanes, D., Blar, A., and Taylor, P., Physical activity and risk of cancer in the NHANES I population, *Am. J. Pub. Health, 79*, 744, 1989.
53. Bernstein, L., et al., Physical exercise and reduced risk of breast cancer in young women, *J. Natl. Cancer Inst., 86*, 1403, 1994.
54. Friedenreich, C.M., Courneya, K.S., and Bryant, H.E., Relation between intensity of physical activity and breast cancer risk reduction, *Med. Sci. Sports Exerc., 33*, 1538, 2001.
55. Lee, I.M., Physical activity and cancer prevention–data from epidemiologic studies, *Med. Sci. Sports Exerc., 35*, 1823, 2003.
56. Bull, F.C., et al., Comparative quantification of health risks: Global and regional burden of disease due to selected major risk factors, *Phys. Activty, 2*, 729, 2004.
57. Rockhill, B., et al., Physical activity and breast cancer risk in a cohort of young women, *J. Natl. Cancer Inst., 90*, 1155, 1998.
58. Colditz, G.A., et al., Physical activity and risk of breast cancer in premenopausal women, *Br. J. Cancer, 89*, 847, 2003.
59. Margolis, K.L., et al., Physical activity in different periods of life and the risk of breast cancer: The Norwegian-Swedish Women's Lifestyle and Health cohort study, *Cancer Epidemiol. Biomarkers Prev., 14*, 27, 2005.

60. McTiernan, A., et al., Recreational physical activity and the risk of breast cancer in postmenopausal women: The Women's Health Initiative Cohort Study, *JAMA, 290*, 1331, 2003.
61. Thune, I., et al., Physical activity and the risk of breast cancer, *N. Engl. J. Med., 336*, 1269, 1997.
62. Shoff, S.M., et. al., Early-life physical activity and postmenopausal breast cancer: Effect of body size and weight change, *Cancer Epidemiol. Biomarkers Prev., 9*, 591, 2000.
63. Patel, A.V., et al., Recreational physical activity and risk of postmenopausal breast cancer in a large cohort of US women, *Cancer Causes Control* 2003, *14*(6), 519–529.
64. Mittendorf, R., et al., Strenuous physical activity in young adulthood and risk of breast cancer (United States), *Cancer Causes Control, 6*, 347, 1995.
65. Marcus, P.M., et al., Physical activity at age 12 and adult breast cancer risk, *Cancer Causes Control, 10*, 293, 1999.
66. Steindorf, K., et al., Case-control study of physical activity and breast cancer risk among premenopausal women in Germany, *Am. J. Epidemiol., 157*, 121, 2003.
67. John, E.M., Horn-Ross, P.L., and Koo, J., Lifetime physical activity and breast cancer risk in a multiethnic population: The San Francisco Bay area breast cancer study, *Cancer Epidemiol. Biomarkers Prev., 12*(11 Pt 1), 1143, 2003.
68. Dorn, J., et al., Lifetime physical activity and breast cancer risk in pre- and postmenopausal women, *Med. Sci. Sports Exerc., 35*, 278, 2003.
69. Matthews, C.E., et. al., Lifetime physical activity and breast cancer risk in the Shanghai Breast Cancer Study, *Br. J. Cancer, 84*, 994, 2001.
70. Friedenreich, C.M., Courneya, K.S., and Bryant, H.E., Influence of physical activity in different age and life periods on the risk of breast cancer, *Epidemiology, 12*, 604, 2001.
71. Yang, D., Bernstein, L., and Wu, A.H., Physical activity and breast cancer risk among Asian-American women in Los Angeles: A case-control study, *Cancer, 97*, 2565, 2003.
72. Pan, S.Y., Ugnat, A.M., and Mao, Y., Physical activity and the risk of ovarian cancer: A case-control study in Canada, *Int. J. Cancer, 117*, 300, 2005.
73. Bertone, E.R., et al., Prospective study of recreational physical activity and ovarian cancer, *J. Natl. Cancer Inst., 93*, 942, 2001.
74. Biesma, R.G., et al., Physical activity and risk of ovarian cancer: Results from the Netherlands Cohort Study (The Netherlands), *Cancer Causes Control, 17*, 109, 2006.
75. Armstrong, B. and Doll, R., Environmental factors and cancer incidence and mortality in different countries, with special reference to dietary practices, *Int. J. Cancer, 15*, 617, 1975.
76. Welsch, C.W., Relationship between dietary fat and experimental mammary tumorigenesis: A review and critique, *Cancer Res., 52*(7 Suppl), 2040s, 1992.
77. Howe, G.R., et al., Dietary factors and the risk of breast cancer: Combined analysis of 12 case-control studies, *J. Natl. Cancer Inst., 82*, 69, 1990.
78. Hunter, D.J., et al., Cohort studies of fat intake and the risk of breast cancer—a pooled analysis, *N. Engl. J. Med., 334*, 356, 1996.
79. Boyd, N.F., et al., Dietary fat and breast cancer risk revisited: A meta-analysis of the published literature, *Br. J. Cancer, 89*, 1672, 2003.
80. Prentice, R., Measurement error and results from analytic epidemiology: Dietary fat and breast cancer, *JNCI, 88(23)*, 1738, 1996.
81. Kipnis, V., et al., Empirical evidence of correlated biases in dietary assessment instruments and its implications, *Am. J. Epidemiol., 153*, 394, 2001.
82. Bingham, S.A., et al., Are imprecise methods obscuring a relation between fat and breast cancer? *Lancet, 362*, 212, 2003.

83. Freedman, L.S., et al., A comparison of two dietary instruments for evaluating the fat-breast cancer relationship, *Int. J. Epidemiol., 35*, 1011, 2006.
84. Wakai, K., et al., Dietary intakes of fat and fatty acids and risk of breast cancer: A prospective study in Japan, *Cancer Sci., 96*, 590, 2005.
85. Engeset, D., et al., Fish consumption and breast cancer risk. The European Prospective Investigation into Cancer and Nutrition (EPIC), *Int. J. Cancer, 119*, 175, 2006.
86. MacLean, C.H., et al., Effects of omega-3 fatty acids on cancer risk: A systematic review, *JAMA, 295*, 403, 2006.
87. Rose, D.P., Boyar, A.P., and Wynder, E.L., International comparisons of mortality rates for cancer of the breast, ovary, prostate, and colon and per-capita food consumption, *Cancer*, 58, 2363, 1986.
88. Li, X.M., Ganmaa, D., and Sato, A., The experience of Japan as a clue to the etiology of breast and ovarian cancers: Relationship between death from both malignancies and dietary practices, *Med. Hypotheses, 60*, 268, 2003.
89. Kato, I., Tominaga, S., and Kuroishi, T., Relationship between westernization of dietary habits and mortality form breast and ovarian cancers in Japan, *Jpn. J. Cancer Res., 78*, 349, 1987.
90. Risch, H.A., et al., Dietary fat intake and risk of epithelial ovarian cancer, *J. Natl. Cancer Inst., 86*, 1409, 1994.
91. Tavani, A., et al., Red meat intake and cancer risk: A study in Italy, *Int. J. Cancer, 86*, 425, 2000.
92. Mori, M. and Miyake, H., Dietary and other risk factors of ovarian cancer among elderly women, *Jpn. J. Cancer Res., 79*, 997, 1988.
93. Bertone, E.R., et al., Dietary fat intake and ovarian cancer in a cohort of US women, *Am. J. Epidemiol., 156*, 22, 2002.
94. Bosetti, C., et al., Olive oil, seed oils and other added fats in relation to ovarian cancer (Italy), *Cancer Causes Control, 13*, 465, 2002.
95. Tzonou, A., et al., Diet and ovarian cancer: A case-control study in Greece, *Int. J. Cancer, 55*, 411, 1993.
96. Kushi, L.H., et al., Prospective study of diet and ovarian cancer, *Am. J. Epidemiol., 149*, 21, 1999.
97. Pirozzo, S., et al., Ovarian cancer, cholesterol, and eggs: A case-control analysis, *Cancer Epidemiol. Biomarkers Prev., 11*(10 Pt 1), 1112, 2002.
98. Larsson, S.C. and Wolk, A., No association of meat, fish, and egg consumption with ovarian cancer risk, *Cancer Epidemiol. Biomarkers Prev., 14*, 1024, 2005.
99. Smith-Warner, S.A., et al., Intake of fruits and vegetables and risk of breast cancer: A pooled analysis of cohort studies, *JAMA, 285*, 769, 2001.
100. Gandini, S., et al., Meta-analysis of studies on breast cancer risk and diet: The role of fruit and vegetable consumption and the intake of associated micronutrients, *Eur. J. Cancer, 36*, 636, 2000.
101. Riboli, E. and Norat, T., Epidemiologic evidence of the protective effect of fruit and vegetables on cancer risk, *Am. J. Clin. Nutr., 78*(3 Suppl), 559S, 2003.
102. van Gils, C.H., et al., Consumption of vegetables and fruits and risk of breast cancer, *JAMA, 293*, 183, 2005.
103. International Agency for Research on Cancer World Health Organization, *IARC Handbooks of Cancer Prevention: Fruits and Vegetables*, IARC Press, Vainio, Harri and Bianchini, Franca; 2003.
104. McCann, S.E., et al., Risk of human ovarian cancer is related to dietary intake of selected nutrients, phytochemicals and food groups, *J. Nutr., 133*, 1937, 2003.

105. Bidoli, E., et al., Micronutrients and ovarian cancer: A case-control study in Italy, *Ann. Oncol., 12*, 1589, 2001.
106. Tung, K.H., et al., Association of dietary vitamin A, carotenoids, and other antioxidants with the risk of ovarian cancer, *Cancer Epidemiol. Biomarkers Prev., 14*, 669, 2005.
107. Bertone, E.R., et. al., A population-based case-control study of carotenoid and vitamin A intake and ovarian cancer (United States), *Cancer Causes Control, 12*, 83, 2001.
108. Bosetti, C., et al., Diet and ovarian cancer risk: A case-control study in Italy, *Int. J. Cancer, 93*, 911, 2001.
109. Cramer, D.W., et al., Carotenoids, antioxidants and ovarian cancer risk in pre- and postmenopausal women, *Int. J. Cancer, 94*, 128, 2001.
110. Kiani, F., et al., Dietary risk factors for ovarian cancer: The Adventist Health Study (United States), *Cancer Causes Control, 17*, 137, 2006.
111. Silvera, S.A., et al., Carotenoid, vitamin A, vitamin C, and vitamin E intake and risk of ovarian cancer: A prospective cohort study, *Cancer Epidemiol. Biomarkers Prev., 15*, 395, 2006.
112. Pan, S.Y., et al., A case-control study of diet and the risk of ovarian cancer, *Cancer Epidemiol. Biomarkers Prev., 13*, 1521, 2004.
113. Koushik, A., et al., Fruits and vegetables and ovarian cancer risk in a pooled analysis of 12 cohort studies, *Cancer Epidemiol. Biomarkers Prev., 14*, 2160, 2005.
114. Smith-Warner, S.A., et al., Alcohol and breast cancer in women: A pooled analysis of cohort studies, *JAMA, 279*, 535, 1998.
115. Hamajima, N., et al., Alcohol, tobacco and breast cancer–collaborative reanalysis of individual data from 53 epidemiological studies, including 58,515 women with breast cancer and 95,067 women without the disease, *Br. J. Cancer, 87*, 1234, 2002.
116. Harvey, E.B., et al., Alcohol consumption and breast cancer, *J. Natl. Cancer Inst., 78*, 657, 1987.
117. Li, C.I., et al., The relationship between alcohol use and risk of breast cancer by histology and hormone receptor status among women 65–79 years of age, *Cancer Epidemiol. Biomarkers Prev., 12*, 1061, 2003.
118. Kinney, A.Y., et al., Alcohol consumption and breast cancer among black and white women in North Carolina (United States), *Cancer Causes Control, 11*, 345, 2000.
119. Terry, P., et al., A prospective study of major dietary patterns and the risk of breast cancer, *Cancer Epidemiol. Biomarkers Prev., 10*, 1281, 2001.
120. Lenz, S.K., et al., Association between alcohol consumption and postmenopausal breast cancer: Results of a case-control study in Montreal, Quebec, Canada, *Cancer Causes Control, 13*, 701, 2002.
121. Feigelson, H.S., et al., Alcohol, folate, methionine, and risk of incident breast cancer in the American Cancer Society Cancer Prevention Study II Nutrition Cohort, *Cancer Epidemiol. Biomarkers Prev., 12*, 161, 2003.
122. Larsson, S.C., Giovannucci, E., and Wolk, A., Folate and risk of breast cancer: A meta-analysis, *J. Natl. Cancer Inst., 99*, 64, 2007.
123. Key, J., et al., Meta-analysis of studies of alcohol and breast cancer with consideration of the methodological issues, *Cancer Causes Control, 17*, 759, 2006.
124. Ginsburg, E.S., Estrogen, alcohol and breast cancer risk, *J. Steroid Biochem. Mol. Biol., 69*, 299, 1999.
125. Dumitrescu, R.G. and Shields, P.G., The etiology of alcohol-induced breast cancer, *Alcohol, 35*, 213, 2005.
126. Sellers, T.A., et al., Dietary folate intake, alcohol, and risk of breast cancer in a prospective study of postmenopausal women, *Epidemiology, 12*, 420, 2001.

127. Baglietto, L., et. al., Does dietary folate intake modify effect of alcohol consumption on breast cancer risk? Prospective cohort study, *Br. Med. J., 331*, 807, 2005.
128. Tjonneland, A., et. al., Folate intake, alcohol and risk of breast cancer among postmenopausal women in Denmark, *Eur. J. Clin. Nutr., 60*, 280, 2006.
129. Stolzenberg-Solomon, R.Z., et al., Folate intake, alcohol use, and postmenopausal breast cancer risk in the Prostate, Lung, Colorectal, and Ovarian Cancer Screening Trial, *Am. J. Clin. Nutr., 83*, 895, 2006.
130. Webb, P.M., et al., Alcohol, wine, and risk of epithelial ovarian cancer, *Cancer Epidemiol. Biomarkers Prev., 13*, 592, 2004.
131. Tavani, A., et al., Coffee and alcohol intake and risk of ovarian cancer: An Italian case-control study, *Nutr. Cancer, 39*, 29, 2001.
132. Genkinger, J.M., et al., Alcohol intake and ovarian cancer risk: A pooled analysis of 10 cohort studies, *Br. J. Cancer, 94*, 757, 2006.
133. Schouten, L.J., et al., Alcohol and ovarian cancer risk: Results from the Netherlands Cohort Study, *Cancer Causes Control, 15*, 201, 2004.
134. Larsson, S.C., Giovannucci, E., and Wolk, A., Dietary folate intake and incidence of ovarian cancer: The Swedish Mammography Cohort, *J. Natl. Cancer Inst., 96*, 396, 2004.
135. Kurzer, M.S., Hormonal effects of soy isoflavones: Studies in premenopausal and postmenopausal women, *J. Nutr., 130*, 660S, 2000.
136. Power, K. and Thompson, L., Flaxseed and Lignans: Effects on Breast Cancer, in *Nutrition and Cancer Prevention*, Awad, A. and Bradford, P., editors; CRC Press: Boca Raton, FL, 2006; Chapter 19, pp. 385–409.
137. Messina, M., McCaskill-Stevens, W., and Lampe, J.W., Addressing the soy and breast cancer relationship: Review, commentary, and workshop proceedings, *J. Natl. Cancer Inst., 98*, 1275, 2006.
138. Petrakis, N.L., et al., Stimulatory influence of soy protein isolate on breast secretion in pre- and postmenopausal women, *Cancer Epidemiol. Biomarkers Prev., 5*, 785, 1996.
139. Henderson, B.E. and Bernstein, L., The international variation in breast cancer rates: An epidemiological assessment, *Breast Cancer Res. Treat., 18 (1 Suppl)*, S11, 1991.
140. Lu, L.J., et al., Effects of soya consumption for one month on steroid hormones in premenopausal women: Implications for breast cancer risk reduction, *Cancer Epidemiol. Biomarkers Prev., 5*(1), 63, 1996.
141. Trock, B.J., Hilakivi-Clarke, L., and Clarke, R., Meta-analysis of soy intake and breast cancer risk, *J. Natl. Cancer Inst., 98*, 459, 2006.
142. Shu, X.O., et al., Soyfood intake during adolescence and subsequent risk of breast cancer among Chinese women, *Cancer Epidemiol. Biomarkers Prev., 10*, 483, 2001.
143. Kilkkinen, A., et al., Serum enterolactone concentration is not associated with breast cancer risk in a nested case-control study, *Int. J. Cancer, 108*, 277, 2004.
144. Zeleniuch-Jacquotte, A., et al., Circulating enterolactone and risk of breast cancer: A prospective study in New York, *Br. J. Cancer, 91*, 99, 2004.
145. McCann, S.E., Moysich, K.B., and Mettlin, C., Intakes of selected nutrients and food groups and risk of ovarian cancer, *Nutr. Cancer, 39*, 19, 2001.
146. Larsson, S.C., Holmberg, L., and Wolk, A., Fruit and vegetable consumption in relation to ovarian cancer incidence: The Swedish Mammography Cohort, *Br. J. Cancer, 90*, 2167, 2004.
147. Qin, L.Q., et al., Milk/dairy products consumption, galactose metabolism and ovarian cancer: Meta-analysis of epidemiological studies, *Eur. J. Cancer Prev., 14*, 13, 2005.

11 Osteoporosis and Osteoarthritis

Wendy E. Ward

CONTENTS

11.1 INTRODUCTION

Osteoporosis and osteoarthritis are among the most common musculoskeletal disorders, and can severely compromise quality of life in both men and women. Recognition of the devastating morbidity and mortality associated with musculoskeletal diseases led to the worldwide initiative, "The Bone and Joint Decade" (2000–2010) [1], which has been endorsed by the United Nations and World Health Organization, with many countries throughout the world participating as National Action Networks. The overall mission of the Bone and Joint Decade is to "promote musculoskeletal health and musculoskeletal science worldwide," with one of the specific objectives being the advancement of understanding of musculoskeletal disorders and improve the prevention and treatment through research. Nutrition has a unique role in preserving and maintaining musculoskeletal health. This chapter aims to build on the specific objective stated above. It will discuss the etiology of osteoporosis, followed by a discussion of sex-based differences in bone health in response to nutritional interventions to aid in the prevention and treatment of this disease. Similarly, osteoarthritis will be discussed, with focus on its etiology and sex-based responses to nutritional interventions as well as weight reduction. Key areas for future research are also indicated.

11.2 OSTEOPOROSIS

11.2.1 Etiology of Osteoporosis

The most recent consensus statement from the National Institutes of Health defines osteoporosis as "a skeletal disorder characterized by compromised bone strength predisposing a person to an increased risk of fracture. Bone strength primarily reflects the integration of bone density and bone quality." [2]. Bone density, often referred to as bone mineral density (BMD), is a measure of the quantity of mineral in the skeleton or at a specific skeletal site. BMD is measured in the clinical setting using dual energy x-ray absorptiometry, and the BMD value of an individual is compared with values for young healthy controls to classify an individual as "normal," "osteopenia," "osteoporosis," or "severe osteoporosis" according to criteria set out by the World Health Organization [3]. For this comparison, *t*-scores are calculated, representing the number of standard deviations that BMD is away from the mean of young, healthy, sex-matched controls. A limitation of a BMD measurement is that it does not fully predict risk of fragility fracture, and thus an active area of research pertains to developing a methodology for assessing fracture risk [4]. The second feature in the definition of osteoporosis is "bone quality," which is influenced by bone microarchitecture, microdamage, and mineralization. At present, arguably the only measure that can be used in the clinical setting to assess bone quality is incidence of fragility fracture. Ideally, safe and effective technologies would image skeletal sites in three dimensions, allow evaluation of both the mineral and matrix in bone, and most importantly the microarchitecture of bone, to more accurately assess risk of fragility fracture. We await safe technologies that can be used in the clinical setting to evaluate bone quality and predict fracture risk.

Osteoporosis in men and women is predominately diagnosed during later life [2,5–7]. In women, it is most commonly observed after menopause as the cessation of endogenous estrogen production leads to a rapid deterioration of BMD. This loss of BMD occurs rapidly during the first 5–10 years postmenopause [5,6]. Men also experience bone loss during aging, but the loss of BMD occurs gradually [8]. In both men and women, osteoporosis results when bone turnover is uncoupled, such that bone resorption occurs at a faster rate than bone formation, leading to the overall loss of bone tissue. While diagnosis of osteoporosis most commonly occurs during later life, often after a fragility fracture has occurred, a growing number of researchers are investigating how nutrition and lifestyle, such as physical activity, help to optimize the attainment of peak bone mass, and the preventive role that these factors may play in maintaining bone health throughout the life cycle [9]. Genetics is estimated to account for about 75% of peak bone mass, indicating that lifestyle factors such as nutrition and physical activity have a role in prevention [9–11]. Life-long nutrition and lifestyle factors are significant contributors to bone health as bone is a dynamic tissue.

Osteoporosis is more common in women than in men, owing to differences in skeletal structure and size, and menopause. Unlike some other diseases and disorders same discussed in this book, osteoporosis in women has been more extensively studied than in men. Similarly, a greater number of studies have investigated the role of nutrition in bone health in women compared with men. Although more women develop osteoporosis and experience a fragility fracture, men have a twofold higher rate of mortality from hip fracture [12]. Data indicate that men who fracture a hip are generally sicker at the time of fracture than women [12]. Thus, more women than men who are otherwise healthy suffer from osteoporosis. Women who fracture a hip commonly have osteoporosis, arthritis, and hypertension whereas men who fracture typically have higher rates of respiratory conditions (i.e., chronic obstructive pulmonary disease, bronchitis, emphysema, asthma), myocardial infarction, and stroke [12]. Moreover, the cause of death postfracture differs from that of women, with men dying because of infections, i.e., pneumonia, influenza, septicemia, and renal failure [12]. In contrast, a woman's cause of death postfracture is wide-ranging [12].

11.2.2 Nutrition

11.2.2.1 Calcium

Calcium (Ca) is widely known to be important for bone health, but the majority of women in North America do not consume recommended levels of Ca established by the Institute of Medicine in 1997 (1000 mg/day for men and women 30–50 years, 1200 mg/day for men and women >50 years) [13]. Since this time, other organizations have recommended higher dietary intakes of Ca to protect against osteoporosis. The Osteoporosis Society of Canada recommends 1500 mg Ca/day for menopausal women and men over age 50 [6], and the National Institutes of Health recommends 1500 mg Ca/day for women not receiving estrogen therapy [14]. The higher requirement for Ca postmenopause is due to decreased Ca absorption and increased resorption of bone after menopause [5,6]. The Position Statement of the North American Menopause Society in 2006 concluded that "adequate Ca intake in the presence of adequate Vitamin D intake has been shown to reduce bone loss in peri- and postmenopausal women older than 60 with low bone mass" [15].

Several recent studies have reported no effect of supplementation with Ca and Vitamin D on bone health, specifically fracture risk, but interpretation of these studies is problematic due to the habitual intakes of women studied, and a lack of reporting of dietary intakes of Ca and Vitamin D in some of these studies [16–19]. Dawson-Hughes [20] commented in an editorial on the findings of the Women's Health Initiative Study [17] that since the habitual intakes of Ca and Vitamin D were similar to current recommended intakes then a dramatic effect would not be expected as there is a threshold after which no further benefit of Ca is observed. Furthermore, pharmacological agents such as calcitonin, bisphosphonates, and hormone replacement therapy (HRT) are prescribed in combination with Ca and Vitamin D supplements to ensure that sufficient substrate is available for bone health. Calcitonin and HRT have been shown to be more effective at maintaining BMD when provided in combination with Ca supplements [21].

To avoid adverse effects due to overconsumption of Ca (i.e., hypercalcemia, kidney stones), the upper tolerable level (UL) of Ca is 2500 mg Ca/day [13], a level that is likely not reached through consumption of foods alone. Use of Ca supplements in combination with a diet abundant in Ca rich foods (particularly dairy foods) means that some individuals could have Ca intakes close to or above the UL. Thus it is important for health professionals to assess dietary intake of Ca when recommending Ca supplements.

11.2.2.2 Vitamin D

The dietary recommended intakes (DRIs) for Vitamin D were published in 1997, and stated that dietary intakes in men and women should be 5 μg/day for under age 50, 10 μg/day for age 50–70, and increased to 15 μg/day over age 70 [13]. Since the establishment of the DRIs, new data on Vitamin D and a variety of diseases and conditions have led leading vitamin experts to encourage higher intakes of Vitamin D for maximal health. These experts have published a thorough review in which they reviewed the evidence that supports the need for higher than currently recommended intakes for Vitamin D [22]. This review eloquently concludes that Vitamin D (specifically 25-hydroxyvitamin D) intakes of 25 μg/day are needed to obtain optimal serum 25-hydroxyvitamin D levels of 90–100 nmol/L. The health benefits are wide-ranging and include improved lower extremity function, decreased risk of falls, decreased risk of fractures, as well as improved periodontal health and decreased risk of colorectal cancer [22].

Vieth et al. [23] recently published an article titled "The urgent need to recommend an intake of Vitamin D that is effective," which further emphasizes the need to reconsider current dietary reference intakes for Vitamin D. This article highlights the fact that it is difficult to achieve the current DRI for Vitamin D and even more challenging to attain the proposed level of Vitamin D (25 μg/day) due to limited quantity of Vitamin D in commonly consumed foods. Vieth et al. [23] suggests that raising Vitamin D levels "can happen only if some or all of the following are implemented: the encouragement of safe, moderate exposure of skin to ultraviolet light; appropriate increase in food fortification with Vitamin D; and the provision of higher dose of Vitamin D in supplements for adults."

The Osteoporosis Society of Canada recommends that postmenopausal women have a Vitamin D intake of 20 μg/day, with the same recommendation for men over age 50 [6]. Many intervention studies investigating Vitamin D and bone health (BMD or fracture) have included both men and women, often with women representing more than 50% of the study population [24]. In some studies, subanalyses have been used to examine sex-specific effects. A meta-analysis evaluating Vitamin D and fracture prevention concluded that the benefit of Vitamin D on fracture prevention was not sex-specific, although the overall number of men studied was somewhat limited [24].

11.2.2.3 n-3 Fatty Acids

Animal studies have consistently demonstrated that bone is responsive to changes in dietary fat [25–27]. In addition, a study in humans undergoing knee replacement has demonstrated that bone marrow in joints reflects dietary intakes of fatty acids (discussed further in Section 11.3.2.2). Of significance is the fact that consuming fish oil with its n-3 LCPUFAs shifts the n-6 pathway towards the n-3 pathway, possibly mediating favorable effects on bone by stimulating production of less inflammatory mediators. The effect of n-3 fatty acids on eicosanoid and proinflammatory cytokine production is discussed in detail in Chapter 12.

There is some evidence that osteoporosis is a state of inflammation, induced by the loss of endogenous estrogen production [28,29]. It is hypothesized that an increase in T-cell activity occurs postovariectomy, and stimulates and perpetuates the loss of BMD by enhancing production of receptor activator of NF-κB ligand and macrophage colony-stimulating factor [28,29]. This hypothesis is based, in part, on the observation that tumor necrosis factor (TNF)-α knockout mice do not experience the rapid loss of BMD that occurs postovariectomy [28,29].

Human studies investigating the effects of n-3 fatty acids on bone health have been conducted in males [30]. Using a prospective study design, healthy young men with a mean age of 16 years at baseline were followed until they reached 22 years of age. This study is unique as it measured serum levels of fatty acids and was able to correlate these measures with BMD. Serum docosahexaenoic acid was positively associated with whole body BMD as well as spine BMD. This finding suggests that consumption of n-3 LCPUFAs may play a role in acquisition of bone mass and attainment of peak bone mass.

A similar study in females has not been reported. Studies designed to evaluate sex-based differences are needed to understand how responses to n-3 fatty acids may differ between men and women. Furthermore, studying effects at critical stages throughout the life cycle will be important.

11.2.2.4 Soy Isoflavones

Over the past decade, there has been considerable research activity in the area of soy isoflavones and bone health in women. The soy isoflavones share a similar chemical structure to endogenous 17-β-estradiol and bind to both estrogen receptor-α and -β. Epidemiological evidence suggests that women consuming soy foods have higher BMD and reduced risk of fracture [31–33]. Findings from human feeding studies and studies using ovariectomized rodent models are less clear [31–33]. Some studies report an attenuation of BMD loss (human and animal studies) and stronger bones (animal studies) while other studies have shown no effects on bone health. Weaver and Cheong [33] published a review in which several possible explanations for variable results are discussed. For example, differences in life stage studied and estrogen status may be a confounder. Isoflavones may also act in a dose-dependent manner or perhaps have synergistic or opposing effects with other components in foods. Moreover, it has been shown that some individuals metabolize isoflavones to a different extent, i.e., metabolize daidzein to equol, which may have greater estrogenic effects than daidzein. Other possible explanations include small sample sizes, duration of studies, differences in the source of isoflavones or extraction techniques, and time since menopause. For more information, the reader is directed to thorough reviews on soy isoflavones and bone health [31–33]. At present, soy isoflavones are not recommended [5,6] as a treatment for maintaining BMD and overall bone health after menopause.

Most research using soy isoflavones has focused on the postmenopausal stage of life, with few data reported in premenopausal women [34] or men [35]. A one year intervention study in young women with regular menses demonstrated that soy isoflavones had no effect on bone mineral content or BMD [34]. A study in older men reported modest effects on BMD at the spine with no effect at the hip [35]. This study compared the effects of consuming a soy beverage over one year between men and women over age 60 [35]. A greater benefit was observed in women compared with men, albeit the effects were modest in both sexes, and likely would not translate into a reduced risk of fracture [35].

As discussed in Chapter 5, epigenetics is an exciting area whereby early exposure to a nutrient or food component can lead to permanent modifications in gene expression without altering the DNA sequence. Studies have shown that the isoflavone genistein can cause epigenetic changes in coat color of a specific mouse strain [36]. Because infants can be exposed to high levels of isoflavones through consumption of soy infant formula [37], researchers are investigating the potential effects, positive or negative, on reproductive and bone health. One study has demonstrated, using a neonatal mouse model, that exposure to the isoflavone genistein, at levels mimicking that experienced by infants, has long-term programming effects on bone metabolism [38]. Both male and female mice that were treated with genistein during the first five days of life had higher BMD at femur and lumbar vertebra at early adulthood, and individual lumbar vertebrae were more resistant to fracture. Whether the higher BMD achieved at early adulthood protects against deterioration of bone tissue after withdrawal of sex steroid hormones (postovariectomy or postorchidectomy) is currently under study using this mouse model.

11.2.3 Conclusion and Future Research

It is essential that recommended intakes of Ca and Vitamin D be achieved for bone health. Several organizations suggest higher intakes of Ca and Vitamin D for postmenopausal women and men over age 50, and it is quite possible that revisions to the DRIs for Vitamin D will occur in the near future. Emerging evidence suggests that n-3 fatty acids have a positive role in bone health, both during acquisition of peak bone mass and during aging, but additional studies in both men and women are needed to confirm its biological benefits. Clarification of the effectiveness of soy isoflavones at preserving bone health postmenopause is needed.

Future studies should focus on elucidating a healthful diet for bone. Since bone is a dynamic tissue, it is likely that a healthy diet throughout the life cycle will ensure that optimal bone health is achieved. While Ca and Vitamin D are proven to be critical for bone health, diets combining these nutrients with other foods such as fish oil and soy protein, containing isoflavones, need to be studied. Prospective studies designed to investigate sex-based differences to combinations of foods or food components would be ideal. It will be important to study various stages of the life cycle, i.e., during acquisition of peak bone mass, and during aging when the greatest losses of BMD occur. Because men have not been studied as extensively as women, sex-based studies will provide useful data regarding nutrition and bone health specific to men.

11.3 OSTEOARTHRITIS

11.3.1 Etiology of Osteoarthritis

Osteoarthritis is a degenerative joint disease in which the protective cartilage around one or more joints is eroded, due in part to a localized inflammation in the joint. With the loss of cartilage at the joint, movement is painful. Osteoarthritis most commonly affects knees, hips, and hands but can occur at any joint in the body. Diagnosis of osteoarthritis is done by assessing radiographical outcomes, a common feature being narrowing of joint space. When assessing effectiveness of treatments a combination of radiographic and clinical outcomes are typically measured. For the studies discussed in this chapter, the clinical outcome most often used is the Western Ontario and McMaster Universities Osteoarthritis Index (WOMAC) with subscales for pain, function, and stiffness [39]. Some studies have also used the Lequesne's indices for hip and knee osteoarthritis [40]. In addition, radiography is often used to confirm the diagnosis of osteoarthritis at the start of an intervention study.

A recent review on sex and gender differences of osteoarthritis concludes that sex-based differences in osteoarthritis exist but that the "understanding of these differences is at a preliminary stage" [41]. It is known that there are sex-based differences in the prevalence of osteoarthritis at various skeletal sites [41]. Women over age 55 have a higher prevalence of osteoarthritis in the knee and hand and a lower prevalence of cervical spine degeneration compared with men, while the prevalence at the hip is similar between sexes [41]. After age 50, the incidence of osteoarthritis in women vs. men increases more rapidly with advancing age. Risk factors for osteoarthritis in both men and women include genetics, advancing age, dysplasia of the hip, excess body weight, and prior knee injury [41]. Possible contributors to sex-based differences in occurrence of osteoarthritis include use of HRT, presence of osteoporosis, anatomical differences, or cartilage thickness. Cartilage thickness is less in women compared with men, and thus may be a contributing risk factor. Estrogen receptors are present in cartilage, demonstrating that cartilage responds to estrogen [42]. Moreover, some studies suggest that use of HRT may reduce the risk of osteoarthritis [43]. Understanding the role of estrogens and potential interactions with osteoporosis is an ongoing area of osteoarthritis research.

While various interventions such as weight loss, physical activity, and nutritional interventions, primarily involving glucosamine and chondroitin, have been studied in relation to relief of symptoms of osteoarthritis, most studies have combined men and women in the trials [44–51]. From review of the distribution of males and females in these studies [44–51], it is clear that most studies have included more women than men, likely due to the fact that more women suffer from osteoarthritis. Sex-based studies that specifically focus on differences in the response to weight reduction and nutritional interventions are needed.

11.3.2 Nutrition

11.3.2.1 Diet, Weight Loss, and Physical Activity

Weight loss in overweight or obese individuals has been shown to alleviate symptoms of osteoarthritis, as reductions in body weight, even small reductions, significantly reduce pressure on diseased joints. In one study, patients with knee osteoarthritis and a mean body mass index (BMI) of 35.9 who were randomized to a low energy diet compared with a control diet lost significantly more body weight (11 kg vs. 4.4 kg) over a 8 week study period [45]. As is common in osteoarthritis intervention trials, most of the subjects were women (89%). Although both groups lost weight, only the group consuming the low energy diet experienced a significant difference in symptoms. The 8 week study period is rather short, and it is possible that the rapid weight loss in the low energy diet group was a major contributor to the overall alleviation of symptoms. An interesting finding was that reduction of body fat was most closely associated with improvements in symptoms (using the WOMAC index). The relationship between body fat and symptoms requires further investigation.

Obese subjects (mean BMI = 51) who underwent bariatric surgery experienced a significant reduction in osteoarthritis symptoms by 6–12 months postsurgery [48]. Although the average BMI of subjects was still classified as overweight or obese (mean BMI = 36) at 6–12 months postsurgery, significant symptomatic relief was observed. The authors comment that weight loss postsurgery often occurs up to 24 months postsurgery so it is possible that with more weight loss, a further improvement would be observed. Another positive finding was that the weight loss improved symptoms at both weight- and nonweight-bearing skeletal sites. This study was primarily conducted in women, as all but 1 of the 48 subjects was female.

The Arthritis, Diet, and Activity Promotion Trial, as the name indicates, included both diet and physical activity in the study design [49]. Patients were mostly women with osteoarthritis of the knee and a BMI $\geq$ 28. Patients were randomized to control (74% female), diet (74% female), physical exercise (74% female), or diet in combination with physical activity (65% female) for 18 months. This study demonstrated that the combination of diet and physical activity was most effective at attenuating self-reported symptoms of osteoarthritis (WOMAC scores), as well as functional measures such as a 6 min walk distance and a stair-climb time. Patients in the diet alone group, who lost a significant amount of body weight in comparison to the control group did not experience improvements in function or lesser symptoms. The fact that weight loss was similar between the diet alone and diet + physical activity group suggests that physical activity itself is important in management of osteoarthritis.

Another aspect of this trial was to determine if changes in BMI were associated with changes in markers of inflammation [52]. Some researchers hypothesize that a low-grade inflammation may be a precursor to developing chronic diseases such as cardiovascular disease [53] and Type II diabetes [54]. Thus, the fact that osteoarthritis is associated with a low-grade inflammation led the authors to measure markers of inflammation including C-reactive protein (CRP), interleukin-6 (IL-6), and soluble TNF-α receptor. The findings demonstrated that it was weight loss and not physical activity that modulated inflammation markers. Weight loss, regardless of physical activity, was associated with significant decreases in CRP, IL-6, and soluble TNR-α. With respect to CRP, a sex-based difference was reported. A greater decrease in CRP due to weight loss was observed in men compared with women, and this finding should be further investigated. The authors conclude that further studies that include larger sample sizes are needed to elucidate sex-based differences in inflammatory markers after weight loss. Moreover, they acknowledge that whether lowering the inflammation markers due to weight loss reduces the risk of cardiovascular disease and Type II diabetes should be investigated.

11.3.2.2 n-3 Fatty Acids

As discussed in Section 11.2.2.3, studies in animals have demonstrated that consumption of n-3 fatty acids can modulate the composition of fatty acids in bone [25–27]. Moreover, these changes in fatty acid profile are likely favorable to musculoskeletal health by shifting the production of proinflammatory mediators away from the arachidonic acid pathway [25]. An 8 week intervention with lyprinol, a 5-lipoxygenase inhibitor extracted from New Zealand green-lipped mussels, was shown to attenuate joint pain and improve function in subjects with osteoarthritis in the knee or hip [44]. When multiple intervention studies are compared, however, findings are inconsistent. A systematic review of the New Zealand green-lipped mussels concluded that because of inconsistent findings these supplements should not be recommended [47]. Randomized controlled trials with large sample sizes and intention to treat design are needed to assess effectiveness.

In humans, dietary fish oil, rich in n-3 LCPUFAs, has been shown to modulate the lipid composition of marrow and joint fluid [55]. In patients undergoing bilateral knee replacement, samples of marrow and joint fluid were analyzed for lipid content before and after supplementation with fish oil for 6 months. Samples were collected from the knee joint at the time of first surgery. Postsurgery, for 6 months, patients received 3 g fish oil/day, containing 11% docosahexaenoic acid (the content of eicosapentaenoic acid was not provided). After the supplementation period, a second set of samples were collected during the knee replacement surgery in the opposite knee. It was shown that consuming fish oil decreased the total amount of marrow lipid, decreased the saturated fatty acids, and increased the unsaturated fatty acids in joint fluid. From a clinical perspective, the author states that the change to an environment that contains more unsaturated fatty acids may enhance lubrication by reducing the surface tension within the joint [55]. This study included 8 men and 12 women but did not analyze data by sex. Randomized controlled trials investigating the effect of diets rich in n-3 LCPUFAs are warranted, to determine if symptoms of osteoarthritis can be lessened.

11.3.2.3 Glucosamine and Chondroitin

Both glucosamine and chondroitin are important constituents in articular cartilage at joints. Glucosamine is a precursor for glycosaminoglycans synthesized by chondrocytes, and chondroitin is a sulfated glycosaminoglycan, often attached to proteins as a proteoglycan. Glucosamine supplements are derived from chitinous exoskeleton of crustaceans [56], while shark cartilage is a common source of chondroitin [57]. Various forms of glucosamine (sulfate or hydrochloride) and chondroitin (sulfate) are aggressively marketed as a safe and effective treatment of osteoarthritis based on the premise that the loss of these compounds from the cartilage, which act as a protective cushion within joints, ultimately resulting in osteoarthritis, can be replaced by consuming oral supplements of glucosamine or chondroitin or both. The science behind such marketing claims is debatable, particularly since bioavailability of oral administration has been shown to be less than optimal based [58]. Moreover, as discussed below, effectiveness at attenuating osteoarthritis has not been proven.

Intervention studies using glucosamine, chondroitin, or the combination of the two have not been designed to elucidate sex-specific responses to these compounds. The most recent Cochrane Review published in 2005 reported on 20 randomized controlled trials in which glucosamine therapy was used for treating osteoarthritis, and notably, 11 of the 20 studies had study populations that were more than 73% women, and only 2 of the 20 studies had study populations that were less than 50% women (5% and 48%) [51]. Thus, women have been represented in the glucosamine intervention studies, but their potentially different biological response compared with men is unknown. Similarly, a randomized controlled trial published since the Cochrane Review also included 64% women [46].

The Cochrane Review, which included findings from 2570 subjects with osteoarthritis at the knee or hip, concluded that intervention with glucosamine for 2–3 months did not alleviate symptoms of osteoarthritis or result in functional improvement [51]. Similarly, a meta-analysis of studies that used chondroitin to attenuate osteoarthritis at the knee or hip concluded that chondroitin had "minimal or nonexistent effects" [50]. The authors of this analysis also commented that of the 20 studies analyzed, only 3 had sufficient strength (i.e., large sample sizes, intention to treat design) [50]. In contrast, they noted that studies with fewer subjects and without the intention to treat design were the studies that, individually, demonstrated some favorable effects.

Most studies to date have studied glucosamine or chondroitin alone rather than in combination. However, a recent study randomized individuals with mild or moderate or severe osteoarthritis of the knee (1583 subjects) to one of five treatments: placebo, glucosamine hydrochloride alone (1500 mg/day), chondroitin sulfate alone (1200 mg/day), glucosamine hydrochloride in combination with chondroitin sulfate (1500 mg/day + 1200 mg/day), or a cycloxygenase-2 inhibitor that served as a positive control (celecoxib, 200 mg) for 24 weeks [46]. Patients were screened for the severity of their disease using radiologic evidence, the WOMAC pain scale, and American Rheumatism Association criteria. Overall analyses did not demonstrate a reduction in symptoms of osteoarthritis with glucosamine or chondroitin alone or in combination. However, a subanalysis revealed that subjects, classified as having moderate or severe osteoarthritis of the knee at the start of the study, did experience significant attenuation of symptoms. As discussed by the authors, these findings suggest that individuals with more severe disease may benefit more, and they are prudent to conclude that future trials are needed to confirm this. Based on this subanalysis, they also comment that a limitation of the study may be the fact that the majority of subjects had mild (70%) vs. moderate or severe (30%) osteoarthritis of the knee. Whether glucosamine and chondroitin act by different mechanisms or synergistically remains to be determined.

The safety of glucosamine is an active area of interest because of concerns that it may impair glucose regulation by stimulating insulin insensitivity. Many studies have reported no adverse effects on glucose metabolism and a recent study with a crossover design showed that 6 week oral administration of glucosamine did not alter insulin resitance or endothelial function in lean or obese individuals [59]. As expected, obese individuals did have some insulin resistance and endothelial dysfunction. Further studies are needed to confirm whether glucosamine is safe in individuals with Type II diabetes.

11.3.3 Conclusion and Future Research

Weight loss among overweight or obese individuals is effective at attenuating symptoms of osteoarthritis. Emerging evidence suggests that the combination of weight loss and regular physical activity may be of greater benefit than weight loss alone. The effectiveness of other interventions, including n-3 fatty acids, and glucosamine and chondroitin, alone and in combination, require further study before being recommended as treatments for osteoarthritis.

Osteoporosis and osteoarthritis are more commonly studied in women and men, but there is still a need to continue to study sex-based differences with respect to the etiology of these diseases and responses to lifestyle interventions such as diet and physical activity.

There is certainly strong evidence supporting that weight loss among overweight and obese individuals significantly lessens pain and improves function. One of the greatest challenges may be in ensuring that patients with osteoarthritis can successfully maintain a healthy body weight and regular physical activity. In our fast-paced, convenience-oriented society that is often contrary to a healthy lifestyle, it will be essential to find supportive ways to assist individuals with osteoarthritis to maintain a healthy lifestyle. Further investigation of types of exercise that are most appropriate and safe in individuals with osteoarthritis is essential. The effectiveness of glucosamine in combination with chondroitin as well as fish oil, and n-3 LCPUFAs should also be pursued. As identified in the reviews of glucosamine and chondroitin, and green-lipped mussels, and studies on n-3 fatty acids, it will be important to design studies with intention-to-treat design and with large sample sizes, allowing efficacy and sex-based differences to be thoroughly assessed.

It is also important to acknowledge that pharmacological agents are available to aid in managing osteoarthritis, and are often necessary for an individual to cope with pain and to function. As with many drugs, adverse effects may occur. Commonly prescribed cycloxygenase-2 inhibitors may potentially increase risk of cardiovascular disease. Having said this, there may be ways in which a healthful diet may attenuate the disease process such that lower doses of drugs are effective at managing osteoarthritis. Future studies should focus on these food–drug interactions in individuals with osteoarthritis.

A more thorough understanding of the etiology of osteoarthritis, including risk factors, is also essential. Particular areas to investigate include the genetic involvement, as well as the potential role of estrogen in protecting against development of osteoarthritis.

REFERENCES

1. Bone and Joint Decade Online, http://www.boneandjointdecade.org/.
2. National Institutes of Health, Osteoporosis prevention, diagnosis, and therapy, *J. Am. Med. Assoc.*, 285, 785–795, 2001.
3. World Health Organization, Assessment of fracture risk and its application to screening for postmenopausal osteoporosis, WHO Technical Report Series 843, 1994.
4. Hernandez, C.J. and Keaveny, T.M., A biomechanical perspective on bone quality, *Bone*, 39, 1173, 2006.
5. North American Menopause Society, Management of osteoporosis in postmenopausal women: 2006 position statement of The North American Menopause Society, *Menopause*, 13, 340, 2006.
6. Brown, J.P. and Josse, R.G., 2002 clinical practice guidelines for the diagnosis and management of osteoporosis in Canada, *Can. Med. Assoc. J.*, 167, S1, 2002.
7. Looker, A.C. et al., Prevalence of low femoral bone density in older U.S. adults from NHANES III, *J. Bone. Miner. Res.*, 12, 1761, 1997.
8. Olszynski, W.P. et al., Osteoporosis in men: Epidemiology, diagnosis, prevention, and treatment, *Clin. Ther.*, 26, 15, 2004.
9. Klein, G.L. et al., The state of pediatric bone: Summary of the ASBMR pediatric bone initiative, *J. Bone Miner. Res.*, 20, 2075, 2005.
10. Davies, J.H., Evans, B.A., and Gregory, J.W., Bone mass acquisition in healthy children, *Arch. Dis. Child*, 90, 373, 2005.
11. Heaney, R.P. et al., Peak bone mass, *Osteoporos. Int.*, 11, 985, 2000.
12. Orwig, D.L., Chan, J., and Magaziner, J., Hip fracture and its consequences: Differences between men and women, *Orthop. Clin. North Am.*, 37, 611, 2006.
13. Standing Committee on the Scientific Evaluation of Dietary Reference Intakes, *Dietary Reference Intakes: Calcium, Phosphorus, Magnesium, Vitamin D, and Fluoride*, Institute of Medicine, National Academy Press, Washington, D.C., 1997.
14. National Institutes of Health, Optimal calcium intake, *NIH Consens. Statement*, 12, 1, 1994.
15. North American Menopause Society, The role of calcium in peri- and postmenopausal women: 2006 position statement of the North American Menopause Society, *Menopause*, 13, 862, 2006.
16. Grant, A.M. et al., Oral vitamin D3 and calcium for secondary prevention of low-trauma fractures in elderly people: A randomised placebo-controlled trial, *Lancet*, 365, 1621–1628, 2005.
17. Jackson, R.D. et al., Calcium plus vitamin D supplementation and the risk of fractures, *N. Engl. J. Med.*, 354, 669, 2006.
18. Porthouse, J. et al., Randomised controlled trial of calcium and supplementation with cholecalciferol (vitamin D3) for prevention of fractures in primary care, *Brit. Med. J.*, 330, 1003, 2005.
19. Prince, R.L. et al., Effects of calcium supplementation on clinical fracture and bone structure: Results of a 5-year, double-blind, placebo-controlled trial in elderly women, *Arch. Intern. Med.*, 166, 869, 2006.

20. Dawson-Hughes, B., Calcium plus vitamin D and the risk of fractures, *N. Engl. J. Med.*, 354, 2285, 2006.
21. Nieves, J.W. et al., Calcium potentiates the effect of estrogen and calcitonin on bone mass: Review and analysis, *Am. J. Clin. Nutr.*, 67, 18, 1998.
22. Bischoff-Ferrari, H.A. et al., Estimation of optimal serum concentrations of 25-hydroxy vitamin D for multiple health outcomes, *Am. J. Clin. Nutr.*, 84, 18, 2006.
23. Vieth, R. et al., The urgent need to recommend an intake of vitamin D that is effective, *Am. J. Clin. Nutr.*, 85, 649, 2007.
24. Bischoff-Ferrari, H.A. et al., Fracture prevention with vitamin D supplementation: A meta-analysis of randomized controlled trials, *J. Am. Med. Assoc.*, 293, 2257, 2005.
25. Watkins, B.A. et al., Modulatory effect of omega-3 polyunsaturated fatty acids on osteoblast function and bone metabolism, *Prostaglandins Leukot. Essent. Fatty Acids*, 68, 387, 2003.
26. Watkins, B.A. et al., Biochemical and molecular actions of fatty acids in bone modeling, *World Rev. Nutr. Diet*, 88, 126, 2001.
27. Watkins, B.A. et al., Omega-3 polyunsaturated fatty acids and skeletal health, *Exp. Biol. Med. (Maywood)*, 226, 485, 2001.
28. Weitzmann, M.N. and Pacifici, R., Estrogen regulation of immune cell bone interactions, *Ann. N.Y. Acad. Sci.*, 1068, 256, 2006.
29. Weitzmann, M.N. and Pacifici, R., Estrogen deficiency and bone loss: An inflammatory tale, *J. Clin. Invest.*, 116, 1186, 2006.
30. Hogstrom, M., Nordstrom, P., and Nordstrom, A., n-3 Fatty acids are positively associated with peak bone mineral density and bone accrual in healthy men: The NO2 Study, *Am. J. Clin. Nutr.*, 85, 803, 2007.
31. Cassidy, A. et al., Critical review of health effects of soyabean phyto-oestrogens in post-menopausal women, *Proc. Nutr. Soc.*, 65, 76, 2006.
32. Reinwald, S. and Weaver, C.M., Soy isoflavones and bone health: A double-edged sword? *J. Nat. Prod.*, 69, 450, 2006.
33. Weaver, C.M. and Cheong, J.M., Soy isoflavones and bone health: The relationship is still unclear, *J. Nutr.*, 135, 1243, 2005.
34. Anderson, J.J. et al., Soy isoflavones: No effects on bone mineral content and bone mineral density in healthy, menstruating young adult women after one year, *J. Am. Coll. Nutr.*, 21, 388, 2002.
35. Newton, K.M. et al., Soy protein and bone mineral density in older men and women: A randomized trial, *Maturitas*, 55, 270, 2006.
36. Dolinoy, D.C. et al., Maternal genistein alters coat color and protects Avy mouse offspring from obesity by modifying the fetal epigenome, *Environ. Health Perspect.*, 114, 567, 2006.
37. Setchell, K.D. et al., Isoflavone content of infant formulas and the metabolic fate of these phytoestrogens in early life, *Am. J. Clin. Nutr.*, 68, 1453S, 1998.
38. Piekarz, A.V. and Ward, W.E., Effect of neonatal exposure to genistein on bone metabolism in mice at adulthood, *Pediatr. Res.*, 61, 48, 2007.
39. Dougados, M., Monitoring osteoarthritis progression and therapy, *Osteoarthritis Cartilage*, 12, S55, 2004.
40. Lequesne, M.G. and Maheu, E., Clinical and radiological evaluation of hip, knee and hand osteoarthritis, *Aging Clin. Exp. Res.*, 15, 380, 2003.
41. O'Connor, M.I., Osteoarthritis of the hip and knee: Sex and gender differences, *Orthop. Clin. North. Am.*, 37, 559, 2006.
42. Richette, P., Corvol, M., and Bardin, T., Estrogens, cartilage, and osteoarthritis, *Joint Bone Spine*, 70, 257, 2003.

43. Reginster, J.Y. et al., Is there any rationale for prescribing hormone replacement therapy (HRT) to prevent or to treat osteoarthritis? *Osteoarthritis Cartilage*, 11, 87, 2003.
44. Cho, S.H. et al., Clinical efficacy and safety of Lyprinol, a patented extract from New Zealand green-lipped mussel (*Perna canaliculus*) in patients with osteoarthritis of the hip and knee: A multicenter 2-month clinical trial, *Allerg. Immunol. (Paris)*, 35, 212, 2003.
45. Christensen, R., Astrup, A., and Bliddal, H., Weight loss: The treatment of choice for knee osteoarthritis? A randomized trial, *Osteoarthritis Cartilage*, 13, 20, 2005.
46. Clegg, D.O. et al., Glucosamine, chondroitin sulfate, and the two in combination for painful knee osteoarthritis. *N. Engl. J. Med.*, 354, 795, 2006.
47. Cobb, C.S. and Ernst, E., Systematic review of a marine nutriceutical supplement in clinical trials for arthritis: The effectiveness of the New Zealand green-lipped mussel *Perna canaliculus, Clin. Rheumatol.*, 25, 275, 2006.
48. Hooper, M.M. et al., Musculoskeletal findings in obese subjects before and after weight loss following bariatric surgery, *Int. J. Obes. (Lond.)*, 31, 114, 2007.
49. Messier, S.P. et al., Exercise and dietary weight loss in overweight and obese older adults with knee osteoarthritis: The Arthritis, Diet, and Activity Promotion Trial, *Arthritis Rheum.*, 50, 1501, 2004.
50. Reichenbach, S. et al., Meta-analysis: Chondroitin for osteoarthritis of the knee or hip, *Ann. Intern. Med.*, 146, 580, 2007.
51. Towheed, T.E. et al., Glucosamine therapy for treating osteoarthritis, *Cochrane Database Syst. Rev.*, CD002946, 2005.
52. Nicklas, B.J. et al., Diet-induced weight loss, exercise, and chronic inflammation in older, obese adults: A randomized controlled clinical trial, *Am. J. Clin. Nutr.*, 79, 544, 2004.
53. Vasto, S. et al., Inflammatory networks in ageing, age-related diseases and longevity, *Mech. Ageing Dev.*, 128, 83, 2007.
54. Duncan, B.B. and Schmidt, M.I., The epidemiology of low-grade chronic systemic inflammation and type 2 diabetes, *Diab. Technol. Ther.*, 8, 7, 2006.
55. Pritchett, J.W., Statins and dietary fish oils improve lipid composition in bone marrow and joints, *Clin. Orthop. Relat. Res.*, 2006. Epub ahead of print.
56. Dahiya, N. et al., Biotechnological aspects of chitinolytic enzymes: A review, *Appl. Microbiol. Biotechnol.*, 71, 773, 2006.
57. Sakai, S. et al., Identification of the origin of chondroitin sulfate in "health foods", *Chem. Pharm. Bull. (Tokyo)*, 55, 299, 2007.
58. Biggee, B.A. et al., Low levels of human serum glucosamine after ingestion of glucosamine sulphate relative to capability for peripheral effectiveness, *Ann. Rheum. Dis.*, 65, 222, 2006.
59. Muniyappa, R. et al., Oral glucosamine for 6 weeks at standard doses does not cause or worsen insulin resistance or endothelial dysfunction in lean or obese subjects, *Diabetes*, 55, 3142, 2006.

12 Rheumatoid Arthritis

Lisa K. Stamp and Leslie G. Cleland

CONTENTS

12.1 INTRODUCTION

Rheumatoid arthritis (RA) is a common, chronic disease characterised by inflammation of the lining of the joint (the synovium), cartilage degradation, and bone erosion. In the early stages of RA, joint pain and swelling are the dominant clinical features. Once acquired, RA persists and over time RA can lead to significant joint destruction with loss of function and disability. RA can also affect areas outside the joints (extra-articular manifestations) including rheumatoid nodules, and lung and cardiac involvement. Characteristic features which aid in the diagnosis of RA include the presence of rheumatoid factor (RF) and antibodies against citrullinated peptides in serum, and erosion of bone and cartilage on radiographs of affected joints.

The pathogenesis of RA has been extensively investigated and a number of the inflammatory pathways and mediators have been defined. Cells found within the rheumatoid synovium include T cells, monocytes/macrophages, neutrophils, and fibroblast-like synoviocytes. These cells are all important sources of inflammatory mediators such as eicosanoids and cytokines. The eicosanoids prostaglandin E_2 (PGE_2), and thromboxane A_2 (TXA_2) have multiple biological activities that are important in mediating the inflammatory response. The cytokines interleukin (IL)-1β and tumour necrosis factor (TNF) are important signalling agents in the tissue destruction seen in RA, which occurs through the actions of matrix metalloproteinases (MMPs). Left unchecked the chronic inflammation that is the hallmark of RA can ultimately lead to cartilage degradation, bone erosion, and failure of joint function.

Like most autoimmune diseases, RA is more common in women. The prevalence of RA is reported to range from 0.5% to 2% with an excess of females to males by 2–4 times [1]. The annual incidence of RA is 36/100,000 in women compared to 14/100,000 in men in the United Kingdom [2]. The sex distribution appears to vary with age with a male:female ratio of incident cases of 1:6 in patients aged <45 years compared with 1:1 in those >60 years of age [2,3]. In females, the incidence of RA increases with age with the peak after the menopause and then a fall after the age of 75 years. In comparison, the incidence of RA in men appears stable until age 45 years and gradually increases thereafter [2].

12.2 ETIOLOGY OF RHEUMATOID ARTHRITIS

12.2.1 General Considerations

In common with other autoimmune diseases, RA appears to have a multifactorial pathogenesis. To understand the general nature of causal factors it is important to recognize that the term "cause" has two related, but in some respects, distinct meanings. In the first, less formal sense, it is used to describe the concurrence or precedence of an event relative to another in a sequence of events (e.g., inflammation is the cause of joint swelling in this person). In the second, more formal sense, a cause is a component of conditions that make an event, of which a disease can be an example, more likely to occur. A cause in this sense is not necessary for the event, unless demanded by definition (e.g., inflammation causes inflammatory swelling), which is a matter of semantics (Sense 1), not probability (Sense 2). Female sex and certain other sex related factors are examples of causes of RA (Sense 2) in that they are preexisting factors that correlate positively with occurrence of RA, even though they may affect only a minority of those bearing the risk factor. Other genetically determined and environmental factors that predispose to rheumatoid arthritis that are discussed below are also causes (Sense 2). Prior factors, occurring by chance or introduced by design, that make an event (e.g., a disease) less likely to occur are preventives.

12.2.2 Genetic Risk Factors in RA

Twin studies provide a means of apportioning the respective influences of genetic and environmental factors upon disease expression. In RA, twin studies have shown monozygotic concordance rates of 12% [4] and 15% [5]. More recently, data from both these cohorts have been the subject of quantitative genetic analysis. The authors report that the "heritability" or extent to which liability to RA is explained by genetic variation in the population is ~60% [6].

A number of different genes have been reported to be associated with increased susceptibility to RA. Commentary will be restricted to polymorphisms of human leukocyte antigen (HLA)-DRβ1 and protein tyrosine phosphatase N22 *(PTPN22)* loci, for which interactions between sex and disease associations have been reported.

12.2.2.1 HLA and the Shared Epitope

RA is associated with certain HLA class II alleles found within the major histocompatibility complex (MHC). The strongest associations are with polymorphisms in the variable β chain of HLA-DR and involve alleles among the HLA-DR4 subtype (e.g., *0401, *0404) and to a lesser extent HLA-DR1 (e.g., *0101) and HLA-DR10. The disease-associated polymorphisms occur in a conserved amino acid sequence in the third hypervariable region of the DRβ chain, which is known as the "shared epitope." Other genes within the MHC are in linkage disequilibrium with HLA-DR genes and alleles of other genes (especially HLA-DQ) linked within MHC haplotypes to disease related DR alleles are also associated with RA. MHC class II molecules are strongly expressed on antigen presenting cells (APCs), most notably the "professional" APC's, dendritic cells. The function of these MHC class II molecules is to present processed peptides to CD4 + T cells. The shared epitope (SE) is situated in the region of the DRβ chain that is important for the formation of the peptide binding groove [7]. The canonical feature of the SE is a positively charged pocket which favors presentation of certain configurations of negatively charged peptide. Presentation of such peptides may be important for both effective protective responses against invasive infections and the nature of the cellular responses to chronic infections [8] and for induction of autoimmunity. An observed compounding risk for RA in subjects with HLA-DR susceptibility alleles and prior intimate exposure to pet cats supports the possibility that latent infection in a genetically susceptible host may predispose to RA through HLA-restricted immune responsiveness or predilection for triggering of autoimmunity [9].

It has been suggested that there is an interaction between sex and genetic association in RA. For example, among the Japanese a stronger association between HLA-DR4 and RA has been found in males compared with females [10]. In a more recent smaller Spanish study comparing males and females with RA, there was an increase in HLA-DR1 in the male group and increases in HLA-DR4 and HLA-DR10 in the female group [11]. However, such sex differences have not been a universal finding [12] and subgroup analyses can be misleading. Meyer et al. have reported sex differences in the penetrance of RA in subjects bearing two HLA-DR susceptibility alleles [13]. One potential explanation for such findings is that non-HLA genes which are closely linked to HLA contribute to the association. In this regard, sex differences in polymorphisms of the TNF gene which is found within the MHC have been reported [14]. Alternatively, hormonal differences may play a role through an interaction between HLA and the prolactin gene, which lies in close proximity to the HLA region [15]. Thus disease-associated haplotypes may contribute multiple genetic factors to disease susceptibility.

The overall genetic associations between RA and HLA are complex and not yet fully understood. It has been estimated that the HLA system is responsible for 30%–50% of the genetic susceptibility to RA. Increasing definition of polymorphisms within the human genome and more informative methods of analysis, including haplotype mapping, offer prospects of deeper understanding of the genetic contributions to RA.

12.2.2.2 Protein Tyrosine Phosphatase N22

PTPN22 encodes the lymphoid protein tyrosine phosphatase (Lyp), which is an important down-regulator of T cell activation. A single nucleotide polymorphism (1858C → T) of *PTPN22*, which results in the substitution of tryptophan (W) for arginine (R) at codon 620 (R620W), has been associated with RA in several different populations [16–18]. Lyp acts to down-regulate T cells and it has been suggested that the disease-associated polymorphism encodes a protein which is less effective in T cell down-regulation, thereby conferring an increased risk for autoimmune diseases, including RA. However, recent evidence suggests that the disease-associated polymorphism results in a protein that is a more potent inhibitor of T cell activation [19]. The authors hypothesize that this increased ability to inhibit T cells results in failure to delete autoreactive T cells or insufficient activity of T regulatory cells which act to down-regulate the immune response [19].

Like HLA-DR, sex differences have been reported in the association between RA and *PTPN22*. Pierer et al. reported that the frequency of the *PTPN22* 1858T allele was disproportionately increased in male compared with female patients with RA (53.8% vs. 33%, $p < 0.001$) [18]. A study of over 4000 RA patients from Sweden and North America also found a higher frequency of *PTPN22* 1858T in RF positive males compared to females [20].

Such differences between genes associated with RA may reflect the differences in disease expression observed between males and females (discussed in Section III) or other hormonal or environmental influences.

12.2.3 Hormones in the Etiology of RA

The female predominance suggests a role for sex hormones in the etiology of RA. The relationship between sex hormones and RA is complex. Both primarily gonadal (estrogen, testosterone) and adrenal (dehydroepiandrosterone [DHEA] and its sulphate [DHEAS]) hormones have been implicated in RA.

In women with RA, serum estradiol and testosterone concentrations do not differ from those in healthy controls [21]. However, serum DHEA and DHEAS concentrations have been reported to be lower in blood and synovial fluid from female patients with RA compared with sex-matched normal controls [21]. In comparison, males with RA have been reported to have lower serum testosterone concentrations but no difference in DHEAS compared with normal controls [21]. Androgens may have a protective effect on pathophysiology and clinical aspects of RA and the reduction of DHEA/DHEAS in women may explain the predominance of RA in women [21].

12.2.3.1 Pregnancy, Breast Feeding, and Risk of RA

Estrogen suppresses cell-mediated immunity [22] and may therefore protect against T cell-mediated diseases such as RA. In mice, excess estrogen suppresses collagen-induced arthritis [23]. Estrogen increases markedly during pregnancy and there is a reduced incidence of the onset of RA during pregnancy with an increased risk postpartum, when the levels of estrogen drop. The risk postpartum seems to be especially marked after the first pregnancy [24]. Nulliparity has been reported to increase the risk of developing RA [25,26], although other studies have found no association between parity and risk of developing RA [27–29]. In addition, women who develop RA within 12 months of their first pregnancy are five times more likely to have breast fed [30]. In contrast, a more recent study reported that longer total lifetime history of breast feeding was associated with a slightly lower risk of developing RA [31]. Increased prolactin, which is pro-inflammatory, has been suggested as explanation for the potential increased risk of RA postpartum [15]. Breast milk is rich in long chain n-3 polyunsaturated fatty acids, which are required for optimal neural development of the fetus and infant. As discussed later in this chapter, n-3 fatty acids have anti-inflammatory effects and the unmet extra demands for maternal dietary n-3 fatty acids during breast feeding may be a contributor to increased risk of RA.

12.2.3.2 Exogenous Estrogens and Risk of RA

The studies examining the risk of RA and use of the oral contraceptive (OC) are also conflicting with some studies suggesting a reduced risk of RA with OC use [26,32] and others finding no effect [33]. Recently, the use of OC has been reported to be inversely associated with RF positivity in women without RA [34]. Although it is not clear that RF has a direct pathogenic role in RA, this finding suggests that if OC use has a protective effect in RA, this occurs early in the development of the disease. Overall, there is no consensus regarding the relationship between the OC and risk of RA. There are similar conflicting data with regard to the use of hormone replacement therapy and the risk of RA [32,35].

12.2.4 Smoking and Risk of RA

Smoking may be an important environmental risk factor for RA. In monozygotic twins, who presumably have the same genetic risk for RA, a strong association between smoking and RA has been observed (odds ratio [OR] 12, 95% confidence interval [CI] 1.78–5.13) [36].

Smoking is associated with the production of RF even in patients without RA [37–39] and the association between smoking and RA appears to be stronger with RF-positive RA than RF-negative RA [40–42]. This association between smoking and RF is stronger the higher the titre of RF. While the exact role of RF in the pathogenesis of RA remains unclear, it may perpetuate the inflammatory process in the synovium [43,44]. However, the association between smoking and RF positivity and the possible role of RF in the pathogenesis of RA provides a potential causal link between smoking and RA.

There also appears to be a compounding risk with smoking and presence of the SE. A recent study reported that the relative risk of RF-positive RA was 2.8 (95% CI 1.6–4.8) in those who had never smoked but carried the SE genes compared to 2.4 (95% CI 1.3–4.6) in current smokers lacking the SE genes and 7.5 (95% CI 4.2–13.1) in current smokers with the SE genes. For those smokers carrying double SE genes the relative risk of RF-positive RA was 15.7 (95% CI 7.2–34.2) [45].

The association between smoking and RA appears to be stronger for men than for women [39,42,46,47], indeed a protective effect of smoking on risk for development of RA has been described in women in one study [48]. However, in women, the association between smoking and RA appears to be stronger after the menopause [41,47,49] and it has been estimated that 18% of RA in postmenopausal women is attributable to smoking [49].

The interaction between smoking and RA in postmenopausal women has reinforced suggestions that sex hormones contribute to RA risk. Smoking has been shown to have antiestrogenic effects, with female smokers having an earlier menopause, increased risk of osteoporosis, and reduced risk of endometrial cancer [50]. As discussed above, estrogen may have a protective effect against RA, which is diminished by smoking.

Recent studies suggest that antibodies against citrullinated peptides may be more directly involved in RA than RF, since antibodies against the synthetic reagent cyclic citrullinated peptide (CCP) are found in RA only slightly less frequently than RF and have greater specificity for RA. Furthermore, citrullinated proteins, including citrullinated fibrin(ogen), are abundant within synovial fluid in RA and antibodies against CCP correlate with progressive radiographic joint damage. Smoking predisposes to presence of anti-CCP antibodies only in patients with the shared epitope [51]. It is conceivable that smoking contributes to citrullinization of proteins, a potentially immunogenic posttranslational modification, which alters charge on peptide fragments, which the shared epitope bearing MHC may be better equipped to present.

12.2.5 Diet and the Risk of RA

The role of diet in the etiology of RA has been examined in a number of epidemiological studies. Obesity has been suggested to be a risk factor for RA especially for women [52]. In this section we discuss the role and potential mechanisms of different food and beverage groups in the etiology of RA.

12.2.5.1 n-3 Fatty Acids

Fatty acids may be grouped into three major classes according to the number of double bonds in the fatty acid chain: (1) saturated fatty acids (no double bond), (2) monounsaturated fatty acids (one double bond), (3) polyunsaturated fatty acids (PUFAs) ($\geq$2 double bonds). The principal PUFAs can be further classified according to the site of the double bond proximal to the methyl terminus as n-6 or n-3. Vertebrates do not have the enzymes required to introduce double bonds in the n-3 and n-6 positions and these fatty acids must therefore be obtained from the diet. Hence they are known as essential fatty acids.

The Western diet generally has an abundance of n-6 fats compared to n-3 fats. This is in large part due to the availability of soybean, safflower, sunflower, and corn oils which contain the n-6 fat linoleic acid (LA; 18:2n-6). The n-3 homologue of LA, α-linolenic acid (ALA; 18:3n-3), is present in flaxseed oil but this is not present in the diet in significant quantities. ALA is present in lesser amounts in rapeseed and canola oils. Once ingested, LA and ALA may be used in energy metabolism or be converted to the C20 fatty acids, arachidonic acid (AA) and eicosapentaenoic acid

TABLE 12.1
Metabolism of n-6 and n-3 Fatty Acids

Fatty Acid Family	n-6	n-3
18 carbon fatty acid	Linoleic acid (LA; 18:2n-6)	α-Linolenic acid (ALA; 18:3n-3)
Dietary sources	Sunflower, corn, and safflower oil	Flaxseed, canola (rapeseed) oil
Dietary intake	Large intake (7%–8% dietary energy)[a] ↓	Minor intake (0.3%–1.0% dietary energy)[a] ↓
Metabolism		Only 5%–10% ALA converted to EPA
C20 fatty acid	Arachidonic acid (AA; 20:4n-6)	Eicosapentaenoic acid (EPA; 20:5n-3)
Sources	Mainly synthesized from ingested linoleic acid, also ingested in red meats	Mainly from ingested EPA (fish, fish oil) ↓ Only 2%–5% converted to DHA
		Docosahexaenoic acid (DHA; 22:6n-3)

[a] In the last 10 years, LA intake decreased and ALA intake increased in some countries where canola oil use has displaced sunflower, safflower, or corn oil use.

(EPA), respectively (Table 12.1). The conversion of ALA to EPA is poor and fish/fish oils are the main dietary source of EPA. These C20 fatty acids are incorporated into cell membranes and tissues and may be further metabolized to eicosanoids, which are mediators and regulators of inflammation. The effects of dietary fatty acids on inflammation are discussed in the section on dietary treatment of RA.

Dietary n-3 fats, which are abundant in fish and fish oils, may have a protective effect against RA. The Japanese diet is rich in n-3 fats as compared with the typical Western diet, and Japanese have approximately one-third the incidence of RA [53] despite a high prevalence of HLA-DR alleles associated with susceptibility for RA [54,55]. The Seattle Women's Health Study has shown a reduced risk for developing RA in subjects consuming two or more fish meals per week with an adjusted OR of 0.57 (95% CI 0.35–0.93) compared to subjects consuming less than one fish meal per week [56]. Consumption of olive oil with dietary vegetables and fish, has also been reported to be associated with a reduced risk of developing RA [57,58]. In a more recent prospective study of diet and RA, neither olive oil nor long chain n-3 fatty acid consumption was associated with a reduced risk of RA [59]. In the same study fish consumption was examined and the authors divided fish into three groups; lean fish (0–2 g fat/100 g fish), medium fat fish (3–7 g fat/100 g fish), and fat fish (≥8 g fat/100 g fish). The authors reported that each additional 30 g of fatty fish consumed per day was associated with a 49% reduction in the risk of RA.

Unexpectedly, intake of medium fat fish was associated with an increased risk of RA with the authors suggesting this may have been a chance finding given lack of biological plausibility [59].

12.2.5.2 Red Meat

High consumption of red meat has been associated with an increased risk of inflammatory polyarthritis (which may evolve into RA) (OR 1.9; 95% CI 0.9–4.0) [60]. However, the authors make no comment on fish consumption during the study period which is a potential confounding factor. Another study using an ecological approach reported that meat and offal (entrails and internal organs of a butchered animal) were associated with an increased risk of developing RA [61] although this association has not been found in another study, albeit using different methodology [59]. Whether the association between red meat consumption and inflammatory arthritis is causative remains unclear although the presence of significant amounts of AA in red meat may provide some explanation for the association (see section on Fatty acids).

12.2.5.3 Antioxidants

Evidence for release of oxygen free radicals (e.g., nitric oxide, superoxide, and hydroxyl radical) has been found in fluid and cells from rheumatoid joints [62,63]. Oxygen free radicals are implicated in the tissue damage observed in RA [64,65]. Antioxidants, such as vitamin E (α-tocopherol), vitamin C (ascorbic acid), β-carotene, and selenium, may have a protective role against tissue damage caused by free oxygen radicals. These observations along with evidence that markers of antioxidant nutritional status are lower in patients with established RA compared to normal controls [66] have led to the suggestion that antioxidants may protect against the development of RA.

Lower serum concentrations of vitamin E, β-carotene, retinol, and selenium have been reported to be weakly associated with an increased risk of developing RA in some but not all studies [67–69]. The strongest association between risk of RA and antioxidants was found for a combined antioxidant index rather than any one specific antioxidant [67].

Results from the Iowa Women's Health Study suggest that a higher dietary intake of β-cryptoxanthin (a carotenoid found in fruit and vegetables) and zinc may protect against the development of RA [70]. This association between β-cryptoxanthin and development of RA has also been reported in a European cohort with evidence that a modest intake of β-cryptoxanthin (equivalent to one glass of freshly squeezed orange juice per day) was associated with a reduced risk of developing inflammatory arthritis even after adjustment for vitamin C intake and smoking (top tertile vs. bottom tertile OR 0.42; 95% CI 0.2–0.88; $p = 0.02$) [71]. Using the same study population, low vitamin C intake was also associated with an increased risk of RA with an adjusted OR of 3.3 (95% CI 1.4–7.9) in the lowest tertile of vitamin C intake (<55.7 mg/day) compared with the highest intake tertile (>94.9 mg/day) [72]. Although the outcome in these studies was inflammatory polyarthritis, rather than RA specifically, many patients with inflammatory polyarthritis will develop RA over time. However, another study with definite RA as the outcome found no association between intake of vitamins C and E, zinc, or selenium and the development of RA [59].

Although, there is a biologically plausible mechanism whereby antioxidants have anti-inflammatory effects, the available data do not provide clear evidence for an effect of dietary intake of antioxidants on the development of RA.

12.2.5.4 Caffeine

Tea and coffee consumption have been examined as potential risk factors for the development of RA in three studies. In the Finnish National Health Study, consumption of four or more cups of coffee per day was associated with an increased risk of RF-positive, but not RF-negative RA even after adjustment for potential confounders such as age, smoking, and sex (relative risk [RR] 2.2; 95% CI 1.13–4.27) [73]. In comparison, there was no association between daily caffeine intake and the risk of RA in the Iowa Women's Health Study. However, compared to noncoffee drinkers, women who consumed four or more cups of decaffeinated coffee per day were at increased risk of RA (RR 2.58; 95% CI 1.63–4.06). Furthermore, women who consumed three or more cups of tea per day had a reduced risk of RA (RR 0.39; 95% CI 0.16–0.97) [74]. An association between tea, coffee, and RA was not found in two more recent studies [59,75].

While the data are conflicting, several theories have been suggested to explain the association between coffee/tea consumption and RA. Tea contains antioxidants, which have been reported to have a protective effect against RA [67,68]. The major catechin in tea inhibits induction of inducible nitric oxidase (iNOS) by macrophages stimulated in vitro [76]. iNOS generates highly reactive free radical products while de-imidating substrate arginine moieties to citrulline. Citrullinated peptides/proteins are immunogens which provide a focus for autoimmunity in RA (as discussed above).

12.2.5.5 Alcohol

There is a conflicting evidence with respect to alcohol consumption and the risk of RA. The Iowa Women's Health Study revealed no association between alcohol consumption and risk of RA [77]. In contrast, two case-controlled studies have reported an inverse association between alcohol consumption and risk of RA. In the first of these studies the relative risk of RA in those who consumed alcohol at least once a day was 0.54 (95% CI 0.35–0.82) even after adjustment for confounders including age, parity, smoking, OC use, and menopausal status [48]. However, the mean time to first clinic visit, when the assessment of alcohol consumption was undertaken, was 1.5 years and information on alcohol consumption prior to or at the onset of symptoms was not collected. It is therefore possible that alcohol consumption may have been modified in the RA cases after symptom onset and prior to the assessment. Voigt et al. reported a reduced risk of RA only in postmenopausal women consuming more than 14 alcoholic drinks per week although this did not reach statistical significance [78]. A biologically plausible mechanism for the role of alcohol in RA has not been established.

12.2.5.6 Vitamin D and Dairy Intake

Vitamin D plays an important role in calcium and bone metabolism. It also has effects on the immune system and dietary supplementation with vitamin D minimizes joint inflammation in animal models of arthritis [79]. In humans, concentrations of the active vitamin D metabolite 1,25 di-hydroxyl cholecalciferol (1,25OHD) are higher in the synovial fluid of patients with RA compared to osteoarthritis [80]. Conversion of 25OH cholecalciferol to 1,25OHD occurs locally under the influence of inflammatory cytokines such as IL-1 [80]. Locally produced 1,25OHD has important autocrine and paracrine effects which include inhibition of maturation of dendritic cells, an effect which in turn may down-regulate T cell responses [81].

In the Iowa Women's Health Study a higher intake of vitamin D was associated with a reduced risk of RA (RR 0.67; 95% CI 0.44–1.00; $p = 0.05$) in women aged 55–69 years [82]. There was no association with calcium intake per se, although there was a reduced risk of RA with higher milk product intake. While this study is by no means definitive, it provides a promising line of investigation into the role of diet in prevention and adjunctive treatment of RA.

12.2.5.7 Conclusion

To date, epidemiological studies provide no clear association between any one single dietary factor and development of RA. However, assessing dietary intake in epidemiological studies is difficult and identifying the effects of a single dietary variable and distinguishing it from other dietary and lifestyle factors such as smoking may not be possible.

12.3 EFFECT OF SEX ON DISEASE EXPRESSION AND OUTCOME IN RA

In addition to being more common in women, sex may influence RA disease expression and severity. In studies of early RA (disease duration <12 months), men tend to be older at disease onset than women [3,83]. RA typically affects the small joints of the hands and feet, although it can affect larger proximal joints such as shoulders, hips, and spine. The pattern of joint involvement has been reported to differ between men and women, with women tending to have more involvement of the small joints of the hands and feet at presentation [3] while men display more involvement of the larger proximal joints [84].

Long-term outcomes may be worse in women with RA compared to men. RA is more likely to remit in men than in women [85]. In a study of early RA, 40% of men were in remission (disease activity score [DAS] 28 < 2.6 see Appendix 1) at 2 years compared with 28% of women ($p < 0.001$) [3]. Women have been shown to have higher disability scores [85] and greater functional limitations than men [86]. Joint erosions are more frequent in men and tend to occur earlier in the disease course [84], although this is not a universal finding [87]. By contrast, structural failure of joints is more common in women, upon whom joint surgery is undertaken more frequently [84,88].

Patients with RA can also display extra-articular manifestations of the disease. In general, these are more common in men, in whom rheumatoid nodules and rheumatoid lung disease are more frequent. By contrast, sicca symptoms (dry eyes and mouth) are more common in women [84].

12.3.1 Cardiovascular Outcomes in Women with RA

RA is associated with increased mortality with a standardized mortality rate of ~2.0 [89]. Cardiovascular disease is increasingly recognised as an important cause of death in patients with RA, especially in those who are RF positive [90]. Women with RA have an increased risk of myocardial infarction (MI) compared to women without RA, even after adjustment for other cardiovascular risk factors (RR 2.0; 95% CI 1.23–3.29). Furthermore, women with RA for >10 years have an RR of MI of 3.1 (95% CI 1.64–5.87) compared with women without RA [91]. Traditional cardiovascular risk factors, including body mass index, diabetes, hypertension, hypercholesterolemia, physical inactivity, and family history of early MI, are similar between women with and without RA [92]. Thus RA is associated with an increased incidence of cardiovascular disease, which is not explained by classical cardiovascular risk factors [93]. Recently several inflammatory markers have been linked to cardiovascular disease including C-reactive protein (CRP) [94], intercellular adhesion molecule (ICAM), and vascular adhesion molecule (VCAM) [95]. These inflammatory markers have been shown to be increased in women with RA compared with women without RA suggesting that the increased risk of cardiovascular disease in RA may be associated with systemic inflammation [92]. Such a link between inflammation and cardiovascular disease is further supported by evidence that disease-modifying antirheumatic agents (DMARDs) such as methotrexate, which suppress the inflammatory process, are associated with lower cardiovascular mortality rates in patients with RA [96]. An increase in carotid intima-media thickness in RA patients has been shown to correlate with raised CRP [97], and a higher risk of cardiovascular death has been found in RA patients with at least three erythrocyte sedimentation rate (ESR) values ≥ 60 mm/h after adjustment for cardiovascular risk factors (hazard ratio 2.03; 95% CI 1.45–2.83) [98]. All nonsteroidal anti-inflammatory drugs (NSAIDs) inhibit the inducible isoform of cyclo-oxygenase (COX)-2, through which the vascular patency factor prostacyclin (PGI_2) is formed. Most NSAIDs appear to increase cardiovascular risk and as these agents are given to most patients with RA [99], they are likely to contribute significantly to increased cardiovascular risk in RA.

12.4 INFLUENCE OF FEMALE REPRODUCTIVE STATUS ON DISEASE ACTIVITY AND OUTCOMES IN RA

The activity of RA varies according to reproductive status and time within the menstrual cycle. There is a tendency for RA to remit during pregnancy and relapse postpartum and disease is often more severe in postmenopausal women. Women with RA also report fewer joint symptoms in the postovulatory phase of the menstrual cycle when levels of estradiol and progesterone are high [100].

12.4.1 Influence of Pregnancy and Breast Feeding on Disease Activity

It has been recognized since the 1800s that RA tends to remit during pregnancy and relapse postpartum. The largest study of 140 pregnant women in the United Kingdom reported that two-thirds of patients experienced an improvement in joint pain and swelling during pregnancy. On the other hand, 16% reported an increase in swelling and 19% an increase in pain. Only 16% of women achieved total remission, defined as no joint swelling and no DMARD therapy [101]. Furthermore, 62% had more swollen or tender joints postpartum compared to during pregnancy. Postpartum disease flare by 6 months appears to be related to breast feeding, especially first-time breast feeders [102].

A number of mechanisms have been implicated in the effects of pregnancy and breast feeding on RA disease activity. Pregnancy induces a change in the maternal immune system so as to prevent the fetus becoming the focus of an immune attack from the mother. T helper (Th) cells can be divided into Th1 and Th2 according to their cytokine secretion profile. Th1 cytokines (e.g., interferon-γ) are considered pro-inflammatory while Th2 cytokines (e.g., IL-4) are considered anti-inflammatory. RA is generally viewed as a Th1 disease while pregnancy induces Th2-like immunological changes. The change in balance from Th1 to Th2 during pregnancy may explain some of the improvement in disease activity [103].

Female sex hormones change during pregnancy with increases in estrogen during pregnancy and reduction postpartum. Estrogens have immunosuppressive effects and the high concentrations during pregnancy could act to suppress RA activity while the reduced levels postpartum may allow the inflammatory process to dominate once again. Prolactin, which has pro-inflammatory actions, increases dramatically postpartum in breast feeding women and may contribute to postpartum flare of RA.

During pregnancy, n-3 fatty acids are transferred from the mother to the fetus. This can result in a negative n-3 fatty acid balance in the mother, which could contribute to the propensity for RA to flare in the postpartum period. Breast milk is rich in n-3 fats [104] and ongoing maternal depletion of n-3 fats associated with breast feeding may also contribute to increased risk of postpartum flare of RA in breast feeding women.

Nelson et al. have suggested that disparity between fetal and maternal HLA-DR alleles may be associated with RA remission during pregnancy [105]. Higher concentrations of fetal DNA in maternal serum have been associated with improved disease control, especially in the third trimester [106]. It is likely that the manner of presentation of the fetal antigens to the maternal immune system promotes immunological tolerance to the fetus.

12.4.2 Influence of Menopause on Disease Activity

Postmenopausal women have been reported to have more severe disease compared with premenopausal women and men of similar age [107]. There is no convincing evidence of benefit on disease activity with the use of hormone replacement therapy in postmenopausal women with RA [108,109].

12.5 ROLE OF NUTRITION IN THE MANAGEMENT OF RA

The role of nutrition in the management of common medical conditions such as ischemic heart disease and diabetes is well accepted and entrenched in standard clinical practice. In comparison, the role of nutrition in the management of RA is less well accepted and not generally considered to be a component of standard clinical practice. Despite this general lack of conviction among physicians as to the role of nutrition, 33%–75% of RA patients believe food plays an important role in their symptom severity and 20%–50% will have tried dietary manipulation in an attempt to relieve their suffering [110,111].

Patients with RA have also been reported to have impaired nutritional status [112]. The term "rheumatoid cachexia" has been coined to describe the loss of body cell mass that occurs in severe RA (for recent review see [113]). Even in those patients with well-controlled disease, body cell mass has been reported to be 13%–14% lower than in healthy controls [114,115]. While patients with RA have adequate intakes of protein and calories, they have increased resting energy expenditure and increased protein catabolism. This is compounded by reduced levels of physical activity. The mechanisms of rheumatoid cachexia are complex and include TNF mediated impairment of protein synthesis and promotion of protein catabolism and enhancement of peripheral insulin resistance which favors muscle loss and fat gain [116].

An evidence-based approach to nutrition is an important aspect of management and can help the patient avoid worthless interventions which are expensive, time consuming, in some cases harmful and which may divert from access to more effective measures. In this section we shall review the evidence for a variety of dietary manipulations in RA. There are no data comparing effects in men and women specifically.

12.5.1 Dietary n-3 Fatty Acids in the Management of RA

Fish oil is a potent source of the anti-inflammatory long chain n-3 fatty acids EPA and docosahexaenoic acid (DHA). Numerous studies have shown the benefits of fish oil in RA (Table 12.2). It is notable that the dose of EPA + DHA needed for an anti-inflammatory effect is 2.7 g/day, which equates to nine or more standard fish oil capsules daily. This is substantially more than doses taken through the common practice of self-medication with fish oil for arthritis. Until recently, all studies of fish oil in RA have been confined to patients with long standing RA. These studies of late disease, in which irreversible joint damage is the norm, show a modest clinical improvement when combined with standard therapies for RA including DMARDs and NSAIDs. Like other DMARDs, there is a latent period of ~12–15 weeks before benefits are observed, which can be shortened somewhat by use of higher doses of fish oil [117–119]. A recent report documents the long-term use of fish oil in early RA [120]. In a longitudinal cohort study, after 3 years of treatment with a standardized

TABLE 12.2
Summary of Clinical Trials of n-3 Supplementation in RA

Number of Patients	Diet and Daily n-3 Fatty Acid Supplement (g/day) or Placebo	Duration	Outcome Measures in Fish Oil Group	DMARD and/or NSAID	Ref.
33/34 patients completed No controls	0.1–0.2 g fish oil/kg IV daily for 7 days (oil contained 2.82 g EPA, 3.09 g DHA per 100 ml) Background diet no change	Outcomes assessed at Day 8 and Day 28	↓DAS28 5.45 (baseline) → 4.51 (Day 8) → 4.73 (Day 28) ($p < 0.001$ baseline—Day 8) ACR20 Day 8 29%, Day 28 18% ACR50 Day 8 12%, Day 28 9% ↓ESR but not CRP ↓Pt pain VAS and physicians global	Continued Change in requirement not assessed	[121]
55/66 patients completed n-3 supplement Placebo	1.4 g EPA + 0.21 g DHA + other micronutrients Water based placebo drink Background diet no change	4 months	No change in any clinical parameter including SJC, TJC, DAS28, CRP, ESR, HAQ	Continued	[173]
60/62 patients completed cross over trial n-3 supplement Placebo	Background diet Western diet or AA < 90 mg/day 30 mg n-3 fatty acids per kg body weight Corn oil 1 g	8 months (3 months on each oil with 2 month washout between)	↓TJC, SJC ↓CRP in those on methotrexate	Continued NSAID could be reduced	[124]

(continued)

TABLE 12.2 (Continued)
Summary of Clinical Trials of n-3 Supplementation in RA

Number of Patients	Diet and Daily n-3 Fatty Acid Supplement (g/day) or Placebo	Duration	Outcome Measures in Fish Oil Group	DMARD and/or NSAID	Ref.
50 patients n-3 supplement Placebo	Background diet n-6 fatty acid <10 g/day 40 mg/kg/day 60% n-3 triglycerides (2.3 g/day n-3 triglycerides) 50/50 corn/olive oil	15 weeks	Overall improvement ↓SJC, morning stiffness, HAQ, pain score, Pt global, physician global No change TJC, CRP, ESR	Continued	[118]
49/66 patients completed n-3 supplement Placebo	Background diet no change 4.6 g EPA + 2.5 g DHA Corn oil	30 weeks	↓TJC, morning stiffness, Pt global, physicians global, physician pain assessment at Week 18 or 22 ↓TJC maintained after stopping diclofenac	Continued DMARD throughout Continued diclofenac until Week 18 or 22	[225]
60/90 patients completed n-3 supplement Placebo	Fish once per week Low dose1.3 g n-3/day (EPA 0.8 and DHA 0.2) High dose 2.6 g n-3/day (EPA 1.7 and DHA 0.4) Olive oil	52 weeks	↓Pt global and pain score as assessed by physician in high dose group only	Continued 47% high dose group able to reduce DMARD and/or NSAID vs. 15% placebo group ($p < 0.05$)	[226]

64 patients n-3 supplement Placebo	Background diet no change 1.7 g EPA + 1.1 g DHA Air filled capsules	52 weeks followed by 12 weeks of placebo	No significant change in clinical or laboratory variables	Continued but stopping NSAID encouraged No patients on DMARDs ↓NSAID requirement (40% n-3 group on NSAIDs vs. 84% placebo group $p < 0.001$)	[128]
43 patients n-3 supplement Placebo	Background diet no change 1.8 g EPA + 1.2 g DHA <2.5% n-3 fatty acids	24 weeks	↓Physicians global	Continued but able to reduce/stop NSAID if able ↓NSAID requirement in n-3 group	[129]
67 patients n-3 supplement Placebo	Background diet no change 3.8 g EPA + 2.8 g DHA Corn oil	16 weeks	↓Morning stiffness, patient and physician global, Ritchie articular index Benefits lost when NSAID stopped	NSAID reduced in some groups	[130]
51 patients n-3 supplement Placebo	Background diet no change 2.0 g EPA + 1.2 g DHA Mixture of n-6 fatty acids	12 weeks	↓Morning stiffness, TJC, CRP No change SJC, pain scores, ESR	Continued	[227]
16 patients n-3 supplement Placebo	Background diet no change 2.0 g EPA + 1.3 g DHA Coconut oil	12 weeks	↓Morning stiffness, SJC	Continued	[228]

(continued)

TABLE 12.2 (Continued)
Summary of Clinical Trials of n-3 Supplementation in RA

Number of Patients	Diet and Daily n-3 Fatty Acid Supplement (g/day) or Placebo	Duration	Outcome Measures in Fish Oil Group	DMARD and/or NSAID	Ref.
49 patients completed n-3 supplement Placebo	Background diet no change Low dose 27 mg/kg/day EPA + 18 mg/kg/day DHA High dose 54 mg/kg/day EPA + 36 mg/kg/day DHA Olive oil	24 weeks	↓TJC, SJC, and mean grip strength in low and high dose groups ↓Morning stiffness and physicians global in high dose group only	Continued—change in DMARD/NSAID required withdrawal from study 6 patients in placebo group vs. 1 in low dose and 0 in high dose withdrawn for DMARD change ($p = 0.008$)	[119]
60 patients n-3 supplement Placebo	Background diet total intake fat 60 g/day including supplements 3.2 g EPA + 2.0 g DHA Olive oil	12 weeks	↓TJC	Continued	[117]
27 patients n-3 supplement Placebo	Background diet no change 2.0 g EPA + 1.3 g DHA Coconut oil	12 weeks	↓SJC, RAI, joint pain index	Continued	[229]
49 patients n-3 supplement Placebo	Background diet no change Evening primrose oil (EPO) (540 mg GLA) EPO + fish oil (540 mg GLA + 240 mg EPA) Liquid paraffin	15 months	Withdrawal from study due to ↑RA disease activity: placebo 10, EPO 1, EPO/fish oil 2 ($p < 0.001$)	NSAID continued for first 3 months then decreased or stopped until month 12 then stable dose 11/15 EPO and 12/15 EPO/fish oil patients reduced or stopped NSAID at 12 months vs. 5/15 Placebo	[127]

30 patients n-3 supplement Placebo	Background diet no change 2.7 g EPA + 1.8 g DHA 10.3 g oleic acid + 2.1 g palmitic acid + 1.8 g LA	36 weeks (14 weeks on each supplement with 4 week washout between)	↓TJC, mean time to fatigue	Continued	[230]
37 patients n-3 supplement Placebo	Ratio of dietary PUFAs to saturated fatty acids in n-3 group 1.4:1. Random dietary changes in placebo group 1.8 g EPA Parrafin oil	12 weeks	↓TJC, morning stiffness	Continued	[122]

Abbreviations: IV—intravenous, EPA—eicosapentaenoic acid, DHA—docosahexanoic acid, DAS28—disease activity score, Pt—patient, ACR—American College of Rheumatology (see Appendix 1), ESR—erythrocyte sedimentation rate, CRP—C-reactive protein, VAS—visual analogue scale, SJC—swollen joint count, TJC—tender joint count, HAQ—health assessment questionnaire, AA—arachidonic acid, NSAID—nonsteroidal anti-inflammatory drug, DMARD—disease modifying anti-rheumatic drug, EPO—evening primrose oil, GLA—gamma-linolenic acid, PUFA—polyunsaturated fatty acids, LA—linoleic acid.

treatment regimen of combination DMARDs, patients taking fish oil, who were in the upper tertile for plasma phospholipid EPA (>5% total fatty acids vs. ~1% at baseline and in controls) were compared with patients who chose not to take supplementary fish oil. The fish oil group was compliant with advice to take 15 ml bottled fish oil daily with juice. At 3 years they displayed better self-reported function in activities of daily living, lower tender joint counts, lower ESR, higher remission rates (72% vs. 31% in controls), and less NSAID requirement (22% vs. 54% in controls) [120] than nonfish oil takers managed according to the same DMARD treatment strategy. A recent open pilot study further demonstrated a reduction in latency when n-3 fats were administered intravenously (IV) [121]. However, long-term IV therapy is impractical and costly. Deterioration in symptoms after discontinuation of the fish oil has been reported [122].

The background diet is important when considering the benefits of n-3 supplementation, especially when lower doses of fish oil are used. Diets lower in n-6 fatty acids favor incorporation of EPA from fish oil supplements into tissues [123] and may thereby enhance the effects of n-3 fatty acid dietary supplementation. A recent placebo controlled crossover trial, compared the effects of n-3 fatty acid supplementation in a diet low in AA and a normal Western diet in patients with RA. The anti-inflammatory effects of n-3 fatty acid supplementation were greater in those on the diet low in AA with a significant reduction in swollen (34% vs. 22%) and tender (28% vs. 11%) joints ($p < 0.01$) [124].

12.5.1.1 Plasma Phospholipid EPA as a Marker of n-3 Nutrition

Like many other standard pharmacotherapies for RA there is a significant degree of inter-individual response to n-3 fatty acid supplementation with respect to their incorporation into tissues. Thus a biochemical marker of n-3 fatty acid supplementation may be useful in assessing its effectiveness and compliance. Plasma phospholipid EPA concentrations have a close linear relationship with peripheral blood mononuclear cell (PBMC) EPA [125]. PBMC EPA concentrations $\geq$1.5% of total fatty acids are associated with significant inhibition of production of the inflammatory cytokines IL-1β and TNF that are important inflammatory mediators in RA [126]. A PBMC EPA concentration $\geq$1.5% of total fatty acids equates to plasma phospholipid concentration of 3.2%, which has therefore been chosen as a nominal marker of effective n-3 fatty acid supplementation.

12.5.1.2 n-3 Fatty Acid Supplements and NSAID Requirement in RA

Dietary supplementation with n-3 fatty acids has been shown to reduce NSAID requirement in patients with RA [127–130]. Long-term NSAID use may have deleterious effects in RA. NSAIDs alter the balance of TXA_2/PGE_2 production in favor of TXA_2, which increases production of the inflammatory cytokines IL-1β and TNF that are associated with tissue damage in RA [131]. In addition, n-3 fatty acids have been shown to reduce IL-1β and TNF production by mononuclear cells [132]. The ability of n-3 fatty acids to reduce NSAID requirement could therefore be beneficial in terms of preventing or reducing tissue damage in the long term. Furthermore, n-3 fatty acid supplements do not have the potentially serious upper gastrointestinal or cardiovascular side effects that are associated with NSAIDs. It is important that patients appreciate that n-3 fatty acid supplements do not afford the immediate analgesic benefits of NSAIDs and that n-3 fatty acid supplementation is a long-term not short-term therapy.

12.5.1.3 n-3 Fatty Acid Supplements and Cardiovascular Risk in RA

In addition to the benefits on disease activity in RA, there may be collateral health benefits of n-3 fatty acid supplementation with regard to cardiovascular disease. As discussed in Section 12.3.1, cardiovascular mortality is increased in women with RA compared with the general population. n-3 Fatty acid supplementation has a number of beneficial effects in cardiovascular disease (for recent review see [133]). n-3 Fatty acid supplementation has been shown to reduce cardiovascular mortality, in particular sudden cardiac death, in studies of primary and secondary prevention [134]. The factors involved in reduction of cardiovascular risk are summarized in Table 12.3. Whether n-3 fatty acid supplementation reduces cardiovascular mortality in patients with RA has not been examined specifically, but a recent study of fish oil in anti-inflammatory doses in early RA has shown reduction in multiple cardiovascular risk factors [120]. Compared with patients not taking fish oil, patients fully compliant with fish oil treatment had lower triglycerides, increased "good" HDL cholesterol, less NSAID use, greater disease suppression, and reduced platelet synthesis of TXA_2, all of which can be expected to reduce cardiovascular risk. The dose of fish oil used was 4.5 g EPA + DHA/day, which is substantially more than the doses of n-3 fatty acids generally recommended for cardiovascular protection (~1 g EPA + DHA/day) [135].

TABLE 12.3
Potential Mechanisms by Which n-3 Fatty Acids Reduce Cardiovascular Risk

Effect	Mechanism
↓Cardiac arrhythmias	Stabilization of the myocardium through alterations in Ca^{2+} and Na^{+} channels (for review see [231])
↓Triglycerides, ↑HDL (favorable lipid profile)	↑Intracellular degradation of apolipoprotein B-100 containing lipoproteins which inhibit secretion of VLDL and thus ↓triglycerides
	↑Chylomicron triglyceride clearance
	↑Conversion of VLDL to LDL
	Decreases LDL synthesis (for review see [232])
↓Blood pressure	Possibly prostacyclin mediated (metanalysis for fish oil in hypertension)
Antithrombotic effects	↓TXA_2 production + ↓platelet derived growth factors but no significant effect on platelet aggregation [232]
Endothelial function	Improved arterial compliance [233]
↑Plaque stability	Evidence from a carotid artery study suggesting n-3 fats increase thickness of fibrous cap and ↓inflammation within the plaque [234]
↓Inflammatory processes	↓TNF and IL-1implicated in atheroma

12.5.1.4 Adverse Effects of n-3 Fatty Acids and Fish Oils

In general, n-3 fatty acids are well tolerated. The most common adverse effects are a fishy after-taste, gastrointestinal upset, and nausea, although these are not serious effects and can be reduced by taking the supplement with food. Cod liver oil, but not fish body oil, contains somewhat high concentrations of the fat soluble vitamins A and D, although clinical hypervitaminosis has not been observed over a period of >3 years of regular cod liver oil consumption at anti-inflammatory doses. With anti-inflammatory doses of fish oil, abdominal discomfort and reflux appears to be more common with ingestion of gelatine coated fish oil capsules (≥ 9 daily required) than of bottled fish oil on juice before a meal according to instructions [136].

More recently there have been concerns regarding potential toxins that accumulate in long-living fish including methylmercury, polychlorinated biphenyls (PCBs), and dioxins. Methylmercury and PCBs have long half lives in the body, therefore, may accumulate with regular consumption of contaminated fish. The amount of PCBs can be reduced by removing the skin and fat from fish, although this has no effect on methylmercury which is distributed throughout the body of the fish. As regards fish oils, PCBs, dioxins, and methylmercury can all be reduced to below detectable and known acceptable limits by processing. Quality control measures are being enacted to ensure adequate processing. The US Federal Drug Administration has accorded "generally regarded as safe" status to intakes of up to 3 g/day of long chain n-3 fatty acids from marine sources. It is important for women to realize that methylmercury risk is essentially limited to certain large carnivorous fish (swordfish, marlin, shark, sea mammals) and that adequate dietary long chain n-3 fatty acids of marine origin (EPA and DHA) are needed for optimal fetal nutrition, especially with regard to long-term neural development. For example, neural function scores were more favorable in offspring of mothers with high fish intakes in a long-term study into the effects of maternal dietary fish intakes on offspring in the Seychelles [137]. A study undertaken in the Faroe Islands showed little evident benefit in neural development from breast feeding; however, pilot whale was a significant component of the usual diet [138]. On balance, avoidance of usual sources of fish other than the specified long-lived carnivorous fish and sea mammals, seems more likely to compromise rather than advantage offspring.

12.5.1.5 Mechanism by Which n-3 Fatty Acids Modulate Inflammation in RA

n-3 Fatty acids have an array of effects on the immune system including alteration in inflammatory eicosanoid and cytokine production, effects on cell adhesion molecule expression, and reduced production of oxygen free radicals (summarized in Table 12.4). These mechanisms may all contribute to the beneficial clinical effects of fish oil observed in RA.

12.5.1.5.1 Effect of n-3 Fatty Acids on Eicosanoid Production

The eicosanoids are a family of biologically active lipids whose synthesis involves the oxidation of the C20 fatty acids AA or EPA which are derived from LA or ALA or obtained from the diet as outlined in Section 12.2.5.1. AA is metabolized via COX to n-6 eicosanoids (prostaglandins [PGs], thromboxanes [TX]) or 5-lipoxygenase

TABLE 12.4
Effects of n-3 Fatty Acids on the Immune System

Effect	Potential Mechanisms
Decreased production of n-6 derived eicosanoids (PGE_2, TXA_2, LTB_4) which have pro-inflammatory effects	Decreased AA compared to EPA and DHA in cell membrane phospholipids Inhibition of AA metabolism by EPA and DHA
Increased production of n-3 derived eicosanoids (PGE_3, TXA_3, LTB_5) which in general are less pro-inflammatory	Increased EPA concentration in cell membrane phospholipids
Increased production of resolvins	Increased EPA and DHA in cell membrane phospholipids
Decreased production of pro-inflammatory cytokines—IL-1β, TNF	Alteration of intra-cellular signalling pathways Differences in the respective activities of n-6 and n-3 eicosanoid inflammatory mediators
Decreased adhesion molecule expression	?Decreased transcription
Decreased MHC II expression by APCs resulting in decreased T cell activation	?Decreased transcription
Decreased expression of MMPs	Decreased transcription

(LOX) to n-6 leukotrienes (LTs). In general the n-6 eicosanoids (PGE_2 and TXA_2) are pro-inflammatory. TXA_2 promotes synthesis by mononuclear phagocytes of the inflammatory cytokines, IL-1β, and TNF [139], while PGE_2 causes vasodilatation, increased vascular permeability, and hyperalgesia (Figure 12.1). PGE_2 can also have potentially desirable regulatory effects on inflammatory cytokine production.

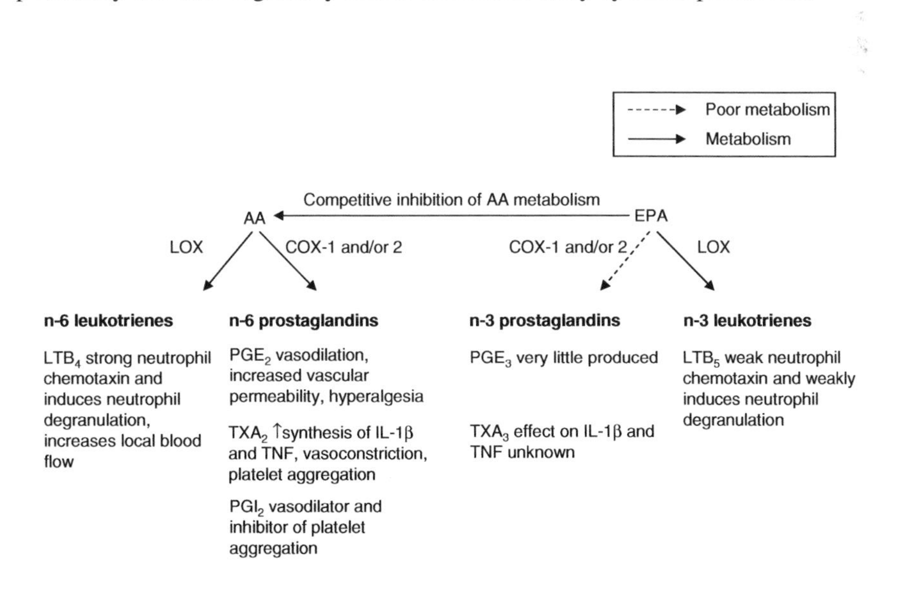

FIGURE 12.1 Metabolism of arachidonic acid (AA) and eicosapentaenoic acid (EPA).

EPA is also a substrate for COX and LOX in the production of n-3 PGs and LTs, respectively. The n-3 eicosanoids are homologous with the n-6 eicosanoids apart from an additional double bond in the n-3 position. In comparison to the n-6 eicosanoids, which are readily produced from AA, EPA is a poor COX substrate such that n-3 PGs are not readily produced. Many of the activities of EPA-derived eicosanoids are similar but less potent than those of their AA-derived counterparts. While PGE_3 is edemogenic, little is actually produced [140,141]. Furthermore, PGE_2 can amplify its own production through positive feedback mechanisms on the expression of the inducible form of COX (COX-2). In comparison, PGE_3 only weakly induces COX-2 expression and may thus result in decreased PGE_2 production [142]. LTB_5 is 10–30 times less potent than LTB_4 as a neutrophil chemotaxin [143,144]. EPA and DHA also competitively inhibit production of n-6 eicosanoids (Figure 12.1).

In human studies, dietary supplementation with n-3 fats has been shown to reduce production of PGE_2 [126,145], TXA_2 [126], and LTB_4 [146] and while there is increased production of TXA_3 [147] and LTB_5 [148], production of PGE_3 has been difficult to demonstrate [140].

12.5.1.5.2 Effect of n-3 Fatty Acids on Pro-Inflammatory Cytokine Production

The inflammatory cytokines IL-1β and TNF have both been implicated in the tissue destruction seen in RA [149–151]. In addition to the effects on eicosanoids, dietary n-3 fatty acids can influence inflammatory cytokine production. Decreased production of IL-1β and TNF has been reported in some, but not all, studies of dietary n-3 fatty acid supplementation in healthy subjects and those with RA [119,126,145,152,153]. At least part of the explanation for these differing findings may lie in genetically determined differences in the effects of n-3 fats on inflammatory cytokine synthesis [154].

The mechanisms by which n-3 fatty acids inhibit cytokine production have not been well elucidated. Recent in vitro studies demonstrate that PGE_2 and PGE_3 have equipotent inhibitory effects on TNF and IL-1β production by human monocytes [155,156]. Differences in the respective activities of other n-6 and n-3 eicosanoid inflammatory mediators may play a role. Fatty acids have been shown to have direct effects on intracellular signalling mechanisms and may thereby affect cytokine production [157–159].

12.5.1.5.3 Effects of n-3 Fatty Acids on MHC Expression

Class II MHC molecules (HLA-DR) are strongly expressed on APCs and present antigen to T cells. The number of MHC molecules expressed on APCs is an important determinant of T cell response to antigen. Patients with RA have high levels of MHC class II expression on synovial fluid mononuclear cells [160]. In vitro studies have shown that human monocyte expression of HLA-DR and HLA-DP molecules is reduced in the presence of the n-3 fatty acids EPA and DHA [161]. Furthermore, human monocytes have a reduced ability to present antigen to autologous lymphocytes after culture with EPA and DHA in vitro [162]. Dietary supplementation with fish oil capsules containing 0.93 g EPA + 0.63 g DHA reduced expression of HLA-DR and HLA-DP on human monocytes ex vivo [163]. Thus in RA, n-3 fatty acids may suppress pathogenic T cell activation through inhibition of the function of APCs and may thereby reduce disease activity.

12.5.1.5.4 *Effect of n-3 Fatty Acids on Adhesion Molecule Expression*

Adhesion molecules are expressed by endothelial cells and leukocytes and mediate the transit of cells from the circulation into tissues. In an animal model of arthritis, the cognate pair, ICAM-1, and leukocyte function associated antigen (LFA)-1 have been implicated in migration of leukocytes into inflamed synovium [164]. Furthermore, ICAM-1 blockade has been reported to reduce disease activity in RA [165]. n-3 Fatty acids have been shown in vitro and ex vivo to decrease expression of ICAM-1 and LFA-1 on human monocytes [161,162].

Dietary supplementation with n-3 fatty acids has been reported to reduce plasma concentrations of soluble ICAM-1 and VCAM-1 in healthy women [166], although whether decreased cell surface expression is also reduced has not been examined. Similar studies in patients with RA have not been undertaken.

12.5.1.5.5 *Effect of n-3 Fatty Acids on Degradative Enzymes*

Matrix metalloproteinases (MMPs) have a pivotal role in cartilage degradation and bone erosion in RA. n-3 Fatty acids added in vitro suppress MMP expression and reduce proteoglycan degradation in IL-1 stimulated bovine chondrocytes [167]. In addition, supplementation of human osteoarticular cartilage explants with n-3 fatty acids reduced expression of MMP-3 and MMP-13 mRNA and also reduced collagenase and aggrecanase proteolytic activity [168]. Thus n-3 fatty acids may have the ability to reduce cartilage damage in inflamed joints.

12.5.1.5.6 *Novel Anti-Inflammatory Mediators Derived from EPA and AA*

More recently a group of novel anti-inflammatory mediators known as resolvins (resolution phase interaction products) have been identified (reviewed in [169]). They are derived from n-3 fatty acids via COX-2. Their proportionate synthesis is increased in the presence of aspirin or NSAIDs. Those derived from EPA are known as E-resolvins while those derived from DHA are known as D-resolvins. The resolvins have anti-inflammatory actions including inhibition of TNF induced transcription of IL-1β [170] and inhibition of human polymorphonuclear leukocyte transendothelial migration [171]. The identification of these resolvins provides a mechanism through which n-3 fatty acids contribute to the inhibition of inflammatory cytokine production.

12.5.1.6 Use of n-3 Fatty Acids during Pregnancy and Lactation

As discussed above, RA often remits during pregnancy and relapses postpartum. Furthermore, standard pharmacotherapies are generally avoided during pregnancy and lactation due to concerns over their potential effects on the fetus and newborn. Use of alternative therapies may thus be considered during these times in order to gain relief from symptoms. There are no studies examining the effects of nutrition in pregnant or breast feeding women with RA. Recently, concerns have been expressed regarding the potential for toxic effects from methylmercury found as a contaminant in large carnivorous fish (e.g., shark, swordfish, king mackerel). This has led to dietary recommendations that these fish should not be eaten in pregnancy, and ingestion should be restricted to one meal fortnightly otherwise [172]. These recommendations regarding pregnancy are controversial as they have led to a general decline in fish consumption during pregnancy with potential adverse effects on neural development of the offspring which is enhanced by dietary n-3 fatty acids found in fish. Anti-inflammatory doses of fish oil are acceptable during pregnancy as they assist in disease control at a time when options for intervention are otherwise limited and medicinal quality fish oils should not contain measurable amounts of methylmercury. The fat soluble vitamins A and D in cod liver oil may be toxic to the fetus at high doses and accordingly anti-inflammatory doses of cod liver oil should be avoided during pregnancy.

12.5.2 Antioxidants

Antioxidants have a protective role against tissue damage caused by oxygen free radicals. However, there is no convincing evidence that dietary supplementation with antioxidants has clinical benefit in RA [173].

12.5.2.1 Vitamin E (α-Tocopherol) and Vitamin C (Ascorbic Acid)

In a transgenic murine model of arthritis (Vβ6TCR/NOD), vitamin E has been shown to reduce IL-1β but not TNF in plasma [174]. In a macrophage cell line vitamin E has been reported to inhibit lipopolysaccharide induced PGE_2 and COX-2 expression [175].

Serum concentrations of vitamin E are similar in patients with RA and controls [176]. A 12 week placebo controlled study of vitamin E supplementation found reduced pain scores but no effect on joint tenderness score, duration of morning stiffness, swollen joint count, or laboratory parameters [177]. In a 3 week study comparing vitamin E supplementation and the NSAID diclofenac in 85 hospitalized RA patients there was similar symptomatic improvement in both groups [178].

Although animal models have shown benefits with vitamin C supplementation [179,180] human studies have not shown any clinical benefit in patients with RA [181].

12.5.2.2 Selenium

Selenium, which is found at the active site of the enzyme glutathione peroxidase, has been reported to have a number of effects on the immune system via eradication of oxygen free radicals (for review see [182]). Plasma concentrations of selenium are reduced in patients with RA compared to healthy controls [183–185]. Furthermore an inverse correlation between serum selenium concentrations and the number of active joints has been reported [186]. However, there are no consistent effects with dietary selenium supplementation. The majority of studies have shown no effect despite increases in serum and red blood cell selenium concentrations [187–190]. However, polymorphonuclear cell selenium concentrations do not increase with dietary supplementation, which may explain the lack of clinical effect [191]. One study has reported a beneficial effect with improvements in swollen and tender joint counts with selenium supplementation. However, n-3 fatty acid supplements were also given during the study and may have contributed to the observed improvements [185].

12.5.2.3 Vitamin B6

The biologically active form of vitamin B6 is pyridoxal 5′-phosphate (PLP). Plasma concentrations of vitamin B6 are lower in patients with RA compared to healthy controls [192,193]. Low plasma PLP levels have also been associated with increased concentrations of TNF [192] and elevated CRP and ESR in RA [193,194]. Morning stiffness and degree of pain have been found to correlate inversely with plasma PLP concentrations [194]. Vitamin B6 supplementation has been shown to improve blood B6 status but in a relatively small pilot study did not yield significant clinical improvement in RA [195].

12.5.3 Vegetarian and Vegan Diets and RA

Vegetarian and vegan diets have been reported to improve clinical symptoms in RA [196–201]. In the majority of these studies the dietary intervention was preceded by a period of fasting. It has also been suggested that combination of vegan diet and diet low in all kinds of fats will provide the most benefit. An uncontrolled study of such a diet showed an improvement in pain, joint swelling, and tenderness but not in duration of morning stiffness, ESR, or CRP [202]. A systematic review of studies examining fasting followed by vegetarian diets concluded that there can be clinically significant long-term benefit in RA with this approach [203]. However, compliance with such a strict dietary regimen is problematic as shown by high dropout rates.

12.5.4 Mediterranean Diet and RA

The Mediterranean diet, which is high in cereals, vegetables, legumes, fruits, olive oil, and monounsaturated and n-3 fatty acids, has been reported to result in clinical improvements with reduction in DAS28 and Stanford Health Assessment Questionnaire scores as well as improvement in the vitality and general health components of the Short Form 36 health assessment questionnaire [204].

12.5.5 Fasting in RA

Fasting reduces disease activity in some patients with RA [196,199,205,206]. The benefits may be superior to those seen with the Mediterranean diet [207]. While, improvements occur within a few days of commencing the fast there is a corresponding deterioration upon reintroduction of food. Despite its short-term benefits, fasting should not be recommended as it can compound the poor nutritional status of patients with RA. Furthermore, RA is a chronic condition requiring long-term therapies and fasting can only be maintained for short periods.

12.5.6 Elimination Diets and RA

Elimination diets remove foods that are thought to exacerbate arthritis. In general, such foods are eliminated from the diet and then gradually reintroduced to determine the effects on disease activity. Given that patients are aware of what foods they ingest, these studies are in general single blind. Two studies have shown benefits in

RA [208,209]. Both of these studies demonstrated that at least some patients improve with such dietary manipulation, that individual responses vary and that compliance is an important limiting factor. Another study compared the "Dong Diet" (contains no red meat, fruit, herbs, spices, dairy products, alcohol, additives, and preservatives) with a "placebo" diet (elimination of certain foods from within each major food group). Overall, there was no evidence of improvement although 2 of 11 patients on the Dong Diet improved dramatically and deteriorated upon returning to their normal diet [210].

12.5.7 Potential Mechanisms of Elimination, Fasting, and Vegetarian Diets

A number of mechanisms have been postulated for the improvements seen with these diets including an alteration of gut flora [211,212] and reduction in IL-6 concentrations [213]. A placebo response or psychological factors may contribute given that patients are aware that their diet has changed. Patients who respond to dietary manipulation are likely to report food allergy and have a higher perceived ability to control their own health and a lower perception that chance affected their health and response to treatment [196]. Furthermore those who respond to dietary therapy may have less belief and confidence in conventional medical treatment compared with diet nonresponders [214].

Weight loss tends to occur with such dietary manipulation, although weight loss per se does not appear to be the main reason for the improvement observed during dietary therapy [215].

Alterations in serum and neutrophil AA and EPA concentrations have been observed after fasting [205]. While plasma phospholipid EPA concentrations were reduced after vegan and lactovegetarian diets in patients with RA, a significant difference between diet responders and nonresponders was not seen [216].

12.5.8 Vitamin D

1,25OHD has been shown to inhibit arthritis induced by experimental infection with the Lyme disease pathogen [79]. 1,25OHD and analogues have been shown to inhibit collagen-induced arthritis in mice [79] and rats [217]. These investigations have shown both preventive and therapeutic effects.

Despite a strong rationale for potentially clinically important immunosuppressive effects, studies into the effect of vitamin D supplementation on RA are lacking. Cod liver oil is a rich source of dietary n-3 fatty acids (typically EPA 10%, DHA 10% w/w) and is also rich in the fat soluble vitamins A and D. Cod liver oil has been used in the management of RA in sufficient doses to deliver anti-inflammatory doses long chain n-3 fatty acids [218]. In this 12 month cohort study, RA patients received 20 ml cod liver oil daily (4 g EPA + DHA). Both serum vitamin D and vitamin A concentrations were observed to rise significantly within the reference range. This study did not allow the respective contributions of vitamin D and co-ingested n-3 fatty acids and vitamin A to benefit on arthritis to be evaluated. In this regard, it should be noted that vitamin A deficiency has been shown to exacerbate experimentally induced polyarthritis [219] and accordingly vitamin A supplementation could contribute to control of polyarthritis.

Vitamin D has been shown to have multiple potential health benefits, which extend from favorable effects on bone metabolism to prevention against some cancers, congestive cardiac failure, and autoimmune disorders [220,221]. By contrast, higher vitamin A intakes have been associated with reduced bone mineral density and increased fracture risk [222]. This effect, which has not been established with cod liver oil [223], in which vitamin D may be counter-active (ibid), is of special concern for women. Fat soluble vitamins partition into body fat, thereby forming a reservoir, which in the case of vitamin D has been shown to allow dosing at intervals of several months, provided that doses given are adequate [224]. This contrasts with the desirability of taking fish oil essentially on a daily basis. Since the cost of quarterly vitamin D (cholecalciferol 100,000 IU every 3 months) is small and fish body oils contain more n-3 fatty acids than cod liver oil (typical fish body oil contains EPA + DHA 30% w/w) and contain little vitamin D or vitamin A, vitamin D supplements are perhaps best given separately from fish oil.

12.6 CONCLUSION

Rheumatoid arthritis is an important health problem for women because of its high prevalence and predilection for women. Also women are more likely to acquire RA early in life with the attendant greater lifetime burden. Female sex can influence disease susceptibility and outcomes through hormonal, physiological, and direct and indirect genetic effects. There are multiple nutritional factors that can potentially influence disease susceptibility and severity. Notable among these in terms of strength of evidence are dietary long chain n-3 fatty acids found in fish and fish oils. On the basis of available evidence, vitamin D is also a candidate for benefit and like dietary n-3 fatty acids, vitamin D delivers a number of collateral health benefits. Diet has an important role in management not only for disease specific benefits, but also for health and well-being more generally, including empowerment through self-directed choices of nonprescription items. Obviously, these choices need to be well informed for safety and cost-effectiveness. As in conventional medicine, achieving an informed choice is inevitably confounded by product marketing that is designed intentionally to skew perceptions. This review is intended to provide a basis for evaluating the options.

12.7 FUTURE RESEARCH

The aim in modern management of RA is to return patients to full health and vitality and to prevent impairment, debility, and cardiovascular risks that result from uncontrolled inflammation and joint damage. Available evidence suggests this objective can be achieved in most cases with combinations of DMARDs applied early, with inclusion of fish oil at anti-inflammatory doses in the regimen. In the context of DMARD therapy, fish oil has been shown to improve disease control and remission rates and to reduce recourse to NSAIDs for analgesia. This latter effect can be expected to reduce risk for serious upper gastrointestinal and cardiovascular events. Fish oil use in RA has also been associated with reduction in multiple "traditional" cardiovascular risk factors. However, further long-term studies are required to determine the extent of reduction of actual cardiovascular events, which are the major cause of the increased mortality seen in RA, that may be achieved from early combination therapy and fish oil treatment in RA. Long-term studies are also needed to document better the extent to which joint damage is contained or slowed by these treatments. These studies are urgently needed in order to place claims regarding the joint protective effects of much more expensive biological agent therapies within the context of outcomes achieved with optimal therapy with combinations of inexpensive low molecular weight therapies and fish oil.

Data from basic and epidemiological studies suggest that vitamin D has important immunomodulatory effects. To date, there have been no reports regarding the effects of vitamin D supplementation in RA. It is notable that vitamin D is inexpensive, well tolerated and, like fish oil, has collateral health benefits. The way forward will be to examine the addition of vitamin D to combination regimens and to evaluate effects on disease control, joint damage, and other health benefits of vitamin D (bone mineral density, muscle function, periodontal disease, colon cancer risk, etc.). These studies will need to be long term and to examine incremental benefits within the context of established best practice combination therapy. Finally, better definition of risk factors for RA and the excellent safety and health benefit profiles of fish oil and vitamin D should make feasible the assessment of their efficacy as preventives for RA. These preventive studies may be focused most productively upon women, who compared to men, carry a substantially higher risk for development of RA.

12.8 APPENDIX 1

Disease Activity Score (DAS)28 [235]

Statistically derived index combining swollen joint counts, tender joint counts, ESR, and global disease activity.

$DAS28 = 0.56\sqrt{(28 \text{ tender joint count})} + 0.28\sqrt{(28 \text{ swollen joint count})} + 0.70 (\ln[ESR])\ 1.08 + 0.16$

ACR 20 response [236]

Twenty percent improvement in five out of seven core set variables, first two required:

1. Tender joint count
2. Swollen joint count
3. Acute phase reactant
4. Patients pain
5. Patients global assessment of disease activity
6. Physicians global assessment of disease activity
7. Physical disability

REFERENCES

1. MacGregor, A. and Silman, A., *Rheumatology*, Mosby, Philadelphia, 1998, Chap 5.2.
2. Symmons, D., et al., The incidence of rheumatoid arthritis in the United Kingdom: results from the Norfolk Arthritis Register, *Br J Rheumatol*, 33, 735, 1994.
3. Tengstrand, B., Ahlmen, M., and Hafstrom, I., The influence of sex on rheumatoid arthritis: a prospective study of onset and outcome after 2 years, *J Rheumatol*, 31, 214, 2004.
4. Aho, K., et al., Occurrence of rheumatoid arthritis in a nationwide series of twins, *J Rheumatol*, 13, 899, 1986.
5. Silman, A., et al., Twin concordance rates for rheumatoid arthritis: results from a nationwide study, *Br J Rheumatol*, 32, 903, 1993.
6. MacGregor, A., et al., Characterizing the quantitative genetic contribution to rheumatoid arthritis using data from twins, *Arthritis Rheum*, 43, 30, 2000.
7. Gregersen, P., Silver, J., and Winchester, R., The shared epitope hypothesis: an approach to understanding the molecular genetics of susceptibility to rheumatoid arthritis, *Arthritis Rheum*, 30, 1205, 1987.
8. Zerva, L., et al., Arginine at positions 13 or 70–71 in pocket 4 of HLA-DRB1 alleles is associated with susceptibility to tuberculoid leprosy, *J Exp Med*, 183, 829, 1996.
9. Penglis, P., et al., Genetic susceptibility and the link between cat exposure and rheumatoid arthritis, *Semin Arthritis Rheum*, 30, 111, 2000.
10. Ohta, N., et al., Association between HLA and Japanese patients with rheumatoid arthritis, *Hum Immunol*, 5, 123, 1982.
11. Gonzales-Escribano, M., et al., Complex associations between HLA-DRB1 genes and female rheumatoid arthritis, *Hum Immunol*, 60, 1259, 1999.
12. Bongi, S., et al., Shared-epitope HLA-DRB1 alleles and sex ratio in Italian patients with rheumatoid arthritis, *Joint Bone Spine*, 71, 24, 2004.
13. Meyer, J., et al., Sex influences on the penetrance of HLA shared-epitope genotypes for rheumatoid arthritis, *Am J Hum Genet*, 58, 371, 1996.
14. Hajeer, A., et al., Tumor necrosis factor microsatellite haplotypes are different in male and female patients with RA, *J Rheumatol*, 24, 217, 1997.
15. Brennan, P., et al., Are both genetic and reproductive associations with rheumatoid arthritis linked to prolactin? *Lancet*, 348, 106, 1996.
16. Begovich, A., et al., A missense single nucleotide polymorphism in a gene encoding a protein tyrosine phosphatase (*PTPN22*) is associated with rheumatoid arthritis, *Am J Hum Genet*, 75, 330, 2004.
17. Simkins, H., et al., Association of the *PTPN22* locus with rheumatoid arthritis in a New Zealand Caucasian cohort, *Arthritis Rheum*, 52, 2222, 2005.
18. Pierer, M., et al., Association of *PTPN22* 1858 single-nucleotide polymorphism with rheumatoid arthritis in a German cohort: higher frequency of the risk allele in male compared to female patients, *Arthritis Res Ther*, 8, R75, 2006.
19. Vang, T., et al., Autoimmune-associated lymphoid tyrosine phosphatase is a gain-of-function variant, *Nat Genet*, 37, 1317, 2005.
20. Plenge, R., et al., Replication of putative candidate-gene associations with rheumatoid arthritis in >4,000 samples from North America and Sweden: association of susceptibility with *PTPN22, CTLA4* and *PADI4, Am J Hum Genet*, 77, 1044, 2005.
21. Masi, A., Feigenbaum, S., and Chatterton, R., Hormonal and pregnancy relationships to rheumatoid arthritis: convergent effects with immunologic and microvascular systems, *Semin Arthritis Rheum*, 25, 1, 1995.
22. Grossman, C., Regulation of the immune system by sex steroids, *Endocr Rev*, 5, 435, 1984.

23. Holmdahl, R., Jansson, L., and Andersson, M., Female sex hormones suppress development of collagen-induced arthritis in mice, *Arthritis Rheum*, 29, 1501, 1986.
24. Silman, A., Kay, A., and Brennan, P., Timing of pregnancy in relation to the onset of rheumatoid arthritis, *Arthritis Rheum*, 35, 152, 1992.
25. Hazes, J., et al., Pregnancy and the risk of developing rheumatoid arthritis, *Arthritis Rheum*, 33, 1770, 1990.
26. Spector, T., Roman, E., and Silman, A., The pill, parity and rheumatoid arthritis, *Arthritis Rheum*, 33, 782, 1990.
27. Heliovaara, M., et al., Parity and risk of rheumatoid arthritis in Finnish women, *Br J Rheumatol*, 34, 625, 1995.
28. Pope, J., Bellamy, N., and Stevens, A., The lack of association between rheumatoid arthritis and both nulliparity and infertility, *Semin Arthritis Rheum*, 28, 342, 1999.
29. Merlino, L., et al., Estrogen and other female reproductive factors are not strongly associated with the development of rheumatoid arthritis in elderly women, *Semin Arthritis Rheum*, 33, 72, 2003.
30. Brennan, P. and Silman, A., Breast feeding and the onset of rheumatoid arthritis, *Arthritis Rheum*, 37, 808, 1994.
31. Karlson, E., et al., Do breast feeding and other reproductive factors influence future risk of rheumatoid arthritis? Results from the Nurses' Health Study, *Arthritis Rheum*, 50, 3458, 2004.
32. Doran, M., et al., The effect of oral contraceptives and estrogen replacement therapy on the risk of rheumatoid arthritis: a population based study, *J Rheumatol*, 31, 207, 2004.
33. del Junco, D., et al., Do oral contraceptives prevent rheumatoid arthritis? *J Am Med Assoc*, 254, 1938, 1985.
34. Bhatia, S., et al., Rheumatoid factor positivity is inversely associated with oral contraceptive use in women without rheumatoid arthritis, *Ann Rheum Dis*, doi:110.1136/ard.2006.060004, 2006.
35. Vandenbroucke, J., et al., Noncontraceptive hormones and rheumatoid arthritis in perimenopausal and postmenopausal women, *J Am Med Assoc*, 255, 1299, 1986.
36. Silman, A., Newman, J., and MacGregor, A., Cigarette smoking increases the risk of rheumatoid arthritis: results from a nationwide study of disease-disconcordant twins, *Arthritis Rheum*, 39, 732, 1996.
37. Tuomi, T., et al., Smoking, lung function and rheumatoid factors, *Ann Rheum Dis*, 49, 753, 1990.
38. Jonsson, T., Thorsteinsson, J., and Valdimarsson, H., Does smoking stimulate rheumatoid factor production in non-rheumatic individuals? *APMIS*, 106, 970, 1998.
39. Krishnan, E., Smoking, gender and rheumatoid arthritis—epidemiological clues to aetiology, *Joint Bone Spine*, 70, 496, 2003.
40. Stolt, P., et al., Quantification of the influence of cigarette smoking on rheumatoid arthritis: results from a population based case-control study, using incident cases, *Ann Rheum Dis*, 62, 835, 2003.
41. Karlson, E., et al., A retrospective cohort study of cigarette smoking and risk of rheumatoid arthritis in female health professionals, *Arthritis Rheum*, 42, 910, 1999.
42. Heliovaara, M., et al., Smoking and risk of rheumatoid arthritis, *J Rheumatol*, 20, 1830, 1993.
43. Edwards, J., Cambridge, G., and Abrahams, V., Do self-perpetuating B lymphocytes drive human autoimmune disease? *Immunology*, 97, 188, 1999.
44. Reparon-Schuijt, C., et al., Functional analysis of rheumatoid factor-producing B cells from the synovial fluid of rheumatoid arthritis patients, *Arthritis Rheum*, 41, 2211, 1998.

45. Padyukov, L., et al., A gene-environment interaction between smoking and shared epitope genes in HLA-DR provides a high risk of seropositive rheumatoid arthritis, *Arthritis Rheum*, 50, 3085, 2004.
46. Uhlig, T., Hagen, K., and Kvien, T., Current tobacco smoking, formal education, and the risk of rheumatoid arthritis, *J Rheumatol*, 26, 47, 1999.
47. Krishnan, E., Sokka, T., and Hannonen, P., Smoking-gender interaction and risk for rheumatoid arthritis, *Arthritis Res Ther*, 5, R158, 2003.
48. Hazes, J., et al., Lifestyle and the risk of rheumatoid arthritis: cigarette smoking and alcohol consumption, *Ann Rheum Dis*, 49, 980, 1990.
49. Criswell, L., et al., Cigarette smoking and the risk of rheumatoid arthritis among postmenopausal women: results from the Iowa Women's Health Study, *Am J Med*, 112, 465, 2002.
50. Baron, J., La Vecchia, C., and Levi, F., The antiestrogenic effect of cigarette smoking in women, *Am J Obstet Gynecol*, 162, 502, 1990.
51. Linn-Rasker, S., et al., Smoking is a risk factor for anti-CCP antibodies only in rheumatoid arthritis patients who carry HLA-DRB1 shared epitope alleles, *Ann Rheum Dis*, 65, 366, 2006.
52. Symmons, D., et al., Blood transfusion, smoking and obesity as risk factors for the development of rheumatoid arthritis, *Arthritis Rheum*, 40, 1955, 1997.
53. Shichikawa, K., et al., A longitudinal population survey of rheumatoid arthritis in a rural district in Wakayama, *Ryumachi*, 21, 35, 1981.
54. Nishimoto, T., et al., Unique associations between HLA-B and HLA-DRB1*04 gene variants in Japanese, *Tissue Antigens*, 42, 497, 1993.
55. Tokunaga, N., et al., Association between HLA-DRB1*15 and Japanese patients with rheumatoid arthritis complicated by renal involvement, *Nephron*, 81, 165, 1999.
56. Shapiro, J.A., et al., Diet and rheumatoid arthritis in women: a possible protective effect of fish consumption, *Epidemiology*, 7, 256, 1996.
57. Linos, A., et al., Dietary factors in relation to rheumatoid arthritis: a role for olive oil and cooked vegetables? *Am J Clin Nutr*, 70, 1077, 1999.
58. Linos, A., et al., The effect of olive oil and fish consumption on rheumatoid arthritis—a case control study, *Scand J Rheumatol*, 20, 419, 1991.
59. Pedersen, M., et al., Diet and risk of rheumatoid arthritis in a prospective cohort, *J Rheumatol*, 32, 1249, 2005.
60. Pattison, D., et al., Dietary risk factors for the development of inflammatory polyarthritis. Evidence for a high level of red meat consumption, *Arthritis Rheum*, 50, 3804, 2004.
61. Grant, W., The role of red meat in the expression of rheumatoid arthritis, *Br J Nutr*, 84, 589, 2000.
62. James, D., Betts, W., and Cleland, L., Chemiluminescence of polymorphonuclear leucocytes from rheumatoid joints, *J Rheumatol*, 10, 184, 1983.
63. Farrell, A., et al., Increased concentrations of nitrite in synovial fluid and serum samples suggest increased nitric oxide synthesis in rheumatic diseases, *Ann Rheum Dis*, 51, 1219, 1992.
64. Halliwell, B., Oxygen radicals, nitric oxide and human inflammatory joint disease, *Ann Rheum Dis*, 54, 505, 1995.
65. McNeil, J., et al., The depolymerization products of hyaluronic acid after exposure to oxy radicals, *Ann Rheum Dis*, 44, 780, 1985.
66. Bae, S., Kim, S., and Sung, M., Inadequate antioxidant nutrient intake and altered plasma antioxidant status of rheumatoid arthritis patients, *J Am Coll Nutr*, 22, 311, 2003.
67. Heliovaara, M., et al., Serum antioxidants and risk of rheumatoid arthritis, *Ann Rheum Dis*, 53, 51, 1994.

68. Comstock, G., et al., Serum concentrations of α-tocopherol, β-carotene, and retinol preceding the diagnosis of rheumatoid arthritis and systemic lupus erythematosis, *Ann Rheum Dis*, 56, 323, 1997.
69. Knekt, P., et al., Serum selenium, serum alpha-tocopherol, and the risk of rheumatoid arthritis, *Epidemiology*, 11, 402, 2000.
70. Cerhan, J., et al., Antioxidant micronutrients and risk of rheumatoid arthritis in a cohort of older women, *Am J Epidemiol*, 157, 345, 2003.
71. Pattison, D., et al., Dietary β-cryptoxanthin and inflammatory polyarthritis: results from a population-based prospective study, *Am J Clin Nutr*, 82, 451, 2005.
72. Pattison, D., et al., Vitamin C and the risk of developing inflammatory polyarthritis: prospective nested case-control study, *Ann Rheum Dis*, 63, 843, 2004.
73. Heliovaara, M., et al., Coffee consumption, rheumatoid factor, and the risk of rheumatoid arthritis, *Ann Rheum Dis*, 59, 631, 2000.
74. Mikuls, T., et al., Coffee, tea, and caffeine consumption and risk of rheumatoid arthritis, *Arthritis Rheum*, 46, 83, 2002.
75. Karlson, E., et al., Coffee consumption and risk of rheumatoid arthritis, *Arthritis Rheum*, 48, 3055, 2003.
76. Lin, Y.-L. and Lin, J.-K., (−)-Epigallocatechin-3-gallate blocks the induction of nitric oxide synthase by down regulating lipopolysaccharide-induced activity of transcription factor nuclear factor-kB, *Mol Pharmacol*, 52, 465, 1997.
77. Cerhan, J., et al., Blood transfusion, alcohol use, and anthropometric risk factors for rheumatoid arthritis in older women, *J Rheumatol*, 29, 246, 2002.
78. Voigt, L., et al., Smoking, obesity, alcohol consumption, and the risk of rheumatoid arthritis, *Epidemiology*, 5, 525, 1994.
79. Cantorna, M., Hayes, C., and DeLuca, H., 1,25-Dihydroxycholecalciferol inhibits the progression of arthritis in murine models of human arthritis, *J Nutr*, 128, 68, 1998.
80. Inaba, M., et al., Positive correlation between levels of IL-1 or IL-2 and 1,25-$(OH)_2D$/25-OH-D ratio in synovial fluid of patients with rheumatoid arthritis, *Life Sciences*, 61, 977, 1997.
81. Griffin, M., et al., Dendritic cell modulation by 1a,25 dihydroxyvitamin D_3 and its analogues: a vitamin D receptor-dependent pathway that promotes a persistent state of immaturity *in vitro* and *in vivo, Proc Natl Acad Sci USA*, 98, 6800, 2001.
82. Merlino, L., et al., Vitamin D is inversely associated with rheumatoid arthritis: results from the Iowa Women's Health Study, *Arthritis Rheum*, 50, 72, 2004.
83. Hallert, E., et al., Comparison between women and men with recent onset rheumatoid arthritis of disease activity and functional ability over two years (the TIRA project), *Ann Rheum Dis*, 62, 667, 2003.
84. Weyand, C., et al., The influence of sex on the phenotype of rheumatoid arthritis, *Arthritis Rheum*, 41, 817, 1998.
85. Harrison, B. and Symmons, D., Early inflammatory polyarthritis: results from the Norfolk Arthritis Register with a review of the literature. II. Outcome at three years, *Rheumatology*, 39, 939, 2000.
86. Sheehan, T., et al., Rate of change in functional limitations for patients with rheumatoid arthritis: effects of sex, age, and duration of illness, *J Rheumatol*, 31, 1286, 2004.
87. Combe, B., et al., Prognostic factors for radiographic damage in early rheumatoid arthritis, *Arthritis Rheum*, 44, 1736, 2001.
88. Gossec, L., et al., Influence of sex on disease severity in patients with rheumatoid arthritis, *J Rheumatol*, 32, 1448, 2005.
89. Wolfe, F., et al., The mortality of rheumatoid arthritis, *Arthritis Rheum*, 37, 481, 1994.

90. Mikuls, T., et al., Mortality risk associated with rheumatoid arthritis in a prospective cohort of older women: results from the Iowa Women's Health Study, *Ann Rheum Dis*, 61, 994, 2002.
91. Solomon, D., et al., Cardiovascular morbidity and mortality in women diagnosed with rheumatoid arthritis, *Circulation*, 107, 1303, 2003.
92. Solomon, D., et al., Cardiovascular risk factors in women with and without rheumatoid arthritis, *Arthritis Rheum*, 50, 3444, 2004.
93. van Doornum, S., Jennings, G., and Wicks, I., Reducing the cardiovascular disease burden in rheumatoid arthritis, *Med J Aust*, 184, 287, 2006.
94. Ridker, P., et al., C-reactive protein and other markers of inflammation in the prediction of cardiovascular disease in women, *N Engl J Med*, 342, 836, 2000.
95. Demerath, E., et al., The relationship of soluble ICAM-1, VCAM-1, P-selectin and E-selectin to cardiovascular disease risk factors in healthy men and women, *Ann Hum Biol*, 28, 664, 2001.
96. Choi, H., et al., Methotrexate and mortality in patients with rheumatoid arthritis: a prospective study, *Lancet*, 359, 1173, 2002.
97. del Rincon, I., et al., Association between carotid atherosclerosis and markers of inflammation in rheumatoid arthritis patients and healthy subjects, *Arthritis Rheum*, 48, 1833, 2003.
98. Maradit-Kremers, H., et al., Cardiovascular death in rheumatoid arthritis. A population based study, *Arthritis Rheum*, 52, 722, 2005.
99. Fries, J., et al., The rise and decline of nonsteroidal-anti-inflammatory drugs-associated gastropathy in rheumatoid arthritis, *Arthritis Rheum*, 50, 2433, 2004.
100. Latman, N., Relation of menstrual cycle phase to symptoms of rheumatoid arthritis, *Am J Med*, 74, 957, 1983.
101. Barrett, J., et al., Does rheumatoid arthritis remit during pregnancy and relapse postpartum? Results from a nationwide study in the United Kingdom performed prospectively from late pregnancy, *Arthritis Rheum*, 42, 1219, 1999.
102. Barrett, J., et al., Breast feeding and postpartum relapse in women with rheumatoid and inflammatory arthritis, *Arthritis Rheum*, 43, 1010, 2000.
103. Straub, R., Buttgereit, F., and Cutolo, M., Benefits of pregnancy in inflammatory arthritis, *Ann Rheum Dis*, 64, 801, 2005.
104. Gibson, R.A. and Kneebone, G.M., Fatty acid composition of human colostrum and breast milk, *Am J Clin Nutr*, 34, 252, 1981.
105. Nelson, J., et al., Maternal-fetal disparity in HLA class II alloantigens and the pregnancy-induced amelioration of rheumatoid arthritis, *N Engl J Med*, 329, 466, 1993.
106. Yan, Z., et al., Prospective study of fetal DNA in serum and disease activity during pregnancy in women with inflammatory arthritis, *Arthritis Rheum*, 54, 2069, 2006.
107. Kuiper, S., et al., Influence of sex, age, and menopausal state on the course of early rheumatoid arthritis, *J Rheumatol*, 28, 1809, 2001.
108. MacDonald, A., et al., Effects of hormone replacement therapy in rheumatoid arthritis: a double blind placebo-controlled study, *Ann Rheum Dis*, 53, 54, 1994.
109. Hall, G., et al., A randomised controlled trial of the effect of hormone replacement therapy on disease activity in postmenopausal rheumatoid arthritis, *Ann Rheum Dis*, 53, 112, 1994.
110. Martin, R.H., The role of nutrition and diet in rheumatoid arthritis, *Proc Nutr Soc*, 57, 231, 1998.
111. Salminen, E., et al., Female patients tend to alter their diet following the diagnosis of rheumatoid arthritis and breast cancer, *Preventative Med*, 34, 529, 2002.

112. Gomez-Vaquero, C., et al., Nutritional status in patients with rheumatoid arthritis, *Joint Bone Spine*, 68, 403, 2001.
113. Rall, L. and Roubenoff, R., Rheumatoid cachexia: metabolic abnormalities, mechanisms and interventions, *Rheumatology*, 43, 1219, 2004.
114. Roubenoff, R., et al., Rheumatoid cachexia: cytokine-driven hypermetabolism accompanying reduced body cell mass in chronic inflammation, *J Clin Invest*, 93, 2379, 1994.
115. Walsmith, J., et al., Tumor necrosis factor-α is associated with less body mass in women with rheumatoid arthritis, *J Rheumatol*, 31, 23, 2004.
116. Svenson, K., et al., Impaired glucose handling in active rheumatoid arthritis: relationship to the secretion of insulin and counter-regulatory hormones, *Metabolism*, 36, 940, 1987.
117. Cleland, L.G., et al., Clinical and biochemical effects of dietary fish oil supplements in rheumatoid arthritis, *J Rheumatol*, 15, 1471, 1988.
118. Volker, D., et al., Efficacy of fish oil concentrate in the treatment of rheumatoid arthritis, *J Rheumatol*, 27, 2343, 2000.
119. Kremer, J.M., et al., Dietary fish oil and olive oil supplementation in patients with rheumatoid arthritis, *Arthritis Rheum*, 33, 810, 1990.
120. Cleland, L., et al., Reduction of cardiovascular risk factors with longterm fish oil treatment in early rheumatoid arthritis, *J Rheumatol*, 33, 1973, 2006.
121. Leeb, B., et al., Intravenous application of omega-3 fatty acids in patients with active rheumatoid arthritis. The ORA-1 trial. An open pilot study, *Lipids*, 41, 29, 2006.
122. Kremer, J., et al., Effects of manipulation of dietary fatty acids on clinical manifestations of rheumatoid arthritis, *Lancet*, 184, 1985.
123. Cleland, L.G., et al., Linoleate inhibits EPA incorporation from dietary fish-oil supplements in human subjects, *Am J Clin Nutr*, 55, 395, 1992.
124. Adam, O., et al., Anti-inflammatory effects of a low arachidonic acid diet and fish oil in patients with rheumatoid arthritis, *Rheumatol Int*, 23, 27, 2003.
125. Cleland, L., et al., A biomarker of n-3 compliance in patients taking fish oil for rheumatoid arthritis, *Lipids*, 38, 419, 2003.
126. Caughey, G.E., et al., The effect on human tumor necrosis factor-α and interleukin-1β production of diets enriched in n-3 fatty acids from vegetable oil or fish oil, *Am J Clin Nutr*, 63, 116, 1996.
127. Belch, J.J., et al., Effects of altering dietary essential fatty acids on requirements for non-steroidal anti-inflammatory drugs in patients with rheumatoid arthritis: a double blind placebo controlled study, *Ann Rheum Dis*, 47, 96, 1988.
128. Lau, C.S., Morley, K.D., and Belch, J.J.F., Effects of fish oil supplementation on non-steroidal anti-inflammatory requirement in patients with mild rheumatoid arthritis—a double blind placebo controlled trial, *Br J Rheumatol*, 32, 982, 1993.
129. Skoldstam, L., et al., Effect of six months of fish oil supplementation in stable rheumatoid arthritis. A double-blind, controlled study, *Scand J Rheumatol*, 21, 178, 1992.
130. Kjeldsen-Kragh, J., et al., Dietary omega-3 fatty acid supplementation and naproxen treatment in patients with rheumatoid arthritis, *J Rheumatol*, 19, 1531, 1992.
131. Penglis, P., et al., Differential regulation of prostaglandin E_2 and thromboxane A_2 production in human monocytes: implications for the use of cyclooxygenase inhibitors, *J Immunol*, 165, 1605, 2000.
132. James, M.J., Gibson, R.A., and Cleland, L.G., Dietary polyunsaturated fatty acids and inflammatory mediator production, *Am J Clin Nutr*, 71, 343S, 2000.
133. Psota, T., Gebauer, S., and Kris-Etherton, P., Dietary omega-3 fatty acid intake and cardiovascular risk, *Am J Cardiol*, 98, 3i, 2006.

134. Wang, C., et al., n-3 Fatty acids from fish or fish-oil supplements, but not a-linoleic acid, benefit cardiovascular disease outcomes in primary- and secondary-prevention studies: a systematic review, *Am J Clin Nutr*, 84, 5, 2006.
135. Deckelbaum, R. and Akabas, S., n-3 Fatty acids and cardiovascular disease: navigating toward recommendations, *Am J Clin Nutr*, 84, 1, 2006.
136. Cleland, L., James, M., and Proudman, S., Fish oil: what the prescriber needs to know, *Arthritis Res Ther*, 8, 202, 2006.
137. Clarkson, T. and Strain, J., Nutritional factors may modify the toxic action of methyl mercury in fish-eating populations, *J Nutr*, 133, 1539S, 2003.
138. Jensen, T., et al., Effects of breast feeding on neuropsychological development in a community with methylmercury exposure from seafood, *J Expo Anal Environ Epidemiol*, 15, 423, 2005.
139. Caughey, G.E., et al., Regulation of tumor necrosis factor-α and IL-1β synthesis by thromboxane A_2 in nonadherent human monocytes, *J Immunol*, 158, 351, 1997.
140. Hawkes, J.S., James, M.J., and Cleland, L.G., Separation and quantification of PGE_3 following derivatization with panacyl bromide by high pressure liquid chromotagraphy with fluormetric detection, *Prostaglandins*, 42, 355, 1991.
141. Hawkes, J.S., James, M.J., and Cleland, L.G., Biological activity of prostaglandin E_3 with regard to oedema formation in mice, *Agents Actions*, 35, 85, 1992.
142. Bagga, D., et al., Differential effects of prostaglandin derived from omega-6 and omega-3 polyunsaturated fatty acids on COX-2 expression and IL-6 secretion, *Proc Natl Acad Sci USA*, 100, 1751, 2003.
143. Prescott, S.M., The effect of eicosapentaenoic acid on leukotriene B production by human neutrophils, *J Biol Chem*, 259, 7615, 1984.
144. Goldman, D.W., Pickett, W.C., and Goetzl, E.J., Human neutrophil chemotactic and degranulating activities of leukotriene B_5 (LTB_5) derived from eicosapentaenoic acid, *Biochem Biophys Res Comm*, 117, 282, 1983.
145. Endres, S., et al., The effect of dietary supplementation with n-3 polyunsaturated fatty acids on the synthesis of interleukin-1 and tumor necrosis factor by mononuclear cells, *N Engl J Med*, 320, 265, 1989.
146. Lee, T.H., et al., Effect of dietary enrichment with eicosapentaenoic and docosahexaenoic acids on *in vitro* neutrophil and monocyte and leucocyte leukotriene generation and neutrophil function, *N Engl J Med*, 312, 1217, 1985.
147. Fischer, S. and Weber, P., Thromboxane A_3 is formed in human platelets after dietary eicosapentaenoic acid, *Biochem Biophys Res Comm*, 116, 1091, 1983.
148. Sperling, R.I., et al., Dietary omega-3 polyunsaturated fatty acids inhibit phosphoinositide formation and chemotaxis in neutrophils, *J Clin Invest*, 91, 651, 1993.
149. Arend, W.P. and Dayer, J.-M., Inhibition of the production and effects of interleukin-1 and tumor necrosis factor-α in rheumatoid arthritis, *Arthritis Rheum*, 38, 151, 1995.
150. Badolato, R. and Oppenheim, J., Role of cytokines, acute-phase proteins and chemokines in the progression of rheumatoid arthritis, *Semin Arthritis Rheum*, 26, 526, 1996.
151. Brennan, F.M., Maini, R.N., and Feldmann, M., TNF-α—a pivotal role in rheumatoid arthritis, *Br J Rheumatol*, 31, 293, 1992.
152. Molvig, J., et al., Dietary supplementation with omega-3 polyunsaturated fatty acids decreases mononuclear cell proliferation and interleukin-1β content but not monokine secretion in healthy and insulin-dependent diabetic individuals, *Scand J Immunol*, 34, 399, 1991.
153. Meydani, S.N., et al., Oral (n-3) fatty acid supplementation suppresses cytokine production and lymphocyte proliferation: comparison between young and older women, *J Nutr*, 121, 547, 1991.

154. Grimble, R.F., et al., The ability of fish oil to suppress tumor necrosis factor-α production by peripheral blood mononuclear cells in healthy men is associated with polymorphisms in genes that influence tumor necrosis factor-α production, *Am J Clin Nutr*, 76, 454, 2002.
155. Dooper, M., et al., The modulatory effects of prostaglandin-E on cytokine production by human peripheral blood mononuclear cells are independent of the prostaglandin subtype, *Immunology*, 107, 152, 2002.
156. Miles, E., Allen, E., and Calder, P.C., In vitro effects of eicosanoids derived from different 20-carbon fatty acids on production of monocyte-derived cytokines in human whole blood cultures, *Cytokine*, 20, 215, 2002.
157. Jump, D. and Clarke, S., Regulation of gene expression by dietary fat, *Ann Rev Nutr*, 19, 63, 1999.
158. Hwang, D. and Rhee, S., Receptor-mediated signaling pathways: potential targets of modulation by dietary fatty acids, *Am J Clin Nutr*, 70, 545, 1999.
159. Deckelbaum, R., Worgall, T., and Seo, T., n-3 Fatty acids and gene expression, *Am J Clin Nutr*, 83, 1520S, 2006.
160. Firestein, G.S. and Zvaifler, N.J., Peripheral blood and synovial fluid monocyte activation in inflammatory arthritis, *Arthritis Rheum*, 30, 857, 1987.
161. Hughes, D.A., Southon, S., and Pinder, A., (n-3) Polyunsaturated fatty acids modulate the expression of functionally associated molecules on human monocytes *in vitro*, *J Nutr*, 126, 603, 1996.
162. Hughes, D.A. and Pinder, A.C., n-3 Polyunsaturated fatty acids inhibit the antigen-presenting function of human monocytes, *Am J Clin Nutr*, 71, 357S, 2000.
163. Hughes, D.A., et al., Fish oil supplementation inhibits the expression of major histocompatibility complex class II molecules and adhesion molecules on human monocytes, *Am J Clin Nutr*, 63, 267, 1996.
164. Liao, H.-X. and Haynes, B.F., Role of adhesion molecules in the pathogenesis of rheumatoid arthritis, *Rheum Dis Clin Nth Am*, 21, 715, 1995.
165. Kavanagh, A.F., et al., Treatment of refractory rheumatoid arthritis with a monoclonal antibody to intercellular adhesion molecule 1, *Arthritis Rheum*, 37, 992, 1994.
166. Lopez-Garcia, E., et al., Consumption of n-3 fatty acids is related to plasma biomarkers of inflammation and endothelial activation in women, *J Nutr*, 134, 1806, 2004.
167. Curtis, C., et al., n-3 fatty acids specifically modulate catabolic factors involved in articular cartilage degradation, *J Biol Chem*, 275, 721, 2000.
168. Curtis, C., et al., Pathological indicators of degradation and inflammation in human osteoarthritis cartilage are abrogated by exposure to n-3 fatty acids, *Arthritis Rheum*, 46, 1544, 2002.
169. Serhan, C., et al., Resolvins, docosatrienes, and neuroprotectins, novel omega-3-derived mediators, and their aspirin-triggered endogenous epimers: an overview of their protective roles in catabasis, *Prostaglandins Other Lipid Mediat*, 73, 155, 2004.
170. Hong, S., et al., Novel docosatrienes and 17S-resolvins generated from docosahexaenoic acid in murine brain, human blood, and glial cells, *J Biol Chem*, 278, 14677, 2003.
171. Serhan, C., et al., Novel functional sets of lipid-derived mediators with antiinflammatory actions generated from omega-3 fatty acids via cyclooxygenase-2 nonsteroidal anti-inflammatory drugs and transcellular processing, *J Exp Med*, 192, 1197, 2000.
172. Federal Drug Administration. 2004 EPA and FDA advice for women who might become pregnant women who are pregnant nursing mothers and young children. www.cfsan.fda.gov.

173. Remans, P.H., et al., Nutrient supplementation with polyunsaturated fatty acids and micronutrients in rheumatoid arthritis: clinical and biochemical effects, *Eur J Clin Nutr*, 58, 839, 2004.
174. De Bandt, M., et al., Vitamin E uncouples joints destruction and clinical inflammation in a transgenic model of rheumatoid arthritis, *Arthritis Rheum*, 46, 522, 2002.
175. Abate, A., et al., Synergistic inhibition of cyclooxygenase-2 expression by vitamin E and aspirin, *Free Radic Biol Med*, 29, 1135, 2000.
176. Paredes, S., et al., Antioxidant vitamins and lipid peroxidation in patients with rheumatoid arthritis: association with inflammatory markers, *J Rheumatol*, 29, 2271, 2002.
177. Edmonds, S., et al., Putative analgesic activity of repeated oral doses of vitamin E in the treatment of rheumatoid arthritis. Results of a prospective placebo controlled double blind trial, *Ann Rheum Dis*, 56, 649, 1997.
178. Wittenborg, A., et al., Effectiveness of vitamin E in comparison with diclofenac sodium in treatment of patients with chronic polyarthritis, *Z Rheumatol*, 57, 215, 1998.
179. Sakai, A., et al., Large dose ascorbic acid administration suppresses the development of arthritis in adjuvant-injected rats, *Arch Orthop Trauma Surg*, 119, 121, 1999.
180. Davis, R., et al., Vitamin C influence on localized adjuvant arthritis, *J Am Podiatr Med Assoc*, 80, 414, 1990.
181. Mangge, H., Hermann, J., and Schauenstein, K., Diet and rheumatoid arthritis—a review, *Scand J Rheumatol*, 28, 201, 1999.
182. Peretz, A., Neve, J., and Famaey, J., Selenium in rheumatic diseases, *Semin Arthritis Rheum*, 20, 305, 1991.
183. O'Dell, J., et al., Serum selenium concentrations in rheumatoid arthritis, *Ann Rheum Dis*, 50, 376, 1991.
184. Kose, K., et al., Plasma selenium levels in rheumatoid arthritis, *Biol Trace Elem Res*, 53, 51, 1996.
185. Heinle, K., et al., Selenium concentrations in erythrocytes of patients with rheumatoid arthritis. Clinical and laboratory chemistry infection markers during administration of selenium, *Med Klin*, 92, 29, 1997.
186. Tarp, U., et al., Low selenium level in severe rheumatoid arthritis, *Scand J Rheumatol*, 14, 97, 1985.
187. Petersson, I., et al., Treatment of rheumatoid arthritis with selenium and Vitamin E, *Scand J Rheumatol*, 20, 218, 1991.
188. Jantti, J., et al., Treatment of rheumatoid arthritis with fish oil, selenium, vitamins A and E and placebo, *Scand J Rheumatol*, 20, 225, 1991.
189. Tarp, U., et al., Selenium treatment in rheumatoid arthritis, *Scand J Rheumatol*, 14, 364, 1985.
190. Peretz, A., Siderova, V., and Neve, J., Selenium supplementation in rheumatoid arthritis investigated in a double blind, placebo-controlled trial, *Scand J Rheumatol*, 30, 208, 2001.
191. Tarp, U., et al., Glutathione redox cycle enzymes and selenium in severe rheumatoid arthritis: lack of antioxidative response to selenium supplementation in polymorphonuclear leukocytes, *Ann Rheum Dis*, 51, 1044, 1992.
192. Roubenoff, R., et al., Abnormal vitamin B_6 status in rheumatoid arthritis. Association with spontaneous tumor necrosis factor α production and markers of inflammation, *Arthritis Rheum*, 38, 105, 1995.
193. Bekpinar, S., et al., The evaluation of C-reactive protein, homocysteine and vitamin B_6 concentrations in Bechet and rheumatoid arthritis disease, *Clin Chim Acta*, 329, 143, 2002.
194. Chiang, E., et al., Abnormal vitamin B_6 status is associated with severity of symptoms in patients with rheumatoid arthritis, *Am J Med*, 114, 283, 2003.

195. Schumacher, H., Bernhart, F., and Gyorgy, P., Vitamin B_6 levels in rheumatoid arthritis: effect of treatment, *Am J Clin Nutr*, 28, 1200, 1975.
196. Kjeldsen-Kragh, J., et al., Controlled trial of fasting and one-year vegetarian diet in rheumatoid arthritis, *Lancet*, 338, 899, 1991.
197. Kjeldsen-Kragh, J., et al., Changes in laboratory variables in rheumatoid arthritis patients during a trial of fasting and one-year vegetarian diet, *Scand J Rheumatol*, 24, 85, 1995.
198. Kjeldsen-Kragh, et al., Antibodies against dietary antigens in rheumatoid arthritis patients treated with fasting and one-year vegetarian diet, *Clin Exp Rheumatol*, 13, 167, 1995.
199. Skoldstam, L., Larsson, L., and Lindstrom, F., Effects of fasting and lactovegetarian diet on rheumatoid arthritis, *Scand J Rheumatol*, 8, 249, 1979.
200. Nenonen, M., et al., Uncooked, lactobacilli-rich, vegan food and rheumatoid arthritis, *Br J Rheumatol*, 37, 274, 1998.
201. Hafstrom, I., et al., A vegan diet free of gluten improves the signs and symptoms of rheumatoid arthritis: the effects on arthritis correlate with a reduction in antibodies to food antigens, *Rheumatology*, 40, 1175, 2001.
202. McDougall, J., et al., Effects of a very low-fat vegan diet in subjects with rheumatoid arthritis, *J Altern Complement Med*, 8, 71, 2002.
203. Muller, H., de Toledo, W., and Resch, K.-L., Fasting followed by vegetarian diet in patients with rheumatoid arthritis: a systematic review, *Scand J Rheumatol*, 30, 1, 2001.
204. Skoldstam, L., Hagfors, L., and Johansson, G., An experimental study of a Mediterranean diet intervention for patients with rheumatoid arthritis, *Ann Rheum Dis*, 62, 208, 2003.
205. Hafstrom, I., et al., Effects of fasting on disease activity, neutrophil function, fatty acid composition, and leukotriene biosynthesis in patients with rheumatoid arthritis, *Arthritis Rheum*, 31, 585, 1988.
206. Uden, A.-M., et al., Neutrophil functions and clinical performance after total fasting in patients with rheumatoid arthritis, *Ann Rheum Dis*, 42, 45, 1983.
207. Michalsen, A., et al., Mediterranean diet or extended fasting's influence on changing the intestinal microflora, immunoglobulin A secretion and clinical outcome in patients with rheumatoid arthritis and fibromyalgia: an observational study, *BMC Complement Altern Med*, 5, 22, 2005.
208. Darlington, L.G., Ramsey, N.W., and Mansfield, J.R., Placebo-controlled, blind study of dietary manipulation therapy in rheumatoid arthritis, *Lancet*, 1 (8475):236–8, 1986.
209. Beri, D., et al., Effect of dietary restrictions on disease activity in rheumatoid arthritis, *Ann Rheum Dis*, 47, 69, 1988.
210. Panush, R., et al., Diet therapy for rheumatoid arthritis, *Arthritis Rheum*, 26, 462, 1983.
211. Kjeldsen-Kragh, J., et al., Decrease in anti-*proteus mirabilis* but not anti-*escherichia coli* antibody levels in rheumatoid arthritis patients treated with fasting and a one year vegetarian diet, *Ann Rheum Dis*, 54, 221, 1995.
212. Peltonen, R., et al., Faecal microbial flora and disease activity in rheumatoid arthritis during a vegan diet, *Br J Rheumatol*, 36, 64, 1997.
213. Fraser, D., et al., Serum levels of interleukin-6 and dehydroepiandrosterone sulphate in response to either fasting or a ketogenic diet in rheumatoid arthritis patients, *Clin Exp Rheumatol*, 18, 357, 2000.
214. Kjeldsen-Kragh, J., et al., Vegetarian diet for patients with rheumatoid arthritis: can the clinical effects be explained by the psychological characteristics of the patients? *Br J Rheumatol*, 33, 569, 1994.

215. Skoldstam, L., et al., Weight reduction is not a major reason for improvement in rheumatoid arthritis from lacto-vegetarian, vegan or Mediterranean diets, *Nutr J*, 4, 15, 2005.
216. Haugen, M.A., et al., Changes in plasma phospholipid fatty acids and their relationship to disease activity in rheumatoid arthritis patients treated with a vegetarian diet, *Br J Nutr*, 72, 555, 1994.
217. Larsson, P., et al., A vitamin D analogue (MC 1288) has immunomodulatory properties and suppresses collagen-induced arthritis (CIA) without causing hypercalcaemia, *Clin Exp Immunol*, 114, 277, 1998.
218. Cleland, L., et al., Fish oil—an example of an anti-inflammatory food, *Asia Pac J Clin Nutr*, 14, 66, 2005.
219. Cantorna, M. and Hayes, C., Vitamin A deficiency exacerbates murine Lyme arthritis, *J Infect Dis*, 174, 747, 1996.
220. Dusso, A., Brown, A., and Slatopolsky, E., Vitamin D, *Am J Physiol Renal Physiol*, 289, F8, 2005.
221. Zittermann, A., et al., Low vitamin D status: a contributing factor in the pathogenesis of congestive heart failure? *J Am Coll Cardiol*, 41, 105, 2003.
222. Crandall, C., Vitamin A intake and osteoporosis: a clinical review, *J Womens Health*, 13, 939, 2004.
223. Barker, M., et al., Serum retinoids and β-carotene as predictors of hip and other fractures in elderly women, *J Bone Mineral Res*, 20, 913, 2005.
224. Wigg, A., et al., A system for improving vitamin D nutrition in residential care, *Med J Aust*, 185, 195, 2006.
225. Kremer, J.M., et al., Effects of high-dose fish oil on rheumatoid arthritis after stopping non-steroidal anti-inflammatory drugs. Clinical and immune correlates, *Arthritis Rheum*, 38, 1107, 1995.
226. Geusens, P., et al., Long-term effect of omega-3 fatty acid supplementation in active rheumatoid arthritis. A 12-month, double-blind, controlled study, *Arthritis Rheum*, 37, 824, 1994.
227. Nielsen, G.L., et al., The effects of dietary supplementation with n-3 polyunsaturated fatty acids in patients with rheumatoid arthritis: a randomized, double blind trial, *Eur J Clin Invest*, 22, 687, 1992.
228. van der Tempel, H., et al., Effects of fish oil supplementation in rheumatoid arthritis, *Ann Rheum Dis*, 49, 76, 1990.
229. Tulleken, J., et al., Vitamin E status during dietary fish oil supplementation in rheumatoid arthritis, *Arthritis Rheum*, 33, 1416, 1990.
230. Kremer, J.M., et al., Fish-oil fatty acid supplementation in active rheumatoid arthritis. A double-blinded, controlled, crossover study, *Ann Int Med*, 106, 497, 1987.
231. Reiffel, J. and McDonald, A., Antiarrhythmic effects of omega-3 fatty acids, *Am J Cardiol*, 98, 50i, 2006.
232. Robinson, J. and Stone, N., Antiathersclerotic and antithrombotic effects of omega-3 fatty acids, *Am J Cardiol*, 98, 39i, 2006.
233. Nestle, P., et al., Arterial compliance in obese subjects is improved with dietary plant n-3 fatty acid from flaxseed oil despite increased LDL oxidizability, *Arterioscler Thromb Vasc Biol*, 17, 1163, 1997.
234. Theis, F., et al., Association of n-3 polyunsaturated fatty acids with stability of atherosclerotic plaques: a randomized, controlled trial, *Lancet*, 361, 477, 2003.
235. Prevoo, M., et. al., Modified disease activity scores that include twenty-eight joint counts, *Arthritis Rheum*, 38, 44, 1995.
236. Felson, D., et al., The American College of Rheumatology preliminary definition of improvement in rheumatoid arthritis, *Arthritis Rheum*, 38, 727, 1995.

13 Irritable Bowel Syndrome

Gerard E. Mullin and Linda A. Lee

CONTENTS

13.1 INTRODUCTION

Irritable bowel syndrome (IBS) is a disorder characterized by chronic abdominal pain or discomfort and altered bowel habits. IBS is the most frequently diagnosed gastrointestinal (GI) condition, with an estimated US prevalence of 5%–25% [1,2]. The diagnosis of IBS is established by fulfilling the symptom-based Rome III criteria (Table 13.1) [3]. IBS accounts for 36%–50% of all referrals to gastroenterologists but is often seen in primary care settings as well [1,2]. In a study to assess the economic burden and health care usage of various GI disorders, IBS accounted for

TABLE 13.1
Rome III Diagnostic Criteria for Irritable Bowel Syndrome[a]

Recurrent abdominal pain or discomfort[b] at least 3 days/month in the last 3 months associated with 2 or more of the following:
- Improvement with defecation
- Onset associated with a change in frequency of stool
- Onset associated with a change in form (appearance) of stool

[a] Criteria fulfilled for the last 3 months with symptoms onset at least 6 months prior to diagnosis.
[b] Discomfort means an uncomfortable sensation not described as pain.

3.7 million annual office visits, being second only to the number of visits for gastroesophageal reflux [4]. IBS and disorders with which it is related has been associated with a significant decrease in quality of life [5,6]. Functional GI disorders that include IBS have been shown to negatively impact quality of life more so than "organic" GI disorders, such as inflammatory bowel disease [7]. Along these lines, IBS is the second leading cause of work absenteeism [2]. IBS appears to have a female predominance, with two-thirds of patients being women [1]. While the greater prevalence among women is well established, the reasons for this sex difference remain elusive. IBS in women appears to be linked to other chronic functional pain disorders that are sex-based, such as fibromyalgia, chronic fatigue syndrome, chronic constipation, interstitial cystitis, and migraine headaches with aura and temporomandibular joint disorder.

Historically, IBS research has not focused on sex comparisons despite that the overwhelming majority of study subjects have been female. In addition, women in past studies were often treated as a homogenous group, with little attention paid to menopausal status, menstrual cycle, use of hormones (i.e., oral contraceptives, hormone replacement therapy), or other sex-related factors [1]. Recent interest in sex differences in IBS has been fueled in part by studies suggesting that new pharmacological therapies for this syndrome are more effective in female than in male IBS patients [1]. There is growing evidence that clinical symptoms differ between male and female IBS patients and are also affected by the menstrual cycle. This review will focus on sex differences in IBS, including epidemiology, clinical presentation, pathophysiology, treatment response, and dietary management.

13.2 ETIOLOGY AND SEX DIFFERENCES

13.2.1 Prevalence of IBS

In the general population, the female-to-male prevalence ratio for IBS varies between 1:1 and 2:1 across a variety of studies [1]. Women are more likely to seek medical care for this condition, as reflected by the even greater female predominance seen in medical clinic populations, as high as 4:1 in one survey [1,8]. Some of this variability can likely be accounted for by cultural factors and sex differences in rates of health care utilization, given that several studies conducted in India and Sri Lanka actually report a male predominance among IBS clinic patients [1,9].

13.2.2 Clinical Symptoms

There have been several studies comparing symptoms between men and women with IBS. Findings have been variable and inconsistent, likely because of differences in sample recruitment sites (community vs. tertiary care clinic) and data collection methodology (daily diary, interview, chart review, questionnaires). However, there is a growing body of evidence for a female predominance in constipation, bloating, and extracolonic manifestations while males appear to have diarrhea as the predominant feature [10].

13.2.2.1 Abdominal Pain and Discomfort

Recurrent abdominal pain is a diagnostic symptom of IBS, in addition to being the single most important determinant for both men and women in deciding to seek treatment for IBS. In one study, "belly pain" was reported by nearly two-thirds of all patients [10]. Interestingly, neither the incidence of pain nor the severity of pain differed between male and female IBS patients. In another study, loose stools associated with the onset of pain, more frequent stools with the onset of pain, pain relieved by defecation, and postprandial exacerbation of symptoms were similar in men and women with IBS [11]. The prevalence of pain and discomfort is due to a heightened perception to colonic contents (visceral hypersensitivity), which is a characteristic finding in patients with IBS [10,12]. However, current measures of enhanced visceral perception (e.g., decreased rectosigmoid pain thresholds) have not been consistently found in IBS patients and therefore are not currently used as a diagnostic marker [13].

13.2.2.2 Altered Bowel Habits

Altered bowel habits are a central feature of IBS. Patients are frequently classified as constipation-predominant, diarrhea-predominant, or alternating diarrhea and constipation. In a relatively large survey of male and female patients with IBS, Lee et al. found women nearly twice more likely to report constipation-predominant bowel habits, while men were more likely to report diarrhea [10]. This observation was reinforced in a community sample, in which Talley et al. similarly found women to be more likely to report constipation and males more likely to have diarrhea [14]. Several physiological factors may play a role in these sex-related differences in bowel habits, including differences in central autonomic control, and enteric nervous system and smooth muscle physiology. In addition, estrogen and progesterone have been postulated to play a role in sex differences in bowel motility (see below).

13.2.2.3 Abdominal Bloating and Distension

Gas and bloating are frequently reported in both men and women with IBS. However, Lee et al. showed that women were significantly more likely than men to complain of bloating and furthermore to report it as their single most bothersome symptom [10]. Several large community and clinic population studies have also confirmed gas, bloating, and distension to be more common among female IBS patients than among male patients [10,14,15]. The cause of these symptoms is likely multifactorial, e.g., dietary factors, slowed transit of gas [16], and visceral hypersensitivity [17–19].

13.2.2.4 Extracolonic Symptoms

Although only colonic symptoms are used in the diagnostic criteria for IBS, patients frequently report extracolonic visceral and somatosensory symptoms. Functional dyspepsia (upper abdominal pain not associated with ulcer) affects 30%–60% of IBS patients [12] and nausea and vomiting is reported in 25%–50% of patients with IBS. Women with IBS are especially prone to increased urinary frequency and urgency, which occurs in 65% of female patients with IBS and are often associated with abnormal urodynamic studies [20]. Sleep disturbances also are more commonly reported by female IBS patients [21–23], although there has been some inconsistency in several studies to show abnormal plysomnographic parameters in IBS patients [24]. Other extracolonic symptoms that have been found to be more likely in women than in men with IBS include alterations in taste and smell, muscle stiffness or aches, headache, back pain, and fatigue [10]. Another important feature of IBS is its high coexistence with other functional pain disorders [25]. Fibromyalgia and other rheumatological symptoms occur in over 60% of female IBS patients [25]. Almost 40% of women with interstitial cystitis, a bladder condition characterized by suprapubic pain and urinary urgency or frequency, also have IBS [26]. In addition, a chronic pelvic pain disorder is another important area of overlap with IBS. Several studies have shown a twofold higher incidence of dyspareunia in female IBS patients, as compared with female inflammatory bowel disease patients [27] or male IBS patients [11,21].

13.2.3 Pathophysiology

The pathophysiology of IBS remains poorly understood, although there are several physiologic processes that appear altered in IBS: (1) alterations in the response of the gut to stimuli such as food (motor response), (2) an altered perception of a visceral stimuli (the afferent sensory pathway or the brain–gut axis), and (3) the perception of a nonnoxious visceral stimulus as noxious (psychological profile and altered cortical processing of visceral stimuli) [2]. Studies have clearly implicated various predisposing and trigger factors that are associated with the onset and exacerbation of IBS and these include genetic predisposition [28,29], chronic stress [30], and inflammation or infection [31]. These factors may be associated with enhanced responsiveness of neural, immune, and neuroendocrine circuits along with brain–gut axis, resulting in altered bowel motility and visceral perception. The neuronal connection between the gut and the central nervous system (CNS) is referred to as the brain–gut axis. This axis is hardwired and involves the stretch receptors in the wall of the gut as well as chemical receptors in the mucosa, the enteric nervous system that relays information from these receptors to the autonomic nervous system, the autonomic pathway

TABLE 13.2
Evidence for Differences in Pathophysiology or Response to Treatment between Men and Women with Irritable Bowel Syndrome

Motility	
	No studies comparing differences in gastrointestinal motility between men and women with IBS
Autonomic nervous system	
	Greater sympathetic and lower vagal activity (by heart rate variability) in response to colorectal distention in men compared with women with IBS
Afferent sensory pathway	
	Lower threshold to rectal distention postprandially in women with IBS compared with men
	Different central nervous system areas activated by colorectal distention in women and men
Postinflammatory or infection IBS	
	Female gender is a risk factor for developing postinfectious IBS. This appears to be associated with psychological profile
Psychological status	
	Greater prevalence of depression, anxiety, and somatization in women compared with men may contribute to presentation or severity of IBS in women
Response to medication	
	Greater efficacy of 5-HT3 antagonist, alosetron, in women with diarrhea-predominant IBS than men with similar condition

and spinal pathways that relay information to the CNS, and the cortices that need to be activated for a stimulus to be perceived consciously. How these pathophysiologic processes are impacted by factors related to sex and gender will be discussed. A framework to conceptualize this is provided in Table 13.2. The evidence for differences in afferent and efferent pathways of the brain–gut axis and in pathophysiology in women and men with IBS is summarized. The main findings reported in the literature related to the effect of gonadal hormones and gender on the physiologic pathways involved in IBS are summarized in Table 13.3.

It is not yet completely understood how the above model of disease can account for the sex differences observed in IBS. Few pathophysiological studies have focused on making sex comparisons, although there has recently been increased interest in this area. Numerous factors need to be considered in the exploration of these differences. These factors include biologic, hormonal, behavioral, psychosocial, and sociophysiological mechanisms of IBS, including any sex-specific finding noted in the literature.

13.2.3.1 Postinfectious IBS

It has long been recognized that IBS-like symptoms may develop in a minority of patients recovering from enteric infection. Up to 17% of all patients with IBS will report their symptoms following an episode of gastroenteritis [32]. Between 7% and 30% of patients recovering from proven bacterial gastroenteritis IBS symptoms have been reported to develop [31]. Organisms that have been associated with postinfectious IBS include *Salmonella, Campylobacter jejuni*, and *Shigella* [32]. A risk factor

TABLE 13.3
Summary of Effects of Sex Hormones or Gender on Physiologic Pathways Controlling the Brain–Gut Axis

Effect of Estrogen or Progesterone
Motility
Impaired gall bladder contraction to progesterone
Decreased lower esophageal sphincter pressure in pregnancy
Visceral afferent pathway
Modulation of response of afferent neurons to substance P (guinea pig)
Lower threshold for visceromotor response in the proestrus compared with estrus phase of estrus cycle in rats
Drug metabolism
Cytochrome P450 pathway is affected by estrogens and progesterone
Gender Effect
Animal studies
Pain pathways
Testosterone
Increases the antinociceptive effect of opiates in somatic pain. Estrogen effect is complex and estrus cycle dependent
Greater potency of opiates to decrease visceromotor response in male compared with female rats
Human studies
Motility
Slower gastric emptying in women compared with men
Response to colonic distention
Conflicting reports of the effect of the menstrual cycle on pain sensation to colorectal distention
Different areas and intensity of brain activation in response to colorectal distention in men and women
Somatic pain response
Women experience greater pain sensation to most levels of pain stimulus
Greater score on a catastrophizing scale in women compared with men
Neurotransmitter uptake pathway
Genetic polymorphism of the 5HT-transporter promoter region is associated with different affective symptom expression in women compared with men

for developing postinfectious IBS appears to be the duration of diarrheal illness greater than 3 weeks [33]. Several studies have found that major, sustained stressful life events occurring either before or immediately following the acute infection are the strongest predictor of IBS development [31,34]. Interestingly, the development of postinfectious IBS appears to have a female predominance. In one study examining equal numbers of men and women with gastroenteritis, IBS symptoms were present at 3 months in 77% of females but only 36% of the males [35].

Exact mechanisms for the association between infection and IBS remain unclear. However, several studies have revealed increased colonic mucosal immune markers (e.g., lymphocytes and mast cells) and enterochromaffin cells in IBS patients, both in postinfectious and unselected patient populations [36,37].

In addition, animal studies demonstrate that low-grade inflammation or immune activation can alter motility and epithelial function of the gut, analogous to changes observed in asthma [38]. The clinical relevance of these findings is not entirely clear and further studies are needed.

13.2.3.2 Altered GI Motility

Given the predominance of altered bowel habits, abnormal gut motility has long been considered a leading etiologic factor of IBS. However, objective findings of motility alterations have been inconsistent, with no distinct pattern distinguishing IBS patients from healthy controls. Two major observations that have been observed are increased gut transit time in some patients with constipation-predominant IBS and decreased transit time in those with diarrhea-predominant IBS. In addition, several studies have shown that IBS patients have increased motility compared with healthy subjects to a variety of stimuli, including psychological stress, meals, and balloon inflation in the gut [39].

Overall, males have shorter intestinal and total GI transit times than their female counterparts. Using ambulatory 24 h colonic manometry in 25 age-matched healthy men and women, Rao et al. found that healthy women showed significantly less pressure activity in the colon than men, and this difference was particularly significant in the transverse or descending colon and during the day [40]. These differences in colon transit and motility may explain the greater vulnerability of developing constipation in women compared with men.

13.2.3.3 Visceral Hypersensitivity

Enhanced perception of visceral stimuli has emerged as an important model IBS pathophysiology and an area of intense GI research. Multiple studies using colonic or rectal balloon distension paradigms have consistently demonstrated lower discomfort thresholds in IBS patients compared with controls [18,19].

Differences in visceral sensitivity between men and women with IBS have not been studied extensively, though evidence thus far shows that women may be more prone to develop hypersensitivity, especially following repeated stimuli. In a study of 52 IBS patients (39 females and 13 males), Ragnarsson et al. [41] found a significant decrease in postprandial rectal thresholds (mmHg) of maximal tolerated distension in women compared with men (i.e., increased rectal sensitivity in women compared with men). Following a standardized meal, thresholds decreased in 50% of the women and 25% of the men and remained unchanged in the remainder of individuals. There were no significant gender differences in symptoms. Another study assessed the presence of sex differences in rectal discomfort thresholds before and after noxious sigmoid distensions in 26 healthy individuals (9 males, 17 females) and 58 IBS patients (34 males and 24 females) [42]. Rectal discomfort thresholds were significantly lower in IBS females compared with IBS males, following noxious stimuli. In addition, though female control subjects had higher rectal discomfort thresholds than IBS females, a significant proportion of both groups demonstrated a decrease in thresholds after noxious sigmoid stimulation.

13.2.3.4 Altered Central Mechanisms

Recent findings in functional neuroimaging studies support the hypothesis that dysregulation of the brain–gut axis plays a key role in IBS. Using neuroimaging techniques such as functional magnetic resonance imaging and positron emission tomography, alterations in regional brain activation have been demonstrated in IBS patients in response to colorectal distension compared with healthy subjects [43,44]. Differences in the activation of several brain regions have been demonstrated and include the anterior and midcingulate cortices, insula, and dorsal pons, which are some of the most consistently activated brain areas in response to visceral as well as somatic nociceptive stimuli [43–46]. These regions are concerned with cognitive and affective aspects of processing of sensory input, including noxious stimuli. These observations suggest that IBS patients have altered central pain modulatory pathways in response to incoming or anticipated visceral pain.

Two studies have examined sex differences in the brain responses to colorectal distension in IBS. Berman et al. reported significantly greater activation of the insula bilaterally in male IBS patients compared with female IBS patients [46]. Naliboff et al. found that men with IBS had greater activation in areas associated with the cognitive processing of painful sensations, including the insula and midcingulate cortex, while women with IBS showed greater activation in limbic regions, including the amygdala and infragenual cingulated cortex, which are associated with the emotional processing of visceral stimuli [45].

13.2.3.5 Hormonal Factors

With women in general, GI symptoms appear to be influenced by female sex hormones; with both upper and lower GI symptoms increasing during the late luteal and early menses phases relative to the follicular phase [1,47]. The effect of menstrual cycle on IBS has been described by several investigators. In one survey, 50.8% of patients reported a worsening of their IBS symptoms at the time of menses [10]. Women with IBS were also found to rate stomach pain, nausea, and diarrhea, but not somatic complaints like backache, as more severe at menses than healthy female subjects, suggesting enhanced visceral sensitivity during the perimenstrual period [11,48]. Other symptoms commonly associated with menstrual cycle function, such as breast tenderness, bloating, and affective symptoms, were found to be elevated in IBS patients across all cycle phases, with a similar increase in severity immediately prior to or at the onset of menses [48,49].

The effect of menstruation on IBS symptoms is thought to be mediated by ovarian hormones affecting bowel function either centrally or peripherally. This is supported by the finding that during pregnancy, a time of very high estrogen and progesterone levels, GI symptoms (nausea, constipation, upper GI distress) increase and intestinal transport decreases [1]. In addition, IBS patients on oral contraceptives that mimic naturally fluctuating ovarian hormones will continue to have amplification of their GI symptoms during menses [47]. Finally, Houghton et al. found that women with IBS had greater rectal sensitivity during menses than other points during menstrual cycle. It is noteworthy that no menstrual cycle phase differences were found in rectal compliance, wall tension, or motility [50].

Interestingly, in addition to a higher prevalence of visceral pain in women patients during the premenstrual phase, the diagnosis of IBS is threefold more common in women with dysmenorrheal (painful menstruation) than in those without [50]. A similar co-morbidity between dysmenorrheal and fibromyalgia has been suggested [11,51]. These findings further support the existence of a more generalized alteration in the perception of visceral and somatic pain in a subset of IBS patients.

13.2.3.6 Gender Role

While recognizing that biologic sex differences exist between male and female IBS patients, Toner and Akman have provided insights into gender-related differences in how symptoms might be experienced and interpreted [52]. They suggest the concept of gender role, which is defined as generalizations about male and female traits that are associated with masculinity and femininity. Gender-related themes such as a history of sexual and physical abuse, gender role socialization, gender role conflict, public embarrassment and humiliation due to GI symptoms, perfectionist views of bodily function, and balancing personal vs. supportive roles may be important components as to how symptoms are interpreted and acted upon. However, there is a lack of available data on how these gender-specific themes participate in a syndrome such as IBS with respect to its physiologic characteristics such as motility, pain sensitivity, and autonomic function.

13.2.3.6.1 Effect of Gender on Psychological Response to Pain: Impact of Abuse History

Patterns of accompanying symptom complaints are different between men and women with symptoms of abdominal distention, anxiety, and depression, being more common in women [53,54]. An interesting study of psychology students demonstrated that the female students tended to score greater on a pain catastrophizing scale than men. This scale incorporates the degree of rumination, magnification, and helplessness that a subject feels when experiencing pain [55]. This study suggests that the affective component to experiencing pain is different between men and women, even when they have no chronic illness.

Recent studies indicate that infection or inflammation contribute to increasing both the nociceptive response to visceral stimulation and the motor activity of the gut [56,57]. Initial studies indicated that women and patients with a psychological profile of neuroticism and anxiety were more at risk for developing postinfectious IBS [58]. Subsequent studies confirm the greater prevalence of these psychological traits, but the female gender appeared to be less of a risk factor [31,59]. In light of the reported predisposing risk factor of infection and the report of a greater number of mucosal mast cells in the colon of subjects with IBS [60], it is of interest that there are more constitutive mast-cell populations in the jejunum and colon in female rats compared with male rats [61]. Whether any similar difference is seen in humans is unknown.

An important factor contributing to the degree of pain experienced by women with IBS is a history of abuse. At a tertiary referral center, the prevalence of a history of abuse was greater in patients presenting with IBS or functional abdominal pain than with organic GI disease [62]. This is clearly more prevalent in female patients than in males, and needs to be identified and addressed if treatment is to be effective.

Gender socialization can impact reporting of pain even without any history of abuse or psychopathology. There is a potential impact of the sex of the patient and of the researcher or physician on pain reporting [63].

13.3 TREATMENT

Given the multiple factors that are altered or contribute to the pathogenesis of IBS, the treatment of this complex disorder requires a biopsychological approach [64]. This multidimensional approach addresses the biology of IBS as well as the psychologic and social factors that are common among affected individuals. A detailed patient history that includes a comprehensive review of the patient's social and psychiatric history is the first step in establishing a treatment plan. The biopsychosocial approach demands more face-to-face patient time and may not be widely available. This may account in part for why only 49% of patients with IBS report a response to medical treatment [65]. Efficacy of specific treatment modalities often is difficult to establish because of the high placebo effect associated with interventions used to treat IBS [66]. It is not surprising that over 50% of IBS patients in an outpatient setting report the use of alternative therapies [67].

It is not the purpose to review every therapy currently available for IBS, but to highlight those whose efficacy, use, or availability are affected by sex or gender.

13.3.1 PHARMACOLOGICAL TREATMENT

Recently, the emergence of new IBS-specific medications has revealed the potential importance of sex-based differences in this disease. Alosetron, a selective 5-HT_3 receptor antagonist, has been FDA approved for use in women with severe diarrhea-predominant IBS. Early clinical trials suggested that alosetron had a greater efficacy in females than in males [68]. The greater efficacy in women may be in part due to the greater change in overall colonic transit in women than in men with IBS [69]. However, there was a more recent study demonstrating that alosetron is effective in men with diarrhea-predominant IBS with respect to adequately relieving abdominal pain and discomfort and improving stool consistency [70]. But there was no significant improvement in stool consistency and urgency with alosetron compared with placebo. The authors postulated that the observed differential treatment effects may be related to a combination of sex-based differences in peripheral as well as central mechanisms.

Similarly, tegaserod, a 5-HT_4 receptor partial agonist, was initially indicated only for female IBS patients with constipation as their primary bowel symptom [71]. However, tegaserod was also recently shown to be effective for the treatment of chronic constipation in men and women and is newly approved for this indication [72].

The initially demonstrated sex difference in response to these serotonergic agents may have been due to the fairly small numbers of males studied in the clinical trials. While there may be some small differences in treatment response to these agents, further studies are needed to substantiate gender differences.

13.3.2 Nonpharmacological Treatment and Complementary Alternative Medicine

In a 1997 survey, 42% of the US population has reported the use of complementary medicine [73] and other studies have indicated that more women than men use such therapy [67]. Most individuals wish to use complementary medicine concurrently with conventional approaches [74]. The reasons why IBS and functional dyspepsia patients report using complementary medicine were dissatisfaction with conventional medicine, a desire to treat digestive symptoms with a more natural approach, to determine whether alternative therapies might help to alleviate the problem, or that complementary medicine was recommended by another individual [75].

The nonpharmacological approaches to the treatment of IBS that have been shown to have documented efficacy are listed in Table 13.4. At this time, there are five nonpharmacological approaches to the treatment of IBS: relaxation alone, hypnotherapy, short-term psychodynamic psychotherapy, cognitive–behavioral combination therapy, and pure cognitive therapy. These therapeutic modalities can be considered in IBS patients with moderate to severe symptoms, when patients have failed medical treatments, or when there is evidence of stress or psychological factors that contribute to GI symptom exacerbation [2]. While many of these studies included men and women, gender differences were not usually determined. The only exception is hypnotherapy, which in a recent study was found to be associated with greater overall improvement in IBS symptoms in females compared with males (52% vs. 33%) [76].

Supplementation with herbal preparations have yielded mixed results except for STW-5 (which is a composite of nine Chinese herbs), standard forms of traditional Chinese medicines, peppermint oil, and artichoke leaf extract, which have proven

TABLE 13.4
Summary of Complementary and Alternative Medicine in Irritable Bowel Syndrome

Herbs	Mind–Body: Best Results
Peppermint oil (p-IBS) (8 studies, benefit)	Psychological
TCM (d-IBS), STW-5 (benefit)	Cognitive behavioral treatment
Diet	Yoga
Elimination diet (15%–71% response, nonsustained)	Reflexology
	Hypnosis
Supplements	Guided imagery
Melatonin (1 study, benefit)	Meditation
Probiotics 8 RCT's (7 benefit)	Biofeedback
Energy medicine	Multicomponent
Acupuncture (2 controlled sham studies 2 benefit)	

TCM, Traditional Chinese medicine; STW, (name of herbal preparation); RCT, randomized controlled trial.

benefits for IBS [77–80]. Melatonin at 3 mg/day was studied specifically in females with IBS [81]. Melatonin is involved in seroterogenic regulation in the gut and thus was studied specifically in females, because serotonin-modifying drugs work best in females. Lu et al. demonstrated that women taking 3 mg of melatonin/day for 8 weeks had significant reductions in global symptoms and pain compared with placebo [81]. These therapeutic modalities can be considered in IBS patients with moderate to severe symptoms, when patients have failed medical treatments, or when there is evidence of stress or psychological factors that contribute to GI symptom exacerbation [1]. The concept that intestinal flora could be responsible for bloating and gassiness associated with IBS was recently bolstered by reports that up to 80% of IBS patients have small intestinal bacterial overgrowth [82]. Other investigators have not been able to substantiate an incidence this high perhaps in part due to the insensitivity of breath hydrogen testing available in most hospitals or centers. A 10 day course of Rifaximin, a nonabsorbable antibiotic, resulted in greater improvement of bloating in IBS patients over a period of 10 weeks after therapy [83], although these results have been challenged due to methodological issues [84]. It has long been speculated that alterations in the normal colonic flora might abate the symptoms of IBS for several reasons. Probiotics, which are ingested substances containing live organisms that have a beneficial effect on the host by altering the body's intestinal microflora, may help to eliminate intestinal pathogens, alter motility, and reduce bacterial fermentation and pathogen-related inflammation. Improvement in bloating and flatulence has been reported from several small studies [85]. Organisms that have been associated with improvement include *L. plantarum, B. infantis*, and *Bifidobacterium.*

While there has been limited evidence of gender differences in response to nonpharmacological treatment, the authors recommend that careful attention to gender issues be given when choosing and providing treatment for IBS patients. Such gender-specific issues were discussed earlier and include history of physical and sexual abuse, gender role socialization or conflict, and perfectionist views of bodily function or image. Mind–body therapies with established efficacy include relaxation, yoga, hypnotherapy, short-term psychodynamic psychotherapy, guided-imagery, cognitive–behavioral combination therapy, and pure cognitive therapy.

13.4 DIETARY MANAGEMENT

Treatment of IBS always involves manipulation of the diet, as it is well known that withdrawal of certain dietary substances can improve IBS symptoms. Foods typically associated with gas production are notorious for provoking IBS symptoms. These include foods rich in fermentable carbohydrates such as beans and cabbage, and foods containing large concentrations of fructose, sorbitol, and lactose [86]. Some IBS patients will report worse bloating after ingesting rich meals, which may be explained by the observation of increased small intestinal gas retention with direct infusion of dietary fat into the small intestine [87,88]. Agents that stimulate colonic motility may precipitate abdominal pain in IBS patients, thus it is generally recommended that IBS patients with bloating, pain, or diarrhea eliminate foods and beverages containing caffeine, a known colonic stimulant [89,90]. Increasing dietary fiber, which is often prescribed as first line therapy for the treatment of IBS because it tends to regulate bowel movements, may also exacerbate IBS symptoms because fiber is not absorbed; indeed, in one study 50% of IBS patients reported an exacerbation of symptoms and only 11% reported an improvement [91]. Both soluble and insoluble dietary fiber are fermented by intestinal flora to produce short-chain fatty acids and gas [89]. A feature of IBS is visceral hypersensitivity to gas distention of the gut, and hence, the association of dietary fiber with increased bloating and gas.

Food hypersensitivities and food intolerances found in IBS patients may also trigger IBS symptoms. Food hypersensitivity, or food allergy, is defined as an immunological response to food proteins and is characterized by alterations in serum antibodies or cellular immunity. The mechanisms responsible for food allergy are now beginning to be discerned and may greatly impact future IBS therapy. Food intolerance on the other hand refers to carbohydrate malabsorption; malabsorption of lactose, fructose, fructans, and sorbitol can produce bloating, abdominal pain, and diarrhea in both IBS patients and normal controls.

It is unknown if the prevalence of food allergy is truly greater in IBS patients compared with normal controls, although 60% of IBS patients suspect they have a food allergy [92]. However, the role of food allergy in IBS symptoms remains unclear since food allergy only affects 4% of American adults [93]. The notion that food allergens could precipitate IBS symptoms is particularly attractive since mast cells and their mediators alter visceral hypersensitivity and gut motility [94,95]. Food allergy may be separated into non-IgE- (cellular) or IgE-mediated reactions. In the worst clinical scenario, food allergies can produce gut anaphylaxis, characterized by acute nausea, vomiting, colicky abdominal pain, and allergic manifestations in other organs [96]. Allergies to peanut, tree nuts, fish, and shellfish account for most adult food allergies. Eosinophilic gastroenteritis, which may be IgE- or non-IgE-mediated, features an eosinophilic infiltration of the GI mucosa and may arise in individuals with atopy or food allergies. Symptoms associated with eosinophilic gastroenteritis depend on which organ is involved, but may include heartburn, nausea, abdominal pain, and vomiting.

A classic example of a non-IgE-mediated allergy is celiac sprue, a disorder of malabsorption caused by an allergy to gluten, a protein found in many grains, including wheat. Celiac sprue has been reported in as many as 20% of IBS patients [97] but this figure has been disputed. Some IBS patients may describe an intolerance to wheat, but this "intolerance" is distinct from a true allergy to gluten. An improvement in symptoms in response to wheat avoidance is often mistakenly interpreted by the patient as evidence that he or she has underlying celiac sprue. The diagnosis of celiac sprue, is more strongly suggested by endoscopic biopsy demonstrating villous flattening and intraepithelial lymphocytosis in the small bowel mucosa in addition to circulating serum IgA antibodies to tissue transglutaminase. The diganosis is ultimately established by demonstrating histologic improvement in response to gluten withdrawal from the diet.

Diagnosing food allergy is a clinical challenge because tests with a high positive predictive value are still lacking [89]. For example, skin prick testing is used extensively, but a positive result does not prove that a specific food is responsible for symptoms. Radioallergosorbent testing (RAST) to identify serum IgE antibodies against potential food allergens has also been proposed; although negative results are effective for ruling out an IgE-mediated reaction to a specific food allergen, the positive predictive value of a positive RAST result is also low. The utility of measuring serum IgG titers has been controversial as well because such food antibodies are common and may even be physiological. But because serum IgG4 and IgE antibodies have been implicated in atopic conditions induced by food hypersensitivity, such as atopic dermatitis, hay fever, and asthma, Zar et al. sought to determine the clinical significance of IgG4 titers to common food antigens in 108 IBS patients and controls [98]. Although they found that serum IgG4 titers to wheat, beef, pork, lamb, and soy bean were higher in IBS patients than in controls, there was no correlation between the titer and degree of symptoms. No significant difference in titers to potatoes, rice, fish, chicken, yeast, tomato, and shrimp was observed. Moreover, in this study no significant difference was observed in IgE antibody response to food antigens or to cutaneous pin-prick testing. These results led the authors to perform another study in which food-specific IgG4 antibody titers >250 mcg/L were used to develop 6 month exclusion diets that improved IBS symptoms and rectal compliance in a small group of patients [99]. Further studies are necessary to elucidate the significance of IgG4 titers in predicting food hypersensitivities.

In the absence of tests with high positive predictive values, the double blind, placebo-controlled food challenge remains the gold standard for the clinical diagnosis of food allergy. After a 2 week withdrawal of suspected food allergens from the diet, encapsulated food substances or placebo are given to patients who are then monitored for symptoms. Most practitioners instead favor the less-cumbersome elimination diet in which symptoms are monitored after potential offenders are withdrawn from the diet for 4–6 weeks and then later reintroduced. The first report that an exclusion diet improved IBS symptoms in a small group of 21 IBS patients was published in 1982 [100]. In Niec's 1998 review of seven studies to determine whether adverse food reactions played a role in IBS symptoms, a positive response to an elimination diet ranged from 15% to 71% [101]. Studies based on subjects with diarrhea-predominant IBS tended to find improvement with elimination diets. The most common offenders were milk, wheat, and eggs, but it should be noted that no included study was free from methodological limitations.

Like food allergy, the diagnosis of food intolerance to carbohydrates is difficult to make given the limitations of current testing. Intolerance to lactose, fructose, fructans (polymerized form of fructose), or sorbitol may contribute to symptoms characteristic of IBS, such as bloating, gassiness, abdominal pain, and diarrhea [102]. Fructose malabsorption leads to the delivery of unabsorbed fructose to the colon where it is fermented by intestinal bacteria to produce gas that can be associated with bloating and abdominal pain. The diagnosis is currently established by breath hydrogen testing, but unfortunately this test is fraught with technical limitations and not well standardized among labs. It appears that fructose, lactose, and sorbitol malabsorption appear to be equally prevalent in healthy volunteers [88]. Hereditary fructose intolerance, due to a deficiency in fructose-1, 6-bisphosphate aldolase, is rare and present in infancy. Thus, most fructose malabsorption may result from a diet high in fructose that overwhelms the absorptive capacity of the normal small intestine, or possibly small bowel bacterial overgrowth in which intestinal bacteria ferment fructose to produce hydrogen gas. It is not certain what is the average consumption of fructose in the daily American diet, but it is likely to be higher than the average 37 g consumed in 1977–78 as a result of the introduction of high fructose corn syrup as a widespread food additive over the past 30 years. It has been estimated that the consumption of high fructose corn syrup has increased more than 1000% in the 20 years spanning 1970–90 [103].

Despite the lack of difference in prevalence in carbohydrate malabsorption, IBS patients may report symptomatic improvement upon withdrawal of fructose, fructans, sorbitol, and lactose. When IBS patients who had fructose malabsorption identified by breath hydrogen testing were given dietary instruction to limit foods containing free fructose and short-chain fructans, reduce dietary fructose load, and to consume foods in which glucose was balanced with fructose, 85% of those adherent to the diet reported symptomatic improvement compared with only 36% who deviated from the diet [104].

13.5 CONCLUSIONS AND FUTURE RESEARCH

IBS is an extremely common GI condition for which there is increasing evidence for sex and gender differences, not only in prevalence, but also in clinical presentation, pathophysiology, and treatment response (Table 13.4). Although there exists a gender bias in diagnostic criteria and rates of general health care utilization, IBS appears to occur in females at about twice the rate of men. While rates of abdominal pain are similar, female IBS patients report more constipation, bloating, and extra-intestinal viscero- and somatosensory symptoms and pain disorders. Both IBS and non-IBS symptoms appear to be influenced by menstrual cycle, presumably through ovarian hormones affecting central and peripheral sensitization. Although there is some evidence that sex and gender differences in treatment response may exist, large clinical trials with sufficient numbers of men and women with IBS are needed to determine if these differences for a specific treatment truly exist.

The physiological basis for the above sex differences in this syndrome is still unclear. There is a growing amount of experimental data that suggest that females may have slower GI transit, exhibit a greater tendency to develop visceral hypersensitivity and postinfectious IBS, and have greater activation of limbic brain regions in response to visceral stimulation than males. Future well-designed studies incorporating sufficient numbers of both males and females with IBS will hopefully lead to a more comprehensive understanding of sex and gender differences in IBS. Other alternatives for treatment and dietary management of IBS, particularly in women, should continue to be explored.

REFERENCES

1. Chang, L. and Heitkemper, M.M. Gender differences in irritable bowel syndrome. *Gastroenterology*, 123, 1686, 2002.
2. Drossman, D.A. et al. AGA technical review on irritable bowel syndrome. *Gastroenterology*, 123, 2108, 2002.
3. Drossman, D., ed. *Rome III: The Functional Gastrointestinal Disorders, 3rd edn.* Degnon Associates, McLean, VA, p. 1048, 2006.

4. Sandler, R.S. et al. The burden of selected digestive diseases in the United States. *Gastroenterology*, 122, 1500, 2002.
5. Spiegel, B.M. et al. Clinical determinants of health-related quality of life in patients with irritable bowel syndrome. *Arch. Int. Med.*, 164, 1773, 2004.
6. Creed, F. et al. Health-related quality of life and health care costs in severe, refractory irritable bowel syndrome. *Ann. Int. Med.*, 134, 860, 2001.
7. Simren, M. et al. Health-related quality of life in patients attending a gastroenterology outpatient clinic: Functional disorders versus organic diseases. *Clin. Gastroenteol. Hep.*, 4, 187, 2006.
8. Drossman, D.A. et al. U.S. householder survey of functional gastrointestinal disorders. Prevalence, sociodemography, and health impact. *Dig. Dis. Sci.*, 38, 1569, 1993.
9. Schuster, M.M. Diagnostic evaluation of the irritable bowel syndrome. *Gastroenterol. Clin. North Am.*, 20, 269, 1991.
10. Lee, O.Y. et al. Gender-related differences in IBS symptoms. *J. Am. Gastroenterol.*, 96, 2184, 2001.
11. Thompson, W.G. Gender differences in irritable bowel symptoms. *Eur. J. Gastroenterol. Hep.*, 9, 299, 1997.
12. Saito, Y.A. et al. The effect of new diagnostic criteria for irritable bowel syndrome on community prevalence estimates. *Neurogastroenterol. Mot.*, 15, 687, 2003.
13. Taub, E. et al. Irritable bowel syndrome defined by factor analysis. Gender and race comparisons. *Dig. Dis. Sci.*, 40, 2647, 1995.
14. Talley, N.J., Boyce, P., and Jones, M. Identification of distinct upper and lower gastrointestinal symptom groupings in an urban population. *Gut*, 42, 690, 1998.
15. Corney, R.H. and Stanton, R. Physical symptom severity, psychological and social dysfunction in a series of outpatients with irritable bowel syndrome. *J. Psycho. Res.*, 34, 483, 1990.
16. Serra, J., Azpiroz, F., and Malagelada, J.R. Impaired transit and tolerance of intestinal gas in the irritable bowel syndrome. *Gut*, 48, 14, 2001.
17. Naliboff, B.D. et al. Evidence for two distinct perceptual alterations in irritable bowel syndrome. *Gut*, 41, 505, 1997.
18. Mertz, H. et al. Altered rectal perception is a biological marker of patients with irritable bowel syndrome. *Gastroenterology*, 109, 40, 1995.
19. Bouin, M. et al. Rectal distention testing in patients with irritable bowel syndrome: Sensitivity, specificity, and predictive values of pain sensory thresholds. *Gastroenterology*, 122, 1771, 2002.
20. Walker, E.A. et al. Chronic pelvic pain and gynecological symptoms in women with irritable bowel syndrome. *J. Psycho. Obst. Gyn.*, 17, 39, 1996.
21. Fass, R. et al. Sexual dysfunction in patients with irritable bowel syndrome and non-ulcer dyspepsia. *Digestion*, 59, 79, 1998.
22. Goldsmith, G. and Levin, J.S. Effect of sleep quality on symptoms of irritable bowel syndrome. *Dig. Dis. Sci.*, 38, 1809, 1993.
23. Jarrett, M. et al. Sleep disturbance influences gastrointestinal symptoms in women with irritable bowel syndrome. *Dig. Dis. Sci.*, 45, 952, 2000.
24. Heitkemper, M. et al. Subjective and objective sleep indices in women with irritable bowel syndrome. *Neurogastroenterol. Mot.*, 17, 523, 2005.
25. Whitehead, W.E., Palsson, O., and Jones, K.R. Systematic review of the comorbidity of irritable bowel syndrome with other disorders: What are the causes and implications? *Gastroenterology*, 122, 1140, 2002.
26. Farthing, M.J., Irritable bowel, irritable body, or irritable brain? *Brit. Med. J.*, 310, 171, 1995.

27. Guthrie, E., Creed, F.H., and Whorwell, P.J. Severe sexual dysfunction in women with the irritable bowel syndrome: Comparison with inflammatory bowel disease and duodenal ulceration. *Br. Med. J. (Clin. Res. Ed.)*, 295, 577, 1987.
28. Kalantar, J.S. et al. Familial aggregation of irritable bowel syndrome: A prospective study. *Gut*, 52, 1703, 2003.
29. Levy, R.L. et al. Irritable bowel syndrome in twins: Heredity and social learning both contribute to etiology. *Gastroenterology*, 121, 799, 2001.
30. Gwee, K.A. et al. The role of psychological and biological factors in postinfective gut dysfunction. *Gut*, 44, 400, 1999.
31. Gwee, K.A. et al. Psychometric scores and persistence of irritable bowel after infectious diarrhoea. *Lancet*, 347, 150, 1996.
32. Spiller, R. and Campbell, E. Post-infectious irritable bowel syndrome. *Curr. Opin. Gastroenterol.*, 22, 13, 2006.
33. Neal, K.R., Hebden, J., and Spiller, R. Prevalence of gastrointestinal symptoms six months after bacterial gastroenteritis and risk factors for development of the irritable bowel syndrome: Postal survey of patients. *Brit. Med. J.*, 314, 779, 1997.
34. Dunlop, S.P. et al. Relative importance of enterochromaffin cell hyperplasia, anxiety, and depression in postinfectious IBS. *Gastroenterology*, 125, 1651, 2003.
35. Spiller, R.C. et al. Increased rectal mucosal enteroendocrine cells, T lymphocytes, and increased gut permeability following acute Campylobacter enteritis and in post-dysenteric irritable bowel syndrome. *Gut*, 47, 804, 2000.
36. Chadwick, V.S. et al. Activation of the mucosal immune system in irritable bowel syndrome. *Gastroenterology*, 122, 1778, 2002.
37. Gwee, K.A. et al. Increased rectal mucosal expression of interleukin 1beta in recently acquired post-infectious irritable bowel syndrome. *Gut*, 52, 523, 2003.
38. O'Sullivan, M. et al. Increased mast cells in the irritable bowel syndrome. *Neurogastroenterol. Mot.*, 12, 449, 2000.
39. Drossman, D.A. Review article: An integrated approach to the irritable bowel syndrome. *Aliment. Pharm. Ther.*, 13 Suppl 2, 3, 1999.
40. Rao, S.S. et al. Ambulatory 24-h colonic manometry in healthy humans. *Am. J. Physiol. Gastrointest. Liver Physiol.*, 280, G629, 2001.
41. Ragnarsson, G., Hallbook, O., and Bodemar, G. Abdominal symptoms are not related to anorectal function in the irritable bowel syndrome. *Scand. J. Gastroenterol.*, 34, 250, 1999.
42. Chang, L. et al. Effect of sex on perception of rectosigmoid stimuli in irritable bowel syndrome. *Am. J. Physiol. Regul. Integr. Comp. Physio.*, 291, R277, 2006.
43. Mertz, H. et al. Regional cerebral activation in irritable bowel syndrome and control subjects with painful and nonpainful rectal distention. *Gastroenterology*, 118, 842, 2000.
44. Naliboff, B.D. et al. Cerebral activation in patients with irritable bowel syndrome and control subjects during rectosigmoid stimulation. *Psycho. Med.*, 63, 365, 2001.
45. Naliboff, B.D. et al. Sex-related differences in IBS patients: Central processing of visceral stimuli. *Gastroenterology*, 124, 1738, 2003.
46. Berman, S. et al. Gender differences in regional brain response to visceral pressure in IBS patients. *Eur. J. Pain*, 4, 157, 2000.
47. Heitkemper, M.M. et al. Daily gastrointestinal symptoms in women with and without a diagnosis of IBS. *Dig. Dis. Sci.*, 40, 1511, 1995.
48. Whitehead, W.E. et al. Evidence for exacerbation of irritable bowel syndrome during menses. *Gastroenterology*, 98, 1485, 1990.
49. Heitkemper, M.M. et al. Symptoms across the menstrual cycle in women with irritable bowel syndrome. *J. Am. Gastroenterol.*, 98, 420, 2003.

50. Houghton, L.A. et al. The menstrual cycle affects rectal sensitivity in patients with irritable bowel syndrome but not healthy volunteers. *Gut*, 50, 471, 2002.
51. Crowell, M.D. et al. Functional bowel disorders in women with dysmenorrhea. *J. Am. Gastrenterol.*, 89, 1973, 1994.
52. Toner, B.B. and Akman, D. Gender role and irritable bowel syndrome: Literature review and hypothesis. *J. Am. Gastroenterol.*, 95, 11, 2000.
53. Halpert, A. and Drossman, D., Gender and irritable bowel syndrome: The male connection. *J. Clin. Gastroenterol.*, 38, 546, 2004.
54. Jarrett, M.E. et al. Anxiety and depression are related to autonomic nervous system function in women with irritable bowel syndrome. *Dig. Dis. Sci.*, 48, 386, 2003.
55. Blanchard, E.B. et al. Gender differences in psychological distress among patients with irritable bowel syndrome. *J. Psycho. Res.*, 50, 271, 2001.
56. D'Eon, J.L., Harris, C.A., and Ellis, J.A. Testing factorial validity and gender invariance of the pain catastrophizing scale. *J. Behav. Med.*, 27, 361, 2004.
57. Khan, W.I. and Collins, S.M. Gut motor function: Immunological control in enteric infection and inflammation. *Clin. Exper. Immun.*, 143, 389, 2006.
58. Akiho, H. et al. Mechanisms underlying the maintenance of muscle hypercontractility in a model of postinfective gut dysfunction. *Gastroenterology*, 129, 131, 2005.
59. Dunlop, S.P., Jenkins, D., and Spiller, R.C. Distinctive clinical, psychological, and histological features of postinfective irritable bowel syndrome. *J. Am. Gastroenterol.*, 98, 1578, 2003.
60. Barbara, G. et al. Activated mast cells in proximity to colonic nerves correlate with abdominal pain in irritable bowel syndrome. *Gastroenterology*, 126, 693, 2004.
61. Bradesi, S. et al. Effect of ovarian hormones on intestinal mast cell reactivity to substance P. *Life Sci.*, 68, 1047, 2001.
62. Drossman, D.A. et al. Sexual and physical abuse in women with functional or organic gastrointestinal disorders. *Ann. Int. Med.*, 113, 828, 1990.
63. Myers, C.D., Riley, J.L. III, and Robinson, M.E. Psychosocial contributions to sex-correlated differences in pain. *Clin. J. Pain*, 19, 225, 2003.
64. Palsson, O.S. and Drossman, D.A. Psychiatric and psychological dysfunction in irritable bowel syndrome and the role of psychological treatments. *Gastroenterol. Clin. North Am.*, 34, 281, 2005.
65. Whitehead, W.E. et al. The usual medical care for irritable bowel syndrome. *Aliment. Pharm. Ther.*, 20, 1305, 2004.
66. Klein, K.B. Controlled treatment trials in the irritable bowel syndrome: A critique. *Gastroenterology*, 95, 232, 1988.
67. Kong, S.C. et al. The incidence of self-prescribed oral complementary and alternative medicine use by patients with gastrointestinal diseases. *J. Clin. Gastrenterol.*, 39, 138, 2005.
68. Camilleri, M. et al. Improvement in pain and bowel function in female irritable bowel patients with alosetron, a 5-HT3 receptor antagonist. *Aliment. Pharm. Ther.*, 13, 1149, 1999.
69. Viramontes, B.E. et al. Gender-related differences in slowing colonic transit by a 5-HT3 antagonist in subjects with diarrhea-predominant irritable bowel syndrome. *J. Am. Gastroenterol.*, 96, 2671, 2001.
70. Chang, L. et al. A dose-ranging, phase II study of the efficacy and safety of alosetron in men with diarrhea-predominant IBS. *J. Am. Gastroenterol.*, 100, 115, 2005.
71. Muller-Lissner, S.A. et al. Tegaserod, a 5-HT(4) receptor partial agonist, relieves symptoms in irritable bowel syndrome patients with abdominal pain, bloating and constipation. *Aliment. Pharm. Ther.*, 15, 1655, 2001.

72. Johanson, J.F. et al. Effect of tegaserod in chronic constipation: A randomized, double-blind, controlled trial. *Clin. Gastroenterol. Hep.*, 2, 796, 2004.
73. Eisenberg, D.M. et al. Trends in alternative medicine use in the United States, 1990–1997: Results of a follow-up national survey. *J. Am. Med. Assoc.*, 280, 1569, 1998.
74. Lackner, J.M. and Gurtman, M.B. Patterns of interpersonal problems in irritable bowel syndrome patients: A circumplex analysis. *J. Psycho. Res.*, 58, 523, 2005.
75. Koloski, N.A., Boyce, P.M., and Talley, N.J. Is health care seeking for irritable bowel syndrome and functional dyspepsia a socially learned response to illness? *Dig. Dis. Sci.*, 50, 153, 2005.
76. Gonsalkorale, W.M., Houghton, L.A., and Whorwell, P.J. Hypnotherapy in irritable bowel syndrome: A large-scale audit of a clinical service with examination of factors influencing responsiveness. *J. Am. Gastroenterol.*, 97, 954, 2002.
77. Bensoussan, A. et al. Treatment of irritable bowel syndrome with Chinese herbal medicine: A randomized controlled trial. *J. Am. Med. Assoc.*, 280, 1585, 1998.
78. Madisch, A. et al. Treatment of irritable bowel syndrome with herbal preparations: Results of a double-blind, randomized, placebo-controlled, multi-centre trial. *Aliment. Pharm. Ther.*, 19, 271, 2004.
79. Simmen, U. et al. Binding of STW 5 (Iberogast)® and its components to intestinal 5-HT, muscarinic M_3, and opioid receptors. *Phytomedicine*, 13 (Suppl 1), 51, 2006.
80. Pittler, M.H. and Ernst, E. Peppermint oil for irritable bowel syndrome: A critical review and metaanalysis. *J. Am. Gastroenterol.*, 93, 1131, 1998.
81. Lu, W.Z. et al. Melatonin improves bowel symptoms in female patients with irritable bowel syndrome: A double-blind placebo-controlled study. *Aliment. Pharm. Ther.*, 22, 927, 2005.
82. Pimentel, M., Chow, E.J., and Lin, H.C. Eradication of small intestinal bacterial overgrowth reduces symptoms of irritable bowel syndrome. *J. Am. Gastroenterol.*, 95, 3503, 2000.
83. Pimentel, M. et al. The effect of a nonabsorbed oral antibiotic (rifaximin) on the symptoms of the irritable bowel syndrome: A randomized trial. *Ann. Intl. Med.*, 145, 557, 2006.
84. Drossman, D.A. Treatment for bacterial overgrowth in the irritable bowel syndrome. *Ann. Int. Med.*, 145, 626, 2006.
85. Camilleri, M. Is there a role for probiotics in irritable bowel syndrome? *Dig. Liver Dis.*, 38 (Suppl 2), S266, 2006.
86. Friedman, G. Diet and the irritable bowel syndrome. *Gastroenterol. Clin. North Am.*, 20, 313, 1991.
87. Serra, J. et al. Lipid-induced intestinal gas retention in irritable bowel syndrome. *Gastroenterology*, 123, 700, 2002.
88. Lea, R. and Whorwell, P.J. The role of food intolerance in irritable bowel syndrome. *Gastroenterol. Clin. North Am.*, 34, 247, 2005.
89. Floch, M.H. and Narayan, R. Diet in the irritable bowel syndrome. *J. Clin. Gastroenterol.*, 35, S45, 2002.
90. Rao, S.S. et al. Is coffee a colonic stimulant? *Eur. J. Gastroenterol. Hep.*, 10, 113, 1998.
91. Francis, C.Y. and Whorwell, P.J. Bran and irritable bowel syndrome: Time for reappraisal. *Lancet*, 344, 39, 1994.
92. Dainese, R. et al. Discrepancies between reported food intolerance and sensitization test findings in irritable bowel syndrome patients. *J. Am. Gastroenterol.*, 94, 1892, 1999.
93. Sicherer, S.H. and Sampson, H.A. Food Allergy. *J. Allergy Clin. Immun.*, 117, S470, 2006.
94. Barbara, G. et al. Mast cell-dependent excitation of visceral-nociceptive sensory neurons in irritable bowel syndrome. *Gastroenterology*, 132, 26, 2007.

95. Barbara, G. et al. Functional gastrointestinal disorders and mast cells: Implications for therapy. *Neurogastroenterol. Mot.*, 18, 6, 2006.
96. Sampson, H.A. Update on food allergy. *J. Allergy Clin. Immun.*, 113, 805, 2004.
97. Wahnschaffe, U. et al. Celiac disease-like abnormalities in a subgroup of patients with irritable bowel syndrome. *Gastroenterology*, 121, 1329, 2001.
98. Zar, S., Benson, M.J., and Kumar, D., Food-specific serum IgG4 and IgE titers to common food antigens in irritable bowel syndrome. *J. Am. Gastroenterol.*, 100, 1550, 2005.
99. Zar, S. et al. Food-specific IgG4 antibody-guided exclusion diet improves symptoms and rectal compliance in irritable bowel syndrome. *Scand. J. Gastroenterol.*, 40, 800, 2005.
100. Jones, V.A. et al. Food intolerance: A major factor in the pathogenesis of irritable bowel syndrome. *Lancet*, 2, 1115, 1982.
101. Niec, A.M., Frankum, B., and Talley, N.J. Are adverse food reactions linked to irritable bowel syndrome? *J. Am. Gastroenterol.*, 93, 2184, 1998.
102. Gibson, P.R. et al. Review article: Fructose malabsorption and the bigger picture. *Aliment. Pharm. Ther.*, 25, 349, 2007.
103. Bray, G.A., Nielsen, S.J., and Popkin, B.M. Consumption of high-fructose corn syrup in beverages may play a role in the epidemic of obesity. *Am. J. Clin. Nutr.*, 79, 537, 2004.
104. Shepherd, S.J. and Gibson, P.R. Fructose malabsorption and symptoms of irritable bowel syndrome: Guidelines for effective dietary management. *J. Am. Diet. Assoc.*, 106, 1631, 2006.

14 Eye Health

Jennifer Evans

CONTENTS

14.1 INTRODUCTION: EYE HEALTH IN CONTEXT

Over 161 million people are visually impaired in the world today, 37 million of whom are blind [1]. Visual impairment is not distributed equally: most people affected are older and they are more likely to be women. Over 90% of visually impaired people live in low or middle-income countries. Eye health is a pressing problem.

The eye has a complex structure (Figure 14.1). Light passes through the cornea and lens, reaches the retina, which then translates the image into signals which are transmitted to the brain via the optic nerve. A wide range of eye-specific and systemic illnesses can affect the eye, often causing visual loss. Fungal and bacterial infections after injury can cause corneal opacities; the lens often becomes cloudy with increasing age, both of which conditions block the passage of light into the eye. Inflammation of the uvea and retina can lead to loss of photoreceptors and optic nerve disease can arise, possibly due to response to pressure in the eye (glaucoma). The causes of these diseases can be congenital, infectious, or nutritional or they can occur as a consequence of aging.

The World Health Organization defines visual impairment as visual acuity in the better eye worse than 6/18 and blindness as visual acuity worse than 3/60 [2]. The prevalence of visual impairment and blindness varies considerably in different parts of the world [1]. The burden of visual loss is much higher in low-income countries. For example, the prevalence of blindness in people aged 50 years and above is ~9% in Africa compared to 0.4% in the United States and 0.5% in the European Union [1].

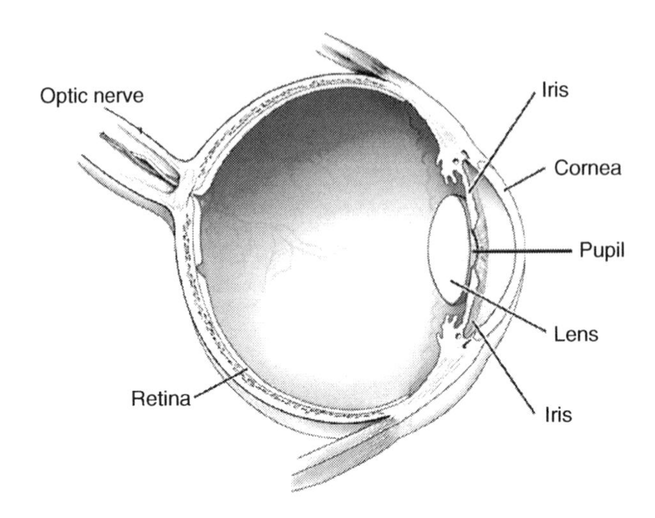

FIGURE 14.1 Structure of the eye. (From National Eye Institute, National Institutes of Health, www.nei.nih.gov/photo/, accessed March 19th 2007.)

Table 14.1 shows the main causes of visual loss worldwide. Cataract and infectious diseases predominate in low-income countries. In high-income countries, where infections are less common and there is better access to cataract surgery, age-related eye disease is more important. In some middle-income countries retinopathy of prematurity (ROP), which is retinal disease of premature babies, has been

TABLE 14.1
Causes of Visual Loss

Cause of Visual Loss		% Cause of Visual Impairment
Cataract	Lens becomes cloudy and light cannot pass through the lens onto the retina.	47.8
Glaucoma	Irreversible optic neuropathy	12.3
Age-related macular degeneration	Degeneration of the macula	8.7
Corneal opacities	Cornea becomes opaque due to fungal or bacterial infection, usually after injury	5.1
Diabetic retinopathy	Due to hyperglycemia in diabetes	4.8
Childhood blindness	Cataract, retinopathy of prematurity, vitamin A deficiency	3.9
Trachoma	Infection with *Chlamydia*	3.6
Others		13.8

Source: From Resnikoff, S., et al., *Bull World Health Organ*, 82, 844, 2004.

increasing [3]. Technology for keeping small babies alive has increased but corresponding skills in the prevention of blindness due to ROP have not kept pace with these developments. As populations in low and middle-income countries become older the burden of age-related eye disease will increase in those countries.

Sex plays an important role in determining the risk of blindness worldwide. In low- and middle-income countries, women are largely at increased risk of visual impairment and blindness due to poverty and limited access to good eye health-care. Poverty is associated with increased risk of malnutrition (e.g., vitamin deficiency in children leading to corneal opacity) and an increased risk of communicable disease (e.g., trachoma and onchocerciasis). Women are also more likely to have problems accessing cataract surgery, a safe, inexpensive, and very effective operation. Research in developing country settings therefore is often focused on the delivery of eye-care programs in resource poor settings. In contrast to developing countries, the main irreversible cause of visual loss in developed countries is age-related macular degeneration (AMD). This chapter focuses on AMD, the role of nutrition in modulating AMD, and highlights sex-specific responses to nutrition.

14.2 ETIOLOGY OF AMD

The retina is the light-sensitive layer at the back of the eye. It consists of photoreceptors which are light-sensitive cells that contain light-absorbing pigments, which change when they are hit by light. As a result of these changes an electric signal is sent to the brain via the optic nerve. The macula or the macula lutea ("yellow spot") is found at the centre of the retina. It is responsible for high acuity and central vision.

AMD is the degeneration of the macula in people aged 50 years and above with no obvious cause. It includes "geographic atrophy" and "neovascular disease." Geographic atrophy is a sharply demarcated area of partial or complete depigmentation reflecting atrophy of the retinal pigment epithelium. Neovascular AMD occurs when new vessels grow under the retinal pigment epithelium and occasionally into the subretinal space. Hemorrhage often results in increased scarring of the retina. In the early stages of the disease lipid material accumulates in deposits underneath the retinal pigment epithelium within Bruch's membrane. These deposits are known as drusen and can be seen as pale yellow spots on the retina. The pigment of the retinal pigment epithelium may become disturbed with areas of hyperpigmentation and hypopigmentation.

AMD is very common in older people in high-income countries. Pooled analysis of seven population-based studies in Europe, North America, and Australia estimated the overall prevalence of AMD in ages 40 years and above to be 1.47% (95% CI 1.38%–1.55%) [4]. The prevalence of neovascular disease (1.02%, 95% CI 0.93%–1.11%) was slightly higher than geographic atrophy (0.81%, 95% CI 0.77%–0.86%). Rates of AMD and large drusen increase with increasing age. People aged 80 years and above had a prevalence of AMD of 11.77% (95% CI 10.69%–12.85%). Figure 14.2 shows the prevalence of AMD in men and women by age using data from this pooled analysis. In the older age groups women had a higher prevalence of all types of AMD than men. This finding is replicated in many prevalence studies [5]. One problem with comparing the prevalence in men and women in older

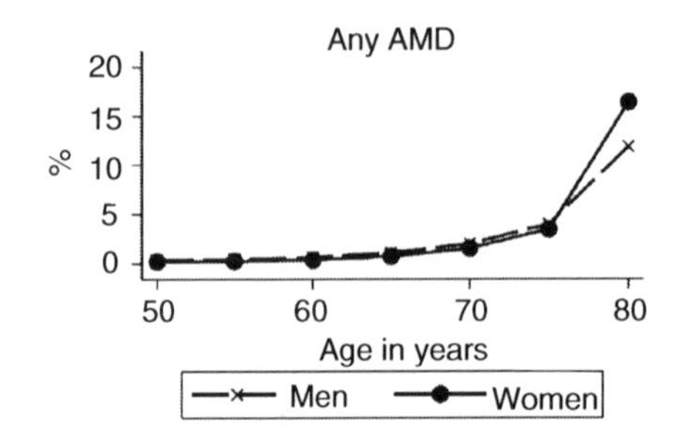

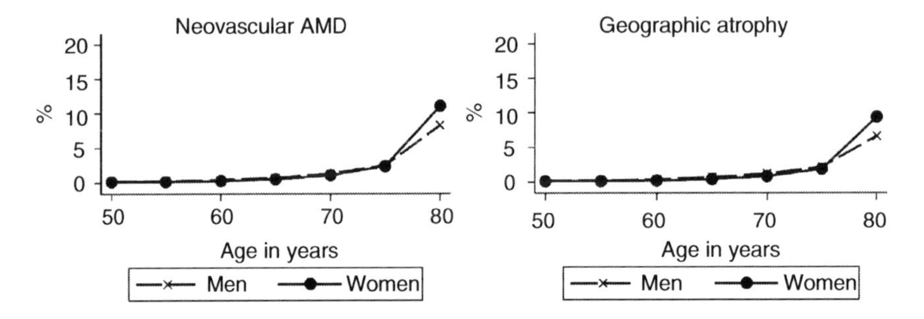

FIGURE 14.2 Prevalence of age-related macular degeneration (AMD) in men and women. Data for these graphs from pooled analysis of seven population-based studies in North America, Europe and Australia [4].

populations is that women tend to live longer and AMD is a strongly age-related disease. Careful examination of the prevalence rates from a wide range of studies suggests that much, if not all, of this increased risk can be attributed to the fact that women live longer. In the pooled analysis overall rates were similar between men and women after adjusting for age (age-adjusted odds ratio for men 1.01 95% CI 0.81–1.25).

Not all cases of AMD are associated with visual loss. The prevalence of visual impairment due to AMD is lower. Pooled data from six large population-based studies in Europe, North America, and Australia estimated the prevalence of visual loss caused by AMD to be 3.5% (95% CI 3.0%–4.1%) in people aged 75 years and above [6]. Sex differences were not statistically significant. This corresponds well with estimates from a large population-based survey in people aged 75 years and above in the UK which found a prevalence of visual impairment due to AMD of 3.7% (95% CI 3.2%–4.2%) [7]. However, this study did find an increased risk in women—age-adjusted odds ratio 1.44 (95% CI 1.22–1.69).

Follow-up of a large population-based study showed that one in four people aged 75 years and above can expect to develop early signs of the disease (e.g., drusen/pigmentary abnormalities) over 15 years and 1 in 12 people aged 75 years and above are likely to develop AMD [8]. This estimate allows for the competing risk of death and gives the probability of developing AMD over 15 years, or before death, whichever comes first. Women in the oldest age group had a significantly higher cumulative incidence of AMD than men.

There are strong genetic determinants of AMD [9]. People with an affected sibling are nearly 20 times as likely to develop AMD. It is likely that multiple genes interacting with environmental factors, such as smoking, are involved. One of the most likely candidate genes is complement factor H gene (CFH) on Chromosome 1. A common polymorphism Y402H in the CFH gene is a major risk factor for AMD [10]. It is estimated that over 50% of people with AMD may have the condition because of this polymorphism [11]. CFH helps to regulate the body's response to inflammation by protecting against uncontrolled complement activation. Inflammation has been implicated in the pathophysiology of AMD [12–15], however, not all studies have found a relationship [16]. There is no evidence for a sex-linked inheritance of AMD. Much research interest is currently focused on the genetic risk factors for AMD, in particular how the genetic factors might interact with environmental factors such as exposure to tobacco smoke. There are two main theories for the development of AMD. Firstly, that it arises due to vascular abnormalities in the choroidal circulation. Secondly, that it arises due to excess oxidative stress in the retina.

14.2.1 Vascular Disease

One of the main hypotheses for the development of AMD is that it is a vascular disease. It is possible that pathogenesis occurs due to problems with the choroidal circulation leading to hypoxia with growth of new vessels (neovascular AMD) and loss of photoreceptors (geographic atrophy). Much research has therefore been focused on risk factors for cardiovascular disease.

There is a well-known socioeconomic gradient in risk of cardiovascular disease. People with lower income and education are at greater risk of the disease [17]. However, this pattern has not been replicated in epidemiological studies of AMD. A number of studies have suggested that increasing years of education are associated with a decreased risk of AMD and early signs of the disease such as drusen [18–20]. However, strong trends were not observed in these studies and several studies have found no association [21,22]. It is unlikely that socioeconomic status is an important factor determining the distribution of AMD in the population.

Cigarette smoking is a well-established risk factor for cardiovascular disease. It is known to increase fibrinogen levels and platelet activity leading to vascular disease as well as increasing levels of oxidative stress in the body. It appears that smoking also plays an important role in AMD [23–27]. Current smokers have a two- to threefold increased risk of developing AMD [28,29] and there is a dose–response relationship with pack-years of smoking [30]. Tobacco smoking is the main modifiable risk for AMD. Public health interventions to help people stop smoking will play an important role in reducing the incidence of AMD in the population [31]. Risks of smoking in men and women appear to be similar [25,26]. The prevalence of smoking in men has decreased, however younger groups of women are smoking more [32]. It may be that cases of AMD in women will increase disproportionately over the next few decades.

Heavy alcohol consumption is an important risk factor for heart disease and moderate consumption is thought to be protective. The results of studies on AMD and heavy alcohol consumption are inconsistent. Analysis of the National Health and Nutrition Survey suggested that moderate wine consumption might be protective [33] as did the Andhra Pradesh Eye Disease Study in South India [34]. Follow-up of the Copenhagen Eye Study found alcohol consumption greater than 250 g/week to be associated with increased odds of early AMD [35]. The Beaver Dam Eye Study found that beer drinking was associated with the development of retinal drusen and neovascular AMD [36,37] and that heavy alcohol consumption of four or more drinks a day was associated with an increased risk of developing neovascular AMD [27]. However, in general, observed associations have been weak and many studies have found little evidence of an association [18,38–42].

Measures of obesity such as body mass index (BMI), waist circumference, and waist–hip ratio have been measured in a number of studies. In general, reported findings suggest an increased risk of AMD with increasing BMI and abdominal obesity [18,43,44]. However, results have been inconsistent. In the Age-Related Eye Disease Study (AREDS), high BMI was associated with neovascular disease at baseline [19] but prospectively with geographic atrophy [45]. Two studies have found evidence of a J-shaped curve with people with low BMI at risk of AMD [46,47]. Inconsistent findings have been seen for men and women. In the Beaver Dam Eye Study, BMI and waist–hip ratio were associated with early AMD in women but not men [48] in contrast to a Finnish study which found high BMI associated with AMD in men and not women [49].

Cardiovascular disease itself is not consistently related to AMD. People with AMD may be at increased risk of coronary heart disease [50], stroke [51], and cardiovascular mortality [52]. However, findings have been inconsistent: some studies have found no association between history of cardiovascular disease and AMD [53,54]. Hypertension may increase the risk of AMD due to its effects on the choroidal circulation [55]. Raised blood pressure has been associated with AMD in some [19,53,56,57] but not all [54,58,59] studies. There is no evidence that anti-hypertensive medication or treatments to lower blood pressure can prevent the development or progression of the disease.

The vascular disease hypothesis for the development of AMD has led to the hypothesis that exposure to estrogen (either endogenous or exogenous) might lead to a reduced risk of AMD in women. There have been a number of cross-sectional [60–66], prospective [67], and case-control studies [18,19,68]. Markers of exposure to estrogen in women, such as age at menarche and menopause, and use of hormone replacement therapy have not been consistently associated with AMD in these studies. However, lifetime exposure to estrogen in these studies is usually measured using rather crude retrospective data collection. It may be that exposure to estrogen during the reproductive ages is more important than postmenopausally when levels of estrogen in men and women become more similar.

Observational studies provide weaker evidence compared to randomized controlled trials in this area as women who choose to take hormone replacement therapy are different to those who do not [69]. There is one randomized controlled trial, the Women's Health Initiative Study, in which hormone therapy and AMD were assessed [70]. Women were randomized to conjugated equine estrogens (CEE), CEE with progestin (CEE + P), or to placebo. Over 4000 women aged 65 years and above in this trial were evaluated for the presence of AMD after an average of 5 years treatment. Overall, there was no association between estrogen supplementation and development of AMD. The group treated with CEE + P had a reduced risk of one early sign (soft drusen) and neovascular disease, however, the study was underpowered to evaluate these associations and the authors were unable to make a definitive statement regarding these effects.

14.2.2 Oxidative Stress

Oxidation refers to the process by which electrons are removed from atoms. This process is a vital part of the means by which animals release energy from dietary carbohydrates. As part of these chemical reactions, reactive oxygen species (ROS) are formed. These are highly reactive molecules and comprise free radicals, hydrogen peroxide, and singlet oxygen. Free radicals contain one or more unpaired electrons in their outer orbits. The production of ROS is increased by irradiation, inflammation, air pollution, and cigarette smoke. Many diseases increase with increasing age, in particular cardiovascular and neurodegenerative diseases. The "free-radical" theory of aging proposes that these age-related degenerative diseases occur because of cumulative exposure to harmful effects of oxygen radicals [71]. It is thought that the degree of oxidative stress is determined by the balance between ROS and antioxidant defenses. The retina is an ideal environment for the generation of ROS because the retina is exposed to high levels of oxygen and high levels of irradiation. As well, the outer segment of the photoreceptor membrane is rich in polyunsaturated fatty acids which can be readily oxidized. Thus considerable interest has focused on the role of antioxidant nutrients (i.e., carotenoids, vitamins C and E, and zinc) in protection against AMD.

14.3 NUTRITIONAL INFLUENCES ON DEVELOPMENT OF AMD

14.3.1 Antioxidant Nutrients

As a result of the oxidative stress hypothesis for the development of AMD, considerable interest has focused on whether foods high in antioxidant nutrients may be protective for the development of AMD. Carotenoids (in particular β-carotene, lutein, and zeaxanthin), vitamins C and E, and zinc are all common in the diet and have antioxidant properties.

A number of studies have investigated the relationship between dietary intake [72–84,111] or serum levels [85–90] of antioxidant nutrients and risk of AMD. Inconsistent results have been found. Few of the studies have compared the effect of dietary intake in men and women separately. This is probably due to sample size considerations or lack of a specific hypothesis that effects may be different in men and women. It is also possible that the sexes have been compared and in the absence of any difference in effect, sex-specific results have not been reported. The exception to this was the follow-up study of women in the Nurses Health Study and men in the Health Professionals Follow-up study [82]. In these studies, fruit and vegetable intake was assessed in over 77,000 women and nearly 41,000 men. The women were followed up for 18 years and the men for 12 years. Fruit intake was found to be protective for neovascular AMD. People who ate three or more servings a day had a reduced risk of developing AMD (relative risk 0.64, 95% CI 0.44–0.93). The results were found to be similar in men and women.

Difficulties with interpreting these studies include the fact that people with diets high in antioxidants are different in many ways from people with diets low in antioxidants [91]. In this area, randomized controlled trials, whereby antioxidant intake is randomly allocated, provide the strongest evidence. There are two regularly updated systematic reviews of controlled trials in this area [92,93]. Although eight trials have been published, the majority of participants have been randomized in one trial—the Age-Related Eye Disease Study (AREDS) [94]. This randomized controlled trial was a large multicentered study based in the United States. Three thousand six hundred and forty study participants aged 55–80 years were followed up for an average of 6 years. They were randomly assigned to receive daily oral tablets containing: (1) antioxidants (vitamin C 500 mg, vitamin 400 IU, and β-carotene 15 mg), (2) zinc 80 mg (zinc oxide and copper 2 mg), (3) antioxidants plus zinc, or (4) placebo. People taking antioxidants or antioxidants plus zinc had a reduced risk of developing advanced AMD compared with people taking placebo (odds ratio 0.72, 99% CI 0.52–0.98). However, this effect was confined to people with signs of AMD (drusen and pigmentary abnormalities). There is not enough evidence to recommend antioxidant supplementation for people in the general population who do not have signs of the disease [95]. Although AREDS was a large study, it did not report any assessment of effect in men and women separately. Fifty-six percent of participants were women.

Although generally regarded as safe, antioxidant supplements may have adverse effects. Two large randomized controlled trials have shown that smokers who take β-carotene may be at increased risk of lung cancer [95,96]. The Heart Outcomes Prevention Evaluation (HOPE) Study found that vitamin E supplementation in people with diabetes or vascular disease increased the risk of heart failure [97]. A recent systematic review identified that regular supplementation with vitamin A, β-carotene, or vitamin E results in a small increased risk of mortality [98]. Taking antioxidant supplements to prevent or slow down the progression of AMD must therefore be considered on an individual basis in both men and women with a clear understanding of the possible benefits and adverse effects of taking supplements.

The macular pigment is composed of two plant-derived carotenoids, lutein and its stereo isomer zeaxanthin. These carotenoids protect the retina by absorbing blue light. They are powerful antioxidants and absorb harmful free radicals generated during light absorption [99]. Levels of macular pigment are influenced by dietary intake of these carotenoids [100,101] which are found in a wide variety of vegetables, in particular green leafy plants such as spinach and kale and in some animal products such as egg yolks [102].

Decreased serum, dietary and retinal levels of these carotenoids have been associated with an increased risk of ARM and AMD in some [72,73,78,81, 85,103–106] but not all observational studies [74,75,79,82,83,87,107]. One small trial showed some benefit of lutein supplementation in people with AMD [108].

Again, the literature has been given little consideration to the possible different effects in men and women.

Currently, there is not enough evidence to recommend lutein and zeaxanthin supplements to prevent or slow down the progression of AMD. A diet rich in fruit and vegetables will have many health benefits, will do no harm, and may reduce the risk of developing AMD. Eating a wide range of vegetables, particularly leafy green vegetables, will improve the levels of macular pigment in the eye and will have other health benefits.

The Age-Related Eye Disease Study 2 (AREDS 2) is currently recruiting 4000 participants in a 5 year controlled trial of supplementation with lutein and zeaxanthin [109]. It would be inadvisable to take supplements of lutein and zeaxanthin before the results of this study become available.

14.3.2 Polyunsaturated Fatty Acids

There are two groups of polyunsaturated fatty acids: n-3 fatty acids and n-6 fatty acids. The retina contains high levels of n-3 fatty acid docosahexaenoic acid (DHA), particularly in the disc membranes of the photoreceptors. The function of DHA in these cells is not clear but it may have a structural effect on the cell membrane. The n-3 fatty acid eicosapentaenoic acid (EPA) has beneficial effects on inflammation which is also implicated in the pathogenesis of AMD.

It is theoretically possible that a reduction in dietary intake of DHA could lead to adverse effects on the photoreceptors so considerable interest has focused on the role of dietary sources of DHA and EPA on the risk for developing AMD. Animal studies have consistently demonstrated that diets poor in DHA lead to visual impairment [110].

One of the largest prospective studies has been the follow-up of the Nurses Health Study and Health Professionals study [111]. Fat intake was assessed by a food frequency questionnaire and participants were followed up for the development of AMD. Total fat intake, particularly linolenic acid, an n-3 fatty acid, was positively associated with risk of AMD (top vs. bottom quintile of relative risk 1.49, 95% CI 1.15–1.94). DHA had a modest inverse relationship with AMD (top vs. bottom quintile 0.70, 95% CI 0.52–0.93). Greater than four servings of fish a week were associated with a 35% reduction in risk of AMD compared with three or less servings a month. Different patterns of risk between men and women were seen in this study, however, as these differences were not statistically significant, only pooled results were reported. For example, the adjusted relative risk of top vs. bottom quintile in total fat intake was 1.61 in women and 1.42 in men, for cholesterol it was 0.98 in women and 1.37 in men, for saturated fat it was 1.53 in women and 1.14 in men, and for polyunsaturated fats it was 1.19 in women and 1.02 in men. These differences are intriguing and indicate that the effects of food components in men and women may be different. However, currently due to low study power these differences cannot be distinguished reliably from random variation.

Currently, evidence for a role of n-3 fatty acids in the pathogenesis of AMD is inconclusive [112]. There are no randomized controlled trials in this area and only six observational studies with inconsistent results. Clear recommendations as to the possible benefits of supplementation with n-3 fatty acid cannot currently be made. The AREDS2 trial (see Section 14.3.1 above) is investigating supplementation with n-3 fatty acids (DHA and EPA) [109]. Including oily fish in the diet is currently advised for other health reasons and may reduce the risk of developing AMD in both men and women.

14.4 CONCLUSIONS

Blindness and visual impairment are common worldwide, and women are at an increased risk due to poverty and lack of access to eye health care services. Age-related eye disease in low- and middle-income countries is likely to become more of a problem as populations age.

In high-income countries, more women are likely to experience age-related conditions such as AMD. Current research points to the fact that this increased risk is associated with the increased longevity of women. However, temporal changes in smoking and nutrition mean that changes in population risk may change over time.

It is possible that specific food components, in particular antioxidant nutrients, zinc, and n-3 fatty acids, modify the disease process leading to AMD in men and women. There is some evidence that fruit and vegetable intake and oily fish in the diet may be protective for the disease. Although the evidence cannot be considered conclusive, given the other health benefits of a diet rich in fruit and vegetables and containing some oily fish, such diets can be recommended. Multivitamin supplementation with β-carotene, vitamins C and E, and zinc slowed down the progression of AMD in people with signs of the disease in one large trial. However, harm from taking supplements cannot be ruled out and given the lack of evidence in the general population, multivitamin supplements cannot be recommended for the general population. However, they may be considered for people at risk of progression to advanced AMD and visual loss.

There is little conclusive evidence for a different response to food or food components in men and women with respect to the development of AMD. Current theories for the development of the disease, for example, a vascular disease hypothesis, suggest that different responses in men and women may exist. For example, hormonal factors in women, including lifetime exposure to estrogen, are very different.

14.5 FUTURE RESEARCH

It is surprising that so little sex-specific research has been reported on nutrition and eye health. There is an extensive literature on risk factors for AMD, but very few studies have used a sex-based approach to study design and interpretation of findings. Future research needs to evaluate the role of different risk factors in men and women separately. In order to do that, predefined hypotheses have to be tested in studies with sufficient sample size. In order for an unbiased picture to emerge, it is important that studies with negative findings, that is, those that find similar effects in men and women, are reported consistently in the literature.

AMD occurs towards the end of a lifetime. Current assessment of nutrition has focused on postmenopausal women, aged 50 years and above, as that is the age after which an increased risk of AMD is observed. However, it may be that nutritional exposures before that time are important. A life course approach to the study of the epidemiology of age-related diseases such as AMD is being increasingly recognized.

REFERENCES

1. Resnikoff, S., et al., Global data on visual impairment in the year 2002, *Bull. World Health Organ.*, 82, 844, 2004.
2. World Health Organization, *International Statistical Classification of Diseases, Injuries and Causes of Death, Tenth Revision*, WHO, Geneva, 1993.
3. Gilbert, C., et al., Retinopathy of prematurity in middle-income countries, *Lancet*, 350, 12, 1997.
4. Friedman, D.S., et al., Prevalence of age-related macular degeneration in the United States, *Arch. Ophthalmol.*, 122, 564, 2004.
5. Evans, J.R., Risk factors for age-related macular degeneration, *Prog. Ret. Eye Res.*, 20, 227, 2001.
6. Owen, C.G., et al., How big is the burden of visual loss caused by age-related macular degeneration in the UK? *Br. J. Ophthalmol.*, 87, 312, 2003.
7. Evans, J.R., Fletcher, A.E., and Wormald, R.P.L., Age-related macular degeneration causing visual impairment in people aged 75 years and above in Britain, *Ophthalmology*, 111, 513, 2004.
8. Klein, R., et al., Fifteen-year cumulative incidence of age-related macular degeneration: the Beaver Dam Eye Study, *Ophthalmology*, 114, 253, 2007.
9. Haddad, S., et al., The genetics of age-related macular degeneration: a review of progress to date, *Surv. Ophthalmol.*, 51, 316, 2006.
10. Sepp, T., et al., Complement factor H variant Y402H is a major risk determinant for geographic atrophy and choroidal neovascularization in smokers and nonsmokers, *Invest. Ophthalmol. Vis. Sci.*, 47, 536, 2006.
11. Despriet, D.D.G., et al., Complement factor H polymorphism, complement activators, and risk of age-related macular degeneration, *JAMA*, 296, 301, 2006.
12. Donoso, L.A., et al., The role of inflammation in the pathogenesis of age-related macular degeneration, *Surv. Ophthalmol.*, 51, 137, 2006.
13. Seddon, J.M., et al., Association between C-reactive protein and age-related macular degeneration, *JAMA*, 291, 704, 2004.
14. Seddon, J.M., et al., Progression of age-related macular degeneration: prospective assessment of C-reactive protein, interleukin 6, and other cardiovascular biomarkers, *Arch. Ophthalmol.*, 123, 774, 2005.
15. Seddon, J.M., et al., C-reactive protein and homocysteine are associated with dietary and behavioral risk factors for age-related macular degeneration, *Nutrition*, 22, 441, 2006.
16. McGwin, G., et al., The relation between C reactive protein and age related macular degeneration in the Cardiovascular Health Study, *Br. J. Ophthalmol.*, 89, 1166, 2005.
17. Pollitt, R.A., Rose, K.M., and Kaufman, J.S., Evaluating the evidence for models of life course socioeconomic factors and cardiovascular outcomes: a systematic review, *BMC Public Health*, 5, 7, 2005.
18. Eye Disease Case-Control Study Group, Risk factors for neovascular age-related macular degeneration, *Arch. Ophthalmol.*, 110, 1701, 1992.

19. Age-Related Eye Disease Study Group, Risk factors associated with age-related macular degeneration: a case-control study in the age-related eye disease study: age-related eye disease study report number 3, *Ophthalmology*, 107, 2224, 2000.
20. Klein, R., et al., The relation of socioeconomic factors to the incidence of early age-related maculopathy: the Beaver Dam Eye Study, *Am. J. Ophthalmol.*, 132, 128, 2001.
21. Klein, R., et al., Age-related maculopathy in a multiracial United States population: The National Health and Nutrition Examination Survey III, *Ophthalmology*, 106, 1056, 1999.
22. Fraser-Bell, S., et al., Sociodemographic factors and age-related macular degeneration in Latinos: the Los Angeles Latino Eye Study, *Am. J. Ophthalmol.*, 139, 30, 2005.
23. Smith, W., et al., Risk factors for age-related macular degeneration: Pooled findings from three continents, *Ophthalmology*, 108, 697, 2001.
24. Mitchell, P., et al., Smoking and the 5-year incidence of age-related maculopathy: the Blue Mountains Eye Study, *Arch. Ophthalmol.*, 120, 1357, 2002.
25. Christen, W.G., et al., A prospective study of cigarette smoking and risk of age-related macular degeneration in men, *JAMA*, 276, 1147, 1996.
26. Seddon, J.M., et al., A prospective study of cigarette smoking and age-related macular degeneration in women, *JAMA*, 276, 1141, 1996.
27. Klein, R., et al., Ten-year incidence of age-related maculopathy and smoking and drinking: the Beaver Dam Eye Study, *Am. J. Epidemiol.*, 156, 589, 2002.
28. Thornton, J., et al., Smoking and age-related macular degeneration: a review of association, *Eye*, 19, 935, 2004.
29. Solberg, Y., Rosner, M., and Belkin, M., The association between cigarette smoking and ocular diseases, *Surv. Ophthalmol.*, 42, 535, 1998.
30. Khan, J.C., et al., Smoking and age related macular degeneration: the number of pack years of cigarette smoking is a major determinant of risk for both geographic atrophy and choroidal neovascularisation, *Br. J. Ophthalmol.*, 90, 75, 2006.
31. Kelly, S.P., et al., Smoking and blindness, *BMJ*, 328, 537, 2004.
32. Ernster, V., et al., Women and tobacco: moving from policy to action, *Bull. World Health Organ.*, 78, 891, 2000.
33. Obisesan, T.O., et al., Moderate wine consumption is associated with decreased odds of developing age-related macular degeneration in NHANES-1, *J. Am. Geriatr. Soc.*, 46, 1, 1998.
34. Krishnaiah, S., et al., Risk factors for age-related macular degeneration: findings from the Andhra Pradesh Eye Disease Study in South India, *Invest. Ophthalmol. Vis. Sci.*, 46, 4442, 2005.
35. Buch, H., et al., Risk factors for age-related maculopathy in a 14-year follow-up study: the Copenhagen City Eye Study, *Acta Ophthalmol. Scand.*, 83, 409, 2005.
36. Ritter, L.L., et al., Alcohol use and age-related maculopathy in the Beaver Dam Eye Study, *Am. J. Ophthalmol.*, 120, 190, 1995.
37. Moss, S.E., et al., Alcohol consumption and the 5-year incidence of age-related maculopathy: the Beaver Dam Eye Study, *Ophthalmology*, 105, 789, 1998.
38. McCarty, C.A., et al., Risk factors for age-related maculopathy: the visual impairment project, *Arch. Ophthalmol.*, 119, 1455, 2001.
39. Smith, W. and Mitchell, P., Alcohol intake and age-related maculopathy, *Am. J. Ophthalmol.*, 122, 743, 1996.
40. Ajani, U.A., et al., A prospective study of alcohol consumption and the risk of age-related macular degeneration, *Ann. Epidemiol.*, 9, 172, 1999.
41. Cho, E., et al., Prospective study of alcohol consumption and the risk of age-related macular degeneration, *Arch. Ophthalmol.*, 118, 681, 2000.

42. Cruickshanks, K.J., et al., The prevalence of age-related maculopathy by geographic region and ethnicity. The Colorado-Wisconsin Study of Age-Related Maculopathy, *Arch. Ophthalmol.*, 115, 242, 1997.
43. Delcourt, C., et al., Associations of cardiovascular disease and its risk factors with age-related macular degeneration: the POLA study, *Ophthalmic Epidemiol.*, 8, 237, 2001.
44. Seddon, J.M., et al., Progression of age-related macular degeneration: association with body mass index, waist circumference, and waist–hip ratio, *Arch. Ophthalmol.*, 121, 785, 2003.
45. Age-Related Eye Disease Study Group, Risk factors for the incidence of advanced age-related macular degeneration in the Age-Related Eye Disease Study (AREDS): AREDS report no. 19, *Ophthalmology*, 112, 533, 2005.
46. Schaumberg, D.A., et al., Body mass index and the incidence of visually significant age-related maculopathy in men, *Arch. Ophthalmol.*, 119, 1259, 2001.
47. Smith, W., et al., Plasma fibrinogen levels, other cardiovascular risk factors, and age-related maculopathy: the Blue Mountains Eye Study, *Arch. Ophthalmol.*, 116, 583, 1998.
48. Klein, B.E., et al., Measures of obesity and age-related eye diseases, *Ophthalmic Epidemiol.*, 8, 251, 2001.
49. Hirvela, H., et al., Risk factors of age-related maculopathy in a population 70 years of age or older, *Ophthalmology*, 103, 871, 1996.
50. Wong, T.Y., et al., Age-related macular degeneration and risk of coronary heart disease: the atherosclerosis risk in communities study, *Ophthalmology*, 114, 86, 2007.
51. Wong, T.Y., et al., Age-related macular degeneration and risk for stroke, *Ann. Intern. Med.*, 145, 98, 2006.
52. Age-Related Eye Disease Study Group, Associations of mortality with ocular disorders and an intervention of high-dose antioxidants and zinc in the Age-Related Eye Disease Study: AREDS report no. 13, *Arch. Ophthalmol.*, 122, 716, 2004.
53. Klein, R., et al., The association of cardiovascular disease with the long-term incidence of age-related maculopathy: the Beaver Dam Eye Study, *Ophthalmology*, 110, 636, 2003.
54. Klein, R., Klein, B.E., and Franke, T., The relationship of cardiovascular disease and its risk factors to age-related maculopathy. The Beaver Dam Eye Study, *Ophthalmology*, 100, 406, 1993.
55. Wong, T. and Mitchell, P., The eye in hypertension, *Lancet*, 369, 425, 2007.
56. Hyman, L., et al., Hypertension, cardiovascular disease, and age-related macular degeneration, *Arch. Ophthalmol.*, 118, 351, 2000.
57. van Leeuwen, R., et al., Blood pressure, atherosclerosis, and the incidence of age-related maculopathy: the Rotterdam Study, *Invest. Ophthalmol. Vis. Sci.*, 44, 3771, 2003.
58. Miyazaki, M., et al., Risk factors for age related maculopathy in a Japanese population: the Hisayama study, *Br. J. Ophthalmol.*, 87, 469, 2003.
59. Klein, R., et al., Early age-related maculopathy in the cardiovascular health study, *Ophthalmology*, 110, 25, 2003.
60. Smith, W., Mitchell, P., and Wang, J.J., Gender, oestrogen, hormone replacement and age-related macular degeneration: results from the Blue Mountains Eye Study, *Aust. N. Z. J. Ophthalmol.*, 25, S13, 1997.
61. Snow, K.K., et al., Association between reproductive and hormonal factors and age-related maculopathy in postmenopausal women, *Am. J. Ophthalmol.*, 134, 842, 2002.
62. Defay, R., et al., Sex steroids and age-related macular degeneration in older French women: the POLA study, *Ann. Epidemiol.*, 14, 202, 2004.

63. Nirmalan, P.K., et al., Female reproductive factors and eye disease in a rural South Indian population: The Aravind Comprehensive Eye Survey, *Invest. Ophthalmol. Vis. Sci.*, 45, 4273, 2004.
64. Abramov, Y., et al., The effect of hormone therapy on the risk for age-related maculopathy in postmenopausal women, *Menopause*, 11, 62, 2004.
65. Freeman, E.E., Bressler, S.B., and West, S.K., Hormone replacement therapy, reproductive factors, and age-related macular degeneration: the Salisbury Eye Evaluation Project, *Ophthalmic Epidemiol.*, 12, 37, 2005.
66. Fraser-Bell, S., et al., Smoking, alcohol intake, estrogen use, and age-related macular degeneration in Latinos: the Los Angeles Latino Eye Study, *Am. J. Ophthalmol.*, 141, 79, 2006.
67. Klein, B.E., Klein, R., and Lee, K.E., Reproductive exposures, incident age-related cataracts, and age-related maculopathy in women: the Beaver Dam Eye Study, *Am. J. Ophthalmol.*, 130, 322, 2000.
68. Vingerling, J.R., et al., Macular degeneration and early menopause: a case-control study, *BMJ*, 310, 1570, 1995.
69. Matthews, K.A., et al., Prior to use of estrogen replacement therapy, are users healthier than nonusers? *Am. J. Epidemiol.*, 143, 971, 1996.
70. Haan, M.N., et al., Hormone therapy and age-related macular degeneration: the Women's Health Initiative Sight Exam Study, *Arch. Ophthalmol.*, 124, 988, 2006.
71. Finkel, T. and Holbrook, N.J., Oxidants, oxidative stress and the biology of ageing, *Nature*, 408, 239, 2000.
72. Goldberg, J., et al., Factors associated with age-related macular degeneration: an analysis of data from the First National Health and Nutrition Examination Survey, *Am. J. Epidemiol.*, 128, 700, 1988.
73. Seddon, J.M., et al., Dietary carotenoids, vitamins A, C, and E, and advanced age-related macular degeneration. Eye Disease Case-Control Study Group, *JAMA*, 272, 1413, 1994.
74. Mares-Perlman, J.A., et al., Association of zinc and antioxidant nutrients with age-related maculopathy, *Arch. Ophthalmol.*, 114, 991, 1996.
75. VandenLangenberg, G.M., et al., Associations between antioxidant and zinc intake and the 5-year incidence of early age-related maculopathy in the Beaver Dam Eye Study, *Am. J. Epidemiol.*, 148, 204, 1998.
76. Christen, W.G., et al., Prospective cohort study of antioxidant vitamin supplement use and the risk of age-related maculopathy, *Am. J. Epidemiol.*, 149, 476, 1999.
77. Smith, W., et al., Dietary antioxidants and age-related maculopathy: the Blue Mountains Eye Study, *Ophthalmology*, 106, 761, 1999.
78. Mares-Perlman, J.A., et al., Lutein and zeaxanthin in the diet and serum and their relation to age-related maculopathy in the third National Health and Nutrition Examination Survey, *Am. J. Epidemiol.*, 153(5), 424, 2001.
79. Flood, V., et al., Dietary antioxidant intake and incidence of early age-related maculopathy: the Blue Mountains Eye Study, *Ophthalmology*, 109, 2272, 2002.
80. Kuzniarz, M., et al., Use of vitamin and zinc supplements and age-related maculopathy: the Blue Mountains Eye Study, *Ophthalmic Epidemiol.*, 9, 283, 2002.
81. Snellen, E.L.M., et al., Neovascular age-related macular degeneration and its relationship to antioxidant intake, *Acta Ophthalmol. Scand.*, 80, 368, 2002.
82. Cho, E., et al., Prospective study of intake of fruits, vegetables, vitamins, and carotenoids and risk of age-related maculopathy, *Arch. Ophthalmol.*, 122, 883, 2004.
83. van Leeuwen, R., et al., Dietary intake of antioxidants and risk of age-related macular degeneration, *JAMA*, 294, 3101, 2005.

84. Moeller, S.M., et al., Associations between intermediate age-related macular degeneration and lutein and zeaxanthin in the Carotenoids in Age-Related Eye Disease Study (CAREDS): ancillary study of the Women's Health Intitiative, *Arch. Ophthalmol.*, 124, 1151, 2006.
85. Eye Disease Case-Control Study Group, Antioxidant status and neovascular age-related macular degeneration, *Arch. Ophthalmol.*, 111, 104, 1993.
86. West, S., et al., Are antioxidants or supplements protective for age-related macular degeneration? *Arch. Ophthalmol.*, 112, 222, 1994.
87. Mares-Perlman, J.A., et al., Serum antioxidants and age-related macular degeneration in a population-based case-control study, *Arch. Ophthalmol.*, 113, 1518, 1995.
88. Delcourt, C., et al., Age-related macular degeneration and antioxidant status in the POLA study. POLA Study Group. Pathologies Oculaires Liees a l'Age, *Arch. Ophthalmol.*, 117, 1384, 1999.
89. Simonelli, F., et al., Serum oxidative and antioxidant parameters in a group of Italian patients with age-related maculopathy, *Clin. Chim. Acta*, 320, 111, 2002.
90. Dasch, B., et al., Serum levels of macular carotenoids in relation to age-related maculopathy: the Muenster Aging and Retina Study (MARS), *Graefes Arch. Clin. Exp. Ophthalmol.*, 243, 1028, 2005.
91. Lyle, B.J., et al., Supplement users differ from nonusers in demographic, lifestyle, dietary and health characteristics, J. *Nutr.*, 128, 2355, 1998.
92. Evans, J.R. and Henshaw, K., Antioxidant vitamin and mineral supplementation for preventing age-related macular degeneration, *Cochrane Database Syst. Rev.*, CD000253, 2000.
93. Evans, J.R., Antioxidant vitamin and mineral supplements for slowing the progression of age-related macular degeneration, *Cochrane Database Syst. Rev.*, CD000254, 2006.
94. Age-Related Eye Disease Study Research Group, A randomized, placebo-controlled, clinical trial of high-dose supplementation with vitamins C and E, β-carotene, and zinc for age-related macular degeneration and vision loss: AREDS report no. 8., *Arch. Ophthalmol.*, 119, 1417, 2001.
95. The Alpha-Tocopherol, The effect of vitamin E and β-carotene on the incidence of lung cancer and other cancers in male smokers., *N. Engl. J. Med.*, 330, 1029, 1994.
96. Omenn, G.S., et al., Effects of a combination of β-carotene and vitamin A on lung cancer and cardiovascular disease, *N. Engl. J. Med.*, 334, 1150, 1996.
97. The HOPE and HOPE-TOO Trial Investigators, Effects of Long-term Vitamin E Supplementation on Cardiovascular Events and Cancer: A Randomized Controlled Trial, *JAMA*, 293, 1338, 2005.
98. Bjelakovic, G., et al., Mortality in randomized trials of antioxidant supplements for primary and secondary prevention: systematic review and meta-analysis, *JAMA*, 297, 842, 2007.
99. Beatty, S., et al., The role of oxidative stress in the pathogenesis of age-related macular degeneration, *Surv. Ophthalmol.*, 45, 115, 2000.
100. O'Connell, E., et al., Macular carotenoids and age-related maculopathy, *Ann. Acad. Med Singap.*, 35, 821, 2006.
101. Trieschmann, M., et al., Changes in macular pigment optical density and serum concentrations of its constituent carotenoids following supplemental lutein and zeaxanthin: The LUNA study, *Exp. Eye Res.*, 84, 718, 2001.
102. Mares-Perlman, J.A., et al., The body of evidence to support a protective role for lutein and zeaxanthin in delaying chronic disease, Overview, J. *Nutr.*, 132, 518S, 2002.
103. Bone, R.A., et al., Macular pigment in donor eyes with and without AMD: a case-control study, *Invest. Ophthalmol. Vis. Sci.*, 42, 235, 2001.

104. Goldberg, J., et al., Age-related macular degeneration and cataract: are dietary antioxidants protective? *Am. J. Epidemiol.*, 128, 904, 1988.
105. Beatty, S., et al., Macular pigment and risk for age-related macular degeneration in subjects from a Northern European population, *Invest. Ophthalmol. Vis. Sci.*, 42, 439, 2001.
106. Gale, C.R., et al., Lutein and zeaxanthin status and risk of age-related macular degeneration, *Invest. Ophthalmol. Vis. Sci.*, 44, 2461, 2003.
107. Sanders, T.A.B., et al., Essential fatty acids, plasma cholesterol, and fat-soluble vitamins in subjects with age-related maculopathy and matched control subjects, *Am. J. Clin. Nutr.*, 57, 428, 1993.
108. Richer, S. et al., Double-masked, placebo-controlled, randomized trial of lutein and antioxidant supplementation in the intervention of atrophic age-related macular degeneration: the Veterans LAST study (Lutein Antioxidant Supplementation Trial), *Optometry*, 75, 216, 2004.
109. AREDS 2. http://www.nei.nih.gov/neitrials/viewStudyWeb.aspx?id=120, accessed 2/15/2007.
110. SanGiovanni, J.P. and Chew, E.Y., The role of omega-3 long-chain polyunsaturated fatty acids in health and disease of the retina, *Prog. Retin. Eye Res.*, 24, 87, 2005.
111. Cho, E., et al., Prospective study of dietary fat and the risk of age-related macular degeneration, *Am. J. Clin. Nutr.*, 73, 209, 2001.
112. Hodge, W.G., et al., Efficacy of [omega]-3 fatty acids in preventing age-related macular degeneration: a systematic review, *Ophthalmology*, 113, 1165, 2006.

15 Alzheimer's Disease and Other Forms of Dementia

Pasqualina Perrig-Chiello, Sara Hutchison, and Hannes B. Staehelin

CONTENTS

15.1 INTRODUCTION

The ongoing demographic changes, namely the increasing longevity of people, have brought new societal challenges. In particular, the longer life expectancy in very old age is associated with a significant higher risk of becoming dependent. One of the main reasons of losing functional autonomy in general is dementia, and in particular, is Alzheimer's disease (AD). Dementia is one of the most disabling health conditions in old age. A central characteristic of dementia is a chronic deterioration of intellectual functions and other cognitive skills severe enough to interfere with the ability to perform activities of daily living [1]. For most people in

Western societies, a possible loss of autonomy is considered very distressing, nowadays more than ever before. In fact, forgetfulness and absentmindedness are among the least desirable and controllable losses anticipated for later life [2]. Complaints of memory loss are among the most frequently reported symptoms of aging by elderly people [3,4]. These complaints are associated with a marked fear of losing control [5]. Surveys indicate that dementia is the condition most feared by older adults in the United States [6]. The reason for this phenomenon is twofold: (a) Establishing and maintaining autonomy is a socially highly valued goal and therefore a central developmental task throughout the life span—thus a loss of autonomy is seen as a painful and sorrowful individual experience. (b) In modern individualistic society, social networks and family ties are not as solid as they were in the past—loss of autonomy means mainly institutionalization [2]. Therefore, functional autonomy and good cognitive functioning are closely related and core conditions of successful aging.

Because of the deep impact of dementia on the well-being and quality of life of the concerned individuals and their families on the one hand, and on the healthcare systems on the other hand, a thorough knowledge of its incidence, prevalence but especially of its etiology is needed. The need for coherent and objective information is especially strong in regard to women's health issues. The demographic and societal changes have definitely created new and often very distinct realities for men and women. However, these diverse realities have only marginally and fragmentally been the topic of research endeavors. There is, for example, a general growing awareness of the societal phenomenon of "feminization of old age," yet the topic and its psychosocial and health-related consequences have not attracted the scientific interest they would deserve. Indeed, population aging has important implications on sex balance since high proportions of the oldest individuals are females. Table 15.1 illustrates the phenomenon of feminization in old age: The older the age group the higher its female:male ratio [7].

Even though life expectancy is used as indicator of successful aging, this parameter can be misleading, disguising some implications of a longer life span. It is known, for example, that the likelihood of disability (especially in connection with dementia) increases with advancing age. It is therefore hardly surprising that

TABLE 15.1
The Phenomenon of Feminization of Old Age

Proportion of Women in Different Age Groups in 2000 in Switzerland						
65–69 years	70–74 years	75–79 years	80–84 years	85–89 years	90–94 years	>95 years
55%	57%	61%	65%	71%	76%	80%

Source: From Swiss Federal Office of Statistics, 2005. Retrieved December 5, 2006 from www.bfs.admin.ch/bfs/portal/de/index/regionen/gleichstellungsatlas/familien_und_haushaltsformen/blank/aeltere_personen.html.

TABLE 15.2
Life Expectancy in Healthy Years in Switzerland, the United Kingdom, and the United States, 2001

	Men		Women	
	Average Life Expectancy	Healthy Life Expectancy	Average Life Expectancy	Healthy Life Expectancy
Switzerland	77.2	71.1	82.8	75.3
The United Kingdom	75.0	69.1	79.0	72.1
The United States	74.4	67.2	79.5	71.3

Source: From WHO, The World Health Report, 2004. Retrieved November 21, 2006 from http://www3.who.int/whosis/hale/hale.cfm?path=whosis,hale&language=English.

national surveys reveal increasing numbers of disabled women among the older populations. Thus the price which women have to pay for their longer life essentially consists of a higher risk of disability. Indeed, if "healthy life expectancy"—that is, expected years of life in relatively good health*—is examined in place of overall life expectancy, women's advantage over men becomes smaller. As can be seen in Table 15.2, the difference between average life expectancy and healthy life expectancy, that is, the number of years with substantial handicaps, is significantly higher among women compared with men in the United Kingdom, the United States, and Switzerland, independent of the different means of longevity in the three nations [8].

It is noteworthy that even a few decades ago, the majority of geriatric and gerontological studies were oriented toward male standards, without considering sex effects. Even though subsequent studies increasingly began to focus on differences between women and men, they referred mainly to the biological sex of a person and not to their gender belonging. Because of these scientific neglects and limitations, the literature on gender, health, and aging is sketchy and often contradictory [9]. Do older women really have more physical and mental health problems than older men, or are these findings influenced by a gender bias, due to a different awareness and understanding of health and illness? Is there truly a higher incidence of Alzheimer's dementia in women than in men, or is the apparently higher incidence simply the consequence of a woman's higher life expectancy? It is impossible to find satisfactory answers to all these questions without considering health behavior as well as the cultural and psychosocial living context of the subjects studied. The inclusion of gender as a social reality in the broadest sense is therefore an absolute prerequisite for gaining valid information.

* Healthy life expectancy is not necessarily life expectancy free of disease. Rather, the concept of healthy life expectancy as normally used refers to life expectancy without limitation of functions that may be the consequence of one or more chronic conditions.

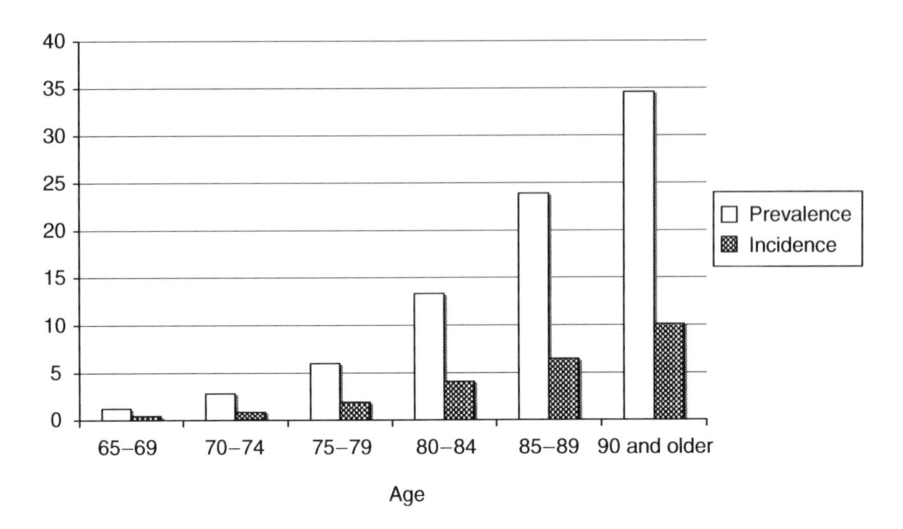

FIGURE 15.1 Incidence and prevalence rates of Alzheimer's disease. (From Bickel, H., *Das Gesundheitswesen*, 62, 211, 2000.)

15.2 DEMENTIA AND AD: DEFINITIONS AND ETIOLOGY

Before delving into the topic of sex differences it is important to first define the central concept of "dementia" and to give some basic information on its epidemiology. Dementia is not a specific disorder or disease, but a syndrome associated with a progressive loss of memory and other intellectual functions that interfere with functional autonomy. The Diagnostic and Statistical Manual of Mental Disorders [10] defines dementia as an overall decline in intellectual function, including difficulties with language, simple calculations, planning and judgment, motor skills, as well as loss of memory. The prevalence of dementia increases rapidly with age; it doubles approximately every five years after age 60 (Figure 15.1) [11]. Dementia affects only 1% of people aged 60–64 but affects 30%–50% of those older than 85.* Although the mean age at the onset of dementia is ~80 years, early-onset disease, defined arbitrarily and variously as occurring before the age of 60–65, can occur but is rare. The overall observed exponential increase between 60 and 90 clearly indicates that dementia is a multifactorial phenomenon resulting from a sum of exogenous and endogenous factors, for example, from genetic predisposition as well as from normal metabolic processes such as free radicals generated during respiration.

There is empirical evidence that dementia can be caused by nearly 40 different diseases and conditions, ranging from dietary deficiencies and metabolic disorders to head injuries and inherited diseases. The possible causes of dementia can be categorized as follows:

* Measures of the prevalence of Alzheimer's disease differ depending on the diagnostic criteria used, the age of the population surveyed, and other factors, including geographic and cultural context.

- *Primary dementia*. These dementias are characterized by damage to or wasting away of the brain tissue itself. They include AD, frontal lobe dementia, and Pick's disease. AD is the most common form of primary dementia, a progressive degenerative brain disorder that results in a profound global dementia characterized by severe amnesia with additional deficits in other areas of functioning such as planning, language, or attention [12]. AD is caused by neuronal cell death characteristically associated with fibrillization and aggregation of proteins in the brain called neuritic plaques and neurofibrillary tangles. The plaques consist primarily of aggregated β-amyloid protein derived from amyloid precursor protein (APP), whereas the tangles contain aggregates of a hyperphosphorylated form of tau protein of broken down microtubules [13]. Frontotemporal dementias are caused by a disorder (sometimes genetic) that affects the frontal and temporal lobe of the brain, and Pick's disease is a rare type of primary dementia that is characterized by a progressive loss of social skills, language, and memory, leading to personality changes and sometimes loss of moral judgment [14].
- *Vascular dementia* (VaD, replaced the term multi-infarct dementia). Neuropathologically VaD is defined as dementia resulting from ischemic or hemorrhagic brain lesions or from cerebral ischemic-hypoxic injuries [15].

There are other manifestations of dementia such as Lewy-body-disease, dementia due to Parkinson's disease, Huntington's disease, infectious diseases (HIV, viral encephalitis, Lyme disease, syphilis, Creutzfeldt-Jakob disease), abnormalities in the structure of the brain (hydrocephalus, tumors, subdural hematoma), to alcoholism or exposure to heavy metals (arsenic, antimony, bismuth), and finally substance-induced dementia. Dementia may also be associated with depression, low levels of thyroid hormone, or niacin or vitamin B12 deficiency. However, the two most frequent types are AD and VaD, with AD accounting for about two-thirds of all dementias (ranging in various studies from 42% to 81% of all dementias), and VaD for another 16% (women) to 36% (men) [16]. Therefore, this chapter will mainly focus on AD, and to some extent on VaD. We want to shed light on the widely discussed questions of whether AD in addition to age is linked to female sex and whether nutritional and socioeconomic factors are associated with AD.

15.3 SEX DIFFERENCES IN THE MANIFESTATION OF AD

One of the most controversially discussed points in regard to risk factors for AD is female sex. For years scientists and practitioners shared the popular hypothesis that women have a higher risk of AD than men, even though the empirical foundation was very weak. Furthermore, it is amazing that even though it was well known in literature that living contexts and lifestyles of men and women diverge substantially, the category "gender" was not taken into account in most of the studies. In the last two decades a large number of research reports showed a rather controversial output. Depending on the methodological approach (incidence or prevalence studies) and on the independent variables studied (socio-economic status, lifestyle variables, etc.), these studies postulated sex differences [17–19] or not (Framingham Study [20]).

15.3.1 Incidence and Prevalence of AD: Sex Differences or Not?

Despite a growing list of potential new risk factors for AD, one of the oldest remains controversial, namely female sex [21]. By reviewing the status quo of the last 20 years of research in this field, one can observe that the same research topic was studied with a rich variety of study designs and sampling. The results of these mostly epidemiological studies gathered in different cultural contexts brought empirical evidence either in favor of sex differences in AD or not. A crucial point in explaining these controversial research results is the study design. A large majority of studies focus on prevalence of dementia rather than on incidence.

An increased prevalence of AD among women has been reported in many studies carried out all over the world [17,18,22–30]. Results from the Framingham Study [20] showed that the prevalence of dementia and probable AD were greater for women than for men. The female:male ratio of prevalence for cohort members 75 years of age and older was 1.8 for all cases of dementia and 2.8 for cases of probable AD. Similar results were found in other US studies [17]. An increased prevalence of AD among women was also found in the Canadian Study of Health and Aging [18]. Here a representative sample of people aged 65 and older (9008 subjects) was screened for possible dementia. Prevalence estimates suggested that 8.0% of all Canadians aged 65 and older met the criteria for dementia, with the female:male ratio being 2:1. European studies came to the same conclusion. In Spain, Manubens et al. [25] assessed the prevalence of dementing disorders in a sample of 1127 subjects. AD was the most common type of dementia. The prevalence of both dementia and AD increased steeply with advancing age and was consistently higher in women. The prevalence of combined vascular and mixed dementia increased less rapidly with age, and was generally higher in men. These results converge with those reported for other regions in Europe and the world ([23] in Italy, [26] Spain, [27] the United Kingdom, [24] Israel, [29] Japan, [30] Korea, or [31] China).

However, there are also prevalence studies with mixed results. Jorm et al. [32] analyzed 22 dementia prevalence studies carried out between 1945 and 1985. They report that the age-correlated prevalence of dementia showed higher rates for AD for women but no differences for VaD. Hofman et al. [33] analyzed age- and sex-specific prevalence rates from European studies carried out between 1980 and 1990. The results show a slightly higher rate of dementia in men for the age group <75 and a higher prevalence of dementia in women for the age group >75.

In contrast to prevalence studies incidence studies generally did not find any sex differences [34–41]. There is a general agreement that for studying risk factors for diseases causing dementia, it is preferable to assess disease incidence rather than prevalence in order to gather valid and reliable information about the phenomenon. The reason for this is that a difference between groups in prevalence may be due to differences in either the duration of the disease or the incidence [42]. Even though it is known that incidence studies guarantee more solid and valid results than prevalence studies, they are much less common because of the considerable resources they require.

Very interesting and differentiated results on this topic were found in several meta-analyses. A first one was carried out by Jorm and Jolley [42]. They analyzed 23 studies published between 1966 and 1997, reporting age-specific incidence rates. Results yielded no sex differences in overall dementia incidence, but women tended to have a higher incidence of AD in very old age, whereas men tended to have a higher incidence of VaD in younger ages.

To study the difference in risk for dementing diseases between men and women, Andersen et al. [43] performed pooled analyses of four population-based prospective cohort studies from Denmark, France, the Netherlands, and the United Kingdom. The sample included persons aged 65 years and older, 528 incident cases of dementia, and 28,768 person-years of follow-up. Incident cases were identified in a two-stage procedure in which the total cohort was screened for cognitive impairment, and screen positives underwent detailed diagnostic assessment. Results show significant sex differences in the incidence of AD after age 85. At 90 years, the rate was 81.7 in women and 24.0 in men. There were no sex differences in rates or risk of VaD. The cumulative risk for 65 year-old women to develop AD by the age of 95 was 0.22 compared with 0.09 for men. The cumulative risk for developing VaD by the age of 95 was similar for men and women.

Different population-based studies did not find any differences in the incidence rate of AD in men and women. Hebert et al. [44] investigated the risk of incidence and prevalence of AD. Beginning in 1982, two stratified random samples of people aged 65 in East Boston, Massachusetts, underwent structured clinical evaluation for prevalent (467 people) and incident (642 people from a cohort previously ascertained to be disease-free) probable AD. The prevalence sample was followed for mortality for up to 11 years. The age-specific incidence of AD did not differ significantly by sex. Controlled for age, prevalence also did not differ significantly by sex. The increase in risk of mortality due to AD did likewise not vary by sex. The odds ratio for women with AD compared with women without AD was 2.07, and for men, the odds ratio was 2.22. These findings suggest that the excess number of women with AD is due to the longer life expectancy of women rather than sex-specific risk factors for the disease. Similarly, Fitzpatrick et al. [45] did not find any sex and racial differences with regard to incidence and prevalence of AD and VaD in a US community sample.

Even though majority of incidence studies did not find any sex differences, there are several studies that report conflicting results to those presented so far, reporting sex differences either for all age strata or only for the oldest old. In a large population-based prospective cohort study (Rotterdam study, 7983 participants) Ruitenberg et al. [46] investigated sex differences in the incidence of AD. The results reveal similar dementia incidence for men and for women, however, after age 90 AD dementia incidence declined in men but not in women. After 90 years of age the incidence of AD is higher for women than for men, whereas the incidence of VaD is higher for men than for women in all age groups. Even more conflicting differences to the studies reported above on incidence of AD were presented by Fratiglioni et al. [47]. Results from a follow-up study with a dementia-free cohort

(1473 subjects, 75 years and older) in Stockholm suggest that for all the age strata the incidence rates of AD and VaD were higher for women than for men, especially in very old age. Similar results are reported by Gao et al. [19]. Based on results from a meta-analysis they conclude that women are at higher risk of developing AD than do men. The odds ratios for women to develop incidence of dementia and AD relative to men are 1.18 and 1.56, respectively. Based on results from a population-based national representative study, Di Carlo et al. [48] report that women in Italy carry a significantly higher risk of developing AD, whereas VaD was more frequent in men.

Summing up the status quo of research, the conclusion is rather sobering. Even though it is generally recognized that the prevalence of AD is higher in women than in men, the incidence of AD remains a controversial issue. However, in a considerable part of those studies reporting no sex differences, there is clearly a trend toward higher incidence among women in the oldest age group. How can the increased prevalence rates of AD in women be explained on the basis of similarly higher incidence rates in old age? There is simply insufficient evidence to support the notion that female sex is per se a risk factor for AD.

Considering the epidemiologic observations made so far, as well as evidence of sex-related differences in cognition and behavior in various other studies [49,50], it must be assumed that there may be important genetic and biological factors related to sex that are operative in the pathogenesis of AD [51]. A thorough look at these factors as well as at possible interactions is most important for developing a more refined and differentiated approach to their treatment.

15.3.2 Possible Explanations for Sex Differences

Different explanations have been proposed to explain the observation of different prevalence and to some extent different incidence rates of AD in women and men. One category of explanations points out possible methodological shortcomings of the studies, a second focuses rather on sociodemographic factors, a third on psychosocial, and a fourth on biological factors. There is empirical evidence that shows that each of these four explanations has its legitimacy to a certain extent.

- *Methodological concerns* have not often arisen, but there is increasing evidence that methodological artifacts, such as selection bias or attrition, could contribute to the observed sex differences in the risk of AD [52]. Results of a study by Bonsignore et al. [53] revealed that the apparent higher risk of AD in women could be attributed to a selection bias during the recruitment of the sample. Sociodemographic factors must also be taken into consideration. The longer life expectancy of women is associated with a higher risk of AD (survival differences). Furthermore, it has been argued that women have longer survival times than men after the initial diagnosis of AD [21,54,55], or that AD has an earlier onset in women than in men [53,56]. Even though these observations are based on empirical evidence, they have only limited explanation value.
- *Psychosocial factors—lifestyle*: Psychosocial risk factors have been identified in different studies, such as negative life events, psychosocial stress,

and personality [57–59]. However, these findings are still contradictory. More conclusive results have been gathered in different studies concerning the positive relation between low educational level and increased risk of AD [31,48,60–62]. Women, especially those who are actually in the age range at risk, on average have a lower education than age-matched men and, consequently, a higher risk of AD. The association between AD and lower education has been found essentially in women, and less in men. Using pooled data from four European population-based follow-up studies Letenneur et al. [63] found that the risk of women with low and middle education to get AD are 4.3 times higher than the risk of women with high education. However, with men, the corresponding risk estimates were close to 1. Consequently, low education can be seen as a potential risk factor for AD in women but not in men. It is possible that these data do not so much reflect a direct causality between education or economic status and AD as reveal factors that condition and determine certain lifestyles (such as nutrition, physical activity), including the degree of stimulation of cognitive capacities throughout an individual's life. Higher levels of stimulation appear to produce a greater resistance to deterioration.

- *Genetic and metabolic factors*: Results from prospective studies show that the risk of AD is associated not only with sociodemographic, psychosocial, and lifestyle factors, but also with genetic factors such as the presence of apolipoprotein E-ε4 (APOE-ε4). The risk of AD increases from 20% to 90%, with increasing numbers of APOE-ε4 alleles in families with late-onset disease [64,65]. However, there is some empirical evidence suggesting that the risk of AD conferred by APOE-ε4, adjusted for age and stratified by sex, is significant only for women [66]. Furthermore, it has been suggested that genetic factors are interlinked with metabolic processes. The results of these interactions can act as protective or as risk factors for AD. Several studies have shown that elevated total cholesterol levels or elevated blood pressure earlier in life could increase the risk for AD. Genetic factors are likely to influence the clinical expression of the disease in addition to influencing the risk. While APOE is prominently involved in neuronal cholesterol metabolism, APOE-ε4 allele and the vascular risk factors independently contribute to the risk for AD [67].
- *Other risk factors*: Use of nonsteroidal anti-inflammatory drugs (aspirin, and other common medications for pain and arthritis), wine consumption, coffee consumption, and past exposure to vaccines are all associated with decreased risk of AD. While hormone replacement therapy is protective in some studies, several studies fail to support this association, including the Canadian Study of Health and Aging (CSHA) [68]. Hormone replacement therapy will be covered in more detail in a later section of this chapter.

Till now there is no compelling evidence that these mechanisms are mutually exclusive. In fact, there are several hypotheses concerning the possible interaction of these factors in the pathogenesis of AD. Considering the uniform single exponential increase of AD with age, with comparable rates in many societies, it is very probable that endogenous genetic–metabolic factors are prominent. However, these factors are highly related to lifestyle, especially to nutrition. In fact, there is empirical evidence that micronutrients may affect the rate of disease via protection against reactive oxygen species, directly as antioxidants or indirectly by stabilizing sensitive structure or improving metabolism [69]. It has been argued that the effect of pro-oxidant nutrients may catalyze the development of disease by interaction with proteins and lipids involved in the pathophysiology of AD. Of potentially far-reaching consequences is the hypothesis that nutritional conditions in early life may program metabolic functions, leading over time to an increasing imbalance and thus favoring the emergence of disease states. Therefore, a closer look on the possible protective function of nutrition should reveal promising insights in prevention strategies for AD.

15.4 NUTRITION AND COGNITIVE FUNCTIONING

The aim of this section is to review the literature on the interaction of nutrition and cognition in general, and then in a second step, to look for empirical evidence for the relation of nutrition and AD in particular, in the context of potential sex differences.

15.4.1 Nutrition and Cognition

It is known that the effective functioning of the central nervous system is dependent on an optimal nutrient supply [70]. Therefore, cognitive functioning may be affected by a deficit in nutrients. It has been shown that a well-balanced diet is associated with lower prevalence of cognitive deficit [71]. There is empirical evidence of the cell-protective effects of antioxidants on brain metabolism [72,73], as well as on the fact that inverse correlations of dietary antioxidant intake or plasma level and subsequent disease have been demonstrated [74–76]. From this fact one might assume that increased oxidative stress is responsible for disturbances in memory functions. In fact, severe lack of vitamins is considered one of the causes of reversible dementia ([77], see later section). The vitamins most often associated with cognitive deficits are folic acid, vitamins B12 and B6. One explanation model is that low folic acid levels or vitamin-B-complex levels raise homocysteine levels. Homocysteine is an amino acid that is produced by the body. However, high homocysteine levels (hyperhomocysteinemia) lead to the production of especially reactive oxides. These free radicals cause damage to the nervous system [78]. Therefore, a deficit in folic acid may contribute to damage to the brain by raising homocysteine levels, which in turn lead to increased oxidative damage.

Antioxidants can inhibit free-radical-mediated chain reactions such as the ones caused by elevated homocysteine levels. Examples of antioxidants are the vitamins E and C, β-carotene, and flavonoids. These antioxidants can be taken either as supplements or stem from high dietary intake. It has long been assumed that high antioxidant levels may be associated with better cognitive performance. Perrig et al. [79] tested this assumption by assessing plasma vitamin levels of vitamin E, β-carotene, and vitamin C and several measures of memory in a sample of elderly Swiss. Four hundred and forty two participants aged 65–94 (mean, 75 years;

312 male, 132 female) were tested for memory. In addition, plasma vitamin levels were measured for the three antioxidants: α-tocopherol, ascorbic acid, and β-carotene. The same vitamin parameters, measured 24 years before, were integrated in the analysis. Furthermore serum cholesterol, ferritin, and systolic blood pressure were taken into account. Results show a high stability of the plasma antioxidants over the time lag of 22 years (for α-tocopherol, β-carotene, and ascorbic acid). Memory functions correlated significantly with ascorbic acid and β-carotene in the cross-sectional data as well as in the longitudinal analysis. These two antioxidants remained significant predictors, especially of long-term memory, after partialing out possible confounding variables like age, education, and sex in multiple regression analyses. None of the memory parameters show significant cross-sectional or longitudinal correlations with systolic blood pressure, serum ferritin, and cholesterin. These results support a role of antioxidants in brain aging and may have implications in prevention of degenerative brain disease.

In a recent study Grodstein et al. [80] investigated the relation of specific vitamin E and vitamin C supplements, including the dose and duration, to the performance on cognitive tests in older women. The Nurses' Health Study cohort, a group of female nurses longitudinally studied in regards to lifestyle and medical history beginning in 1976, was used in the present investigation. Collection of dietary information regarding vitamin supplements began in 1980. A total of 22,213 women completed the interview. Results revealed that long-term, current users of vitamin E with vitamin C had significantly better mean performances, as judged by a global score that combined the individual cognitive test scores, than did women who had never used vitamin E or C. There was a trend for increasingly higher mean scores with increasing durations of use. These associations were found to be strongest among women with low dietary intakes of α-tocopherol. The benefits were less consistent for women taking vitamin E alone, with no evidence of higher scores with longer durations of use. Additionally, use of vitamin C supplements alone had little relation to performance on the cognitive tests. It appears that the use of specific vitamin E supplements, especially when combined with vitamin C supplements, may be beneficial in maintaining cognitive function during later adult years.

These results from correlational studies were confirmed by various intervention studies. Bryan et al. [70] supplied 211 women of various ages with either folate, vitamins B12 and B6, or placebo during 35 days. Folate supplementation was associated with an improvement in reaction time, memory, and fluency. vitamins B12 and B6 supplementation was associated with improved memory performance. A review of intervention studies concerned with folate supplementation (vitamin B9) comes to the conclusion that "folate treatment was effective in lessening cognitive deficits" [77]. The same authors conducted a study in which they treated elderly patients with cognitive deficits with folic acid [77]. After 60 days, they found a significant improvement in both memory and attention. Furthermore, the magnitude of memory improvement was positively associated with the initial severity of folic acid deficiency.

Manders et al. [81] performed a systematic review of randomized controlled studies on the effectiveness of nutritional supplementation on cognitive functioning. Twelve studies of the 21 analyzed found significant positive effects of nutritional intervention on cognitive functioning, whereas 9 studies did not. None of the studies found a significantly negative effect of nutritional intervention. Despite the heterogeneity in trial design, the results of this review suggest that nutritional supplements may improve the cognitive functioning of elderly persons and do no harm. Further well-designed studies are needed to support these findings.

In summary, there is strong scientific evidence linking deficits in certain nutrients, especially folic acid and vitamins B12 and B6, to reduced cognitive performance. None of the studies we examined mentioned any sex effects. The question remains whether lack of nutrients may also be associated with increased risk of dementia, and whether supplementation of certain nutrients may stave off the cognitive deterioration associated with dementia. These questions will be dealt with in the next section.

15.4.2 Nutrition and Dementia

There are various lines of evidence linking dietary components as well as nutrition-related disorders to a general cognitive decline, and in particular, AD and VaD. Most often mentioned are hypercholesterolemia, homocysteine, folic acid, vitamins B6 and B12 [82], vitamins E and C, total caloric intake, as well as several metals such as zinc, copper, iron, aluminum, selenium, and mercury [69]. The differential relation of these parameters with dementia in general and with AD in particular will be examined, starting with the vitamins.

15.4.2.1 Vitamins and Polyphenols

The vitamins of the B group as well as vitamins E and C are most frequently mentioned in research concerned with dementia. The vitamins A, C, and E are considered to be antioxidants, that is, they can bind free oxygen radicals, which may otherwise cause oxidative damage. Oxidative damage plays an important role in aging (e.g., [83]). The brain, in particular, is susceptible to free-radical damage, as it only has low levels of endogenous antioxidant enzymes [82]. Most of the free radicals originate in the mitochondria. The repair capacity of the mitochondria is not as efficient as the nuclear repair mechanisms. Furthermore, most neuronal cells are postmitotic and can only be replaced by neuronal stem cells in a very limited way. Therefore, oxidative damage has especially grave consequences for the brain. There is evidence that oxidative damage may be involved in the pathogenesis of AD and other neurodegenerative diseases [84]. In view of these findings, it is not surprising that many research projects examined the role of vitamins or antioxidants in dementia. Three approaches are most commonly used: first, one can measure the nutrient status in healthy elderly and compare it to the nutrient status of patients with dementia; a second option is to conduct a prospective study and follow which participants develop dementia over the following years; whereas the third approach would be an intervention study in which some participants are supplied with vitamins and others with placebo.

The PAQUID study, a large French prospective cohort study of normal and pathological brain aging (Personnes Âgées Quid) [85], followed the first approach by using a prospective nested case-control design. Each participant who developed dementia within 10 years of the first examination was matched to two other, nondemented participants by age and sex. The final study sample consisted of 46 demented and 136 healthy participants. Plasma concentrations of vitamin E were lower among the demented than among the healthy participants. Furthermore, when the plasma concentrations were split into tertiles, logistic regression analyses showed that the participants belonging to the lowest tertile had a significantly increased risk of dementia. The authors conclude that participants who had lower plasma levels of vitamin E had an increased risk of developing dementia [85]. In addition to the vitamin E plasma levels, plasma malondialdehyde concentration was also assessed. Plasma malondialdehyde is the end product of lipid peroxidation caused by free radicals and can therefore be considered an indicator of oxidative damage. Even though the results did not reach statistical significance, there was nevertheless a tendency for subjects with a high plasma malondialdehyde concentration to have an increased risk of dementia. These results show that oxidative stress may play a role in the development of dementia.

This view is supported by a review [82] that comes to the conclusion that "oxidative damage may be central to the neurodegenerative process in both VaD and AD." However, the question remains whether a nutrient deficient diet leads to an increase of oxidative stress, which promotes dementia, or whether an increase in oxidative stress is actually the first sign of dementia.

The Rotterdam study is another prospective study that examined, among other things, the determinants of dementia in the elderly [86]. Results yielded that high vitamin E and vitamin C intake was associated with a lower risk of AD, after adjustments for age, sex, education, body mass index, and caloric intake. The association between vitamin intake and risk of dementia did not vary by apolipoprotein E genotype. However, in another prospective study [87], the protective effect of vitamin E was only found in people who were APOE-ε4 negative. In the same study, high vitamin C intake failed to result in a reduced risk of dementia. Furthermore, only vitamin E that came from food and not from supplements appeared to have a protective effect [87]. The Rotterdam study did not discriminate between dietary and supplemented vitamin E; however, the authors state that the results did not alter when supplement users were excluded from the analysis [86].

Apart from these cross-sectional studies, there are also intervention studies with longitudinal design to be considered. The Vital Trial Collaboration [88] for example supplied participants with either aspirin, folic acid plus vitamin B12, vitamins E plus C, or placebo, and measured the effect of this intervention on cognition and certain physiological parameters. All participants had a diagnosis of either dementia or mild cognitive impairment. None of the treatments had any effect on cognition, however, the supplementation of folic acid in combination with vitamin B12 significantly lowered plasma homocysteine concentration (by 30%). Therefore, even though the interventions did not have a direct effect on cognition, the combination of folic acid and vitamin B12 was "effective in reducing biochemical factors associated with cognitive impairment in people at risk of dementia" [88].

Another intervention study, which has been considered to be "the one published trial of acceptable methodology" [89], was carried out by Sano et al. [90]. They conducted a double-blind, placebo-controlled, and randomized intervention study in patients with moderate severity AD. For 2 years, patients were given either vitamin E, selegiline (a monoamine oxidase inhibitor), a combination of vitamin E and selegiline, or placebo. The authors then assessed how much time passed until the patients either died, were institutionalized, lost the capability to perform simple activities of daily living, or were classified as suffering from severe dementia. When the baseline mini-mental score was used as a covariate, patients treated with vitamin E took the longest to deteriorate (median 670 days), followed by the selegiline group (655 days), and the combination group (585 days). In comparison, the median time for deterioration in the control group was 440 days. Treatment with vitamin E therefore seemed to slow the progression of the disease. The doses of vitamin E used in this study were 2000 IU. Vitamin E can act as an anticoagulant and may increase the risk of bleeding problems. The Food and Nutrition Board of the Institute of Medicine has set an upper tolerable intake level (UL) for vitamin E at 1000 mg (1500 IU) for any form of supplementary α-tocopherol per day [91]. Therefore, the recommended doses were exceeded by Sano et al. A review from 2006 [89] concludes that this one study by Sano et al. is an insufficient evidence for the effectiveness of vitamin E in the treatment of AD, especially as the people treated with vitamin E in Sano et al.'s study had a higher incidence of falls than the participants in the other groups. The results by Sano et al. will need to be confirmed by further research, especially in terms of the safety of such doses of vitamin E.

Not only vitamins have antioxidant properties. Another substance that has been in the spotlight for its antioxidant characteristics is fruit polyphenols. Polyphenols are a group of chemical substances found in plants. A certain kind of polyphenols has antioxidant properties. This type of polyphenols is found, for example, in strawberries, spinach, cranberries, blueberries, or dark chocolate [84]. It has been shown that fruits that are rich in polyphenols are beneficial to brain function. Animal studies with rats came to the conclusion that a polyphenol-supplemented diet prevented "a variety of age-related deficits including cognitive performance" [92], and may even reverse age-related cognitive deficits [93]. Other experiments (also with rats) indicate that supplementation with blueberries may increase hippocampal plasticity and cognitive performance [94]. In summary, fruit polyphenols appear to be promising, but there is need for studies with humans and Alzheimer patients before any conclusion can be drawn.

15.4.2.2 Metals

Apart from vitamins and polyphenols, certain metals have also been associated with dementia, especially copper, zinc, iron, aluminum, selenum, and mercury. Alzheimer patients have been shown to have significantly changed copper and zinc levels in the brain, a finding that was confirmed in mouse models [95,96]. The APP binds copper and zinc. Certain experiments indicate that a high copper content may stabilize the APP [69], thus leading to less β-amyloid. The role of zinc appears to be more negative. Religa et al. [96] conclude that "brain zinc accumulation is a prominent feature of advanced AD and is biochemically linked to brain amyloid β-peptide accumulation and dementia severity in AD."

- *Aluminum* is known to affect neuronal structures. It leads to cell death in vivo as well as in vitro [97]. High aluminum blood levels can result in dementia that is similar to AD [98]. Furthermore, there is evidence from epidemiological studies that the risk of AD is increased in areas where there is a high concentration of aluminum in the drinking water [99].
- *Iron* levels appear to play a role in AD in connection with cholesterol. Transferrin saturation is an indicator of body iron stores. The risk of developing AD is markedly higher when a person has both elevated transferrin saturation and elevated cholesterol (both levels above the 75th percentile resulted in a risk ratio for developing AD of 3:19). The risk for AD increased only for people who had elevated scores in both factors; one alone did not suffice [100].
- *Selenium* is an essential micronutrient for all mammals but is toxic at high levels. Mammals need selenium to produce a certain enzyme (glutathione peroxidase), which protects against oxidation-induced cancer. Considering its key role in the production of antioxidant enzymes, selenium could be important in connection with AD; however, up to this point there is little information regarding this topic [69].
- *Mercury* has been associated with various negative effects on health. When mercury is washed into rivers or other bodies of water, it is converted to methylmercury by certain bacteria. Methylmercury is lipophilic and tends to accumulate in tissue [98]. Methylmercury is particularly toxic because 95% of an ingested dose is absorbed into the bloodstream and can cross the blood–brain and placental barriers, causing adult and fetal neurotoxicity. Besides damaging the brain and peripheral nervous system, methylmercury may also adversely affect the adult and fetal cardiovascular systems. However, a relationship between AD and mercury has so far not been confirmed [69].

15.4.2.3 Caloric Intake

Apart from certain substances, total caloric intake has also been implicated to affect the risk for AD. A longitudinal study by Luchsinger et al. [101] assessed the daily caloric intake of 980 healthy elderly over 4 years. The individuals in the lowest quartile of caloric intake showed a significantly lower risk to develop AD compared with the persons in the highest quartile of caloric intake. However, this relation proved true only for people who were carriers of the APOE-ε4. For people who were not carriers of that allele, the relationship was not significant [101]. Animal studies yield further evidence of the role of caloric restriction in AD. For example, Wang et al. [102] were able to show in a mouse model that "caloric restriction may prevent AD-type amyloid neuropathology" in the brain.

15.4.2.4 Cholesterol

In a review from 2006, Kivipelto et al. [64] examined five longitudinal studies concerned with midlife serum cholesterol and subsequent dementia or AD. Four of the five studies found a positive association, while the fifth found no association.

Some studies yielded contradictory results: Mielke et al. [103] concluded that "high total cholesterol levels in late life associated with a reduced risk of dementia," whereas Li et al. [104] state that "the data do not support an association between serum total cholesterol or high density lipoprotein in late life and subsequent risk of dementia or Alzheimer disease."

A possible reconciliation of the contradictory results can be derived from a study conducted by Mainous et al. [100]. This study yielded the result that the risk of developing AD is higher when a person has both elevated transferrin saturation and elevated cholesterol [100]. Cholesterol alone had no effect. In a review from 2006, Panza et al. conclude that "the prevailing wisdom is that high total cholesterol is a risk factor for dementia. However, the relationship between total cholesterol and dementia may vary considerably depending on when cholesterol is measured over the life course, or, alternatively, in relation to the underlying course of the disease" [105].

15.4.2.5 Insulin

Nutrition is a key factor in the development of diabetes mellitus. Even though there are also genetic factors involved, obesity is one risk factor for developing insulin resistance (diabetes mellitus type 2). An association between diabetes and AD was found in several large epidemiological studies, which revealed an increased incidence of dementia among diabetic patients [106]. The mechanism involved is not quite clear yet. Frequently mentioned concepts are "cerebral insulin resistance" and "insulin-induced amyloid pathology" [107].

The cerebral insulin resistance theory is based on the fact that insulin and its receptors can be found throughout the brain. Insulin is involved in the regulation of body weight and acts also as neuromodulator, influencing the release and reuptake of neurotransmitters. With increasing age, the amount of insulin and also the amount of insulin receptors in the brain decreases. In patients with AD, insulin receptor signaling appears also to be disturbed, resulting in an insulin resistance of the brain [107].

The second theory is concerned with the connection between insulin and β-amyloid. β-amyloid is a building block of amyloid plaques, which is a neuropathological indicator of AD. Excessive β-amyloid can be cleared through several processes; one of them involves the insulin-degrading enzyme. Insulin may stimulate β-amyloid secretion and may also inhibit its degradation by competing for the same degrading enzyme [107]. In the context of this chapter it is important to mention that none of the studies mentioned above calculated sex effects.

15.4.2.6 Omega-3 Fatty Acids

Omega-3 fatty acids are essential fatty acids that the body cannot manufacture by itself. They need to be supplied over the diet. Omega-3 fatty acids can be found for example in oily fish or in flaxseed. Some studies indicate that a high consumption of omega-3 fatty acids is associated with a lower risk of AD. Patients suffering from AD have furthermore been shown to have lower plasma levels of omega-3 fatty acids than healthy controls, lending additional support for the proposed link between AD and polyunsaturated fatty acids [108]. One likely mechanism is that a high intake of omega-3 fatty acids can reduce serum cholesterol levels. A study using a transgenic mouse model showed that supplementation with omega-3 fatty acids reduced amyloid and oxidative damage [109].

None of the studies on metals, insulin, caloric intake, cholesterol, or omega-3 fatty acids mentioned any sex effects, or reported results by sex.

15.4.2.7 Hormone Replacement Therapy

Estrogen receptors have been found in the central nervous system, suggesting a role for estrogens in cognitive function [110,111]. This finding stimulated studies that showed a positive effect of estrogen replacement therapy (ERT) [112,113] on memory, executive functioning, and risk of AD [112,114]. However, ERT is not innocuous and its use has been related to increased risk of breast cancer, recurrent vaginal bleeding [115], and lately also increased risk of cardiovascular disease [116]. Moreover, opposite results were found concerning the effect on cognition. The Women's Health Initiative Memory Study, for example, found that hormone replacement therapy led to a significantly increased risk of dementia (hazard ratio 2:1) [117].

There have been various explanation attempts for the conflicting results. One line of reasoning is that hormone replacement therapy increases the risk of strokes, and that such microinfarcts may contribute to AD [118]. Another line of reasoning is that not all hormones used in hormone replacement therapy may have the same effect. As an example, one study implied a positive trend on cognition for estrogen-only users, whereas there was a significant cognitive decline in estrogen–progestin users [119]. Medroxyprogesterone acetate has been shown to counteract the positive effect estrogen has on hippocampal neurons [120].

Another explanation attempt is that testosterone may protect against AD. Estrogen treatment in women leads to a decrease in free testosterone, thus negating the protective effect [121]. It is also possible that hormone replacement therapy in women leads to a downregulation of estrogen receptors on cholinergic neurons. This could reduce cholinergic activity [122]. It is as yet unclear which of the mechanisms described is responsible for the findings.

Parallel to the various studies on hormone replacement theory and cognitive performances, there has been an increasing interest in alternative forms of estrogen supply, namely phytoestrogens in the last years. This interest in the effects of phytoestrogens as dietary components that may share the benefits of estrogens has been also promoted by results on the relation of nutrition and cognitive decline (see above, [123]). Phytoestrogens are natural compounds found in plants, with a diphenolic structure similar to that of natural and synthetic estrogens [124]. There are three major categories of phytoestrogens: isoflavones, lignans (as found in plant food and as produced by intestinal microflora), and coumestans [125,126]. Isoflavones, like genistein, daidzein, and formononetin, are found, especially in soy products, beans, peas, nuts, tea, and coffee. The main dietary sources of lignans are oilseeds, flaxseed, and berries. Coumestans are found mainly in alfalfa and sprouts [125,126]. The three major types of phytoestrogens are all considered agonists of estrogen receptors, especially the β-form, and may thus mimic the effects of estrogens [127]. A recent study suggested that isoflavones might indeed positively affect cognition without substantial side effects [128]. However, data on the relation between phytoestrogens and cognitive function are still sparse and far from sufficient to become conclusive.

Franco et al. [129] conducted a community-based survey among 394 postmenopausal women with the aim to examine the relation between the dietary intake of phytoestrogens and cognitive function in healthy postmenopausal women consuming a Western diet. Isoflavone and lignan intake was calculated from a validated food frequency questionnaire. Cognitive function was evaluated using the Mini-Mental State Examination (MMSE). Data were analyzed using logistic regression with intact cognitive function defined as a score of 26 as the outcome variable. After adjustment for confounders, increasing dietary lignans intake was associated with better performance on the MMSE. Results were most pronounced in women who had been postmenopausal for 20–30 years. The results of this study provide evidence that higher dietary intake of lignans is associated with better cognitive function in postmenopausal women. This association was not observed for isoflavones.

15.5 CONCLUSIONS AND FUTURE RESEARCH

The observed gain in individual life expectancy can not only be seen as a success, but also as a challenge, namely to cope with the functional decline associated with very old age. This is especially true for women [130]. Since a high proportion of the oldest individuals are females and the likelihood of disability, especially in connection with dementia, increases exponentially with advancing age, it is hardly surprising that national surveys reveal increasing numbers of disabled women among the older populations.

Among the types of disability, dementia and especially AD are currently acknowledged as one of the most important quality of life and public health concerns of older women. As we have seen, the longer life expectancy of women is indeed associated with a higher risk of AD. Women have higher prevalence rates for AD; however, incidence rates tend to be higher only in the oldest age group. The question whether sex per se is a determinant of AD or not is still the subject of scientific debates. The most prominent explanations of the increased risk of AD in women focus on sociodemographic factors (longer life expectancy of women) and methodological concerns (selection bias, sex-specific attrition), psychosocial factors (more psychosocial stress, lower education of women), genetic and metabolic factors (presence of apolipoprotein E-ε4, which is involved in cholesterol metabolism). There are several hypotheses concerning the possible interaction of these factors on the differential pathogenesis of AD. Considering the uniform single exponential increase with age of AD, with comparable rates in many societies, it is very probable that endogenous genetic–metabolic factors are prominent. However, since these factors are highly related to lifestyle, especially to nutrition, they deserve special attention with regard to primary and secondary prevention of AD.

There is indeed empirical evidence that a multitude of factors related to nutrition as well as essential and nonessential food components, including a growing list of bioactive secondary plant components may, over a long time period, modify neuronal function and regeneration in subtle but important ways. These changes take effect either directly or by slowing or accelerating cerebrovascular disease [131]. Some of the most important factors are the following:

- Nutrition has a long-lasting effect on brain aging and brain function.
- Antioxidants may diminish oxidative stress.
- Fatty acids affect intracellular and extracellular signaling by cytokines.
- Cholesterol influences the Aβ-amyloid formation related to AD.

Since a curative treatment of cognitive impairment such as AD is currently impossible, the treatment of nutrition-related risk factors may have great implications for the prevention of dementia in general and in women in particular. The recommendations made by several scholars in the field point in the same direction: lower caloric intake, a diet with less fat, especially saturated fat and cholesterol, more vitamins, especially folate, vitamins C and E and β-carotenes, more minerals, especially zinc, may be advisable not only to improve the general health of the elderly but also to improve, or at least maintain, cognitive function. In addition, the relationship between polyunsaturated fatty acid intake and lower risk of dementia, including AD, should encourage greater consumption of oils rich in omega-3 fatty acids and of fish or seafood [132]. These dietary recommendations are also aimed at preventing obesity, diabetes, hypertension, coronary artery disease, and stroke, which have been pointed out to be risk factors of dementia.

There is great need for action concerning the aforementioned risk factors. As recent study results have impressively demonstrated, these nutrition-related risk factors are very common in Western society. A population-based multidisciplinary study (NAME-study, $N = 300$ community-based elders aged 60 and older from the Boston area) [133] revealed the high risk status of this population: 31% have either probable or possible AD or VaD, 31% are diabetic, 92% have hypertension, over half are obese (BMI > 30), 36% have renal insufficiency, 16% have deficiency of vitamin B12, 33% have vitamin B6 deficiency, and 42% have elevated plasma homocysteine concentrations. The fact that there is extensive empirical evidence that these risk factors are associated with low education shows the necessity for specific prevention strategies.

Indeed, it has been suggested that the most important prevention of cognitive decline is probably education and the continued use of intellectual faculties [69]. This is not only explained by a greater neuronal functional reserve but also by much more general phenomena relating education to better coping styles, less cardiovascular risk, better nutrition, and more control over life. The importance of education is well documented in aging research. It has been shown that the rate of chronic disability is less than half in individuals with a college or university degree compared with those with less schooling [134]. This has implication for a gender-specific view on AD prevention strategies. As we know, even in Western society, women are still disadvantaged with regard to education, and low education has been identified as a main risk factor for AD especially in women. It has been argued that the relation between AD and low education does not so much result from a direct causality, but reveals factors that condition and determine certain lifestyles—such as malnutrition and decreased physical activity—leading to an increased risk of AD. These lifestyles mirror the still different living contexts of women and men. One basic health-relevant consequence of differential life expectancy is that women have a high likelihood of being caregivers of their frail partners and are far more likely to be widowed or to live alone than older men. This is associated with the fact that women tend to have partners older than themselves. Both conditions imply important health risks such as more psychosocial stress, higher medication rate, loneliness, and mal- or even undernutrition [135,136].

Knowledge of the differential effects of these risk factors for AD is necessary to develop prevention and intervention programs that respond to the specific needs of women and men. However, there are many open questions concerning the gender-specificity of these risk factors. Gender analyses, that is, analyses of the different implications and context of a given disease for men as compared with women, are still often left out of research studies. Another shortcoming of actual research on gender differences in aging and health is the lack of gender-specific prospective and intervention studies. Considering that lifestyles and socialization have a deep impact on cognitive functioning and health, research with a lifespan perspective that takes into account gender aspects should be promoted with high priority.

REFERENCES

1. Beers, M.H. and Berkow, R. (Eds.), *The Merck Manual of Diagnosis and Therapy*, Merck Research Laboratories, Whitehouse Station (NJ), 1999.
2. Heckhausen, J., Dixon, R.A., and Baltes, P.B., Gains and losses in development throughout adulthood as perceived by different adult age groups, *Developm. Psych.*, 25, 109, 1989.
3. Zarit, S.H., Cole, K.D., and Guider, R.L., Memory training strategies and subjective complaints of memory in the aged, *Gerontologist,* 21, 158, 1981.
4. Dobbs, A.R. and Rule, B.G., Prospective memory and self-reports of memory abilities in older adults, *Can. J. Psychol.*, 41, 209, 1987.
5. Perrig-Chiello, P., Perrig, W.J., and Staehelin, H.B., Differential aspects of memory self-evaluation in old and very old people, *Ageing & Mental Health*, 4, 2, 2000.
6. MetLife Foundation Alzheimer's Survey: What America Thinks. Retrieved December 5, 2006, from www.metlife.com/Applications/Corporate/WPS/CDA/PageGenerator/4773, P12046,00.html.
7. Swiss Federal Office of Statistics, 2005, Retrieved December 5, 2006, from www.bfs.admin.ch/bfs/portal/de/index/regionen/gleichstellungsatlas/familien_und_haushaltsformen/blank/aeltere_personen.html.
8. WHO, The World Health Report, 2004. Retrieved November 21, 2006, from http://www3.who.int/whosis/hale/hale.cfm?path=whosis,hale&language=English.
9. Perrig-Chiello, P. and Hoepflinger, F., *Jenseits des Zenits. Frauen und Männer in der zweiten Lebenshälfte*, 2nd edn., Haupt, Bern, 2004.
10. American Psychiatric Association, *Diagnostic and Statistical Manual of Mental Disorders DSM-IV-TR* (4th edn., text revision), American Psychiatric Association, Washington, DC, 2000.
11. Bickel, H., Demenzsyndrom und Alzheimer Krankheit: Eine Schätzung des Krankenbestandes und der jährlichen Neuerkrankungen in Deutschland, *Das Gesundheitswesen*, 62, 211, 2000.

12. Salmon, D.P. and Bondi, M.W., Neuropsychology of Alzheimer disease, in *Alzheimer Disease*, 2nd edn., Salmon, D.P. and Bondi, M.W., Eds., Lippincott Williams & Wilkins, Philadelphia, 1999, p. 39.
13. Munoz, D.G. and Feldman, H., Causes of Alzheimer's disease, *CMAJ*, 162, 65, 2000.
14. Diehl-Schmid, J. et al., Behavioral disturbances in the course of frontotemporal dementia, *Dement. Geriatr. Cogn. Disord.*, 22, 352, 2006.
15. McPherson, S.E. and Cummings, J.L., Neuropsychological aspects of vascular dementia, *J. Cogn. Neurosci.*, 9, 534, 1997.
16. Nussbaum, R.L. and Ellis, C.E., Genomic medicine: Alzheimer's disease and Parkinson's disease, *New Engl. J. Med.*, 348, 1356, 2003.
17. Folstein, M.F. et al., Dementia: Case ascertainment in a community survey, *J. Gerontol.*, 46, M132, 1991.
18. Canadian Study of Health and Aging Working Group, Canadian Study of Health and Aging: Study methods and prevalence of dementia, *Can. Med. Assoc. J.*, 150, 899, 1994.
19. Gao, S. et al., The relationships between age, sex, and the incidence of dementia and Alzheimer's disease: A meta-analysis, *Arch. Gen. Psychiatry*, 55, 809, 1998.
20. Bachman, D.L. et al., Incidence of dementia and probable Alzheimer's disease in a general population: The Framingham Study, *Neurology*, 43, 515, 1993.
21. Swanwick, G. and Lawlor, B.A., Is female sex a risk factor for Alzheimer's disease? *Int. Psychogeriatr.*, 11, 219, 1999.
22. Bachman, D.L. et al., Prevalence of dementia and probable senile dementia of the Alzheimer type in the Framingham Study, *Neurology*, 42,115, 1992.
23. Corso, E.A. et al., Prevalence of moderate and severe Alzheimer's dementia in the population of southeastern Sicily, *Ital. J. Neurol. Sci.*, 13, 215, 1992.
24. Friedland, R.P. et al., Alzheimer's disease prevalence is high in Israeli Arabs, *Neurobiol. Aging*, 19(suppl), S139, 1998.
25. Manubens, J. et al., Prevalence of Alzheimer's disease and other dementing disorders in Pamplona, Spain, *Neuroepidemiology*, 14, 155, 1995.
26. Lopez Pousa, S. et al., The prevalence of dementia in Girona, *Neurologia*, 10, 189, 1995.
27. Kay, D., Beamish, P., and Roth, M., Old age mental disorders in Newcastle-upon-Tyne. Part I: A study of prevalence, *Br. J. Psychiatry*, 110, 146, 1964.
28. Graves, A.B. et al., Prevalence of dementia and its subtypes in the Japanese American population of King County, Washington State: The Kame Project, *Am. J. Epidemiol.*, 144, 760, 1996.
29. Kiyohara, Y. et al., Changing patterns in the prevalence of dementia in a Japanese community: The Hisayama Study, *Gerontology*, 40(suppl 2), 19, 1994.
30. Woo, J.I. et al., Prevalence estimation of dementia in a rural area of Korea, *J. Am. Geriatr. Soc.*, 46, 983, 1998.
31. Zhang, Z., Sex differentials in cognitive impairment and decline of the oldest old in China, *J. Gerontol.*, 61B (2), 107, 2006.
32. Jorm, A.F., Korten, A.E., and Henderson, A.S., The prevalence of dementia: A quantitative integration of the literature, *Acta Psychiatr. Scand.*, 76, 465, 1987.
33. Hofman, A. et al., The prevalence of dementia in Europe: A collaborative study of 1980–1990 findings. Eurodem Prevalence Research Group, *Int. J. Epidemiol.*, 20, 736, 1991.
34. Nilsson, L.V., Incidence of severe dementia in an urban sample followed from 70 to 79 years of age, *Acta Psychiatr. Scand.*, 70, 478, 1984.
35. Jarvik, L.F., Ruth, V., and Matsuyama, S.S., Organic brain syndrome and aging, *Arch. Gen. Psychiatry*, 37, 280, 1980.

36. Brayne, C. et al., Incidence of clinically diagnosed subtypes of dementia in an elderly population: Cambridge Project for Later Life, *Br. J. Psychiatry*, 167, 255, 1995.
37. Bachman, D.L. et al., Incidence of dementia and probable Alzheimer's disease in a general population: The Framingham Study, *Neurology*, 43, 515, 1993.
38. Hagnell, O. et al., Senile dementia of the Alzheimer type in the Lundby Study. I. A prospective, epidemiological study of incidence and risk during the 15 years 1957–1972, *Eur. Arch. Psychiatry Clin. Neurosci.*, 241, 159, 1991.
39. Åkesson, H.O., A population study of senile and arteriosclerotic psychoses, *Hum. Hered.*, 19, 546, 1969.
40. Yoshitake, T. et al., Incidence and risk factors of vascular dementia and Alzheimer's disease in a defined elderly Japanese population: The Hisayama Study, *Neurology*, 45, 1161, 1995.
41. Aevarsson, O. and Skoog, I., A population-based study on the incidence of dementia disorders between 85 and 88 years of age, *J. Am. Geriatr. Soc.*, 44, 1455, 1996.
42. Jorm, A.F. and Jolley, D., The incidence of dementia: A meta-analysis, *Neurology*, 51, 728, 1998.
43. Andersen, K. et al., Sex differences in the incidence of AD and vascular dementia: The EURODEM studies, *Neurology*, 53, 1992, 1999.
44. Hebert, L.E. et al., Age-specific incidence of Alzheimer's disease in a community population, *JAMA*, 273, 1354, 1995.
45. Fitzpatrick, A.L. et al., Incidence and prevalence of dementia in the Cardiovascular Health Study, *J. Am. Geriatr. Soc.*, 52, 195, 2004.
46. Ruitenberg, A. et al., Incidence of dementia: Does sex make a difference? *Neurobiol. Aging*, 22, 575, 2001.
47. Fratiglioni, L. et al., Very old women at highest risk of dementia and Alzheimer's disease: Incidence data from the Kungsholmen Project, Stockholm, *Neurology*, 48, 132, 1997.
48. Di Carlo, A. et al., Incidence of dementia, Alzheimer's disease, and vascular dementia in Italy. The ILSA study, *J. Am. Geriatr. Soc.*, 50, 41, 2002.
49. Deary, J.A. et al., The impact of childhood intelligence on later life: Following up the Scottish Mental Survey of 1932 and 1947, *J. Pers. Soc. Psych.*, 86, 130, 2004.
50. Meinz, E.J. and Salthouse, T.A., Is age kinder to females than to males? *Psychon. Bull. Rev.*, 5, 56, 1998.
51. Ott, B.R. and Cahn-Weiner, D., Sex differences in Alzheimer's disease, *Geriatric Times*, II, 2001.
52. Gerstorf, D., Herlitz, A., and Smith, J., Stability of sex differences in cognition in advanced old age: The role of education and attrition, *J. Gerontol. B Psychol. Sci. Soc. Sci.*, 61, 245, 2006.
53. Bonsignore, M., Barkow, K., and Heun, R., Possible influences of selection bias on sex differences in the risk of Alzheimer's disease, *Arch. Women's Mental Health*, 5, 73, 2002.
54. Barclay, L.L. et al., Survival in Alzheimer's disease and vascular dementias, *Neurology*, 35, 834, 1985.
55. Jagger, C., Clarke, M., and Stone, A., Predictors of survival with Alzheimer's disease: Community-based study, *Psychol. Med.*, 25, 171, 1995.
56. Breitner, J.C. et al., Familial aggregation in Alzheimer's disease: Comparison of risk among relatives of early- and late-onset cases, and among male and female relatives in successive generations, *Neurology*, 38, 207, 1988.
57. Bauer, J. et al., Premorbid psychological processes in patients with Alzheimer's disease and in patients with vascular dementia, *Z. Gerontol. Geriatr.*, 28, 179, 1995.

58. Shen, Y., A case-control study of risk factors on Alzheimer's disease. Multicenter collaborative study in China, *Chung Hua Shen Ching Ching Shen Ko Tsa Chih*, 25, 284, 1992.
59. Shimamura, K. et al., Environmental factors possibly associated with onset of senile dementia, *Nippon Koshu Eisei Zasshi*, 45, 203, 1998.
60. Katzman, R., Education and the prevalence of dementia and Alzheimer's disease, *Neurology*, 43, 13, 1993.
61. Ott, A. et al., Prevalence of Alzheimer's disease and vascular dementia: Association with education. The Rotterdam Study, *BMJ*, 310, 970, 1995.
62. Evans, D.A. et al., Education and other measures of socioeconomic status and risk of incident Alzheimer disease in a defined population of older persons, *Arch. Neurol.*, 54, 1399, 1997.
63. Letenneur, L. et al., Education and risk for Alzheimer's disease: Sex makes a difference. EURODEM pooled analyses, *Am. J. Epidem.*, 151, 1064, 2000.
64. Kivipelto, M. and Solomon, A., Cholesterol as a risk factor for Alzheimer's disesase—epidemiological evidence, *Acta Neurol. Scand.*, 114(suppl 185), 50, 2006.
65. Corder, E.H. et al., Gene dose of apolipoprotein E type 4 allele and the risk of Alzheimer's disease in late onset families, *Science*, 261, 921, 1993.
66. Molero, A.E., Pino-Ramirez, G., and Maestre, G.E., Modulation by age and sex of risk for Alzheimer's disease and vascular dementia associated with the apolipoprotein E-ε4 allele in Latin Americans: Findings from the Maracaibo Aging study, *Neurosci. Lett.*, 307, 5, 2001.
67. Hofman, A. et al., Atherosclerosis, apolipoprotein and prevalence of dementia and Alzheimer's disease. The Rotterdam Study, *Lancet*, 349, 151, 1997.
68. Lindsay, J. and Anderson, L., Dementia and Alzheimer's disease, *Women's Health Surv. Rep.*, 4(suppl 1), S20, 2004.
69. Staehelin, H.B., Micronutrients and Alzheimer's disease, *Proc. Nutr. Soc.*, 64, 565, 2005.
70. Bryan, J., Calvaresi, E., and Hughes, D., Short-term folate, Vitamin B12, or Vitamin B6 supplementation slightly affects memory performance but not mood in women of various ages, *J. Nutr.*, 132, 1345, 2002.
71. Corrêa Leite, M.L. et al., Nutrition and cognitive deficit in the elderly: A population study, *Europ. J. Clin. Nutr.,* 55, 1053, 2001.
72. Tucker, D.M. et al., Nutrition status and brain function in aging. *Am. J. Clin. Nutr.*, 52, 93, 1990.
73. Bell, I.R. et al., Vitamin B12 and folate status in acute geropsychiatric inpatients: Affective and cognitive characteristics of a vitamin nondeficient population, *Biol. Psychiatry*, 27, 125, 1990.
74. Kozlowski, B.W., Megavitamin treatment of mental retardation in children: A review of effects on behavior and cognition, *J. Child Adol. Psychopharmacol.*, 2, 307, 1992.
75. Volicer, L. and Crino, P.B., Involvement of free radicals in dementia of the Alzheimer type: A hypothesis, *Neurobiol. Aging*, 11, 567, 1990.
76. Evans, P.H., Free radicals in brain metabolism and pathology, *Br. Med. Bull.*, 49, 577, 1993.
77. Fioravanti, M. et al., Low folate levels in the cognitive decline of elderly patients and the efficacy of folate as a treatment for improving memory deficits, *Arch. Gerontol. Geriatr.*, 26, 1, 1997.
78. Salerno-Kennedy, R. and Cashman, K.D., Relationship between dementia and nutrition-related factors and disorders: An Overview, *Int. J. Vit. Nutr. Res.*, 75, 83, 2005.
79. Perrig, W.J., Perrig, P., and Staehelin, H.B., The relation between antioxidants and memory performance in the old and very old, *J. Am. Geriatr. Soc.*, 45, 718, 1997.

80. Grodstein, F., Chen, J., and Willett, W.C., High-dose antioxidant supplements and cognitive function in community-dwelling elderly women, *Am. J. Clin. Nutr.*, 77, 975, 2003.
81. Manders, M. et al., Effectiveness of nutritional supplements on cognitive functioning in elderly persons: A systematic review, *J. Gerontol. A Biol. Sci. Med. Sci.*, 59, M1041, 2004.
82. Gonzalez-Gross, M., Marcos, A., and Pietrzik, K., Nutrition and cognitive impairment in the elderly, *Brit. J. Nutr.*, 86, 313, 2001.
83. Harman, D., Free-radical theory of aging. Increasing the functional life span, *Ann. NY Acad. Sci.*, 717, 1, 1994.
84. Lau, F.C., Shukitt-Hale, B., and Joseph, J.A., The beneficial effects of fruit polyphenols on brain aging, *Neurobiol. Aging*, 26S, 128, 2005.
85. Helmer, C. et al., Association between antioxidant nutritional indicators and the incidence of dementia: Results from the PAQUID prospective cohort study, *Europ. J. Clin. Nutr.*, 57, 1555, 2003.
86. Engelhart, M.J. et al., Dietary intake of antioxidants and risk of Alzheimer disease, *JAMA,* 287, 3223, 2002.
87. Morris, M.C. et al., Dietary intake of antioxidant nutrients and the risk of incident Alzheimer disease in a biracial community study, *JAMA*, 287, 3230, 2002.
88. Vital Trial Collaboration Group, Effect of vitamins and aspirin on markers of platelet activation, oxidative stress and homocysteine in people at high risk of dementia, *J. Int. Med.*, 254, 67, 2003.
89. Tabet, N. et al., Vitamin E for Alzheimer's disease, *The Cochrane Library*, 3, 2006.
90. Sano, M. et al., A controlled trial of selegiline, α-tocopherol, or both as a treatment for Alzheimer's disease, *New Engl. J. Med.*, 336, 1216, 1997.
91. Institute of Medicine, Food and Nutrition Board, Dietary reference tables, Retrieved December 5, 2006, from http://www.iom.edu/?id=15072.
92. Joseph, J.A. et al., Long-term dietary strawberry, spinach, or Vitamin E supplementation retards the onset of age-related neuronal signal transduction and cognitive behavioral deficits, *J. Neurosci.*, 18, 8047, 1998.
93. Jospeh, J.A. et al., Reversals of age-related declines in neuronal signal transduction, cognitive and motor behavioral deficits with blueberry, spinach or strawberry dietary supplementation, *J. Neurosci.*, 19, 8114, 1999.
94. Casadeus, G. et al., Modulation of hippocampal plasticity and cognitive behavior by short-term blueberry supplementation in aged rats, *Nutr. Neurosci.*, 7, 309, 2004.
95. Kessler, H. et al., Zur Bedeutung von Kupfer für die Pathophysiologie der Alzheimer-Krankheit, *Nervenarzt*, 76, 581, 2005.
96. Religa, D. et al., Elevated cortical zinc in Alzheimer disease, *Neurology*, 67, 69, 2006.
97. Kawahara, M., Effects of aluminum on the nervous system and its possible link with neurodegenerative diseases, *J. Alzheimers Dis.*, 8, 171, 2005.
98. Carpenter, D.O., Effects of metals on the nervous system of humans and animals, *Int. J. Occup. Med. Environm. Health*, 14, 209, 2001.
99. Martyn, C.N. et al., Geographic relation between Alzheimer's disease and aluminium in drinking water, *Lancet*, 1, 59, 1989.
100. Mainous III, A.G. et al., Cholesterol, transferrin saturation, and the development of dementia and Alzheimer's disease: Results from an 18-year population-based cohort, *Fam. Med.*, 37, 36, 2005.
101. Luchsinger, J.A. et al., Caloric intake and the risk of Alzheimer disease, *Arch. Neurol.*, 59, 1258, 2002.

102. Wang, J. et al., Caloric restriction attenuates β-amyloid neuropathology in a mouse model of Alzheimer's disease, *FASEB J.*, 19, 659, 2005.
103. Mielke, M.M. et al., High total cholesterol levels in late life associated with a reduced risk of dementia, *Neurology*, 64, 1689, 2005.
104. Li, G. et al., Serum cholesterol and risk of Alzheimer disease: A community-based cohort study, *Neurology*, 65, 1045, 2005.
105. Panza, F. et al., Lipid metabolism in cognitive decline and dementia, *Brain Res. Rev.*, 51, 275, 2006.
106. Stewart, R. and Liolitsa, D., Type 2 diabetes mellitus, cognitive impairment and dementia, *Diabet. Med.*, 16, 93, 1999.
107. Biessels, G.J. and Kapelle, L.J., Increased risk of Alzheimer's disease in type II diabetes: Insulin resistance of the brain or insulin induced amyloid pathology? *Biochem. Soc. Trans.*, 33, 1041, 2005.
108. Greenwood, C.E. and Winocur, G., High-fat diets, insulin resistance and declining cognitive function, *Neurobiol. Aging*, 26S, 42, 2005.
109. Cole, G.M. et al., Prevention of Alzheimer's disease: Omega-3 fatty acids and phenolic anti-oxidant interventions, *Neurobiol. Aging*, 26S, 133, 2005.
110. Keenan, P.A. et al., Prefrontal cortex as the site of estrogen's effect on cognition, *Psychoneuroendocrinology*, 26, 577, 2001.
111. McEwen, B.S., Estrogen's effects on the brain: Multiple sites and molecular mechanisms, *J. Appl. Physiol.*, 91, 2785, 2001.
112. Smith, Y.R. et al., Long-term estrogen replacement is associated with improved nonverbal memory and attentional measures in postmenopausal women, *Fertil. Steril.*, 76, 1101, 2001.
113. Zec, R.F. and Trivedi, M., The effects of estrogen replacement therapy on neuropsychological functioning in postmenopausal women with and without dementia: A critical and theorietical review, *Neuropsych. Rev.*, 12, 65, 2002.
114. Tang, M.X. et al., Effect of oestrogen during menopause on risk and age at onset of Alzheimer's disease, *Lancet*, 348, 429, 1996.
115. Van Gorp, T. and Neven, P., Endometrial safety of hormone replacement therapy: Review of literature, *Maturitas*, 42, 93, 2002.
116. Rossouw, J.E. et al., Risks and benefits of estrogen plus progestin in healthy postmenopausal women: Principal results from the Women's Health Initiative randomized controlled trial, *JAMA*, 288, 321, 2002.
117. Shumaker, S.A. et al., Estrogen plus progestin and the incidence of dementia and mild cognitive impairment in postmenopausal women: The Women's Health Initiative Memory Study: A randomized controlled trial, *JAMA*, 289, 2651, 2003.
118. Writing Group for the Women's Health Initiative Investigators, Risks and benefits of estrogen plus progestin in healthy postmenopausal women: Principal results from the women's health initiative randomized controlled trial, *JAMA*, 288, 321, 2002.
119. Rice, M.M. et al., Postmenopausal estrogen and estrogen-progestin use and 2-year rate of cognitive change in a cohort of older Japanese American women: The Kame Project, *Arch. Intern. Med.*, 160, 1641, 2000.
120. Nilsen, J. and Brinton, R.D., Impact of progestins on estrogen-induced neuroprotection: Synergy by progesterone and 19-norprogesterone and antagonism by medroxyprogesterone acetate, *Endocrinology*, 143, 205, 2002.
121. Morley, J.E., Testosterone and behavior, *Clin. Geriatr. Med.*, 19, 605, 2003.
122. Baum, L.W., Sex, hormones and Alzheimer's disease, *J. Gerontol. A Biol. Sci. Med. Sci.*, 60A, 736, 2005.

123. Chiechi, L.M., Dietary phytoestrogens in the prevention of long-term postmenopausal diseases, *Int. J. Gynaecol. Obstet.*, 67, 39, 1999.
124. Miksicek, R.J., Estrogenic flavonoids: Structural requirements for biological activity, *Proc. Soc. Exp. Biol. Med.*, 208, 44, 1995.
125. de Kleijn, M.J. et al., Intake of dietary phytoestrogens is low in postmenopausal women in the United States: The Framingham study (1–4), *J. Nutr.*, 131, 1826, 2001.
126. Knight, D.C. and Eden, J.A., Phytoestrogens—A short review, *Maturitas*, 22, 167, 1995.
127. Kuiper, G.G. et al., Interaction of estrogenic chemicals and phytoestrogens with estrogen receptor-β, *Endocrinology*, 139, 4252, 1998.
128. File, S.E. et al., Eating soya improves human memory, *Psychopharmacology* (Berl.), 157, 430, 2001.
129. Franco, O.H. et al., Higher dietary intake of lignans is associated with better cognitive performance in postmenopausal women, *J. Nutr.*, 135, 1190, 2005.
130. Perrig-Chiello, P. et al., Impact of physical and psychological resources on functional autonomy in old age, *Psych. Health Med.*, 11, 470, 2006.
131. Staehelin, H.B., Role of nutrition in prevention or delay of Alzheimer's disease, in *Alzheimer's Disease—A physician's Guide to Practical Management*, Richter R.W. and Zoeller Richter B., Eds., Humana Press, Totowa, New Jersey, 2004.
132. Salerno-Kennedy, R. and Cashman, K.D., The role of nutrition in dementia: An overview, *J. Brit. Menopause Soc.*, 12, 44, 2006.
133. Scott, T.M. et al., The nutrition, aging, and memory in elders (NAME) study: Design and methods for a study of micronutrients and cognitive function in a homebound elderly population, *Int. J. Geriatr. Psychiatry,* 21, 519–528, 2006.
134. Manton, K.G. et al., Education-specific estimates of life-expectancy and age-specific diability in the US elderly population: 1982 to 1991, *J. Aging Health*, 9, 419, 1997.
135. Callen, B.L. and Welsh, T.J., Screening for nutritional risk in community-dwelling old–old, *Public Health Nurs.*, 22, 138, 2005.
136. Castel, H., Shahar, D., and Harman-Boehm, I., Sex differences in factors associated with nutritional status of older medical patients, *J. Am. Coll. Nutr.*, 25, 128, 2006.

16 Depression and Psychiatric Disorders

Christina P.C. Borba and David C. Henderson

CONTENTS

16.1 INTRODUCTION

Diet and nutrition is a well-studied, critical part of many disease states that commonly affect women including obesity, hypertension, diabetes mellitus, and cardiovascular disease. However, much less is known regarding the role of diet and nutrition in psychiatric disorders such as depression and other mood disorders, schizophrenia, and anxiety disorders. This chapter will review the available data on diet and nutrition and psychiatric disorders, with a specific focus on women.

16.2 ETIOLOGY OF MENTAL ILLNESS AND ROLE OF NUTRITION

Diet has the potential to affect mental health and well-being at every stage of life. The development of the brain at conception, during pregnancy, and throughout the first 3 years of life is a critical stage in this process [1]. Infants born at full term and at a healthy weight have physical and cognitive advantages over other preterm or low-weight babies, with differences recorded in IQ, language, and reading ability [2–4]. Studies have also shown that infants with low birth weights are less cooperative, less active, less alert, and less happy than normal weight infants [5]. Diet and nutrition continue to play a critical role in childhood development and have a contributory influence on mental health. Researchers have stated that the changes in nutrition provided in school and at home over the past 20 years may be a contributing factor to the rise of mental health problems in childhood and adolescence [6].

16.2.1 DEPRESSION

Problems in mental health have been increasing, with depression predicted to become the second highest cause of global disease [7]. Research indicates that food plays an important role in the development, management, and prevention of mental health illnesses such as depression, bipolar disorder, and schizophrenia [8–14]. The brain requires different amounts of complex carbohydrates, essential fatty acids, amino acids, vitamins and minerals, and water to remain healthy [15]. Food can have an immediate and lasting effect on mental health and behavior because of the way it affects the structure and function of the brain [15]. For example, rates of depression have been shown to be higher in countries with low intakes of fish [15]. Lack of folic acid, omega-3 fatty acids, selenium, and the amino acid tryptophan are thought to play an important role in mental illness and deficiencies of essential fats and antioxidant vitamins are also thought to be a contributory factor [15]. Fish consumption is reported to have an association with better moods and a higher self-reported mental health [16]. Evidence also suggests that unequal or insufficient intakes of omega-3 and omega-6 fats are implicated in a number of mental health problems [17].

16.2.2 SCHIZOPHRENIA

A cross sectional study was conducted examining the dietary intake of 88 patients with schizophrenia [18]. The data was compared to the general population from the National Health and Nutrition Examination Survey (NHANES). Patients with schizophrenia had higher body mass indexes; however, they consumed significantly fewer calories, carbohydrates, protein, total fat, saturated fat, monounsaturated fatty acid, polyunsaturated fatty acid, fiber, folate, sodium, and alcohol but consumed significantly more caffeine than the NHANES group [18]. Overall, patients with schizophrenia consumed less food than those in the general population; however, the data suggests that their diet is of poor nutritional quality. In this study, patients with schizophrenia did not meet the USDA's recommendations for vegetables, fruits, and grains [18]. Patients with mental illness tend to consume more convenience foods and snacks and a pattern of missed meals may account for the reduction in total caloric intake [18].

A community-based study of 102 schizophrenia patients in Scotland, assessed diet, smoking, weight, and exercise habits to determine cardiovascular disease (CVD) risk and compared them with the general population [19]. Results indicated that patients with schizophrenia made poorer dietary choices, consumed fewer servings of fruits and vegetables, were less physically active, were more obese or overweight, and smoked more compared to the general population [19]. Another study of 102 schizophrenia patients found that they consumed diets higher in fat and lower in fiber than the reference population [20].

Although mental illness results from a complex interplay of biological, psychological, social, and environmental factors, diet should be an everyday component of mental health care. The role for nutrition is currently being examined in the etiology and treatment of neurological and psychiatric disorders. Some researchers believe that the future of psychiatry is in nutrition. Additionally, investigators have hypothesized that fatty acids can play a role in the etiology of psychiatric disorders, specifically, lower levels of n-3 and n-6 essential fatty acids [21].

Deficiencies in vitamins and minerals are sometimes implicated in a number of mental health problems [22–24]. Vitamins work as antioxidants, which protect the brain from the damaging process of oxidation. Vitamins and minerals also play a critical role in the conversion of carbohydrates into glucose, and fatty acids into components of healthy brain cells such as amino acids and neurotransmitters. As such, they are vital in promoting and maintaining positive mental health. This has also been observed for vitamins C, B12, and B2 and has led to research on the mood effects of depleting or supplementing various nutrients [22–24].

16.2.3 Mood

One double blind, placebo-controlled trial supplemented 129 participants' diet with nine separate vitamins, at over 10 times the recommended daily level, for 1 year [25]. After 12 months, the mood of females taking the vitamin supplement was significantly improved in that they felt more composed and reported better mental health. Their baseline thiamine status was associated with poor mood and an improvement in thiamine status after 3 months was associated with improved mood [25]. The same study also found that female attention levels improved in those taking the supplements versus males who were taking the supplements [26].

Thiamine, or vitamin B1, has also been the subject of a number of studies. Several placebo-controlled trials have demonstrated that subjects with low thiamine levels experienced low mood, irritability and fatigue, and their mood improved when their thiamine levels were increased [27–30]. A low selenium status has also been associated with poor mood [31] and selenium supplementation has led to improvements in mental health [32]. Another study, which removed selenium from some of the study participants' diets, recorded increased levels of hostility and depressed moods when the selenium status decreased, compared with subjects with normal selenium levels [33]. Similar results have been found in studies examining iron deficiency [34].

16.3 MENTAL HEALTH ILLNESSES AND SPECIFIC DIET COMPONENTS

16.3.1 Depression and Bipolar Disorder

Depression is one of the most common mental health problems and the incidence has increased over recent decades [6] which has been accompanied by a decrease in the age of onset. Significant increases have been reported in children, adolescents, and young adults [35].

16.3.1.1 Essential Fatty Acids

A number of studies have linked the intake of certain foods and nutrients with the reported prevalence of different types of depression. Several depression studies have examined the intake of essential fatty acids (EFAs) by measuring intake and the amount of fish or seafood consumed. Correlations have been found between low intake of fish and high levels of depression. The reverse has been shown for major depression [9], postnatal depression [10], seasonal affective disorder [8], and bipolar disorder [11]. Another study examined the change in diets of people living in the Arctic and Subarctic regions and observed that levels of depression rose at the same time that traditional diets, which were high in EFAs, were being abandoned for more processed foods [36]. These findings have prompted many studies investigating the effectiveness of EFAs in treating depression and bipolar disorder. A number of case studies show effects of omega-3 supplementation on depressive symptoms. One of the studies supplied eicosapentaenoic acid (EPA), an n-3 fat, as an additional treatment to an individual who had previously not shown improvement with antidepressants [37]. Nine months after beginning treatment with EPA, all depressive symptoms had disappeared. This study also found that the EPA treatment was accompanied by a reduction in the lateral ventricular volume of the brain [37]. Similar results have been found in controlled trials of EPA for bipolar disorder [38] and clinical depression [39,40].

Another study conducted by Mischoulon and Fava [41] examined the consumption of docosahexaenoic acid (DHA) and the association with depression. Individuals with major depression had marked depletions in n-3 fatty acids, especially DHA, compared with controls. This data suggests that a low level of DHA may be associated with depression and that supplementation with DHA or other n-3 fatty acids has beneficial psychotropic effects [41].

16.3.1.2 Vitamins and Minerals

One study of over 2000 subjects found a correlation between dietary intake of folate or folic acid and depression. Those with low intakes of folate were significantly more likely to be diagnosed with depression than those with higher intakes [42]. These findings have been replicated in other populations [43]. However, recently many countries have added folate additives to many food products to offset the low folate levels in the general population [43]. Similarly, studies have examined the association of depression with low levels of zinc and vitamins B1, B2, and C [44,45].

Supplementing standard treatments with these nutrients resulted in greater relief of symptoms of depression and bipolar disorder and in some cases by as much as 50% [44,45].

16.3.1.3 Amino Acids

There is evidence that consuming tryptophan leads to an increase of brain serotonin and removing it from the diet reduces serotonin [46]. Tryptophan, one of the eight essential amino acids, is present in protein foods and plays a role in a number of biochemical reactions in the body. Tryptophan is used in protein synthesis, is converted into niacin (vitamin B3), and enters the brain to be transformed into the neurotransmitter serotonin. Serotonin, a key brain chemical, is responsible for producing, among other things, a feeling of calm and well-being and has a major impact on depression and anxiety disorders [47].

16.3.2 Schizophrenia

Schizophrenia is a severe mental illness characterized by hallucinations, delusions, and disordered thinking. It occurs in approximately 1% of the population. High rates of medical morbidity and excess mortality have long been associated with chronic mental illness, particularly schizophrenia. Medical morbidity remains the domain least improved by recent treatment advances, at least in part due to unhealthy lifestyles, medication side effects, and inadequate medical care. Whereas a meta-analysis of 18 international studies published in 1997 found a mean 1.5-fold elevation in mortality rates for people with chronic mental illness [48], some reports suggest that mortality rates have been increasing in recent decades, possibly as a result of deinstitutionalization [49–51]. Nutrition plays a major role in this. Symptoms of schizophrenia may influence dietary intake and dietary intake may also influence symptoms. Additionally, medications commonly used to treat schizophrenia may increase appetite, cravings for carbohydrates or fatty foods, and impair satiety [18,52,53].

16.3.2.1 Fats

In a Danish study that compared the amount of fat in the average national diet, the researchers found significant correlations between low intakes of saturated fats and lower rates of schizophrenia [12]. Also, where there were higher percentages of fat from vegetables, fish, and seafood, there were reduced rates of schizophrenia [12]. This evidence is consistent with the observation that people with schizophrenia have lower levels of polyunsaturated fatty acids (PUFAs) in their bodies than those without schizophrenia [54,55]. As with depression and bipolar disorder, one of the primary contributors is omega-3 fatty acid [56]. A number of studies observed reductions in symptoms with higher intakes of this fatty acid [57–59]. These studies have led to larger randomized placebo-controlled trials. Peet et al. [58] attempted to distinguish between the effect of the two fatty acids, EPA and DHA. A total of 45 schizophrenic patients on stable antipsychotic medication were still symptomatic when treated with EPA, DHA, or placebo for 3 months. However, subjects receiving

EPA showed statistically significant improvement in their symptoms measured by the Positive and Negative Syndrome Scale (PANSS) total score compared to patients receiving DHA or placebo [58].

16.3.2.2 Antioxidants and Vitamins

Clinical trials testing the efficacy of treating schizophrenia with antioxidants and vitamins have proved inconclusive. One double blind, placebo-controlled trial testing vitamin B6 showed no improvement in schizophrenia symptoms [60]. Another trial that tested supplementation with vitamins showed no improvement in symptoms or behavior over 5 months in spite of raising vitamin levels in the body [61]. However, a controlled trial supplementing folate-deficient schizophrenia patients with folate did show improvements in symptoms over the 6 month trial [62]. Food intake was assessed in 44 patients with a diagnosis of schizophrenia or schizoaffective disorder using a 4 day dietary record [52]. Estimated intake of individual nutrient totals were calculated by the Minnesota Nutrient Database. Psychopathology was assessed using the PANSS. Schizophrenia patients' folate intake correlated with their serum folate levels and their serum folate levels also correlated with the PANSS negative symptoms subscale score. Smoking status was found to have a significant impact on serum folate levels. These results suggest that food intake and smoking may play a role in low folate levels in patients with schizophrenia [52].

In addition to folate status, vitamin D may have an important role in the etiology of schizophrenia. A birth cohort study in Finland found an association with vitamin D supplementation during early life and a lower incidence of schizophrenia in males, but not females [63].

16.3.3 Conclusion

There is extensive evidence linking diet to mental health. The scientific evidence points to the important role nutrition has in the prevention and treatment of specific mental health problems. It is imperative that individuals are given the resources that enable them to incorporate dietary changes alongside their other care options.

16.4 WOMEN, MENTAL ILLNESS, AND NUTRITION

Women's health concerns cover a wide spectrum. While many health conditions affect both men and women, a number of health issues affect only women and some are more prevalent in women. In addition, a number of medical conditions may cause different symptoms in women, affect women differently than men, and require different treatment or prevention approaches.

Besides conditions such as menopause, ovarian and cervical cancer, and pregnancy, which are unique to women, other medical conditions play a large role in women's health. Breast cancer and osteoporosis are thought of as women's health concerns, although they do occur in men. Heart disease is a serious concern to both men and women, but risk factors and preventive strategies differ in women and women may experience different symptoms of an impending heart attack than men.

Mental illness is associated with a significant burden of morbidity and disability. Sex is a critical determinant of mental health and mental illness. Sex differences occur particularly in the rates of common mental disorders such as depression, anxiety, and somatic complaints. These disorders, in which women predominate, affect approximately one in three people in the community and constitute a serious public health problem [64].

Major depression is twice as common in women and is more persistent in women than in men. There are no marked sex differences in the rates of severe mental disorders such as schizophrenia and bipolar disorder. However, sex differences have been reported in areas such as age of onset of symptoms, frequency of psychotic symptoms, course of the disorders, social adjustment, and long-term outcomes [64].

16.4.1 Depression

Most studies have found clear sex differences in the prevalence of depressive disorders. Typically, studies report that women have a prevalence rate for depression up to twice that of men and sex differences in depression appear to be at their greatest during reproductive years [65]. For example, Kessler et al. [66] conducted the National Co-Morbidity Survey to examine psychiatric disorders among noninstitutionalized civilian population aged 15–54 in the United States. Approximately 50% of respondents reported one or more lifetime psychiatric disorders, with the most common being major depressive episode, alcohol dependence, social phobia, and simple phobia. Women were approximately two-thirds more likely than men to experience affective disorders and anxiety disorders, while men had elevated rates of substance abuse and antisocial personality disorder [66].

Because women have special requirements for specific micronutrients, further attention should be given to the role of minerals such as calcium and iron. Low calcium intake appears to be one important factor in the development of osteoporosis which women have a greater risk than men of developing [67]. Additionally, a number of studies have observed a reduced quality of life in women with osteoporosis, with or without fractures [68–70]. Bianchi et al. [70] found that women affected by osteoporosis perceived it as a disease resulting in undesirable consequences on their personal life, including chronic pain (66% of women with fractures and 40% of women without fractures), impaired physical ability, reduced social activity, poor well-being (21% of women without fractures), and depressed mood (42% of women irrespective of fractures). Forty-one percent of the women showed a reduced quality of life compared with only 11% in the control group. Additionally, women require more iron intake than men, as they lose an average of 15–20 mg of iron each month during menstruation. Anemia, caused by iron deficiency, can develop and cause symptoms that include fatigue and headaches which can mimic symptoms of depression [67].

16.4.2 Schizophrenia

A study conducted by Hafner et al. [71] indicates that men and women have an equal lifetime risk for schizophrenia. However, schizophrenia tends to strike women 3–4 years later than men. Most men develop schizophrenia between 15 and 25 years of age.

For women, the period of maximum onset is between 15 and 30 with a smaller increase between 45 and 50 (after menopause). Women also tend to have milder forms of the disease in their younger years than their male counterparts do. But, in the postmenopausal years, women often have a renewed onset of psychotic symptoms and a worse course of the disease where symptoms in men tend to decrease in severity [71].

Hafner et al. [71] attributes the delayed onset of schizophrenia in women to the protective effects of estrogen. Higher levels of estrogen in women than in men may delay the onset and decrease the severity of schizophrenia. After menopause, women's estrogen levels decrease and disease symptoms that were delayed manifest themselves [71].

There is no difference, other than age, in the symptom-related course of the disease between men and women. However, when interviewed about the social course of the disease and life satisfaction, women tended to have a better prognosis than men [71] and some positive factors such as family involvement are more common in women. Schizophrenia is a debilitating disease and its onset tends to halt or severely hinder social and emotional development. Girls tend to mature faster during childhood than boys and tend to develop schizophrenia several years later. So even though social development decreases equally in women and men, women have higher baseline of development when they become ill.

16.4.3 Conclusion

Science is just beginning to comprehend the complex relationship between sex and mental illness. In addition, women's unique life circumstances, for example, pregnancy, postpartum, and postmenopausal periods need closer examination in how they relate to the management and treatment of mental illness. Recently, there has been growing evidence supporting the relationship between diet and mood and behavior. It is clear that a healthy and balanced diet contributes to the stable maintenance of the brain's vital function. Nutrients play a critical role in mental health, however, mental illnesses affect women and men differently and furthermore, the field of nutrition, mental illness, and their relationship to sex is not well understood.

16.5 FUTURE RESEARCH

Nutrition and mental illness is starting to receive the attention it warrants, however, sex specific research on nutrition and the promotion of mental health is an area of much needed future work. Due to sex bias, women are more likely to be prescribed mood altering psychotropic drugs [64] and doctors are more likely to diagnose depression in women compared with men. This bias exists even when men and women have similar scores on standardized measures of depression or present with identical symptoms [64]. Women are also more likely to seek help from and disclose mental health problems to their primary health care physician while men are more likely to seek specialist mental health care and are the principal users of inpatient care [64]. If we are to promote nutrition as a form of prevention and treatment of mental illness, then the field must move in the direction of sex-based research so both women and men can benefit in having a better mental health. While studies examining the role of nutrition and psychiatric disorders, including schizophrenia, depression and bipolar disorder, are ongoing with many focusing on omega-3 fatty acid, studies investigating the potential benefits of supplementation with various vitamins and amino acids are warranted.

REFERENCES

1. Lanphear, B.P., Vorhees, C.V., and Bellinger, D.C., Protecting children from environmental toxins, *Proc. Med.*, 2, e61, 2005.
2. Rubin, R.A., Rosenblatt, C., and Balow, B., Psychological and educational sequelae of prematurity, *Pediatrics*, 52, 352, 1973.
3. Osmond, C. and Barker, D.J., Fetal, infant, and childhood growth are predictors of coronary heart disease, diabetes, and hypertension in adult men and women, *Environ. Health Perspect.*, 3, 545, 2000.
4. Middle, C., et al., Birthweight and health and development at the age of 7 years, *Child Care Health Dev.*, 22, 55, 1996.
5. Grantham-McGregor, S.M., Small for gestational age, term babies, in the first six years of life, *Eur. J. Clin. Nutr.*, 52, S59, 1998.
6. WHO, Mental health context: mental health policy and service guidance package, in Geneva, *World Health Organization*, 2003.
7. Murthy R.S., et al, Mental health: new understanding, new hope, *The World Health Report,* 2001.
8. Cott, J. and Hibbeln, J.R., Lack of seasonal mood change in Icelanders, *Am. J. Psychiatry*, 158, 328, 2001.
9. Hibbeln, J.R., Fish consumption and major depression, *Lancet*, 351, 9110, 1998.
10. Hibbeln, J.R., Seafood consumption, the DHA content of mothers' milk and prevalence rates of postpartum depression: a cross-national, ecological analysis, *J. Affect Disord.*, 69, 15, 2002.
11. Noaghiul, S. and Hibbeln, J.R., Cross-national comparisons of seafood consumption and rates of bipolar disorders, *Am. J. Psychiatry*, 160, 2222, 2003.
12. Christensen, O. and Christensen, E., Fat consumption and schizophrenia, *Acta. Psychiatr. Scand.*, 78, 587, 1988.
13. Peet, M., International variations in the outcome of schizophrenia and the prevalence of depression in relation to national dietary practices: an ecological analysis, *Br. J. Psychiatry*, 184, 404, 2004.
14. Hintikka, J., et al., High vitamin B12 level and good treatment outcome may be associated in major depressive disorder, *BMC Psychiatry,* 3, 17, 2003.
15. Lawrence, F., Rise in mental illness linked to unhealthy diets, *The Guardian*, 2006.
16. Silvers, K.M. and Scott K.M., Fish consumption and self-reported physical and mental health status, *Public Health Nutr.*, 5, 427, 2002.
17. Kalmijn, S., et al., Dietary intake of fatty acids and fish in relation to cognitive performance at middle age, *Neurology*, 62, 275, 2004.
18. Henderson, D.C., et al., Dietary intake profile of patients with schizophrenia, *Ann. Clin. Psychiatry*, 18, 99, 2006.
19. McCreadie, R.G., Diet, smoking and cardiovascular risk in people with schizophrenia: descriptive study, *Br. J. Psychiatry*, 183, 534, 2003.
20. Brown, S., et al., The unhealthy lifestyle of people with schizophrenia, *Psychol. Med.*, 29, 697, 1999.

21. Fenton, W.S., Hibbeln, J., and Knable, M., Essential fatty acids, lipid membrane abnormalities, and the diagnosis and treatment of schizophrenia, *Biol. Psychiatry*, 47, 8, 2000.
22. Sterner, R.T. and Price, W.R., Restricted riboflavin: within-subject behavioral effects in humans, *Am. J. Clin. Nutr.*, 26, 150, 1973.
23. Hector, M. and Burton, J.R., What are the psychiatric manifestations of vitamin B12 deficiency? *J. Am. Geriatr. Soc.*, 36, 1105, 1988.
24. Kinsman, R.A. and Hood, J., Some behavioral effects of ascorbic acid deficiency, *Am. J. Clin. Nutr.*, 24, 455, 1971.
25. Benton, D., Haller, J., and Fordy, J., Vitamin supplementation for 1 year improves mood, *Neuropsychobiology*, 32, 98, 1995.
26. Benton, D., Fordy, J., and Haller, J., The impact of long-term vitamin supplementation on cognitive functioning, *Psychopharmacology*, 117, 298, 1995.
27. Benton, D., Selenium intake, mood and other aspects of psychological functioning, *Nutr. Neurosci.*, 5, 363, 2002.
28. Benton, D., Griffiths, R., and Haller, J., Thiamine supplementation mood and cognitive functioning, *Psychopharmacology*, 129, 66, 1997.
29. Smidt, L.J., et al., Influence of thiamin supplementation on the health and general well-being of an elderly Irish population with marginal thiamin deficiency, *J. Gerontol.*, 46, M16, 1991.
30. Brozek, J. and Caster W.O., Psychologic effects of thiamine restriction and deprivation in normal young men, *Am. J. Clin. Nutr.*, 5, 109, 1957.
31. Benton, D. and Cook, R., The impact of selenium supplementation on mood, *Biol. Psychiatry*, 29, 1092, 1991.
32. Hawkes, W.C. and Hornbostel, L., Effects of dietary selenium on mood in healthy men living in a metabolic research unit, *Biol. Psychiatry*, 39, 121, 1996.
33. Rangan, A.M., Blight, G.D., and Binns, C.W., Iron status and non-specific symptoms of female students, *J. Am. Coll. Nutr.*, 17, 351, 1998.
34. Leyton, M., et al., Effects on mood of acute phenylalanine/tyrosine depletion in healthy women, *Neuropsychopharmacology*, 22, 52, 2000.
35. Klerman, G.L., The current age of youthful melancholia. Evidence for increase in depression among adolescents and young adults, *Br. J. Psychiatry*, 152, 4, 1988.
36. McGrath-Hanna, N.K., et al., Diet and mental health in the Arctic: is diet an important risk factor for mental health in circumpolar peoples?—a review, *Int. J. Circumpolar Health*, 62, 228, 2003.
37. Puri, B.K., et al., Eicosapentaenoic acid in treatment-resistant depression associated with symptom remission, structural brain changes and reduced neuronal phospholipid turnover, *Int. J. Clin. Pract.*, 55, 560, 2001.
38. Stoll, A.L., et al., Omega 3 fatty acids in bipolar disorder: a preliminary double-blind, placebo-controlled trial, *Arch. Gen. Psychiatry*, 56, 407, 1999.
39. Nemets, B., Stahl, Z., and Belmaker, R.H., Addition of omega-3 fatty acid to maintenance medication treatment for recurrent unipolar depressive disorder, *Am. J. Psychiatry*, 159, 477, 2002.
40. Peet, M. and Horrobin, D.F., A dose-ranging study of the effects of ethyl-eicosapentaenoate in patients with ongoing depression despite apparently adequate treatment with standard drugs, *Arch. Gen. Psychiatry*, 59, 913, 2002.
41. Mischoulon, D. and Fava, M., Docosahexanoic acid and omega-3 fatty acids in depression, *Psychiatr. Clin. North Am.*, 23, 785, 2000.
42. Tolmunen, T., et al., Dietary folate and the risk of depression in Finnish middle-aged men. A prospective follow-up study, *Psychother. Psychosom.*, 73, 334, 2004.

43. Ramos, M.I., et al., Plasma folate concentrations are associated with depressive symptoms in elderly Latina women despite folic acid fortification, *Am. J. Clin. Nutr.*, 80, 1024, 2004.
44. Nowak, G., et al., Effect of zinc supplementation on antidepressant therapy in unipolar depression: a preliminary placebo-controlled study, *Pol. J. Pharmacol.*, 55, 1143, 2003.
45. Kaplan, B.J., et al., Effective mood stabilization with a chelated mineral supplement: an open-label trial in bipolar disorder, *J. Clin. Psychiatry*, 62, 936, 2001.
46. Delgado, P.L., et al., Serotonin function and the mechanism of antidepressant action. Reversal of antidepressant-induced remission by rapid depletion of plasma tryptophan, *Arch. Gen. Psychiatry,* 47, 411, 1990.
47. Christensen, L., Diet–behavior relationships: focus on depression, Washington, *American Psychological Association*, 1996.
48. Brown, S., Excess mortality of schizophrenia. A meta-analysis, *Br. J. Psychiatry*, 171, 502, 1997.
49. Hansen, V., Jacobsen, B.K., and Arnesen, E., Cause-specific mortality in psychiatric patients after deinstitutionalisation, *Br. J. Psychiatry,* 179, 438, 2001.
50. Osby, U., et al., Time trends in schizophrenia mortality in Stockholm county, Sweden: cohort study, *BMJ*, 321, 483, 2000.
51. Osby, U., et al., Mortality and causes of death in schizophrenia in Stockholm county, Sweden, *Schizophr. Res.*, 45, 21, 2000.
52. Borba, C.P., et al., Correlation of food intake, serum folate levels and negative symptoms in patients with schizophrenia, *in New Clinical Drug Evaluation Unit (NCDEU)*, Boca Raton, Florida, 2005.
53. Henderson, D.C., et al., Clozapine, diabetes mellitus, weight gain, and lipid abnormalities: a five-year naturalistic study, *Am. J. Psychiatry*, 157, 975, 2000.
54. Glen, A.I., et al., A red cell membrane abnormality in a subgroup of schizophrenic patients: evidence for two diseases, *Schizophr. Res.*, 12, 53, 1994.
55. Peet, M., et al., Depleted red cell membrane essential fatty acids in drug-treated schizophrenic patients, *J. Psychiatr. Res.,* 29, 227, 1995.
56. Mellor, J.E., Laugharne, J.D., and Peet, M., Schizophrenic symptoms and dietary intake of n-3 fatty acids, *Schizophr. Res.*, 18, 85, 1995.
57. Puri, B.K., et al., Eicosapentaenoic acid treatment in schizophrenia associated with symptom remission, normalisation of blood fatty acids, reduced neuronal membrane phospholipid turnover and structural brain changes, *Int. J. Clin. Pract.,* 54, 57, 2000.
58. Peet, M., et al., Two double-blind placebo-controlled pilot studies of eicosapentaenoic acid in the treatment of schizophrenia, *Schizophr. Res.*, 49, 243, 2001.
59. Emsley, R., et al., Randomized, placebo-controlled study of ethyl-eicosapentaenoic acid as supplemental treatment in schizophrenia, *Am. J. Psychiatry*, 159, 1596, 2002.
60. Lerner, V., et al., Vitamin B6 as add-on treatment in chronic schizophrenic and schizoaffective patients: a double-blind, placebo-controlled study, *J. Clin. Psychiatry*, 63, 54, 2002.
61. Vaughan, K. and McConaghy, N., Megavitamin and dietary treatment in schizophrenia: a randomized, controlled trial, *Aust. N. Z. J. Psychiatry*, 33, 84, 1999.
62. Godfrey, P.S., et al., Enhancement of recovery from psychiatric illness by methylfolate, *Lancet*, 336, 392, 1990.
63. McGrath, J., et al., Vitamin D supplementation during the first year of life and risk of schizophrenia: a Finnish birth cohort study, *Schizophr. Res.*, 67, 237, 2004.
64. WHO, Gender and women's mental health, 2006.
65. Bebbington, P., The origins of sex differences in depressive disorder: bridging the gap, *International Review of Psychiatry*, 8, 295, 1996.

66. Kessler, R.C., et al., Lifetime and 12-month prevalence of DSM-III-R psychiatric disorders in the United States. Results from the National Comorbidity Survey, *Arch. Gen. Psychiatry,* 51, 8, 1994.
67. FDA, Women and nutrition: a menu of special needs, *FDA Consumer Magazine*, 1991.
68. Lips, P., et al., Quality of life in patients with vertebral fractures: validation of the Quality of Life Questionnaire of the European Foundation for Osteoporosis (QUALEFFO). Working Party for Quality of Life of the European Foundation for Osteoporosis, *Osteo-poros. Int.*, 10, 150, 1999.
69. Iqbal, M.M., Osteoporosis: epidemiology, diagnosis, and treatment, *South Med. J.*, 93, 2, 2000.
70. Bianchi, M.L., et al., Quality of life in post-menopausal osteoporosis, *Health Qual. Life Outcomes*, 3, 78, 2005.
71. Hafner, H., Gender differences in schizophrenia, *Psychoneuroendocrinology*, 2, 17, 2003.

17 Eating Disorders

Richard E. Kreipe and Sophie Bucher Della Torre

CONTENTS

17.1 INTRODUCTION

This chapter focuses on conditions characterized by severe disturbances in eating behavior that are grouped within the category of "eating disorders" in the *Diagnostic and Statistical Manual*, 4th edn. [1]. This reference text, popularly known as the DSM-IV, had a "text revision" in 2000, but there were no changes for eating disorder criteria. The purpose of the DSM-IV is to define diagnostic categories for clinicians and researchers to treat and study individuals with "mental disorders," a poorly defined term applied to conditions that have prominent emotional, behavioral, and psychological symptoms. Although evidence points toward a strong biological component to the initiation and maintenance of eating disorders, with emerging evidence of a genetic predisposition that may be triggered by developmental and environmental factors, eating disorders are still considered "psychiatric" conditions by many professionals, resulting in many limitations to both treatment and research beyond the scope of this chapter.

In the following sections, diagnostic criteria for eating disorders will be detailed, followed by an exploration of the epidemiology (distribution and determinants) and then the etiology of these conditions as a foundation to understand the role of nutrition in the development, maintenance, and recovery from eating disorders. A discussion of how foods or food components modulate eating disorders will be followed by an exploration of future areas of study to help elucidate remaining questions.

17.2 FORMAL DIAGNOSTIC CRITERIA

The formal, DSM-IV criteria for eating disorders are included in Tables 17.1 through 17.3. Briefly, the two main categories of eating disorders are (1) anorexia nervosa, in which dieting and weight loss predominate, with two subtypes: restrictive or binge eating (or purging), depending on the presence or absence of features of bulimia nervosa, and (2) bulimia nervosa, in which binge eating is the predominant behavior in association with behaviors to minimize weight gain, also with two subtypes: purging or nonpurging, depending on the presence or absence of behaviors intended to rid the body of the effects of ingested food. Patients not meeting full criteria for either of these diagnoses are categorized as "Eating Disorder, Not Otherwise Specified (EDNOS)," and may represent the largest number of patients in practice, since at present binge eating disorder (BED) is included in this poorly defined category [2].

TABLE 17.1
DSM-IV Criteria for Anorexia Nervosa

A. Refusal to maintain body weight at or above a minimally normal weight for age and height (e.g., weight loss leading to maintenance of body weight less than 85% of that expected; or failure to make expected weight gain during period of growth, leading to body weight less than 85% of that expected).
B. Intense fear of gaining weight or becoming fat, even though underweight.
C. Disturbance in the way in which one's body weight or shape is experienced, undue influence of body weight or shape on self-evaluation, or denial of the seriousness of the current low body weight.
D. In postmenarcheal females, amenorrhea, i.e., the absence of at least three consecutive menstrual cycles. (A woman is considered to have amenorrhea if her periods occur only following hormone, e.g., estrogen, administration.)

Specify Type

Restricting Type: During the current episode of anorexia nervosa, the person has not regularly engaged in binge eating or purging behavior (i.e., self-induced vomiting or the misuse of laxatives, diuretics, or enemas).

Binge Eating or Purging Type: During the current episode of anorexia nervosa, the person has regularly engaged in binge eating or purging behavior (i.e., self-induced vomiting or the misuse of laxatives, diuretics, or enemas).

Source: From *Diagnostic and Statistical Manual of Mental Disorders*, 4th ed., American Psychiatric Association, 1994. With permission.

TABLE 17.2
Diagnostic Criteria for Bulimia Nervosa

A. Recurrent episodes of binge eating. An episode of binge eating is characterized by both:
   1) eating, in a discrete period of time (e.g., within any 2 h period), an amount of food that is definitely larger than most people would eat during a similar period of time and under similar circumstances, and
   2) a sense of lack of control over eating during the episode (e.g., a feeling that one cannot stop eating or control what or how much one is eating)

B. Recurrent inappropriate compensatory behavior in order to prevent weight gain, such as self-induced vomiting; misuse of laxatives, diuretics, enemas, or other medications; fasting; or excessive exercise.

C. The binge eating and inappropriate compensatory behaviors both occur, on average, at least twice a week for 3 months.

D. Self-evaluation is unduly influenced by body shape and weight.

E. The disturbance does not occur exclusively during episodes of anorexia nervosa.

Specify type

Purging Type: During the current episode of bulimia nervosa, the person has regularly engaged in self-induced vomiting or the misuse of laxatives, diuretics, or enemas.

Nonpurging Type: During the current episode of bulimia nervosa, the person has used other inappropriate compensatory behaviors, such as fasting or excessive exercise, but has not regularly engaged in self-induced vomiting or the misuse of laxatives, diuretics, or enemas.

Source: From *Diagnostic and Statistical Manual of Mental Disorders*, 4th ed., American Psychiatric Association, 1994. With permission.

TABLE 17.3
Diagnostic Criteria for Eating Disorder Not Otherwise Specified

The eating disorder not otherwise specified (EDNOS) category is for disorders of eating that do not meet the criteria for any specific eating disorder. Examples include:

1. For females, all of the criteria for anorexia nervosa are met except that the individual has regular menses.
2. All of the criteria for anorexia nervosa are met except that, despite significant weight loss, the individual's current weight is in the normal range.
3. All of the criteria for bulimia nervosa are met except that binge eating and inappropriate compensatory mechanisms occur at a frequency of less than twice a week or for a duration of less than 3 months.
4. The regular use of inappropriate compensatory behavior by an individual of normal body weight after eating small amounts of food (e.g., self-induced vomiting after the consumption of two cookies).
5. Repeatedly chewing and spitting out, but not swallowing, large amounts of food.
6. Binge eating disorder (BED): recurrent episodes of binge eating in the absence of the regular use of inappropriate compensatory behaviors characteristic of bulimia nervosa.

Source: From *Diagnostic and Statistical Manual of Mental Disorders*, 4th ed., American Psychiatric Association, 1994. With permission.

17.3 CLINICAL FEATURES

Although formal criteria are important for research purposes, clinical profiles better capture some of the nuances of these extremely complex disorders and will be presented before discussing epidemiology and etiology. Clinically, anorexia nervosa is a syndrome in which caloric intake insufficient to maintain weight or normal growth is associated with a delusion of being fat, and an obsession to be thinner, that do not diminish with weight loss. Patients with anorexia nervosa truly believe they are fat, even when emaciated (delusion). Likewise they are driven to lose weight (obsession) through a variety of means (compulsions), including dieting to reduce energy intake and a variety of means to increase energy losses. Exercise, often ritualistic and unrelenting, is used by more than three-fourths of patients with anorexia nervosa, while vomiting and laxatives are uncommonly used means of losing calories. A feature that differentiates simple dieting from an anorexia nervosa is the difficulty of an affected individual to identify, or to be satisfied with, a healthy weight goal. An initial weight goal of 110 lb cascades down to 105 lb, then to 100 lb, then to 95 lb, and so on. Anorexia, true loss of appetite, does not occur until there has been extreme weight loss. Prior to that, there is a refusal to acknowledge, or to "give in" to, one's appetite, since this is perceived as a loss of will power or strength [3].

The key clinical feature of bulimia nervosa is not, as is often assumed, vomiting. Binge eating is the *sine qua non* for bulimia. An awareness of abnormal eating patterns is associated with depressed moods and self-deprecating thoughts. Temporary relief of this distress is sought through methods that are intended to rid the body of the effects of calories. Over 80% of patients with bulimia nervosa engage in self-induced vomiting, laxative, or diuretic abuse for this purpose. However, fasting, exercise, or both may be the primary methods used to avoid weight gain, often unsuccessfully, as many patients with bulimia nervosa are normal to slightly overweight. Patients with bulimia are more likely than patients with anorexia nervosa to be impulsive, not only in eating behavior, but also in their use of drugs and alcohol, self-mutilation or self-harm, sexual promiscuity, lying, stealing, and other manifestations of personality disturbance [4].

The two disorders are not mutually exclusive, however. Approximately 40% of patients with anorexia nervosa have a bulimic phase in the course of their illness or recovery [5], and, as previously noted, there are more individuals who fit into the EDNOS category than either anorexia nervosa or bulimia nervosa formal categories. Outside of the scope of this chapter, both anorexia and bulimia nervosa are associated with a variety of medical complications and significant mortality over time [6].

The underlying conflicts in eating disorders often relate to a fear of growing up, difficulty in achieving independence or autonomy, confusion regarding an emerging identity, or various inter- and intrapersonal disconnections. Patients with bulimia nervosa have sometimes been traumatized in interpersonal relationships. The most common accompanying mental health issues are depression, anxiety, or obsessive–compulsive traits. Also, the label of "dysfunctional" is often attached to the family because of enmeshment, poorly defined interpersonal boundaries, rigidity, and ineffective conflict resolution. However, such labels often divert attention away from the considerable strengths that these individuals and their families exhibit.

17.4 EPIDEMIOLOGY

17.4.1 Distribution in the Population

Eating disorders are not distributed uniformly in the population. Over 90% of patients are female and White, and more than three-quarters are adolescents when they first develop their eating disorder. Most patients are from middle to upper middle socioeconomic status families. However, it should be emphasized that this stereotyping can lead to underidentification of the condition, since patients can be of any sex, race, age, or social stratum. There is an increasing awareness of these conditions, especially bulimia nervosa, among females in minority groups and among males. Prevalence is estimated at between 0.5% and 5% of adolescent females [7]. Certain groups, such as athletes or dancers whose performance may be perceived as weight-related, may have a higher risk for developing an eating disorder.

17.4.2 Sex Differences

Compared with males, self-esteem tends to be much more closely related to body dissatisfaction for females. In a study of adolescents by Furnham et al. [8], boys were as likely to want to be heavier as lighter, whereas very few girls desired to be heavier. Although the "body image ideal" tends to be thin for females and more muscular for males, in a study comparing the two sexes, this study found that, unlike females, male self-esteem was not affected by body dissatisfaction. However, if males are dissatisfied with their body image, behaviors directed at improving body image generally focus on increasing the muscle mass, definition, and tone through intense physical training or through the use of anabolic products.

In a study of adolescents and young adults, Elgin and Pritchard [9] found, not surprisingly, that females experienced more symptoms of disordered eating, as well as body dissatisfaction than did their male counterparts. While mass media exposure, low self-esteem, and perfectionism related to disordered eating for women, only perfectionism and mass media exposure were related to disordered eating behaviors. Thus, risk factors for disordered eating and body dissatisfaction for men and women may be different, which has implications for understanding the etiology of body dissatisfaction and disordered eating and for possible treatment interventions.

17.4.3 Age

Females are most likely to develop an eating disorder that corresponds, chronologically, between the onset of puberty and the peak of fertility. Thus, menstruation, ovulation, and childbearing can all be affected by eating disorders [10]. The loss of menstrual periods in anorexia nervosa and the menstrual irregularities in bulimia nervosa and eating disorders not otherwise specified have a significant impact on the health care and childbearing outcomes of the female population. Even when menstruation is fairly regular, women with eating disorders may not ovulate regularly. Our group found that once adolescent females with anorexia nervosa recovered from their disorder, and gained to and maintained a normal weight, their fertility and childbearing outcomes were not adversely affected [11].

17.4.4 Nutrition-Related Characteristics

Neumark-Sztainer's group [12] conducted a longitudinal study of more than 2500 adolescents and found that dieting and unhealthful weight-control behaviors predicted outcomes related to obesity and eating disorders 5 years later, leading them to conclude that a shift away from dieting and drastic weight-control measures toward the long-term implementation of healthful eating and physical activity behaviors is needed to prevent obesity and eating disorders in adolescents. Their findings are echoed by other investigators who have found that unsupervised dieting by girls is a strong risk factor in the development of an eating disorder [13,14].

In females with anorexia nervosa, meals are typically restricted to small amounts of a monotonously narrow range of low-calorie, low-fat foods and beverages [15]. Not surprisingly, eating disorders are disproportionately found among vegetarian women [16], more likely the result of their desire to limit fat and calories than as a cause of the eating disorder. Breakfast is generally avoided, as are snacks. If not entirely vegetarian, the intake of meat is typically severely restricted and eaten primarily at dinner, often confined to small amounts of grilled skinless poultry or broiled fish. Desserts are assiduously avoided. If "forbidden foods" are ingested, there is generally tremendous guilt and emotional upheaval followed by fasting, exercise, or vomiting. In a controlled study, Sysko et al. [17] found that females hospitalized for the treatment of anorexia nervosa consumed substantially less of a single-item test meal that did control subjects, both before and after weight gain. Thus, the expected dysfunctional eating habits while women were severely underweight persisted after weight restoration and significant improvements in eating-disordered and psychological symptoms were realized.

In females with bulimia nervosa, binge eating is most likely with the co-occurrence of both emotional triggers (e.g., feeling bored, depressed, anxious, tense, or sad) and physiological triggers (e.g., hunger and the urge to eat sweets) [18]. Binge eating (eating a large amount of food in a brief period of time) is characteristic of both bulimia nervosa and BED; in the former there is some kind of compensatory behavior to limit the effect of the overeating while in BED there is not, often resulting in obesity. Binges typically consist of high-carbohydrate, high-fat, energy-dense forbidden foods considered to be fattening, and tend to occur in the evening or at night. Binge eating is less common in anorexia nervosa.

Binge eating and vomiting have a peculiarly addictive pattern. After an episode, individuals often go to bed at night vowing to be good the next morning. This translates into avoiding breakfast and limiting lunch to save calories. They then find themselves very hungry and their dietary restraint gives way to disinhibition. Even in the absence of an eating disorder, we found that young adult women may highly restrain caloric intake and consistently diet, only to become disinhibited and overeat when a female is emotionally distressed when thinking about dieting [19]. In bulimia nervosa, binge eating leads to self-deprecation, which is relieved by purging, but this is soon followed by depression and negative self-evaluation. This vicious cycle results in patients with bulimia nervosa more likely to seek treatment than those with anorexia nervosa. Although there is tremendous shame, guilt, and embarrassment associated with this repetitive behavior, often labeled by patients as "disgusting," the emotional pain that they experience makes help-seeking more likely.

Cooke et al. [20] compared women with BED to weight-matched women without BED and to normal weight controls during binge eating with respect to temporal patterns of food selection. Although the subjects with BED consumed significantly more calories than the obese subjects who did not have BED, the dessert, vegetable, or carbohydrate consumption did not differ significantly between the two groups. They also found that women with BED consumed significantly more meat than subjects without BED. Most notable was the contrast in temporal pattern during the binge in subjects with BED compared with the patients with bulimia nervosa. When served the same meal as the subjects with BED, these investigators found that patients with bulimia nervosa spent more of their meal time eating dessert and snack foods, began eating these foods earlier, and distributed their meat consumption more evenly across their meals than did control subjects in the same weight category [21]. While females with bulimia nervosa ate dessert foods earlier in the meals, all other groups ate meat toward the beginning of their meal and ate more dessert foods toward the end of the meal. Thus, foods ingested during binges in females with BED tend to differ from those eaten by females with bulimia nervosa, suggesting that binge eating episodes between different groups of eating-disordered populations are qualitatively different. Patients with bulimia nervosa spent more of their meal time eating dessert and snack foods, began eating these foods earlier, and distributed their meat consumption more evenly across their meals than did weight-matched controls.

17.5 ETIOLOGY

17.5.1 Gene–Environment Interactions

There is a genetic predisposition to eating disorders [22], with chromosomes 1, 2, and 13 revealing regions of interest [23] for restrictive anorexia nervosa. Relatives of patients with eating disorders have about a 10-fold greater lifetime risk of developing an eating disorder compared with relatives of unaffected individuals [23], with the highest risk occurring for a monozygotic twin of a person with anorexia nervosa. However, emerging data indicate that the strongest association is with mood or anxiety disorders [24]. That is, eating disorders are not inherited directly. Rather, "inheritance" is best considered as a "vulnerability" to developing an eating disorder, based on being depressed or anxious, both of which are recognized familial genetic traits. Prevalence rates that include the entire population as the denominator grossly underestimate the prevalence of eating disorders in target groups. Females in late childhood and adolescence may feel a need to diet or lose weight and therefore be at-risk of adopting potentially harmful weight-loss habits. Of concern for the future is that the rapidly rising incidence of obesity worldwide may trigger some vulnerable individuals to develop an eating disorder in an effort to lose weight (if they are or perceive themselves to be overweight) or in an effort to prevent becoming overweight.

Two lines of research are especially promising with respect to genetics (immutable) and the environment (modifiable) in relation to both external and internal environmental factors [25,26]. Caspi [27] points out that a better understanding of genetic susceptibility to environmental factors will help explain why some individuals react to environmental stressors and why their genetic makeup makes them susceptible. Especially noteworthy is the rapidly emerging science of imaging genomics, which combines brain imaging and human genome identification. A basic principle of this line of inquiry is that environmental pathogens can cause the expression of genes that result in demonstrable differences in brain imaging in the face of behavior pathology. Replacing environmental pathogens with beneficial environmental conditions, such as occurs in nutritional and psychological therapy, could hold promise in suppressing gene expression, in the overall treatment of eating disorders.

Equally intriguing are recent studies demonstrating that ovarian hormones may have important links to the development of eating disorders. Data from the Minnesota Twin study, which included 1200 female twins and their parents, that examined genetic and environmental factors involved in the etiology of eating disorders are providing insights into the reasons why adolescent females going through the changes of puberty may be most susceptible to developing an eating disorder [28]. This study of 11 and 17 year-old twins showed that at age 11 (corresponding to early puberty), genetic influences accounted for 0% of the variability of eating disorder symptoms, while environmental influences made up 100% of variability of eating disorder symptoms. Among the 17 year-olds, the genetic or environmental influence changed to 60% or 40%. These findings suggest that in early adolescence, environmental influences of peers, media messages, and the like are strongly related to the onset of eating disorder behaviors. By the time an adolescent female has largely completed puberty and ovarian hormones are generally at adult levels, genetic influences are stronger than environmental ones. This suggests that sex hormones may influence the expression of genes that would make an individual susceptible to develop an eating disorder. Furthermore, when 14 year-old twins (mid puberty) were studied, the genetic or environmental influences accounting for symptoms were very similar to 17 year-olds. This dramatic change in the risk of developing eating disorder symptoms seen in mid-adolescence—recognized clinically—suggests that the initiation of puberty activates genes that make an individual susceptible to develop an eating disorder [29]. In animal studies, ovarian hormones have a direct effect on ingestion of food, but it is important to not overestimate the interaction between puberty and genes in the development of an eating disorder as a purely biological phenomenon [29]. Eating disorders are much more complex, clearly having psychological and social triggers.

17.6 ETIOLOGY OF EATING DISORDERS RELATED TO NUTRITION

17.6.1 Energy Amount

Most models of eating disorders identify various predisposing, precipitating, and perpetuating factors. Nutritional factors tend to be the result, rather than the cause, of clinical findings with respect to the first two elements. When weight control behaviors occur in a vulnerable individual (most likely a female), they can trigger the onset of an eating disorder, if they become habitual and entrenched. Such entrenchment usually occurs because the eating disorder helps the person to cope with problems that were previously unresolved, and to the patient's perception unresolvable [30]. It is precisely because these behaviors *do* help the person to cope that they are also likely to be perpetuated. However, energy prescription is important [31], with attention to avoiding refeeding syndrome while also acknowledging the limits that a woman with an eating disorder will tolerate.

17.6.2 Energy Distribution

Although it is often assumed that patients with anorexia nervosa become protein deficient, this is unusual unless there is some concomitant bizarre eating pattern, such as eating pickles and drinking vegetable juice cocktail as the predominant sources of nutrition. A 3 oz fat-free sliced turkey and 8 oz glass of skim milk contains 30 g of high-quality protein, but no fat. Until recently, it would have been difficult to be able to maintain a diet that was adequate in protein and carbohydrate, but deficient in fat. However, the daily intake of patients with restrictive anorexia nervosa who ingests predominantly fat-free foods frequently falls below 10 g of fat. It would not be possible to design a study to determine the effects of a fat-deficient diet due to ethical restrictions, and so scientists cannot say with certainty how these diets affect individuals with eating disorders.

With respect to energy distribution in treatment, our group studied adolescent and young adult women with anorexia nervosa in a General Clinical Research Center and found no difference in weight gain or recovery for patients on a 10% compared with a 20% protein-diet [32]. However, Latner [33] found that adding protein to the diets of women with bulimia nervosa and BED resulted in reduced food intake and binge eating over a 2 week period.

17.6.3 Vitamins and Minerals

As is true of the balance of protein, fat, and carbohydrates in the diet, vitamin and mineral disturbances are generally the result, rather than the cause of the pathological behaviors. Elevated plasma levels of retinol (the primary form of vitamin A in plasma) and retinyl esters (a transient form of vitamin A associated with chylomicrons) have been reported by some investigators [34]. These changes are not typical of protein-energy malnutrition and may be due to altered metabolism (low triodothyroxine levels) or delayed clearance of chylomicrons. It is not clear why individuals with anorexia nervosa tend to become hypercarotenemic. The intake of β-carotene can be quite high in patients whose diet consists largely of yellow vegetables. However, Rock and Curran-Celentano [35] pointed out that elevated plasma carotenoids in anorexia nervosa may also indicate a diminished ability to clear or metabolize these compounds. However, there is little evidence for these increased levels posing a risk of hypervitaminosis A.

Investigators have reported increased, decreased, and normal plasma concentrations of tocopherol [34]. Because vitamin E is known to be associated with lipoproteins, levels may reflect the effects of binding to blood lipids rather than tissue concentrations. Vitamin E deficiency has been related to cognitive and neuropsychological problems, even though there is no consistent pattern of deficiency yet recognized. Further investigation is required to elucidate the circumstances in which alteration of vitamin E status might be expected. Thiamin, riboflavin, and vitamin B-6 may also contribute to cognitive problems and physiological features associated with semistarvation in many patients with anorexia nervosa [36]. The dietary requirements for these vitamins are determined by substrate utilization, the severity of malnutrition, the refeeding process, and the stage of recovery. Measurements of blood levels are of little clinical use unless the history and physical examination suggest the presence of a specific deficiency.

The minerals of primary concern in anorexia nervosa are calcium and zinc [36]. Although calcium intake is typically much less than the RDA, serum levels are usually normal and urinary excretion is often increased. This is most likely due to the resorption of bone associated with the low estrogen and high cortisol levels typically found in anorexia nervosa. There is little evidence that variation in calcium intake has measurable effects on bone density over the short term, possibly because the high resorptive state makes skeletal calcium available, even if dietary calcium is reduced. On the other hand, adequate calcium and vitamin D need to be included in the daily intake because it is impossible to predict how long the patient will engage in the dysfunctional eating habits. Ideally, this should be in the form of high nutritional-value foods and beverages, including dairy products and calcium-fortified foods or beverages. If these sources are low in vitamin D, then another source of vitamin D is needed to provide the adequate intake (AI) [36]. For example, orange juice can also be fortified with both calcium and vitamin D. Calcium intake is of concern for all adolescent females, since only 40% of them achieve the recommended adequate dietary intake of calcium of 1300 mg/day [37].

Zinc is lost in catabolic states, such as occurring in anorexia nervosa, but serum levels are difficult to measure and interpret; balance studies are probably more useful clinically than serum levels. There is a theoretical link between zinc deficiency and some of the symptoms of anorexia nervosa, but little evidence to suggest that it is clinically relevant. Lask's group conducted a double-blind, placebo-controlled clinical trial of zinc supplementation and found that zinc levels returned quickly without supplementation [38]. Furthermore, it is important to note that excessive zinc supplementation may aggravate marginal copper deficiency [39].

Tannhauser [40] proposed that childhood zinc deficiency, aggravated in puberty by high energy need with low zinc intake in the diet and aggravated by stresses of various kinds, can influence both mental and physical development and ultimately lead to the development of anorexia nervosa.

Birmingham and Gritzner [41] conducted a randomized controlled trial of zinc supplementation in anorexia nervosa, and reported a twofold increase of the rate of increase of body mass index in the zinc group. They proposed that although zinc is inexpensive, readily available and free of significant side effects, oral zinc supplementation is infrequently prescribed as an adjunctive treatment for anorexia nervosa, even though low zinc intake, common in anorexia nervosa, adversely affects neurotransmitters in various parts of the brain, including γ-amino butyric acid and the amygdale, which are abnormal in anorexia nervosa. They concluded that oral administration of 14 mg of elemental zinc daily for 2 months in all patients with anorexia nervosa should be routine.

17.6.4 Nutrition Prescription

"Food is medicine" is a central nutritional theme in the treatment of females with eating disorders [31]. The initial caloric prescription is generally between 1000 and 1400 kcal/day, although the use of 130% of resting energy expenditure as determined by indirect calorimetry or adjusted Harris-Benedict equation are more precise methods of determining actual resting energy requirements. These values need to be adjusted for estimated energy expenditure in daily activity, especially for females involved in sports or vigorous physical exercise. The nutrition prescription should work toward gradually increasing weight at the rate of about 1/2 to 1 lb/week, by increasing energy intake at 100–200 kcal increments every few days. In addition, the gradual inclusion of "forbidden foods" should be part of the nutrition prescription once the patient shows evidence of being able to eat adequately to gain weight. A standard nutritional balance of 45%–65% carbohydrate and total fat 20%–35% fat is appropriate [42]. However, the fat content may need to be lowered to 15%–20% early in treatment because of continued fat phobia.

Rock and Curran-Celentano note that if refeeding is accomplished with an increasing energy-containing diet consisting of a variety of regular foods, sufficient amounts of vitamins and minerals will be provided, so that correction of deficiencies without supplementation is anticipated [36]. Treating the nutritional problems with nutrient-dense foods will also help to correct the multitude of metabolic and physiological abnormalities associated with semistarvation in addition to reversing specific micronutrient deficiencies. Low-dose multiple vitamins with minerals at RDA levels may be appropriate for chronically ill adolescents who are unable to maintain adequate nutrition. On the other hand, the use of high-dose supplements can have unfavorable effects either through excessive levels of the micronutrient itself or through adverse interactions with other elements (such as may occur between excessive zinc supplementation and copper deficiency) [39].

Most females with severe anorexia nervosa, who require hospitalization because of low weight, require at least 1500 cal/day to maintain weight [31]. Their reduced basal metabolic rate (BMR) may be as low as 800–1000 cal/day, and maintenance requirements are 130%–150% of BMR. Our group has demonstrated that ~1 g of weight is gained for every 5 cal of intake in excess of output; to accrue 100 additional grams of weight requires an excess of 500 cal. At low weight, few calories are expended in exercise than at higher weights; even with one hour of vigorous exercise the patient expends ≤400 cal. If a female appears to eat >3500 cal daily and still does not gain weight, it is likely that food is being vomited or discarded or that unrecognized exercise is occurring. On a pound for pound basis, younger females require more energy to gain weight than older patients, since some of their intake is required for growth. For example, the recommended AI of energy is about 2400 cal for both 14 and 24 year-old females [43], even though the younger individual weighs, on average, about 15 lb less.

First, many malnourished adolescents are hypovolemic and gain weight in the form of extracellular fluid. Second, their BMR can be half of normal. This reduction in energy expenditure enables calories ingested to exceed calories expended even at low levels of intake, resulting in weight gain in the form of body tissues. Third, these newly formed tissues are two-thirds lean [32], not entirely fat as presumed by most patients, regardless of the protein content of the diet. It requires much less energy to produce protein-rich lean tissues than it does to produce fat-rich storage tissues (that are formed in quantity only after restoration of the lean body mass). Thus, more weight is gained initially for each excess calorie over expenditure than will be gained later as the patient approaches normal weight and body composition.

Therefore, although the daily requirement may eventually exceed 2500 cal, one should not attempt to prescribe an increase of more than 50% over present average daily intake of energy [31]. Not only is the patient unlikely to respond favorably to a "normal" diet, but also it is unnecessary and can be physically and psychologically dangerous if the patient gains weight too quickly. Parents, especially, need to recognize that "more" is not necessarily "better" with respect to eating and weight gain. By focusing on a gradual, monitored increased intake, the dietitian can often lessen the adolescent's resistance to changing her eating habits.

The minimal daily caloric intake can begin at about 1000–1200 calories, but may need to be lower if the patient was ingesting only a few hundred cal/day prior to admission [31]. Intake is increased, as necessary, at 250–500 cal increments every 2 days. In severely malnourished patients, fluid retention, congestive heart failure [44], hypophosphatemia [45], and other manifestations of the "refeeding syndrome" can occur with too rapid replacement. Rarely is it advisable to decrease the daily caloric minimum, once it is established at a higher level. Only if the patient has demonstrated consistent weight gain not attributable to fluid should lowering energy intake be considered.

17.7 CONCLUSION

Eating disorders are extremely complex conditions with biological, psychological, and social aspects. Although a key feature is unhealthy eating patterns, they should not be the sole focus of either prevention or treatment interventions. A common sense approach is most likely to be helpful in optimizing women's health in this domain. That is, there does not appear to be any particular nutrient that needs to be increased or decreased insofar as nutrition is concerned. Although the caloric content needs to be modified depending on the need to gain, maintain, or lose weight, a well-balanced meal plan, spread out over the day in three meals and one or two snacks, is indicated for anorexia nervosa, bulimia nervosa, and BED. In addition, balancing the intake with healthy energy expenditure in regular physical activity that is enjoyable and sustaining over time needs to be part of both prevention and treatment. As Neumark-Sztainer points out in her book [46], the present obesity epidemic tends to shift the focus away from eating disorders, since obesity is often considered at the other end of the spectrum of nutritional disturbance. However, she emphasizes that balancing intake and output will also address the energy balance problems seen in obesity. Obviously, if the diet is deficient in any nutrient, efforts should be directed at mitigating those, but this should be accomplished with food and beverage rather than through supplements.

17.8 FUTURE RESEARCH

Several research questions deserve further exploration with respect to sex-based nutrition. First, what is the relationship to dieting among females relative to the onset of eating disorders insofar as the type of diet followed? Does a small reduction in calories in a balanced manner put a female at the same risk of developing an eating disorder as does drastic reduction in calories? Also, what is the relationship of various diet aids, often termed "fat burners," but marketed as "nutritional supplements" and are therefore not subject to the same regulatory oversight as drugs? Second, what is the influence of a diet that is marginally adequate with respect to energy, but deficient in fat? It would be unethical to design a clinical trial to answer this question, but naturalistic longitudinal studies could be designed to determine the effect of such restrictions. Third, larger studies of zinc seem indicated, since some researchers have found a positive correlation between zinc supplementation and weight gain in anorexia nervosa. Likewise, given the tendency for the diet of adolescent females to be deficient in calcium, we need better studies to determine the role of calcium and vitamin D in health, beyond that of bone health.

Most intriguing is the possibility of including nutrition in longitudinal studies that determine gene–environment–pubertal interactions in the development of eating disorders. These would be extremely difficult to tease out, but it may be that nutritional interventions would be more likely to be beneficial at different times in female puberty with respect to moderating the effect of the external environment on gene expression. Such studies would best be conducted as large, multicenter trials. However, as technology advances and our understanding of the effect of normal nutrition and eating behavior on healthy development, opportunities may arise.

REFERENCES

1. American Psychiatric Association, *Diagnostic and Statistical Manual of Mental Disorders*, 4th edn., American Psychiatric Association, 1994.
2. Hudson, J.I. et al., The prevalence and correlates of eating disorders in the National Comorbidity Survey Replication, *Biol. Psych.*, 61, 348, 2007.
3. Kreipe, R.E. and Higgins, L.A., Anorexia Nervosa, *Rickert VI Adolescent Nutrition: Assessment and Management*, New York, NY: Chapman & Hall, pp. 159–180, 1995.
4. Kreipe, R.E. and Mou, S.M., Eating disorders in adolescents and young adults, *Obstet. Gynecol. Clin. N. Am.*, 27, 101, 2000.
5. Kreipe, R.E., Churchill, B.H., and Strauss, J., Long-term outcome of adolescents with anorexia nervosa, *Am. J. Dis. Child.*, 143, 1322, 1989.
6. Rome, E.S. et al., Children and adolescents with eating disorders: The state of the art, *Pediatrics*, 111, 98, 2003.
7. Committee on Adolescence, AAP, Identifying and treating eating disorders, *Pediatrics*, 11, 204, 2003.
8. Furnham, A., Badmin, N., and Sneade, I., Body image dissatisfaction: Gender differences in eating attitudes, self-esteem, and reason for exercise. *J. Psych.*, 136, 581, 2002.
9. Elgin, J. and Pritchard, M., Gender differences in disordered eating and its correlates, *Eat. Weight Dis.*, 11, e96, 2006.
10. Mitchell, A.M. and Bulik, C.M., Eating disorders and women's health: An update, *J. Midwifery Women's Health*, 51, 193, 2006.

11. Kreipe, R.E. and Dukarm, C.P., Outcome of anorexia nervosa related to treatment utilizing an adolescent medicine approach, *J. Youth Adolesc.*, 25, 483, 1996.
12. Neumark-Sztainer, D. et al., Obesity, disordered eating, and eating disorders in a longitudinal study of adolescents: How do dieters fare 5 years later? *J. Am. Diet. Assoc.*, 106, 559, 2006.
13. Spear, B.A., Does dieting increase the risk for obesity and eating disorders? *J. Am. Diet. Assoc.*, 106, 523, 2006.
14. Butryn, M.L. and Wadden, T.A., Treatment of overweight in children and adolescents: Does dieting increase the risk of eating disorders? *Int. J. Eat. Dis.*, 37, 285, 2005.
15. Gwirtsman, H.E. et al., Energy intake and dietary macronutrient content in women with anorexia nervosa and volunteers, *J. Am. Diet. Assoc.*, 89, 54, 1989.
16. Berg, F.M. and Rosencrans, K., *Women Afraid to Eat: Breaking Free in Today's Weight-Obsessed World*, Healthy Weight Publishing Network, Hettinger, ND, 2000.
17. Sysko, R. et al., Eating behavior among women with anorexia nervosa, *Am. J. Clin. Nutr.*, 82, 296, 2005.
18. Vanderlinden, J. et al., Which factors do provoke binge eating? An exploratory study in eating disorder patients, *Eat. Weight Dis.*, 9, 300, 2004.
19. Strauss, J., Doyle, A.E., and Kreipe, R.E., The paradoxical effect of diet commercials on reinhibition of dietary restraint, *J. Abnorm. Psychol.*, 103, 441, 1994.
20. Cooke, E.A. et al., Patterns of food selection during binges in women with binge eating disorder, *Int. J. Eat. Dis.*, 22, 187, 1997.
21. Hadigan, C.M., Kissileff, H.R., and Walsh, B.T., Patterns of food selection during meals in women with bulimia, *Am. J. Clin. Nutr.*, 50, 7759, 1989.
22. Rankinen, T. and Bouchard, C., Genetics of food intake and eating behavior phenotypes in humans, *Ann. Rev. Nutr.*, 26, 413, 2006.
23. Bulik, C.M., Exploring the gene-environment nexus in eating disorders, *J Psych. Neuro.*, 30, 335, 2005.
24. Keel, P.K. et al., Shared transmission of eating disorders and anxiety disorders, *Int. J. Eat. Dis.*, 38, 99, 2005.
25. Caspi, A. and Moffitt, T.E., Gene–environment interactions in psychiatry: Joining forces with neuroscience, *Nat. Rev. Neuro.*, 7, 583, 2006.
26. Moffitt, T.E. et al., Strategy for investigating interactions between measured genes and measured environments, *Arch. Gen. Psych.*, 62, 473, 2005.
27. Caspi, A., Gene–environment interactions, *Eat. Dis. Rev.*, 17, 2, 2005.
28. Klump, K.L. et al., Preliminary evidence that gonadal hormones organize and activate disordered eating, *Psych. Med.*, 36, 539, 2006.
29. Klump, K., Gene–environment interactions, *Eat. Dis. Rev.*, 17, 2, 2006.
30. Kreipe, R.E. and Yussman, S.M., The role of the primary care practitioner in the treatment of eating disorders, In Fisher M., Golden N., Jacobsen M. (Eds.). *The Spectrum of Disordered Eating: Anorexia Nervosa, Bulimia Nervosa, and Obesity in Adolescent Medicine*, 14, p. 133, 2003.
31. Marcason, W., Nutrition therapy and eating disorders: What is the correct calorie level for clients with anorexia? *J. Am. Diet. Assoc.*, 102, 644, 2002.
32. Forbes, G.B. et al., Body composition changes during recovery from anorexia nervosa: Comparison of two dietary regimes, *Am. J. Clin. Nutr.*, 40, 1137, 1984.
33. Latner, J.D., Binge eating and satiety in bulimia nervosa and binge eating disorder: Effect of macronutrient intake, *Int. J. Eat. Dis.*, 36, 402, 2004.
34. Vaisman, N., Wolfhart, D., and Sklan, D., Vitamin A metabolism in plasma of normal and anorectic women, *Eur. J. Clin. Nutr.* 46, 873, 1992.
35. Rock, C.L. and Curran-Celentano, J., Nutritional disorder of anorexia nervosa: a review, *Int. J. Eat. Dis.*, 15, 187, 1994.

36. Rock, C.L. and Curran-Celentano, J., Nutritional management of eating disorders, *Psych. Clin. N. Amer.*, 19, 701, 1996.
37. Fiorito, L.M. et al., Girls' dairy intake, energy intake, and weight status, *J. Am. Diet. Assoc.*, 106, 1851, 2006.
38. Lask, B., Fosson, A., Rolfe, U., and Thomas, S., Zinc deficiency and childhood-onset anorexia nervosa, *J. Clin. Psych.*, 54, 63, 1993.
39. Kleinman, R.E. (Ed.), Trace elements, In *Pediatric Nutrition Handbook*, 5th edn., Committee on Nutrition, American Academy of Pediatrics, Elk Grove, Illinois, pp. 313–337, 2003.
40. Tannhauser, P.P., Anorexia nervosa: A multifactorial disease of nutrition origin? *Int. J. Adolesc. Med. Health*, 14, 185, 2002.
41. Birmingham, C.L. and Gritzner, S., How does zinc supplementation benefit anorexia nervosa? *Eat. Weight Dis.*, 11, e109, 2006.
42. U.S. Department of Health and Human Services and U.S. Department of Agriculture, Dietary Guidelines for Americans, Washington, D.C., 2005.
43. Stang, J. and Story, M. (Eds.), *Guidelines for Adolescent Nutrition Services*, Division of Epidemiology and Community Health, School of Public Health, University of Minnesota, 2005.
44. Kohn, M.R., Golden, N.H., and Shenker, I.R., Cardiac arrest and delirium: Presentations of the refeeding syndrome in severely malnourished adolescents with anorexia nervosa, *J. Adolesc. Health*, 22, 239, 1998.
45. Fisher, M., Simpser, E., and Schneider, M., Hypophosphatemia secondary to oral refeeding in anorexia nervosa, *Int. J. Eat. Dis.*, 28, 181, 2000.
46. Neumark-Sztainer, D., *"I'm, Like, SO Fat!": Helping Your Teen Make Healthy Choices about Eating and Exercise in a Weight-Obsessed World*, Guilford Publishing, NY, 2005.

18 Oral Health

Peter C. Fritz and Wendy E. Ward

CONTENTS

18.1 INTRODUCTION

Oral health is inextricably and positively linked with nutritional status. Maintaining oral health throughout the life cycle is critical to ensure that a maximum number of functional teeth are maintained into old age. Of all the conditions affecting oral health, periodontal disease is a major reason why an individual's oral health, and thus nutritional status is compromised. Both men and women develop periodontal disease. There are limited data comparing the prevalence of periodontitis in males and females and one study has shown that, in general, the prevalence is lower among women compared with men. However, since the development of periodontal disease often corresponds to stages of the life cycle in which fluctuations in hormones occur, women experience an elevated risk of developing periodontal disease at specific life stages, such as pregnancy or postmenopause. As well, periodontal health can vary depending on the stage of the menstrual cycle. There are a significant number of studies suggesting that, in addition to compromising oral health and causing tooth loss, periodontal disease may have systemic manifestations or be influenced by other disease states such as type II diabetes and cardiovascular disease.

This chapter will discuss the etiology of periodontal disease, as well as the specific life stages in which periodontal disease is most common, and the potential interrelationships with other chronic diseases. This will be followed by discussion of the different nutritional interventions that have been studied in relation to periodontal disease. The chapter concludes with a discussion of important areas for future research.

18.2 ETIOLOGY OF PERIODONTAL DISEASE

Periodontal disease encompasses gingival diseases, chronic periodontitis, aggressive periodontitis, periodontitis as a manifestation of systemic disease, necrotizing periodontitis, abscesses of the periodontium, periodontitis associated with endodontic lesions, and developmental or acquired deformities and conditions [1,2]. Gingival diseases are the mildest form of periodontal disease, in which gums are reddened, swollen, and bleed easily. Plaque-induced gingivitis, the most common form of the gingival diseases, is fully reversible through proper oral hygiene, and routine dental appointments in which teeth are cleaned. If gingivitis is left untreated, bacterial plaque spreads, growing below the gum line. Proinflammatory mediators, including a variety of inflammatory prostaglandins and cytokines, are released into the gum tissue, stimulating and propagating an inflammatory reaction. Depending upon the host response, this inflammatory reaction can result in the erosion of the gum tissue around individual teeth, simultaneously forming a pocket around the teeth and eroding bone in the jaw, resulting in attachment loss and tooth loss. The result is periodontitis. It is termed chronic periodontitis if the process occurs over a longer period of time in comparison to aggressive periodontitis in which a rapid loss of clinical attachment occurs. The other forms of periodontal diseases are relatively rare compared to gingivitis and chronic periodontitis. Emerging evidence suggests that periodontitis may be a manifestation of other chronic, systemic diseases, particularly type II diabetes and cardiovascular disease. Known risk factors for periodontal disease are shown in Table 18.1 [1,3].

Individuals with periodontitis leading to tooth loss are vulnerable to nutritional insults as they age. Functional teeth are critical for chewing, and thus it is not surprising that studies have reported a significant relationship between the oral health status of an individual, often assessed as the number of functional teeth, and their overall nutritional status [4–7]. This relationship has been most extensively studied in the elderly. Studies have shown that oral health, particularly the number of teeth an older individual has, is related to overall nutritional status [4–7]. Intakes of protein, carbohydrates, iron, vitamin B1, vitamin C, fiber, and total energy are reported to be lower among elderly with fewer or no teeth [4–7].

18.3 PERIODONTAL DISEASE IN WOMEN

Prevalence data from two of the National Health and Nutrition Examination Survey (NHANES) studies suggest that periodontitis has decreased from 7.3% (NHANES

TABLE 18.1
Risk Factors for Periodontal Disease

Genetics
Smoking
Medications
Hormonal fluctuations: puberty, pregnancy, menopause
Stress
Systemic conditions: diabetes, rheumatoid arthritis
Physical trauma: clenching and grinding of teeth
Poor oral hygiene
Inadequate nutrition: calcium, vitamin D, vitamin C
Obesity

Source: From Burt, B., *J. Periodontol.*, 76, 1406, 2005.

III 1988–1994) to 4.2% (NHANES 1999–2000) for all ethnic groups in the United States when both sexes are combined [8]. This study included non-Hispanic black, non-Hispanic white, and Mexican-American, with subjects being older than 18 years of age, and included a similar number of women and men for each ethnic group [8]. The authors commented that the lower prevalence from the NHANES 1999–2000 study may be due, in part, to an overall reduction in smoking, a strong risk factor for periodontal disease [8]. Based on data from NHANES 1999–2000, women had a lower overall prevalence of periodontal disease than males for all ethnic groups studied (non-Hispanic black 8.9 versus 4.9, Mexican-American 6.5 versus 2.5, and non-Hispanic white 4.8 versus 2.7). Further analyses of the NHANES data, in which specific ages, smoking or disease states such as diabetes, are considered, are needed to identify specific prevalence rates in women at different stages of the life cycle and in specific disease states, particularly type II diabetes.

18.3.1 Menstrual Cycle and Oral Contraceptive Use

Changes in estrogen and progesterone levels during the menstrual cycle have been shown to affect periodontal health [9]. In this study, healthy women with no periodontal disease were assessed at three different stages of the menstrual cycle (ovulation, premenstruation, menstruation), and at each stage, specific markers of periodontal health that were measured included (1) plaque index, (2) gingival index, (3) probing depth, and (4) clinical attachment level. A higher gingival index was observed during premenstruation and ovulation compared to menstruation. Although these women did not have periodontal disease, gingival scores worsened at specific stages of the menstrual cycle. Moreover, because some women experience significant changes in their measures of periodontal health during their menstrual cycle, the investigators prudently recommend that the stage of menstrual cycle be taken into consideration when studying epidemiological data relating to the periodontal health of women [9].

Divergent data exist with regard to use of oral contraceptives and periodontal health [10–12]. Some studies report an increased prevalence of gingivitis among oral contraceptive users [12]. Specific outcomes such as plaque index, gingival index, and periodontal attachment were measured, and women who had used contraceptives for 2–4 years or <2 years had less healthy gingival compared with nonusers [12]. Women taking contraceptives for 2–4 years had greatest periodontal attachment loss. In contrast, a recent study based on two sets of the NHANES data (1971–1974 and 1998–1994) did not demonstrate a negative relationship, despite the marked differences in the doses of estrogen and progesterone in the formulations of oral contraceptives between these two studies [11]. A study of experimental gingivitis in women using oral contraceptives is in agreement with the NHANES data [10]. In this study, users and nonusers of oral contraceptives who served as their own control, were instructed to maintain normal oral hygiene in one quadrant of the mouth and to stop oral hygiene of the contralateral quadrant. Plaque index, gingival index, and gingival crevicular fluid volume were measured at baseline and at the end of the 21 day study. As expected, plaque index, gingival index, and crevicular fluid volume were higher in the quadrants receiving no oral hygiene within both users and nonusers. Interestingly, the periodontal health did not differ between users and nonusers, suggesting that oral contraceptive use did not enhance the inflammatory response and stimulate disease progression [10].

18.3.2 Adverse Pregnancy Outcomes Including Premature Birth

With respect to periodontal disease and women's health, a large proportion of research has focused on whether periodontal disease affects pregnancy outcomes, including risk of premature birth. A recent review of 25 published studies concluded that "periodontal disease may be associated with an increased risk of adverse pregnancy outcome" [13]. Adverse pregnancy outcomes included miscarriage, pregnancy loss, preeclampsia, preterm birth, low birthweight due to preterm birth, and birthweight by gestational age. The authors of the review commented that there is a paucity of randomized controlled trials, and that variation in periodontal disease definitions and socioeconomic status as well as small sample sizes (<100 subjects) may confound study findings [13]. They further commented that studies that have shown the strongest link between periodontal disease and adverse pregnancy outcomes have included greater numbers of women with low socioeconomic status [13].

Based on the substantial body of evidence suggesting a link between periodontal disease, studies are focused on determining if treatment of periodontal disease protects against adverse pregnancy outcomes (as defined earlier). A recently reported randomized controlled trial failed to demonstrate a difference in rates of preterm birth, low birth-weight, or fetal growth restriction with nonsurgical periodontal treatment [14]. The treatment consisted of periodontal scaling and root planning with the use of ultrasonic and hand instruments with up to four visits for treatment. In addition, subjects had tooth polishing on a monthly basis, were instructed in oral hygiene, and underwent scaling and planing as needed until delivery. In the interpretation of their study findings, the authors carefully determined whether women who had most severe disease (i.e., subjects with greatest bleeding on probing or periodontal pocketing) or were most responsive to treatment (i.e., experienced a 40% reduction in bleeding on probing) had improved pregnancy outcomes [14]. However, these subanalyses did not demonstrate a relationship. The authors commented that the timing of intervention may be critical, and that earlier intervention may result in a reduction of adverse pregnancy outcomes [14]. Women received treatment prior to 21 weeks of gestation, being recruited prior to 17 weeks of gestation.

A few other studies have investigated whether periodontal treatment has favorable effects on pregnancy outcomes [15,16]. Of the studies reporting improved pregnancy outcomes, a large proportion of subjects are of a lower socioeconomic status than the study by Michalowicz et al. [14], and effectiveness of periodontal treatment was not consistently assessed. Future research is required to determine if adverse pregnancy outcomes can be reduced by modifying treatment of periodontal disease.

18.3.3 Menopause and Aging

Data from the NHANES III and NHANES 1999–2000 study reported that the overall prevalence of periodontal disease, without differentiating between men and women, increases with older ages [8]. This pattern is similar to the prevalence patterns of osteoporosis in men and women. It is known that tooth loss is directly correlated with changes in bone mineral density (BMD) at common sites of fragility fracture such as the hip and lumbar spine in men and women [17]. See Chapter 11 for further discussion of osteoporosis.

18.3.4 Obesity and Type II Diabetes

While obesity and insulin resistance are precursors to the development of type II diabetes, obesity and insulin resistance have more recently been linked with periodontal disease [18] (Figure 18.1). It is widely known that obesity, particularly

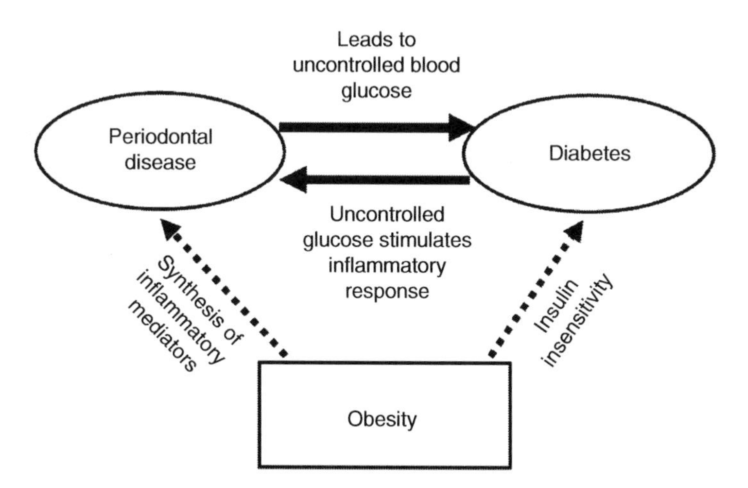

FIGURE 18.1 The interrelationship among periodontal disease and diabetes. Obesity may also modulate this relationship by leading to insulin insensitivity and release of inflammatory mediators by adipocytes.

childhood obesity, is a leading health issue facing developed countries. Using data from the NHANES III study, obese subjects between the ages of 18 and 34 years were shown to be at an elevated risk for periodontal disease [19]. Males and females were analyzed together and not separately. Adipocytes secrete a wide range of factors, many of which are proinflammatory such as tumor necrosis factor-α and its receptor, and thus may propagate the inflammatory aspect of periodontal disease [18].

The American Academy of Periodontics refers to periodontal disease and type II diabetes as a "two-way street" [20]: type II diabetes may make an individual more susceptible to periodontal disease while periodontal disease may make it more difficult for a patient to control their blood glucose. Glycemic control, assessed as glycated hemoglobin (HbA1c), was shown to be a marker of periodontal health in patients with diabetes [21]. Patients with higher HbA1c, indicative of uncontrolled blood glucose, had greater probing depths ($\geq$5 mm) and a greater number of sites with these probing depths. Moreover, an unfavorable blood lipid profile including elevated total and LDL cholesterol and triglycerides was associated with uncontrolled blood glucose [21]. In contrast, individuals demonstrating controlled blood glucose had fewer sites that bled upon probing and fewer probing depths that were $\geq$5 mm. The study by Lim et al. [21] studied males and females together, and thus further study delineating sex-based differences is warranted. Periodontal treatment has also been shown to aid in metabolic control of blood glucose at 3 and 6 months of posttreatment [22]. Significant reductions in HbA1c are reported [22]. Because periodontal disease may occur in part due to obesity and type II diabetes, the reader is referred to Chapters 7 and 8 on obesity and type II diabetes, respectively, for further information on their etiology.

18.3.5 Cardiovascular Disease

Epidemiological studies suggest that cardiovascular disease may, at least in part, result from an inflammatory-mediated process such as periodontal disease [23–26]. This leads to the question of whether periodontal disease, an inflammation of the gums, contributes directly to the development of cardiovascular disease. A study that measured and compared endothelial function in male and female subjects with advanced periodontal disease versus healthy controls demonstrated that periodontal disease resulted in endothelial dysfunction (i.e., flow mediated dilation) accompanied by elevated levels of C-reactive protein, a sensitive marker of inflammation [27]. Thus, the study concluded that periodontal disease may be a risk factor for developing cardiovascular disease [27]. This study population represented a smaller number of women compared with men in the control (29% women) and periodontal disease (39% women) groups and did not analyze data for sex [27]. The findings from this study lead one to question if treatment of periodontal disease leads to improved endothelial function. A study published this year reports that 6 months after intensive treatment for periodontitis, improved oral health was accompanied by improved endothelial function [28]. Whether men and women have sex-specific responses to such interventions remains to be determined.

18.4 ROLE OF NUTRITION IN PERIODONTAL DISEASE

Based on what is known about the etiology of periodontal disease and the emerging interrelationships among multiple diseases and periodontal disease, nutrition has a unique role in modulating periodontal disease. While studies specifically designed to examine sex-based responses to nutritional interventions for periodontal disease treatments are rare, several nutrients and novel food components have been studied in relation to periodontal disease.

18.4.1 Calcium and Vitamin D

Among females aged 20–39 years, low (2–499 mg/day) and moderate (500–799 mg/day) levels of calcium were associated with an increased risk of periodontal disease based on data from the NHANES III [29]. Interestingly, there was no association among older women but the association was present in males aged 20–39 and 40–59 years [29]. These findings emphasize the fact that intakes of calcium below the dietary reference intake (DRI) are associated with poor oral health.

Because loss of BMD occurs at multiple sites throughout the skeleton, including the jaw, it is biologically plausible that nutritional interventions aimed at slowing bone loss at common sites of fragility fracture (i.e., hip, spine) will also result in improved oral health, such as tooth retention. It has been reported that men and women, over age 65 years, who received a combination of calcium (500 mg/day as calcium citrate malate) and vitamin D (700 I.U./day) supplementation retained more teeth than individuals not receiving the supplemental calcium and vitamin D [30]. The study involved a 3 year supplementation period followed by a period of 2 years in which no supplementation was provided but subjects were free to choose to take supplements. At the start of the study, ~60% of subjects were women. During the supplementation phase of the study, 27% versus 13% of subjects lost one or more teeth in the placebo versus the supplemented group, respectively, suggesting that supplementation was effective at reducing tooth loss. However, it is unclear whether vitamin D, calcium, or both mediated the positive effect. During the 2 year follow-up study, supplementation was not provided but subjects could choose to take supplements. A greater number of subjects consuming the lower levels of calcium (59%) lost one or more teeth compared to subjects consuming higher levels of calcium (40%) [30]. An interesting finding was that dietary vitamin D was not independently related to tooth loss in this study. This finding may be due to weaknesses in the study design to answer the specific question of whether calcium and vitamin D are important for oral health. The authors acknowledged that because the study was not specifically designed to look at oral health outcomes, and ultimately tooth retention, further studies are needed to confirm the efficacy of supplementation with calcium and vitamin D alone and in combination on oral health [30].

There is currently much discussion about the DRI for vitamin D and whether it should be higher than the current recommendation for optimal health, including oral health. Based on data showing that higher levels of serum 25(OH)D are associated with lesser gingivitis and clinical attachment loss [31,32], it is proposed that serum

25(OH)D concentrations between 90 and 100 nmol/L are optimal for periodontal health and suggest that intakes of vitamin D should be >25 μg/day (>1000 I.U.), considerably higher than the current recommendation of 10 μg/day for age 50–70 years and 15 μg/day for over 70 years of age [33]. The relationship existed for both men and women over the age of 50. It is possible that vitamin D, in addition to positive effects on bone metabolism, may act via anti-inflammatory mechanisms as the relationship between vitamin D and clinical attachment loss was independent of changes in hip BMD. These findings require further investigation.

18.4.2 Fatty Acids

As discussed in several other chapters in this book (Chapters 8 through 12, Chapters 14 through 16), n-3 long chain polyunsaturated fatty acids such as those found in fish oil have potential anti-inflammatory effects, and a balance between n-3 and n-6 pathways is likely critical for many aspects of health. A few small studies have investigated the relationship between fish oil and the ratio of n-3 or n-6 fatty acids and periodontal health. One study postulated that periodontal bone loss may result from an imbalance between n-3 and n-6 fatty acids [34]. This study showed that subjects with periodontal disease had an elevated quantity of fatty acids from the n-6 pathway compared with healthy controls. The study did not specifically analyze sex but 60 out of 78 subjects with periodontal disease were women, and 22 out of 27 controls were women [34]. Route of delivery may be an important consideration as another study used a rinse, containing either n-3 or n-6 fatty acids. However, this treatment did not prevent gingivitis [35]. Using a rat model of experimental periodontal disease, intervention with n-3 fatty acids attenuated osteoclastic activity and overall bone resorption [36]. Larger, randomized controlled trials designed to elucidate sex-based differences in response to specific fatty acids in periodontal disease are warranted.

18.4.3 Antioxidants

Antioxidant vitamins such as vitamin C have been shown to be inversely related with periodontal disease based on data from male and female subjects (over 20 years of age) in the NHANES III [37]. Vitamin C has an important role in collagen synthesis and is also known to reduce oxidant stress. Perhaps not surprisingly, the inverse relationship between serum vitamin C and periodontal disease was strongest among individuals with the most severe periodontal disease. Whether individuals with periodontal disease would benefit from higher intakes of vitamin C remains to be determined, and such a study should examine sex-based differences in the response to vitamin C. Moreover, whether vitamin C status improves in individuals who are successfully treated for periodontal disease should be determined. An interesting finding was that this relationship persisted regardless of smoking status (i.e., smokers, former smokers, never-smokers).

In addition to compromised antioxidant status, there is further evidence that total antioxidant capacity and superoxide dismutase activity may be compromised in periodontal disease, and further exacerbated by a menopausal state [38]. The study compared postmenopausal women without periodontitis to postmenopausal women with periodontitis, and also included a group of premenopausal women without periodontitis [38]. Total antioxidant capacity, which measured the ability of antioxidants in serum and gingival crevicular fluid to inhibit a classic free-radical pathway (Fenton reaction), showed that total antioxidant activity was lower among women with periodontitis, and also that menopause in combination with periodontitis resulted in a further reduction in total antioxidant activity [38]. Serum superoxide dismutase activity was significantly lower among all postmenopausal women regardless of periodontal health, while gingival crevicular fluid superoxide dismutase activity was lower in menopausal women with periodontitis. Thus, periodontitis and menopausal status both altered antioxidant defense mechanisms.

A more recent study has demonstrated that treatment of periodontal disease increased total antioxidant capacity in gingival crevicular fluid, but not in plasma, to the levels in healthy control subjects [39]. This study included a sex analysis and noted that plasma total antioxidant capacity was higher in males compared with females at baseline and posttherapy, but that these sex differences did not exist for total antioxidant capacity in gingival crevicular fluid [39].

18.4.4 Folate

Data from the NHANES (2001–2002), that included both older men and women (>60 years of age), showed that serum folate is inversely related with periodontal disease [40]. Sex was considered in the model and was reported to have no effect on the relationship between serum folate and periodontal disease [40]. Folate deficiency is associated with increased oxidative stress, endothelial dysfunction, genomic instability, defective DNA repair, and apoptosis [40]. Thus, low folate status, in particular, may modulate periodontal disease by one or more of these mechanisms, or yet unknown mechanisms.

The authors acknowledge that a prospective trial is needed to more clearly establish low levels of folate as a risk factor for periodontal disease. It is possible that a diet low in folate occurs due to a poor diet. It is also possible that due to folate fortification of the food supply in Canada and the United States the relationship reported in this study may be weakened as dietary folate intakes have increased [41]. While this study uses folate intakes from surveys done in 2001 and 2002, a time when the food supply was already fortified, individuals studied in prospective studies started in the future will have likely had a significant greater intake of dietary folate for a longer proportion of their lives.

18.4.5 Whole Grains

To date, one study has specifically assessed whether intakes of whole grains and fiber reduce risk of periodontal disease in men as part of the Health Professionals Follow-Up Study [42]. Men who consumed the highest versus the lowest intakes of whole-grains had a much lower risk of developing periodontal disease [42]. It is postulated that the whole grains resulted in better glucose control through slowing digestion and absorption of carbohydrate, maintaining lower serum glucose over time, and ultimately improving insulin sensitivity. The authors further propose that with improved insulin sensitivity, inflammatory response is reduced (i.e., lower oxidative stress, cytokine production) which may subsequently lower the risk of periodontal disease. Although the study was conducted only in men, it provides a basis for conducting a similar study in women. It is important to note that the men included in this study did not have preexisting cardiovascular disease (myocardial infarction, stroke), diabetes, or periodontal disease as it clearly shows that even among healthy individuals, periodontal risk may be reduced by prudent dietary choices.

18.4.6 Weight Management

Achieving and maintaining a healthy weight reduces the risk of developing type II diabetes. Since obesity and subsequent development of type II diabetes may make some individuals more susceptible to developing periodontal disease (see Section 18.3.4), one strategy is to advise individuals to have a healthy body weight. The reader is referred to Chapters 7 and 8 for specific information on nutritional recommendations for a healthy body weight and prevention and/or treatment of type II diabetes.

18.4.7 Cardiovascular Disease

Studies to date suggest that periodontal disease may be a risk factor for cardiovascular disease. Thus, maintenance of periodontal health is critical for lowering this risk. The reader is referred to Chapter 9 for specific lifestyle guidelines for lowering the risk of developing cardiovascular disease and managing the disease.

18.5 CONCLUSION

In conclusion, our understanding of how foods and food components promote and enhance periodontal and oral health, and ultimately overall health, is in its infancy. Data to date have identified calcium, vitamin D, fish oil, antioxidants, folate, and whole grains as modulators of periodontal health, with varying degrees of scientific strength, but studies have not been specifically designed to delineate potential sex-based responses to nutritional interventions. With the growing body of evidence identifying periodontal disease as a risk factor for adverse pregnancy outcomes, as well as its interrelationships with chronic diseases such as type II diabetes and cardiovascular, there is much opportunity for investigators to elucidate the unique role of nutrition in whole body health.

18.6 FUTURE RESEARCH

Future research is needed to clearly establish how women differ from men in their response to nutritional interventions with respect to oral health, and to further elucidate the interrelationships with other chronic diseases such as cardiovascular disease, obesity, and type II diabetes. It will also be important to identify whether stage of the life cycle is an important consideration in determining when a nutritional intervention may be most effective for optimal oral health. Without question, the dental profession aims for each patient to have optimal oral health, and ultimately to not experience tooth loss during their life. The reality is that a proportion of individuals will lose teeth at some point during the life cycle. Ideally, these individuals will be able to have a dental implant placed to maintain normal eating patterns, facilitating healthy dietary intakes, and to prevent resorption of bone in the jaw. With the aging demographic in developed countries, an increasing number of patients are replacing lost teeth with dental implants. Thus, an emerging area of interest is whether nutritional interventions may aid in healing of periodontium after surgical procedures such as placement of dental implants as well as other procedures such as grafts. Some dentists make recommendations to patients about nutritional or complimentary therapies to aid with healing and recovery after surgical procedures including placement of dental implants; however, randomized controlled trials have not been conducted. Clinical dental practice is based on evidence-based dentistry, and thus it will be essential for these studies to be completed with the highest scientific standards and rigor if they are to be incorporated into patient management.

REFERENCES

1. Dye, B.A. and Selwitz, R.H., The relationship between selected measures of periodontal status and demographic and behavioural risk factors. *J. Clin. Periodontol.*, 32, 798, 2005.
2. Armitage, G.C., Development of a classification system for periodontal diseases and conditions. *Ann. Periodontol.*, 4, 1, 1999.
3. Burt, B., Position paper: epidemiology of periodontal diseases. *J. Periodontol.*, 76, 1406, 2005.
4. Fontijn-Tekamp, F.A., et al., The state of dentition in relation to nutrition in elderly Europeans in the SENECA Study of 1993. *Eur. J. Clin. Nutr.*, 50, S117, 1996.
5. Hashimoto, M., et al., Oral condition and health status of elderly 8020 achievers in Aichi Prefecture. *Bull. Tokyo Dent. Coll.*, 47, 37, 2006.
6. Sheiham, A. and Steele, J., Does the condition of the mouth and teeth affect the ability to eat certain foods, nutrient and dietary intake and nutritional status amongst older people? *Public Health Nutr.*, 4, 797, 2001.
7. Suzuki, K., et al., Relationship between number of present teeth and nutritional intake in institutionalized elderly. *Bull. Tokyo Dent. Coll.*, 46, 135, 2005.
8. Borrell, L.N., Burt, B.A., and Taylor, G.W., Prevalence and trends in periodontitis in the USA: the [corrected] NHANES, 1988 to 2000. *J. Dent. Res.*, 84, 924, 2005.
9. Machtei, E.E., et al., The effect of menstrual cycle on periodontal health. *J. Periodontol.*, 75, 408, 2004.
10. Preshaw, P.M., Knutsen, M.A., and Mariotti, A., Experimental gingivitis in women using oral contraceptives. *J. Dent. Res.*, 80, 2011, 2001.
11. Taichman, L.S. and Eklund, S.A., Oral contraceptives and periodontal diseases: rethinking the association based upon analysis of National Health and Nutrition Examination Survey data. *J. Periodontol.*, 76, 1374, 2005.
12. Tilakaratne, A., et al., Effects of hormonal contraceptives on the periodontium, in a population of rural Sri-Lankan women. *J. Clin. Periodontol.*, 27, 753, 2000.
13. Xiong, X., et al., Periodontal disease and adverse pregnancy outcomes: a systematic review. *BJOG*, 113, 135, 2006.
14. Michalowicz, B.S., et al., Treatment of periodontal disease and the risk of preterm birth. *N. Engl. J. Med.*, 355, 1885, 2006.

15. Jeffcoat, M.K., et al., Periodontal disease and preterm birth: results of a pilot intervention study. *J. Periodontol.*, 74, 1214, 2003.
16. Lopez, N.J., Smith, P.C., and Gutierrez, J., Periodontal therapy may reduce the risk of preterm low birth weight in women with periodontal disease: a randomized controlled trial. *J. Periodontol.*, 73, 911, 2002.
17. Krall, E.A., Garcia, R.I., and Dawson-Hughes, B., Increased risk of tooth loss is related to bone loss at the whole body, hip, and spine. *Calcif. Tissue Int.*, 59, 433, 1996.
18. Genco, R.J., et al., A proposed model linking inflammation to obesity, diabetes, and periodontal infections. *J. Periodontol.*, 76, 2075, 2005.
19. Al-Zahrani, M.S., Bissada, N.F., and Borawskit, E.A., Obesity and periodontal disease in young, middle-aged, and older adults. *J. Periodontol.*, 74, 610, 2003.
20. American Academy of Periodontology, A patient page. Diabetes and Periodontal Diseases: A Two-Way Street. www.perioorg. 3, 2002.
21. Lim, L.P., et al., Relationship between markers of metabolic control and inflammation on severity of periodontal disease in patients with diabetes mellitus. *J. Clin. Periodontol.*, 34, 118, 2007.
22. Faria-Almeida, R., Navarro, A., and Bascones, A., Clinical and metabolic changes after conventional treatment of type 2 diabetic patients with chronic periodontitis. *J. Periodontol.*, 77, 591, 2006.
23. Beck, J.D., et al., Relationship of periodontal disease to carotid artery intima-media wall thickness: the atherosclerosis risk in communities (ARIC) study. *Arterioscler. Thromb. Vasc. Biol.*, 21, 1816, 2001.
24. Demmer, R.T. and Desvarieux, M., Periodontal infections and cardiovascular disease: the heart of the matter. *J. Am. Dent. Assoc.*, 137, 14S, 2006.
25. DeStefano, F., et al., Dental disease and risk of coronary heart disease and mortality. *Brit. Med. J.*, 306, 688, 1993.
26. Mattila, K.J., et al., Dental infections and coronary atherosclerosis. *Atherosclerosis*, 103, 205, 1993.
27. Amar, S., et al., Periodontal disease is associated with brachial artery endothelial dysfunction and systemic inflammation. *Arterioscler. Thromb. Vasc. Biol.*, 23, 1245, 2003.
28. Tonetti, M.S., et al., Treatment of periodontitis and endothelial function. *N. Engl. J. Med.*, 356, 911, 2007.
29. Nishida, M., et al., Calcium and the risk for periodontal disease. *J. Periodontol.*, 71, 1057, 2000.
30. Krall, E.A., et al., Calcium and vitamin D supplements reduce tooth loss in the elderly. *Am. J. Med.*, 111, 452, 2001.
31. Dietrich, T., et al., Association between serum concentrations of 25-hydroxyvitamin D3 and periodontal disease in the US population. *Am. J. Clin. Nutr.*, 80, 108, 2004.
32. Dietrich, T., et al., Association between serum concentrations of 25-hydroxyvitamin D and gingival inflammation. *Am. J. Clin. Nutr.*, 82, 575, 2005.
33. Bischoff-Ferrari, H.A., et al., Estimation of optimal serum concentrations of 25-hydroxyvitamin D for multiple health outcomes. *Am. J. Clin. Nutr.*, 84, 18, 2006.
34. Requirand, P., et al., Serum fatty acid imbalance in bone loss: example with periodontal disease. *Clin. Nutr.*, 19, 271, 2000.
35. Eberhard, J., et al., Local application of n-3 or n-6 polyunsaturated fatty acids in the treatment of human experimental gingivitis. *J. Clin. Periodontol.*, 29, 364, 2002.
36. Iwami-Morimoto, Y., Yamaguchi, K., and Tanne, K., Influence of dietary n-3 polyunsaturated fatty acid on experimental tooth movement in rats. *Angle Orthod.*, 69, 365, 1999.

37. Chapple, I.L., Milward, M.R., and Dietrich, T., The prevalence of inflammatory periodontitis is negatively associated with serum antioxidant concentrations. *J. Nutr.*, 137, 657, 2007.
38. Baltacioglu, E., et al., Total antioxidant capacity and superoxide dismutase activity levels in serum and gingival crevicular fluid in post-menopausal women with chronic periodontitis. *J. Clin. Periodontol.*, 33, 385, 2006.
39. Chapple, I.L., et al., Compromised GCF total antioxidant capacity in periodontitis: cause or effect? *J. Clin. Periodontol.*, 34, 103–110, 2007.
40. Yu, Y.H., Kuo, H.K., and Lai, Y.L., The association between serum folate levels and periodontal disease in older adults: data from the National Health and Nutrition Examination Survey 2001/02. *J. Am. Geriatr. Soc.*, 55, 108, 2007.
41. Dolega-Cieszkowski, J.H., Bobyn, J.P., and Whiting, S.J., Dietary intakes of Canadians in the 1990s using population-weighted data derived from the provincial nutrition surveys. *Appl. Physiol. Nutr. Metab.*, 31, 753, 2006.
42. Merchant, A.T., et al., Whole-grain and fiber intakes and periodontitis risk in men. *Am. J. Clin. Nutr.*, 83, 1395, 2006.

Section IV

Conclusion

19 Conclusion: What We Know, and Where Do We Go from Here

Lilian U. Thompson and Wendy E. Ward

CONTENTS

19.1 INTRODUCTION

There are differences in the biology, physiology, and disease risks between sex. Chapters 1 and 2 described several examples of these differences that may explain the differences in susceptibility of men and women to diseases, and nutrient requirements for maintainance of health and management of diseases. Sex hormones, which differ between men and women (higher testosterone in men, higher estradiol in women), appear to be a major driving force in determining the characteristics of the digestive system. This then may affect how the other organs function. In women, the monthly fluctuation in hormones and the special state of pregnancy further modify those characteristics. Clearly there is a need to separately identify the needs of women from those of men and we focused here on the needs of women for optimum health.

19.2 NUTRIENT NEEDS IN THE LIFE CYCLE

It is evident that women have different nutrient needs at distinct stages of the life cycle and in recent years nutrient requirements have been modified for the different age groups in various countries.

19.2.1 Adolescence

Adolescence is a life stage of rapid physical growth and development and thus their total energy and nutrient requirements are more than at other stages of the life cycle. The peak growth and hence peak nutrient requirements tend to occur earlier in adolescent women than in men. This is an important period because eating behaviors may develop during this time, and continue through adulthood. Nutrient requirements of adolescents for healthy living have been described in Chapter 3, but a large proportion of adolescents do not meet these requirements. Western practices promote unhealthy eating practices that could lead to overweight and obesity, poor bone mineralization, nutrient deficiencies such as iron-deficiency anemia and eating disorders, including anorexia nervosa, bulimia, and binge eating.

To optimize adolescent health, the home, school, and community should provide a stable and positive environment for the promotion of good nutrition. As discussed in Chapter 3, at *home*, parents can positively influence the adolescent behavior by (a) serving as role models in healthy eating and weight-related behaviors, (b) providing an environment with ample opportunity to choose nutritious foods and beverages, for example, kitchen filled with healthy foods and beverages, and (c) avoiding negative comments about weight as this has been related to increases in binge eating, dieting, and unhealthy weight control behaviors. *Schools* may impact eating behaviors of female adolescents through their food services, food policies, and classroom nutrition education. School meal programs must meet nutritional standards. The school should promote healthy eating by (a) developing nutrition guidelines for foods and beverages sold beyond these school meals, (b) limiting the access to foods with minimal nutritional value to certain times, that is, no access during meal times, and not using them as incentives, (c) providing nutrition education on how to follow nutrition guidelines and prepare healthy meals, and (d) involving students themselves in the promotion of healthy eating. The physical environment and resources in the *community* where adolescents live can also influence healthy eating behavior. Food outlets, including fast food restaurants, convenience stores, and vending machines, can provide access to unhealthy high-fat, high-sugar snack foods and beverages. Creation of a community coalition or task force with members from food outlets, youth groups, recreation facilities, religious organizations, and families to evaluate the need for and develop a nutrition program for adolescents will help in the development of healthy eating behavior and optimum health at an early age.

19.2.2 Premenopause

Premenopausal women are of childbearing age and it is essential that they maintain a healthy diet for optimum health. Recommended nutrient intakes have been described in Chapter 4. Among other nutrients, adequate intakes of iron, to compensate for menstrual cycle losses, and folic acid, to prevent neural tube defect in pregnancy are essential. However, further research is needed to differentiate the independent effects of age and luteal phase length on the susceptibility of the reproductive system to disruption by energy deficiency. Certain chemicals found in plant foods (phytochemicals) with estrogenic or antiestrogenic effect are of interest because they may suppress certain types of cancer but their effect in the reproductive systems is not fully explored and should be further studied.

Overnutrition and high energy intake that lead to overweight and obesity should particularly be controlled in premenopausal women. Optimum health during premenopausal years will help in maintaining health during the postmenopausal period. Short-term studies have already suggested the efficacy of low-fat diets in weight loss, but long-term studies with years of follow-up still need to be conducted to establish the efficacy and safety of low-fat diets. However, because of the burden of chronic diseases associated with excess weight and obesity, it is prudent to already encourage women at the population level to adopt a low-fat diet regimen with exercise for maintenance of optimal body weight.

19.2.3 Pregnancy and Lactation

The maternal requirement for nutrients is increased during pregnancy and lactation to support the needs for fetal and infant growth and development as well as the deposition and maintenance of maternal tissues. Chronic disease prevention starts at an early age and a mother's poor nutrition during pregnancy and lactation affects not only maternal health but also the long-term health and susceptibility of the offspring to adult diseases such as cardiovascular disease (CVD) and cancer. The needs of women during preconception, pregnancy and lactation are well described in Chapter 5. Additional references for healthy pregnancy can also be found in the following reports: Nutrition for a Healthy Pregnancy:National Guidelines for the Childbearing Years [1] and the American Dietetic Association Position on Nutrition and Lifestyle for a Healthy Pregnancy Outcome [2]. During preconception, the significance of folate supplements cannot be overemphasized in order to reduce neural tube defects and other malformations in the offspring, and of iron supplemennts to meet the needs of the fetus and for maternal expansion of blood volume. However, excessive intake of multivitamin and mineral supplementation is controversial and it is advisable to consume levels that do not exceed the recommended daily allowance.

19.2.4 Menopause and Midlife

Menopause is a period when the ovaries stop producing the hormones estrogen and progesterone that leads to many bodily changes, including cessation of menstruation, increased risk of heart disease and osteoporosis, and many symptoms such as hot flashes, depression, and anxiety. However, with proper diet and exercise as described in Chapter 6, it is possible to combat these undesirable conditions during menopause and midlife and to have healthy lives.

Menopausal women have special nutritional requirements that may be met through a healthy diet rich in whole grains, fruits, vegetables, a small amount of fat from n-3 fatty acids, and low levels of trans fatty acids, n-6 fatty acids, sugar, and salt. In addition, dietary supplements, including vitamins, minerals, and certain botanicals, may be beneficial, particularly for women at risk of specific chronic diseases (i.e., calcium and vitamin D supplementation if at risk for osteoporosis). Few long-term, large-scale randomized clinical trials have assessed the efficacy and safety of dietary interventions involving combinations of different food sources, vitamin and mineral supplements, and botanical supplements, on health maintenance and the prevention and management of disease. Some botanical supplements commonly consumed by menopausal women have not undergone rigorous testing for safety and efficacy in various doses. These types of studies need attention in future research.

19.3 NUTRITION NEEDS IN OTHER CONDITIONS AND CHRONIC DISEASE

19.3.1 Obesity

Overweight and obesity are increasing in epidemic proportion with higher rates in women than in men and there is a recognition that increased energy intake and decreased activity are responsible. This is serious because they are closely associated to other major chronic diseases, including metabolic syndrome, Type 2 diabetes, CVD, and cancer.

The body composition differs between sexes, e.g., with women having more total and subcutaneous fat while men have more visceral fat and lean tissue. However, the response to energy restriction in terms of weight loss does not differ between men and women, regardless of diet macronutrient composition. Popular weight loss diets include low-fat diets such as the Atkins diet (low fat, high carbohydrate), and the South Beach Diet (modified from the Atkins diet with replacement of saturated with unsaturated fat); and high protein and moderate carbohydrate diets such as the Zone, Protein Power, and CSIRO diet; and meal replacement diet such as Optifast diets. The effectiveness and safety of these diets over the long term has not been studied. As discussed in Chapter 7, weight loss that is achieved through long-term lifestyle changes to healthful dietary habits together with regular physical activity is best for optimizing health.

19.3.2 Metabolic Syndrome and Type 2 Diabetes

Metabolic syndrome is characterized by a group of metabolic risk factors in an individual, with many affected individuals also having insulin resistance that often develops into Type 2 diabetes. The prevalence of diabetes in both men and women continues to increase, with a considerable increase occurring over the last 10–15 years.

The role of nutrition in attenuating metabolic syndrome and Type 2 diabetes has been extensively studied and overall guidelines for treating each condition are presented in Chapter 8, and include a focus on dietary strategies in combination with lifestyle aspects (i.e., weight reduction, physical activity). Of note is the fact that the weight management and dietary modifications would benefit many aspects of health beyond metabolic syndrome and Type 2 diabetes. Studies to date suggest that sex-based differences with respect to risk of or treatment of these conditions do not exist, but as discussed by the authors of this chapter, future studies designed to definitely answer this question are needed.

19.3.3 Cardiovascular Disease

The leading cause of death of women in the United States and most developed countries is CVD, particularly coronary heart disease and stroke. Although the death rate from CVD in men has recently declined, no decline has been reported in women. More women die of heart disease than do men and about twice as many women die of heart disease than of cancer. The risk factors for CVD are well known to include high cholesterol, high blood pressure, and obesity, with diabetes, hypertriglyceridemia, and low HDL being greater risk factors in women than in men. The National Cholesterol Education Program and American Heart Association (AHA) have published recommendations for the prevention and treatment of CVD, which have been outlined in Chapter 9. The AHA has defined a heart healthy diet as one that includes a variety of vegetables, fruits, whole grains, low-fat or nonfat dairy products, fish, legumes, and protein source low in saturated fatty acids such as poultry, lean meat, and plant sources. The saturated fatty acid should be $<10\%$ calories, the cholesterol <300 mg/day, and trans fatty acid $<1\%$ calories. In addition to dietary modification, increased physical activity and smoking cessation are strongly encouraged.

19.3.4 Breast and Ovarian Cancer

Cancer is the second leading cause of death in the United States and breast and ovarian cancers are two cancers of particular concern to women. In particular, breast cancer is the leading cause of cancer death among women, second only to lung cancer. Although incidence of ovarian cancer is less than that of breast cancer, the survival after ovarian cancer diagnosis is less than that of breast cancer. As described in Chapter 10, there are many risk factors for breast and ovarian cancer that can be classified as genetic or demographic, nutritional or behavioral, and hormonal. Family history and reproductive indices such as early onset of menarche, nulliparity, late stage of first birth, and late natural menopause have been established as breast cancer risk factors but their role in ovarian cancer is less clear. Body size is also a risk factor but it depends on menopausal status. No specific nutrient, food group, or dietary pattern has convincingly been shown in epidemiological studies to reduce breast or ovarian cancer but there is general agreement that minimizing lifetime weight gain, regular moderate to vigorous physical activity, and limited alcohol intake may reduce breast cancer. In addition, a healthy lifestyle should include consumption of more plant-based diet rich in fruits and vegetables, whole grains, and reduced fat coming more from n-3- and monounsaturated fatty acid-rich foods and less from animal fat and trans fatty acids. Further information can be found in the American Cancer Society Guidelines on Nutrition and Physical Activity for Cancer Prevention [3] and the forthcoming revision of the American Institute for Cancer Research and the World Cancer Research Fund in Food Nutrition and the Prevention of Cancer: A Global Prospective [4].

Because the relationship between specific food components and breast and ovarian cancer is still inconclusive, further work beyond case control and cohort studies should be conducted to establish their efficacy. More mechanistic-based intervention trials emphasizing the whole diet rather than single nutrient or bioactive component may provide a better understanding of the role of diet on cancer prevention. Longitudinal intervention studies to determine the effect of in utero or prepubescent exposure to certain diets on breast and ovarian cancer remains to be further explored in the future.

19.3.5 Osteoporosis and Osteoarthritis

Osteoporosis and osteoarthritis are among the most common musculoskeletal disorders, and both are more common in women than in men, owing to differences in skeletal structure and size, and menopause. Bone is a dynamic tissue, and thus nutrition plays an important role throughout the life cycle. Unlike many other diseases and disorders discussed in this book, nutritional responses of women with osteoporosis have been more extensively studied than in men. Because of an increased risk of osteoporosis after menopause, as discussed in Chapter 11, general recommendations for women over age 50 include 1500 mg calcium and 800 IU vitamin D/day (in contrast to the DRIs for calcium and vitamin D); however, experts suggest that optimal vitamin D intakes for musculoskeletal health should be >1000 IU/day, higher than the current DRI. Bone is known to be responsive to changes in dietary fat; therefore, some studies support the fact that modulating the n-6 pathway towards the n-3 pathway may have favorable effects on bone metabolism. Adequate protein is important, particularly during fracture healing. There are divergent findings on the effectiveness of soy protein (containing isoflavones) or purified isoflavones at attenuating bone loss, and fracture trials have not been performed. With respect to osteoarthritis, weight management is critical to prevent or relieve symptoms of osteoarthritis. In general, a balanced diet and maintenance of a healthy body weight throughout the life cycle are important for musculoskeletal health.

19.3.6 Rheumatoid Arthritis

Rheumatoid arthritis is a painful, inflammatory disease of the joints resulting in cartilage degradation and erosion of bone. It most commonly occurs in premenopausal women, and thus has a long-term impact on health. As described in Chapter 12, the etiology is multifactorial, having a genetic basis as well as being linked to hormones, such as estrogen, obesity, and various dietary factors. Dietary factors have been associated with an increased or decreased risk of the disease, with the strongest evidence being a decreased risk of rheumatoid arthritis with n-3 fatty acid consumption. A less substantial body of evidence suggests that antioxidants may be helpful, possibly via attenuation of free radicals present in fluid and cells of joints. With respect to nutritional interventions, the n-3 fatty acids have been most extensively studied because of their potential anti-inflammatory effect, and thus potential for attenuating the disease process. Clinical benefits are observed with intakes of 2.7 g/day of eicosapentaenoic acid and docosahexaenoic acid (~9 or more standard fish oil capsules). Specifically, n-3 fatty acids in fish oil favorably modulate eicosanoid, cytokine, and adhesion molecule production. Fish oil supplementation has also been shown to reduce nonsteroid anti-inflammatory drug usage in patients. To date, there is no clear evidence that antioxidants have a clinical benefit in patients with rheumatoid arthritis but requires further study. Emerging interest in vitamin D and its potential anti-inflammatory activity should also be investigated in future studies.

19.3.7 Irritable Bowel Syndrome

Irritable bowel syndrome (IBS) is the most common gastrointestinal disorder that is characterized by chronic abdominal pain or discomfort, altered bowel habits, abdominal bloating, and distention. Its prevalence in the United States is about 5%–25% and there is evidence that there is gender or sex difference not only in prevalence (about twice in women than men) but also in clinical presentation, pathophysiology, and treatment response as discussed in Chapter 13. In women, the symptoms have been associated with female sex hormones as it usually worsens at the time of menses.

A biopsychological approach has been suggested for the treatment of IBS because of the multiple factors that contribute to this disorder. Pharmacological and nonpharmacological treatments as well as complementary alternative medicine, including the use of herbs, melatonin or probiotic supplements, and acupuncture, have been used for alleviation of IBS. Dietary management may reduce IBS symptoms by eliminating foods associated with gas production such as beans, and those that stimulate colonic motility such as caffeine rich foods and beverages. Although dietary fiber has been prescribed to regulate bowel movements of IBS patients, its fermentation by colonic flora produce short-chain fatty acids and gas that can cause bloating. Allergy, hypersensitivities, or intolerance to certain foods or components such as lactose, fructose, fructans, gluten or wheat, and peanuts can also precipitate IBS symptoms. Excluding such foods in the diet may improve IBS symptoms. Other alternative treatments and dietary management of IBS have yet to be explored. There are sex differences in response to treatment, but large clinical trials with both males and females still need to be conducted to further establish whether response to specific treatments really differ between sex or gender.

19.3.8 Eye Health

Visual impairment is common throughout the world, particularly in developed countries, as increased longevity among women means that greater numbers of women develop the disease. Studies to date suggest that vascular disease and oxidative stress may be key contributors to age-related macular degeneration (AMD), and thus diets that are rich in antioxidants and n-3 fatty acids may protect against disease development (Chapter 14). Specific dietary recommendations for prevention of AMD include high consumption of fruits, vegetables, and fatty fish. There is some evidence that progression of AMD may be slowed from multivitamin supplementation (B-carotene, vitamins C and E, zinc) but it is prudent not to recommend such supplementation for individuals without AMD. Studies have primarily focused on older adults and further research into the timing of exposure to specific nutrients and foods is critical for determining when a nutritional intervention may be most effective at preventing AMD.

19.3.9 Dementia and Alzheimer's Disease

Dementia includes a variety of cognitive diseases such as Alzheimer's disease, and is one of the most disabling health conditions in old age. Since women live longer, and dementia is largely a disease of aging, more women than men are at risk of developing dementia. Multiple mechanisms may contribute to the etiology of the disease and include oxidative stress, to which the brain is particularly sensitive. Dementia is characterized by plaque formation and impaired intra- and extracellular signaling in the brain. Evidence regarding the effect of nutritional interventions on dementia is inconclusive but data suggest specific nutrients may attenuate the disease process. The major dietary factors that may attenuate the progression of dementia include antioxidants (vitamins C and E, B-carotene, zinc), and polyunsaturated fatty acids from fish oil that may improve cell signaling. Diets low in fat, particularly saturated fat and cholesterol, as well as low calorie diets may protect against dementia. A recurrent theme throughout the book is the health consequence of obesity; the etiology of dementia may be stimulated by insulin insensitivity resulting from obesity. As stated in Chapter 15, there is an urgent need for sex-specific prospective and intervention studies, which are specifically designed to identify how nutrition may modulate the disease process.

19.3.10 Depression and Psychiatric Disorders

Mental health disorders are increasing throughout the world, and constitute a major cause of global disease. The most common mental health disorders are depression, bipolar disorder, and schizophrenia (Chapter 16). Adequate nutrition in utero and during the first several years of life is critical for healthy brain development and, may possibly, along with social and behavioral factors, determine adult mental health. Nutrition at later stages of the life cycle is also critical for mental health. The strongest evidence regarding a relationship between nutrition and mental health pertains to fish oil, possibly due to it being a rich source of long-chain polyunsaturated fatty acids such as eicosapentaenoic acid. Countries with low fish intake have higher rates of depression, and higher fish consumption is associated with better moods and self-reported mental health. Similarly, a high fish intake has been associated with decreased risk of multiple mental health disorders such as postnatal depression, seasonal affective disorder, and bipolar disorder. Among aboriginals, an increase in depression occurred along with changes in traditional diet, including a decline in fish intake. Schizophrenia may also be favorably modulated by fish oil.

In patients with uncontrolled symptoms, but who were receiving antipsychotic medications, improvements were observed with supplementation of eicosapentaenoic acid. Furthermore, schizophrenic patients may be particularly vulnerable to poor nutritional status as they consume fewer calories, and their overall diet is nutritionally inadequate. Sex-based differences in response to fish oil and n-3 fatty acids, as well as other less understood nutrients such as vitamins and amino acids, need to be investigated to develop strategies that result in improved mental health.

19.3.11 Eating Disorders

Eating disorders, including anorexia and bulimia are a complex psychiatric conditions, with biological, psychological, and social aspects. As discussed in Chapter 17, it is characterized by atypical food intake and behavior and preoccupation with body image, weight, and shape. About 90% of patients with this disorder are females and White with more than 75% developing it during adolescence. Studies suggest that environmental influences of peers and media messages are related to the onset of eating disorders in early adolescence. However, genetics play a more important role than environmental factors by the time the adolescent female has completed puberty, suggesting that sex hormones may trigger the gene expression that affect susceptibility to development of eating disorder.

For primary prevention, nutrition education is suggested particularly to those at preadolescent age and those who may have genetic predisposition to an eating disorder. For those suffering from eating disorder, there are no specific nutrients that need to be increased or decreased. Rather, it is suggested that a well-balanced meal plan may be spread out throughout the day with the total caloric content adjusted depending on the need to lose, gain, or maintain weight. A registered dietitian with specialized training should be a member of the health care team to help in the normalization of the patient's eating behavior and body weight as well as in counseling regarding acceptance of certain body size.

19.3.12 Oral Health

Periodontal disease, an inflammatory disease that ultimately can result in erosion of jaw bone and tooth loss, often compromises nutritional status. In women, susceptibility to periodontal disease is somewhat dependent on hormonal status, with pregnancy and menopause representing vulnerable stages of the life cycle. For this reason, regular hygiene appointments are recommended, particularly prior to pregnancy. Newer evidence suggests that periodontal disease is a complex state, and is interrelated with Type II diabetes, and possibly cardiovascular disease. Thus, nutritional strategies that prevent or treat these chronic diseases may also improve oral health. As stated in Chapter 18, a combination of calcium and vitamin D supplementation has been suggested to slow tooth loss in both older men and women, and moreover, vitamin D may have anti-inflammatory effects in addition to specific effects on bone metabolism. Other studies suggest that the balance of n-3 and n-6 fatty acids is important for periodontal health, and antioxidant requirements may be elevated in individuals with periodontal disease. Emerging evidence suggests that folate may be important for oral health, with low levels of folate associated with greater risk of periodontal disease. Other newer information suggests that consumption of whole grains is associated with a decreased risk of periodontal disease, possibly linked to better glucose control. There are many areas of research that must be investigated to fully understand the role of nutrition in periodontal health and disease. It will be critical to also assess sex-based differences in response to nutrition in periodontal disease, both from a prevention and treatment perspective.

19.4 OVERALL CONCLUSION AND FUTURE WORK

It is evident that the dietary and lifestyle recommendations stated within the individual chapters can lead to a wide range of health benefits with potential to protect against multiple chronic diseases. An overall dietary pattern based on those recommendations for healthy living is summarized in Table 19.1.

TABLE 19.1
Recommendations for Healthy Lifestyle

Follow Healthy Dietary Pattern
Dietary fat
Select healthy foods with healthy fats:
Fish, avocado, nuts, seeds (i.e., flaxseed)
Incorporate healthier oils:
Olive, flaxseed, canola
Use nonfat salad dressings and sauces
Reduce fat intake from animal sources:
Select lean cuts of meat and poultry
Use low or no-fat dairy products
Consume more servings of fish
Avoid consumption of trans fats
Dietary Carbohydrate
Increase fiber by choosing whole grains, beans, and legumes more often
Dietary Protein
Choose poultry, fish, soy, nuts more often than red meat
Consider "Plant-Based" Diet
Vegetables are the main course with meat as a side dish
Consume vegetables at each meal or snack
Choose colorful vegetables
Maintain Healthy Weight with Physical Activity
Have healthy food choices (as above)
Adhere to suggested serving size and number of servings per day (most countries have specially designed food guide that will help with this)
Consume less processed and "fast" foods
Have regular physical activities with realistic goals to ensure they can be successfully incorporated into the lifestyle over the long term
Limit Alcohol Intake
Quit or Do not Start Smoking
Minimize Stress

In addition to healthy food choices, a lifestyle that includes regular physical activity will contribute to optimum health in women. A recurrent theme throughout this book is the role of maintaining a healthy body weight for prevention of metabolic syndrome, Type 2 diabetes, cardiovascular disease, osteoarthritis, and possibly breast cancer and periodontal disease. Thus, it is prudent to consider maintaining a healthy body weight as integral to optimal health (Table 19.1).

While it is important to select healthy foods, there is still a danger of consumption of such healthy foods at levels that will contribute to weight gain and obesity. The importance of serving size, no matter how healthy a food, is critical to achieving a healthy body weight. Regular physical activity has an important role in various chronic diseases such as cardiovascular disease, osteoporosis, and osteoarthritis where individualized exercises can have positive effects on cardiovascular and musculoskeletal health, while also ensuring a healthy body weight. Limiting alcohol intake, minimizing stress, and avoiding smoking are other key components of a healthy lifestyle.

To encourage attainment of optimum health in women, the government, food industry, researchers, and health professionals should continue to play an active role. How each of these groups can potentially participate is summarized in Table 19.2. The government can play a significant role by regulating the manufacturing and labeling of healthy foods, requiring nutrition education in the school system and providing funds for encouraging healthy lifestyle and research. The *food industry* can assist in providing a healthy eating environment not only through processing of healthy foods but also through adjustment of serving sizes and appropriate incentives and advertisements. Several specific areas for future research have been mentioned above and in the individual chapters. In addition, researchers should continue to determine the biological, physiological, and behavioral basis of sex and gender differences. How sex modifies cellular and signalling pathways and gene expression should be studied to provide an understanding of how and why men and women differ in response to diet and certain therapeutic drugs. Other less explored diseases and conditions that affect women's health through the lifespan should also be investigated. Many recommendations have been made regarding specific foods or nutrients for optimum health. However, large, long-term, randomized controlled trial has yet to be conducted in a large population using both men and women (to differentiate sex differences in response) to test the effectiveness of such foods or nutrient in combinations or their combination with drugs. Research results should be widely communicated. Health professionals should educate and train others and try to integrate the research results into health practice considering the sex differences in response to diet and drugs, alone and in combination, for disease treatment and prevention. Further information on emerging issues and trends in women's health can be found in the document Women's Health USA 2005 [5] and other documents published by the Office of Women's Health within the US Department of Health and Human Services [6] and the Society of Women's Health Research [7].

Great strides have been made in the last decade but with continued efforts, it is possible to optimize women's health through application of nutrition principles based on sound scientific evidence and cooperation of everyone interested in healthy living. Imperative to the success of optimizing women's health is communication among all

TABLE 19.2
Some Suggestions for Future Action

Government
Provide guidelines for labeling of healthy foods
Provide incentives to industry to develop healthy foods
Encourage "farm to table" practices—e.g., increase availability of fresh fruits and vegetables to all members of society (local markets etc.)
Regulate the manufacture of healthy foods, e.g., trans-fatty acid free
Fund research
Require nutrition education in school curriculum
Encourage overall healthy lifestyle: help build playgrounds, recreation centers, swimming pools (accessibility, 24 h/day)
Encourage mandatory physical activity breaks in the workplace
Industry
Process foods that are more nutrient dense
Carefully consider package serving size (make it easier for consumer to purchase single serving foods)
Use easy to understand nutrition labels
Advertise healthy foods
Reduce grocery shelves for unhealthy food products
Adjust serving size (no supersizing) in restaurants and other food outlets
Provide incentives for purchase of healthy foods
Researchers
Study biological and behavioral basis of sex and gender differences
Determine sex and gender differences in response to foods and drugs for prevention and treatment
Further study diseases and conditions that affect women's health through the lifespan
Conduct large randomized controlled trials or prospective trials in men and women to determine effectiveness of food or nutrient or component combinations rather than of single food or food components
Always include women in clinical trials
Study food interactions with drugs and determine whether dietary interventions may reduce drug doses
Focus on emerging areas of research, e.g., nutrition and mental health
Work as multidisciplinary team
Disseminate research results
Health Professionals and Educators
Develop training and education programs to update and disseminate knowledge
Integrate research results into health practice
Consider sex differences in disease prevention and treatment
Consider food–drug combination for therapies

parties involved, including researchers, government, food industry, health professionals, educators, and consumers. The last and most important step in this process will be the effective communication of clear and concise messages about health and nutrition to the consumer. Success will be achieved if our daughters and future generations live longer, healthier lives, in which they are active and fruitful participants in society.

REFERENCES

1. http://www.hc-sc.gc.ca/fn-an/nutrition/prenatal/national_guidelines_tc-lignes_directrices_nationales_tm_e.html
2. Kaiser, L.L., Allen, L., American Dietetic Association. Position of the American Dietetic Association: nutrition and lifestyle for a healthy pregnancy outcome, *J. Am. Diet. Assoc.*, 102, 1479, 2002.
3. Kushi, L. H. et al., American Cancer Society Guidelines on Nutrition and Physical Activity for cancer prevention: Reducing the risk of cancer with healthy food choices and physical activity, *CA Cancer J. Clin.*, 56, 254, 2006.
4. American Institute for Cancer Research and World Cancer Research Fund, *Food, Nutrition and the Prevention of Cancer: A Global Perspective*, American Institute for Cancer Research: Washington, DC, 1997.
5. US Department of Health and Human Services, Health Resources and Services Administration, *Women's Health USA 2005*, Rockville, Maryland, 2005.
6. http://www.4women.gov/OWH/multidisciplinary/reports/GenderBasedMedicine
7. http://www.womenshealthresearch.org

Index

A

B

C

D

E

F

G

H

I

J

K

L

M

N

O

P

R

S

T

U

V

W

Z